Risk Management Handbook

American Society for Healthcare Risk Management

Series Editor: Roberta Carroll

Volume I Editors: Peggy Nakamura & Roberta Carroll

JB JOSSEY-BASS

Risk Management Handbook

FOR HEALTH CARE ORGANIZATIONS

Fifth Edition

VOLUME I

The Essentials

BICENTENNIAL
BICENTENNIAL
1807
WILEY
2007
BICENTENNIAL
BICENTENNIAL

John Wiley & Sons, Inc.

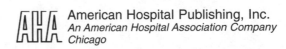

American Hospital Publishing, Inc.
An American Hospital Association Company
Chicago

Library of Congress Cataloging-in-Publication Data

Risk management handbook for health care organizations. — 5th ed.
    p. ; cm.
 Includes bibliographical references and index.
 ISBN-13: 978-0-7879-8672-8 (v. 1 : alk. paper)
 ISBN-10: 0-7879-8672-0 (v. 1 : alk. paper)
 ISBN-13: 978-0-7879-8708-4 (v. 2 : alk. paper)
 ISBN-10: 0-7879-8708-5 (v. 2 : alk. paper)
 ISBN-13: 978-0-7879-8724-4 (v. 3 : alk. paper)
 ISBN-10: 0-7879-8724-7 (v. 3 : alk. paper)
1. Health facilities—Risk management. I. Nakamura, Peggy. II. Carroll, Roberta.
 [DNLM: 1. Health Facilities—economics. 2. Health Facilities—organization & administration.
3. Risk Management. WX 157 R59533 2006]
 RA971.38.R58 2006
 362.11'068—dc22   2006023722

FIFTH EDITION
HB Printing   10 9 8 7 6 5 4 3 2 1

Contents

List of Exhibits, Figures, Tables, and Appendices

EXHIBITS

FIGURES

TABLES

APPENDICES

About the Contributors

Geraldine Amori, Ph.D., ARM, CPHRM, FASHRM, Director of the Professional Development and Education Center for The Risk Management and Patient Safety Institute, develops, coordinates, and delivers educational programs in all aspects of patient safety and risk management. She has previously served as principal of Communicating Health-Care, and risk manager for Fletcher Allen Health Care in Burlington, Vermont. Dr. Amori is a nationally known speaker, facilitator, and consultant on risk management, focusing on communication issues in health care and patient safety. She is a past president of ASHRM, and past president of the Northern New England Society for Healthcare Risk Management. In 2004, she received ASHRM's coveted Distinguished Service Award. She has a master of science degree in counseling and human systems from Florida State University and a Ph.D. in counselor education from the University of Florida. She serves on the Board of Consumers Advancing Patient Safety board of directors, and as an advisor to Partnership for Patient Safety. She is a lifetime member of the American Society for Healthcare Risk Management.

Ellen L. Barton, JD, CPCU, DFASHRM, Independent Risk Management Consultant, served as president of Neumann Insurance Company and director of risk management of Franciscan Health System in Aston, Pennsylvania, from May 1987 to December 1996. She also served as general counsel for Franciscan Health System from July 1993 to July 1996 and as senior vice president, legal services, from July 1994 to July 1996. In addition to those responsibilities, Barton sat on the boards of several insurance companies and a captive insurance company management firm. Other past positions include: vice president, Risk Management for Med Star Health, Inc., Columbia, Maryland; vice president and health care practice leader, Aon Risk Services, Inc. of Maryland; vice president, legal services, American Radiology Services, Inc., Baltimore, Maryland; chief operating officer and general counsel of New American Health, LLC, Glen Burnie, Maryland; director of risk management at the University of Pennsylvania; associate director and director of risk management at the University of Cincinnati; assistant editor of the FC&S Bulletins at the National Underwriter Company, Cincinnati, Ohio; and independent claims adjuster for Lloyd R. Deist Insurance Adjusters, Inc., Cincinnati, Ohio. Barton received her J.D. degree from the University of Cincinnati in 1978. She has written numerous articles and book chapters on risk management issues and has conducted seminars on national and regional levels. Barton is admitted to the Bars of Ohio, Maryland, and Pennsylvania, and holds membership in the Maryland Bar Association, the

Society of Chartered Property and Casualty Underwriters, the American Health Lawyers Association, and the Maryland Society for Healthcare Risk Management (of which she was president 2002–2003), and American Society for Healthcare Risk Management, of which she was president for 1990–1991. Barton was the recipient of ASHRM's Distinguished Service Award in 1993 and was honored in 2001 to have the Certificate in Healthcare Risk Management named after her.

Roberta L. Carroll, RN, ARM, CPCU, MBA, CPHRM, CPHQ, LHRM, HEM, DFASHRM, Senior Vice President, Aon Healthcare, based in Tampa, Florida. Previously she was Director of Risk Management Consulting Services and senior vice president and manager of the health care unit, Aon Risk Services of Northern California. She has held a variety of positions, including vice president of risk and insurance management for Uni-Health in Burbank, California; senior vice president and manager of the health care unit for Corroon & Black of Illinois; vice president of risk management, claims and marketing for Premier Alliance Insurance Company; trust administrator and risk manager for Premier Hospitals Alliance in Chicago, Illinois, and director of risk management at Mount Sinai Medical Center, Miami Beach, Florida. Carroll served on the ASHRM board for six years and was president 1995–1996. She has been on the Board of the Southern California Association for Healthcare Risk Management and was one of the founding members, first president, and board member of the Florida Society for Healthcare Risk Management and Patient Safety (FSHRMPS). In addition, Carroll was one of the founders and officers of the Florida Medical Malpractice Claims Council, Inc. (FMMCCI). She is a Licensed Healthcare Risk Manager (LHRM) in the State of Florida and faculty member for the health care risk management course at the University of South Florida. Carroll is also a faculty member for the ASHRM-sponsored Barton certificate program "Essentials" module. Previously, she was a faculty member for Module 1-The Fundamentals of Health Care Risk Management: Constructing the Comprehensive Program, for eight years. Carroll received a bachelor of science degree in health services administration and a certificate in emergency medical services systems administration from Florida International University and a master of business degree from Nova Southeastern University. She is editor of the *Risk Management Handbook for Health Care Organizations* 2nd (1997), 3rd (2000), 4th (2004) editions, and the series editor for the 5th edition (2006). Carroll has received the following awards: in 1997, ASHRM's highest honor, the Distinguished Service Award (DSA), 1998 Distinguished Alumni Achievement Award from the School of Business and Entrepreneurship, Nova Southeastern University, Most Contributing Member to Risk Management in 1996 from the Southern California Association of Healthcare Risk Management (SCAHRM), and the Most Valuable Contribution to the Field of Risk Management in 1993 from SCAHRM. She is a member of ASHRM, FSHRMPS, the Society of CPCU, and the Risk Management Affinity Group of the American Health Lawyers Associations (AHLA). She is an expert and educator in the health care risk management areas of risk financing, loss control, claims administration, early intervention programs, enterprise risk management (ERM), strategic planning, and reengineering. She is a well-known speaker on risk management issues on a national level. Her professional and committee activities are numerous.

Dominic A. Colaizzo, MBA, is managing director of Aon's National Healthcare Alternative Risk Practice, based in Philadelphia. He is responsible for directing Aon resources for the development, implementation, and servicing of alternative risk transfer programs for the health care industry. His sixteen years of experience in health care administration and nineteen years of broking and consulting experience with Aon have provided him with a broad understanding of the issues faced by all health care providers. He had served as chief operating officer and senior vice president of a community hospital and has held various administrative positions in a major teaching hospital. He has extensive experience in developing and servicing alternative risk financing and innovative insurance programs for profit and not-for-profit health systems, health insurers, managed care organizations, extended care organizations, and physicians' groups. Colaizzo also serves as a key advisor for Aon's National Healthcare Practice. He has earned a master of business administration for the Leonard Davis Institute for Health Economics at the Wharton School of the University of Pennsylvania. He has also earned a bachelor of arts degree in economics and mathematics from Washington and Jefferson College. Colaizzo is a diplomat of the American College of Health Care Executives and holds memberships in the American Society for Healthcare Risk Management (ASHRM), The American Hospital Association, and the Health Care Financial Association. He serves on the faculty for professional development seminars and has written two chapters for ASHRM's *Risk Management Handbook for Health Care Organizations.* He has co-authored an article for the *ASHRM Journal* entitled, "Integrating Quality With Risk Financing Through A Risk Retention Group."

Mary Lynn Curran, RN, MS, CPHRM, FASHRM is the Director of Clinical Risk Management for Thilman Filippini, Chicago, Illinois. Curran has been working in the health care risk management field as a consultant to health care organizations and insurance companies for many years. Her background includes nursing practice in acute and clinical settings. Before working with Thilman Filippini, Curran was consultant with AIG Consulting, Inc.–Healthcare Management Division, Chicago, Illinois, where she worked as consultant to hospitals, long-term care organizations, and miscellaneous health care facilities. She also worked for Premier, Inc., Chicago, Illinois, in the insurance division and hospital relations division. Currently, she is responsible for working directly with Thilman Filippini's health care and senior housing clients as a consultant to their risk management and safety programs. Specifically, Curran is responsible for development of prevention and control programs; education and training of client staff, and on-site consultation surveys with the agency's clients. She served on the executive board of the Chicago Healthcare Risk Management Society (CHRMS) in 2002–2004 and sits on various committees. She has sat on various committees of the American Society for Healthcare Risk Management (ASHRM) including bylaws and editorial review. She is a contributing author of numerous risk management-related articles for CHRMS and ASHRM publications including *Pearls–Risk Management Advice for the Long Term Care Organization, Pearls For Physicians* and a chapter on "Healthcare Enterprise Organizational Staffing" for the fourth edition of *Risk Management Handbook for Healthcare.* Curran earned her nursing degree from St. Francis School of Nursing, Evanston, Illinois, and her bachelor's in science and master's in healthcare administration from the University of St. Francis, Joliet, Illinois. She earned the designation of Certification in Professional Healthcare Risk Management (CPHRM) in 2002 and in 2005. She was awarded the Designation of Fellow from the American Society of HealthCare Risk Management (FASHRM) in 2005.

Kirk S. Davis, J.D., is a Florida Bar board certified health care attorney. He is head of the health care group of Akerman & Senterfitt. Davis is President of the Florida Academy of Healthcare Attorneys for the 2004–2006 term. He is ranked Number One for Florida Healthcare in *Chambers USA: America's Leading Lawyers for Business* in 2005. He is listed in Florida Trend's Legal Elite in 2004 and 2005, Best Lawyers in America from 1997 to present, and Best Healthcare Attorney in Tampa by Florida Medical Business in 2001. He was appointed as an inaugural member of the Health Law Certification Committee and was its chair in 1998–1999. He served as chair of the Florida Bar Health Law Section in 1992–1993. His health law practice includes representation of hospitals and other health care providers in general health care matters, primarily of a civil and administrative trial nature. He has extensive experience in the medicolegal aspects of the health care practice, and in all aspects of medical staff matters from both the physician and hospital perspectives, including hospital-based physician contracting. He has been practicing law in the area of civil litigation and health care since 1983. He received his bachelor of science in biology *magna cum laude* from Stetson University and his J.D. from Stetson University College of Law.

Harlan Y. Hammond, Jr., MBA, ARM, CPHRM, DFASHRM, is the Assistant Vice President for Risk Management Services at Intermountain Health Care (IHC) in Salt Lake City, Utah. His responsibilities include oversight for IHC's risk financing, loss prevention, loss control, claims administration efforts, safety, security, and system-wide emergency response. Hammond received his bachelor's degree in business administration from the University of Utah, followed by a master's of business administration degree from the University of Washington. Hammond has served in various capacities with ASHRM, including twice as a member of the ASHRM board of directors and as a faculty member for the Barton Certificate in Healthcare Risk Management Program. He received ASHRM's Distinguished Service Award in 2000.

Monica Hanslovan, Esq., is an associate of Horty, Springer & Mattern, P.C., in Pittsburgh, Pennsylvania. She focuses her practice exclusively on hospital and health care law, with particular emphasis on medical staff matters. She advises clients on a wide range of medical staff issues, including development of, analysis, and proposed revisions to medical staff bylaws, and related documents; development of hospital and medical staff policies; and management of issues related to protection of peer review documents and sharing of confidential peer review and credentialing information. Hanslovan received her J.D., *magna cum laude,* from Widener University School of Law and her B.A., *with high distinction,* from Pennsylvania State University. She is a member of the Allegheny County, Pennsylvania, and American Bar Associations, and the American Health Lawyers Association.

Judy Hart is executive vice president of Endurance Specialty Insurance, Ltd. and heads the company's health care practice. Hart has more than thirty years of experience in the insurance industry and has been dedicated to health care risk financing for the past twenty-six years. She spent most of her career at Alexander & Alexander Services, where she was a managing director and deputy national director of their health care practice. During that period of time she participated in the development of alternative risk financing programs for health care organizations across the United States. Before joining Endurance, she spent four years as vice president, Employers Reinsurance Corporation, where she was responsible for marketing, new product development, and the development of health care strategies. At ERC she was a member of the health care senior leadership team. She is the current president of the Bermuda Society for Healthcare Risk Management. She is a frequent speaker and author on risk management issues associated with risk financing, managed care, and the evolving risks facing health care providers. She attended Southeast Missouri State University and Washington University in St. Louis, Missouri.

Peter J. Hoffman, Esq. is a partner of the Philadelphia law firm of McKissock & Hoffman, P.C. He received his B.A. from Washington and Jefferson College, his M.A. from State University of New York Graduate School of Public Affairs, and his J.D., *cum laude,* from Temple University School of Law, where he was the executive editor of the *Law Review.* Hoffman was a member of the Pennsylvania Select Committee on Medical Malpractice from 1984–1986. He was a member of Governor Edward Rendell's Medical Malpractice Task Force, and is currently counsel to the Commonwealth of Pennsylvania Patient Safety Authority. He is a past president of the Pennsylvania Defense Institute. He was the recipient of the Defense Research Institute Exceptional Performance Citation in 1989 and the Fred H. Sievert Award in 1989. Hoffman was a co-author of the book *Laws and Regulations Affecting Medical Practice.* He was the Chairman of Hearing Committee 1.15, Supreme Court of Pennsylvania Disciplinary Board from 1993 to 1998, and serves on the faculty for the Temple University School of Law, Masters of Laws in Trial Advocacy and Academy of Advocacy. He has been listed as a top attorney in *Philadelphia Magazine* each time the article appears and has been listed in *Best Lawyers in America* since 1995. He was listed as one of the top 100 lawyers in Pennsylvania in *Pennsylvania Super Lawyers 2004* and *2005.* Hoffman was a member of the Temple Inns of Court. He is a member of ASHRM, a Fellow of the International Academy of Trial Lawyers, and Fellow of the American College of Trial Lawyers, and of the American Board of Trial Advocates.

John Horty, Esq., is the managing partner of Horty, Springer & Mattern, P.C., and the editor of all HortySpringer publications. He presently serves as chair of the board and a faculty member of the Estes Park Institute in Englewood, Colorado, and president and chair of the Indigo Institute in Washington, D.C. He is an honorary fellow of the American College of Hospital Executives, a recipient of the Award of Honor of the American Hospital Association, and an Honorary Life Member of the American Hospital Association. He is a founding member of the American Academy of Hospital Attorneys, a past board member of the Hospital Association of Pennsylvania, the Health Alliance of Pennsylvania, the Hospital Council of Western Pennsylvania, and was chair of St. Francis Central Hospital in Pittsburgh, Pennsylvania, from 1971–1999.

Sandra K. Johnson, RN, ARM, LHRM, FSHRM, is Director of Risk Services for the North Broward Hospital District in Fort Lauderdale, Florida. She began her career in risk management twenty-five years ago, working for PHICO Insurance Group, Inc. in Mechanicsburg, Pennsylvania. Past positions include Director, Risk and Insurance for Keystone Health System in Drexel Hill, Pennsylvania; Director, Risk and Insurance at Holy Cross Hospital in Fort Lauderdale, Florida, and System Director of Risk Management at Intracoastal Health System, West Palm Beach, Florida. She has served on many ASHRM committees, as a faculty member of the 1988 Annual Conference and nominations committee. She has served two terms on the ASHRM Board of Directors. While in Philadelphia, she held various officer and committee positions with the Philadelphia Area Society for Healthcare Risk Management and the Pennsylvania Society for Health Care Risk Management. She has also been recognized on three occasions for outstanding contribution to the field of Risk Management by the Philadelphia Area Society for Healthcare Risk Management and the Pennsylvania Healthcare Risk Management Society. She currently serves on the Florida Society for Healthcare Risk Management and Patient Safety Board of Directors as president. Additionally, she is a member of the Advisory Board for the publication *Healthcare Risk Management,* published by American Health Consultants, and has held positions on the Broward County Risk and Insurance Management Society board of directors. She was awarded the ARM designation in 1990 and the FASHRM designation in 1991. She is a licensed healthcare risk manager (LHRM) in the State of Florida.

Trista Johnson, Ph.D., MPH, is the Director of Performance Measurement and Analysis for Allina Hospitals & Clinics. Johnson provides coordinated, accurate analysis and results to drive organizational improvement. Previously, she served as the Director of Patient Safety and coordinated initiatives and measurements across the eleven hospitals and forty-four clinics within the Allina system. She was involved in the creation of a standard data collection tool and taxonomy for patient safety events, and continues to work with this system through analysis of the data and utilization of the results in safety collaboratives. A few examples of collaboratives conducted while leading patient safety include falls prevention, teamwork and patient safety, insulin safety, and the IHI trigger tool analysis. Johnson serves as a member of the Minnesota Alliance for Patient Safety (MAPS), which is involved in implementing the mandatory statewide reporting of the twenty-seven National Quality Forum events. She completed her doctoral work on the application of epidemiology to the study of medical errors.

Mark A. Kadzielski is the partner in charge of the West Coast Health Law practice at Fulbright & Jaworski, L.L.P. He represents hospitals, medical staffs, managed care enterprises, and institutional and individual health care providers throughout the United States in a broad spectrum of matters, including government regulatory investigations, contracting issues, credentialing, licensing, medical staff bylaws, Joint Commission accreditation, and Medicare certification. Kadzielski has served on the board of directors of both the American Academy of Healthcare Attorneys and the American Health Lawyers Association. He has also served on many advisory bodies in the health care industry. Kadzielski is a member of the California Bar, the American Health Lawyers Association and the California Society for Healthcare Attorneys. Since 1991, on the basis of peer evaluations, he has been selected for the Healthcare Law Section of *The Best Lawyers in America.* In 2004 and again in 2005 he was selected as a Southern California "Super Lawyer" in Health Law. In 2005, he was named to the American Health Lawyers Association's inaugural class of Fellows, one of only four attorneys in California and forty attorneys nationwide to receive this honor. Also in 2005 he was selected as one of a few leading Healthcare Lawyers in California by Chambers USA as a result of extensive interviews with clients and peers. Kadzielski has written numerous articles and chapters in health care publications, and is a nationwide speaker on a wide range of health-related subjects. Kadzielski is a 1976 graduate of the University of Pennsylvania Law School.

Leilani Kicklighter, RN, ARM, MBA, DFASHRM, CPHRM, is corporate director, patient safety & risk management services, for the Miami Jewish Home & Hospital for the Aged, Inc. in Miami, Florida. The MJHHA is the only teaching nursing home in the southeastern United States. Kicklighter began her health care career as a registered nurse. Her career in health care risk management of more than twenty-eight years has afforded her experience in the large university-based teaching hospital environment, in the medical school setting, and in several other health care provider settings, including the large multi-specialty medical clinic, the for-profit community hospital, the not-for profit integrated acute care multi-facility system, and a large HMO. She was a health care risk management consultant for a large international insurance broker, and has consulted in many countries. Kicklighter is an instructor for the Florida Risk Management Institute and the University of South Florida, preparing students to take the examination for the Florida health care risk management license. She has been active in state and local health care risk management organizations and a member of ASHRM since its inception, serving on various committees and its board of directors. She is a past president of ASHRM and of the Florida (FSHRM) and Greater Houston, Texas (GHSHRM) chapters and president of the Florida Society for Healthcare Risk Management and Patient Safety (FSHRMPS) for the 2006 term. In addition to earning the ARM and a master of business administration, she has been awarded the DFASHRM and the CPHRM.

Jane J. McCaffrey, MHSA, DFASHRM, is Director of Safety and Risk Management at Self Regional Healthcare in Greenwood, South Carolina. She has developed risk management programs at several South Carolina hospitals over the last twenty years. McCaffrey has served twice as the President of American Society for Healthcare Risk Management (1985 and 2003). She participates on several state-level patient safety and risk committees, and was a faculty member for "Fundamentals of Risk Management" for over a decade. McCaffrey received ASHRM's "Distinguished Service Award" in 1994. She also serves on the editorial advisory boards for ECRI's newsletter *Risk Management Reporter* and American Healthcare Consultant's *Healthcare Risk Management*. In 2005 she became a member of Health Research and Educational Trust's 2005–2006 Patient Safety Leadership Fellowship Class.

Jane C. McConnell, RN, MBA, JD, is executive director of the Maryland Medicine Comprehensive Insurance Program, a joint venture between the University of Maryland Medical System and University Physicians, Inc. Past positions include, vice-president, insurance and risk management, for the Franciscan Sisters of Allegany Health System, Inc. in Tampa, Florida, vice-president for risk management for FOJP Service Corporation in New York City, deputy director of New York County Professional Review Organization, director of nursing at the Brooklyn Cumberland Medical Center, and director of quality assurance with the New York City Health Department. She received her law degree from Fordham University School of Law, two master's degrees from New York University, an RN from St. Vincent's Hospital in New York, and an ARM from the Insurance Institute of America. McConnell is a past president of ASHRM and is a member of the Maryland Society for Healthcare Risk Management, AAHA and the ABA.

Peggy L. B. Nakamura, RN, MBA, JD, DFASHRM, CPHRM, is Assistant Vice President, Chief Risk Officer, and Associate Counsel of Adventist Health, a multi-state and multi-hospital health care system in the western United States. Nakamura is a past president of ASHRM and the California Chapter (CSHRM) and served on the boards of ASHRM and CSHRM. She has more than thirty years of experience in the health care field, including critical care nursing, nursing administration, medical malpractice defense attorney, and developing multi-hospital system risk management programs. In her current position, she oversees a comprehensive risk management department, including self-administered and self-insured programs in workers' compensation and professional, general, and managed care liability. In 2001, Nakamura was named to the Business Insurance's Risk Management Honor Roll and, in 1997, was awarded the Outstanding Advocate Award from the American Association of Nurse Attorneys (TAANA). She lectures frequently on risk management topics to a variety of audiences.

Judith Napier is Corporate Director Risk Management and Patient Safety for Allina Hospitals and Clinics in Minnesota. Before joining Allina, Napier was Senior Director, Patient

Safety and Risk Management Services, for Children's Hospitals and Clinics in Minnesota. Napier has held the past position of Senior Vice President for MMI Companies, an international health care risk management company, where she was responsible for an international consulting division and product innovation and customization for the company, specifically introducing new risk management strategies and products to the health care industry. Before her work with MMI Companies, she practiced nursing in high-risk perinatal units and taught maternal child nursing in several academic accredited nursing programs at both the baccalaureate and associate degree level. Her career includes clinical practice, consultation, teaching and more than twenty years as an executive in the health care industry. Napier holds a bachelor's degree in Nursing from Niagara University and a master's degree in Maternal Child Clinical Specialty Nursing from California State University at Los Angeles. She has recently received a certificate of completion from HRET and the Health Forum Patient Safety Leadership Fellowship 2004–2005. Napier has been a frequent national and international speaker in the area of patient safety, quality, and risk management.

Gisele Anne Norris, DrPH, is Senior Consultant, Aon National Healthcare, Alternative Risk Practice, Aon Healthcare, San Francisco, California. Norris has spent fifteen years in the health care industry focusing on issues of health care finance. She currently directs Aon's Alternative Risk (ART) Practice in the western United States, where she assists clients with the formation, restructuring, and management of all types of alternative risk financing vehicles. Before accepting her role with the ART team, she was responsible for the development of new health care product opportunities for Aon internationally. Before joining Aon seven years ago, she provided consultation to various governments on issues of health finance policy on behalf of a contractor for the United States State Department's Agency for International Development. Norris is widely published in various insurance industry publications. She received her B.A. from the University of California at Berkeley in 1988; Master of Public Health and Master of Public Administration degrees from Columbia University in 1994; and a Doctorate in Public Health from the University of California at Berkeley in 2000. She worked full time in the insurance industry while completing her doctorate.

Pamela J. Para, RN, MPH, CPHRM, FASHRM is the director of professional and technical services for the American Society for Healthcare Risk Management of the American Hospital Association in Chicago, Illinois. In this role, Para is responsible for responding to member inquiries and compiling member feedback on relevant risk management issues of importance to health care organizations, managing the development and production of ASHRM education programs, and developing and administering the society's advocacy activities. Para's prior experience includes evaluating a variety of health care organizations, nationwide and in Puerto Rico, for potential medical professional, general, and workers' compensation liability exposures for a major commercial insurance carrier. She has also performed medical-legal reviews of potential and litigated claims, negotiated settlements for a major pharmaceutical recall, managed workers' compensation claims, and served as advisor to risk managers and other corporate claims coordinators of various self-insured health care facilities in the metropolitan Chicago area and nationwide for a third-party claims administrator. Para has more than twenty years of professional health care experience, including fourteen years in health care risk management and nursing experience in both civilian and military maternal-child clinical settings. She received a Bachelor of Science degree in nursing with a minor in Spanish from DePauw University and a master of public health degree from the University of Illinois at Chicago. Para is a published author and has been a frequent presenter of risk management and workers' compensation topics.

Madelyn S. Quattrone, Esq., is a Senior Risk Management Analyst for ECRI, Plymouth Meeting, Pennsylvania. She is editor of ECRI's publication Continuing Care Risk Management, and is a regular contributor to ECRI's Healthcare Risk Control System. She has been a panelist in ECRI audio conferences discussing risk management and legal issues involving the health information privacy regulations and the security regulations of the Health Insurance Portability and Accountability Act of 1996 (HIPAA). Before joining ECRI, Quattrone was a shareholder in the law firm of George, Koran, Quattrone, Blumberg & Chant, P.A., in Woodbury, New Jersey, concentrating on the defense of medical malpractice cases from 1982 to 1999. A member of the bars of the Commonwealth of Pennsylvania, New Jersey, the U.S. District Court of New Jersey, the Third Circuit Court of Appeals, and the U.S. Supreme Court, Quattrone achieved certification by the New Jersey Supreme Court as a civil trial attorney in 1990 and was selected for membership in the American Board of Trial Advocates in 1993. Quattrone also provided risk management consultation to physicians, hospitals, and professional liability insurers, and contributed to the development of a clinicolegal correspondence course for the Medical Inter-Insurance Exchange of New Jersey. She wrote regularly for numerous publications, including the *Emergency Physician Legal Bulletin*, the *Emergency Nurse Legal Bulletin*, and the *Emergency Medical Technician Legal Bulletin*. For many years, Quattrone co-authored a column on legal and risk management issues affecting emergency nurses in the *Journal of Emergency Nursing*. She developed case scenarios and participated in mock medical malpractice trials for audiences of physicians, medical students, residents, and clinical engineers, and has been a frequent speaker in numerous risk management areas, including informed consent, ethical and legal issues involving human reproduction, obstetrics, the provision of emergency care, and medical record documentation. Quattrone earned a J.D. degree from Rutgers University School of Law, Camden, New Jersey, in 1981 and a B.A. degree in anthropology from Temple University, Philadelphia, Pennsylvania.

Michael L. Rawson is the Corporate Director of Safety, Security, and Environmental Health for Intermountain Health Care (IHC) in Salt Lake City, Utah, where he has been employed for the past twenty-six years. Responsibilities include management of safety, security, and environmental health issues and compliance with regulatory activities specific to these areas. Rawson holds a Bachelor of Science degree in Sociology with a Certificate in Law Enforcement from the University of Utah and a master's degree in Administration of Justice from Wichita State University. He is a Certified Healthcare Safety Professional (CHSP), a Certified Healthcare Environmental Manager (HEM), and a Senior American Society for Healthcare Engineering (SASHE). Rawson has served on various committees with the American Society for Healthcare Engineering (ASHE), The National Fire Protection Association (NFPA), Department of Homeland Security (DHS), and Department of Veterans Affairs–Facilities (VA), and as president of the Mountain States Society for Healthcare Engineering (MSSHE). Rawson is a faculty member for ASHE-sponsored *Environment of Care JCAHO Survey Process Preparation* programs and has presented throughout the United States programs on hospital security, safety, and emergency preparation and management.

Sheila Hagg-Rickert, JD, MHA, MBA, CPCU, DFASHRM, PHRM is Chief Risk Officer and Senior Vice President, Sun Healthcare Group, Irvine, California. Hagg-Rickert has more than twenty years experience in health care risk management, including insurance program development and administration, claims management, loss control, and regulatory compliance. Her experience includes senior positions with individual hospitals, long-term care providers, not-for-profit and proprietary multi-hospital systems, and national insurance brokerage organizations. Hagg-Rickert has written and spoken extensively on risk management and health care legal topics and has served on the Board of Directors of ASHRM. She holds a law degree from the University of Iowa and master's degrees in both business administration and health care administration. She has earned the Distinguished Fellow and Certified Professional in Healthcare Risk Management designations from ASHRM and is a Chartered Property and Casualty Underwriter (CPCU).

Jeannie Sedwick, ARM, Vice President, Relationship Management, is a health care broker for Aon Risk Services, Inc. and is based in Winston-Salem, North Carolina. Previously she was Director of Risk Management for Wake County Hospital System, Inc., in Raleigh, North Carolina for more than twenty years. She held the position of Vice President of Marketing for The Medical Protective Company/Employers Reinsurance Company and was responsible for production of health care accounts for the southern United States. She served as Managing Director for Property Casualty for Insurance Resource, Inc. a division of the American Hospital Association, in Chicago, Illinois. She served on the ASHRM board for six years and was president, 1996–1997. She is a founding member of the North Carolina Chapter of ASHRM and has served as its president and board member and on many committees. She was recognized for her contributions to the NC ASHRM Chapter and was awarded the Distinguished Service Award in 1996. She has been an author in the *Risk Management Handbook for Health Care Organizations,* 2nd (1997), 3rd (2000) and 4th (2004) editions. Sedwick was selected to the Business Insurance, Risk Manager of the Year Honor Roll in 1997 for her contributions to the field of risk management and for her achievements as Risk Manager at Wake County Hospital System, Inc.

Elizabeth D. Shaw, RN, BSN, MSA, JD, is an associate with the law firm of Akerman Senterfitt in Jacksonville, Florida, practicing health care and corporate law. She is also a licensed health care risk manager and a registered nurse in the State of Florida. Shaw received her law degree from Florida Coastal School of Law (J.D. with honors), a Master of Science in Administration, specializing in general health services, from Central Michigan University, and a Bachelor of Science in Nursing from Florida State University. Shaw is a member of the Florida Bar, the Health Law Section of the American Bar Association, and the American Health Lawyers Association. She is a frequent lecturer on various health care law topics.

Ronni P. Solomon, JD, is executive vice president and general counsel at ECRI, a non-profit health services research agency in suburban Philadelphia that focuses on the safety, quality, and cost-effectiveness of patient care. Solomon has approximately twenty years' experience in health care risk management, patient safety, law, and regulation. She works with leaders at hospitals, health systems, government agencies, continuing care organizations, and insurance providers to implement patient safety and quality assessment systems. She has published numerous articles and book chapters, and has lectured frequently in the United States and abroad. Solomon serves as the Center Director for ECRI's Collaborating Center for the World Health Organization in patient safety, health care technology and risk management. She is a past member of ASHRM's board of directors and has served in many other leadership roles for ASHRM. She received ASHRM's first Award for Writing Excellence.

John C. West, JD, MHA, DFASHRM, is a senior health care consultant with AIG Consultants Inc., Healthcare Management Division. He holds a bachelor's degree from the University of Cincinnati, a law degree from Salmon P. Chase College of Law, and a master's degree in health services administration from Xavier University. He received the Distinguished Service Award from ASHRM in 2001, the highest honor bestowed by that society. He also received the designation of distinguished fellow of the American Society for Healthcare Risk Management (DFASHRM) in 1999. West has been a frequent speaker at national and regional educational programs and has published numerous articles on various aspects of health care risk management. He currently writes the "Case Law Update" column on a quarterly basis for the *Journal of Healthcare Risk Management*.

Kimberly Willis, MBA, CPCU, ARM currently serves as Vice President, Field Underwriting for Berkley Medical Excess. In this capacity, she is responsible for risk evaluation, marketing strategy, and product positioning. Before joining BerkleyMed, Willis served as Managing Director, Healthcare Syndication, for Aon Risk Services. She managed a team responsible for the design, negotiation, and broking of over $500 million in health care professional liability premium. Willis earned her bachelor of science in Business Administration at the University of Missouri and a master of business administration at Maryville University. She holds the Chartered Property and Casualty Underwriter (CPCU) and Associate in Risk Management (ARM) designations. She has taught the economics and accounting modules of the CPCU designation, and is currently a faculty member for ASHRM's Barton Certificate in Healthcare Risk Modules. She is a member of the Professional Liability Underwriting Society, Society of Chartered Property and Casualty Underwriters, American Society for Healthcare Risk Management, and Missouri Society for Healthcare Risk Managers.

Sheila Cohen Zimmet, BSN, JD, is Associate Dean (Research Compliance) at Weill Medical College of Cornell University, where she serves as the course director for the Tri-Institutional Responsible Conduct of Research course for Weill Cornell Medical College, Rockefeller University, and Memorial Sloan-Kettering Institute. She previously served as Director of Research Assurance and Compliance and as senior counsel for Georgetown University Medical Center. She started her professional career as a neonatal intensive care nurse after earning her undergraduate nursing degree from Georgetown University in 1971. After she received her law degree (JD) from Georgetown in 1975, Zimmet pursued a legal career with the federal government in the fields of occupational and mine safety and health. She returned to Georgetown University in 1984, where her health law practice focused on clinical, bioethical, and biomedical research issues, professional liability and risk management, and other hospital and higher education legal issues involving patients, students, faculty, and staff that are common to academic medical centers. Zimmet also serves as a member of the National Advisory Research Resources Council of the National Institutes of Health.

Preface

As health care risk management continues to evolve as a profession, the opportunities abound for astute risk management professionals to advance their careers while adding value to their organizations. Risk management professionals are in a unique position to enhance organizational efforts to ensure patient safety and minimize risk, while creating an atmosphere that is conducive to teaming and trust. They work within an environment that is complex, changing, and burdened with increasing regulations and laws. They have never been more needed.

Health risk management today requires a well-seasoned, dedicated professional with the requisite skill set to recommend and facilitate change. These committed professionals are valued by their organization for the strategies and solutions that they offer to enhance the culture of the work environment, and by initiating techniques to reduce the exposures to risk inherent in all health care operations. Risk management professionals are generalist; and while not expert in all areas, they are familiar with all aspects of the organization and readily see the "big picture" of how risks interact and are synergistic. *The risk management professional understands how risk represents not only the potential for loss but also the opportunity for gain and profit.*

Enterprise risk management, while slow for health care to grasp, is nonetheless making headway. An analogy can be made to current efforts in patient safety. Both are organization-wide initiatives requiring the commitment and attention of every employee, and both emanate from the top of the organization. Neither of these initiatives is easily accomplished. Both represent a life commitment on the part of the organization if they are to be successful.

The fifth edition of the *Risk Management Handbook for Health Care Organizations* has tried to capture that essential knowledge crucial for the risk management professional in health care today and translate the information into a useful reference resource. Very little in risk management ever seems to go away. We just keep adding to this vast wealth of information by way of new requirements, statutes, standards, best practices, and so on. What has changed is how we evaluate organizational risks, the impact that one risk has on another, and our approach to eliminate or manage those risks.

Our goal with this handbook is to educate the risk management professional on an enterprise-wide basis offering discussion on a variety of risk topics, both clinical and non-clinical, representative of different care settings. Where possible, we have discussed the risk issue, developed a strategy to eliminate or minimize specific risks, and offered solutions. We have continued, as with other editions, to offer an extensive variety of tools such as policies and procedures, checklists, tables, graphs, figures, and the like. It is anticipated that this information will be supplemented by material from the Internet, an invaluable resource for any risk management professional. Many contributing authors have suggested Web sites and readings to augment their chapter information.

The sheer volume of information that was felt to be important to communicate to the health care risk management professional (or other interested parties) necessitated that we revise the format. No longer could the information be contained in one book. Therefore, this edition has been written as a three-volume series. Although many chapters are new to this edition, others have simply been updated or revised. Many of the chapters refer the reader to other chapters within the series. We have highlighted those references for you to make it easier to find additional information within the series. The three volumes in the series are:

Volume I   The Essentials
Volume II   Clinical Risk
Volume III Business Risk: Legal, Regulatory, & Technology Issues

New chapters on medication safety, risk management information systems, risk in the operating room, pediatrics, ICU, radiology, and emergency departments, and chapters on Enterprise Risk Management ~ The Basics, and Basic Claims Administration represent just some of the new material presented in this fifth edition.

This series embodies the collective work of eighty-seven authors and fifty-eight chapters, and represents the better part of two years to finalize from the initial author contact until publication. It was no easy feat on an all-volunteer basis. I want to thank all the contributing authors for their dedication and their willingness to give up personal time to advance the profession of risk management. They all have an abiding commitment to our educational efforts, for which we are appreciative. Please give a resounding and well-deserved "thank you" the next time you see one of the authors. Each volume has a beginning section, "About the Contributors," where you will see every author listed with a brief biographical sketch. I think you will agree that the diversity and expertise of our author panel is unsurpassed by any other risk management text. In this edition we have also added the writing of several new physician authors and experts from the ISMP, IHI, and many other organizations dedicated to risk management and patient safety, all adding to the credibility of this reference series.

An undertaking of this magnitude requires the assistance of a dedicated team. I want to personally express my gratitude and thanks to each volume editor for an outstanding job. Without them this project would not have been done.

Volume I   Peggy Nakamura and Roberta Carroll
Volume II   Sylvia Brown
Volume III Glenn Troyer

Peggy, Sylvia, and Glenn each worked with a dedicated task force to assist with their specific volume. Please take a moment to look in the "About this Book" section in the front of each volume for a listing of those individuals. Again, they are entitled to a well-deserved "thank you" and our gratitude.

The support of ASHRM staff with our publication efforts is very much appreciated. We anticipate that this new series will quickly be a best seller and a big hit with the attendees at the 2006 ASHRM annual educational conference.

Even with the best of intentions not to compete with the holiday season, this series was prepared for the publisher by the beginning of 2006. I want to thank my family for their patience while I disappeared into my office over the holidays to read and edit. A special thank you, once again, to my brother Terrance (Red) Carroll for his production assistance in preparing the manuscript for the publisher. I'll make him a risk manager yet!

We hope you find this series easy to use, thorough, convenient, and an invaluable resource that becomes a mainstay in your risk management library. Share it with others in your organization, so that they can better understand and support the role of the health care risk management professional.

Thank you,
Roberta Carroll
Series Editor

About This Book

The field of health care risk management continues to evolve, mature, and expand as the concept of enterprise risk management (ERM) takes hold in health care organizations. Volume I of the fifth edition of the *Risk Management Handbook for Health Care Organizations* is a risk management primer covering the essential core elements of a successful risk management program, regardless of the type of health care organization or the experience level of the risk management professional charged with administering such programs.

This volume begins by addressing basic considerations, such as ERM, legal concepts, and effective governance. From there, the reader can learn, or review, how to develop a risk management program, grow as a risk management professional, and use metrics in developing and evaluating the program's success.

The remainder of the book addresses several critical areas for risk management programs. In the risk financing area, the reader will find excellent information on claims administration, insurance principles, and coverage concepts, and an introduction to risk financing as a distinct program component. Additional chapters address ethics, patient communication, credentialing of providers, contract review concepts, information technology, documentation and health information management, occupational health, organizational staffing, and emergency management.

The majority of the chapters were revised and updated from the fourth edition of the *Risk Management Handbook*. For reviewing and editing hundreds of pages, it was a pleasure to work with Fran Kurdwanoski, Harlan Hammond, Terie Zimmerman, and the always present Roberta Carroll on this project.

The readers of this volume benefit from their caring, commitment, and sharing of their knowledge for the advancement of the health care risk management profession.

Peggy Nakamura
Volume I, Co-Editor

1

Enterprise Risk Management in Health Care ~ The Basics

Roberta L. Carroll
Gisele A. Norris

INTRODUCTION

The Committee of Sponsoring Organizations of the Treadway Commission (COSO) defines Enterprise Risk Management (ERM) in the Executive Summary of "Enterprise Risk Management—Integrated Framework" as:

". . . a process, effected by an entity's board of directors, management and other personnel, applied in strategy setting and across the enterprise, designed to identify potential events that may affect the entity, and manage risk to be within its risk appetite, to provide reasonable assurance regarding the achievement of entity objectives."[1]

This chapter applies the principles and concepts of enterprise risk management to health care. The intent is to provide a basic overview for those new to the concept of ERM. For a more comprehensive treatment of ERM, please see the chapter on "Enterprise Risk Management" in Volume III of this series.

ERM is an ongoing series of interrelated activities, designed to identify, assess, manage, and monitor the events and risk facing an organization. The risks identified by an ERM process may be insurable or uninsurable and may traditionally be handled by different divisions within a given organization. Once all risks are identified, evaluated, and measured, the organization can develop prioritized, organization-wide solutions and strategies for dealing with those risks. Because ERM takes a broad, high-level view of risk, it requires the commitment of various professionals throughout an organization, including those in the "C-Suite" (Chief Executive Officer, Chief Financial Officer, Chief Nursing Executive, Chief Medical Executive, and so on).

. . . .

THE SHORTCOMINGS OF TRADITIONAL RISK MANAGEMENT

Traditionally, risk management has focused on specific categories of risk (silos) and how a particular risk might affect one aspect of organizational health (insurance costs, for example). Although identifying such risks is a step in the right direction, stopping the analysis once a particular risk is acknowledged might paint an incomplete picture. For example, let's imagine that a clinical risk manager identifies wrong-site surgery as a risk and estimates the impact of wrong-site surgery on professional liability costs by evaluating filed claims and insurance premiums. This provides some information about the consequences of wrong-site surgery. However, this risk might have other important effects (financial and otherwise) that could also be identified and measured. Examples include: a negative impact on reputation leading to decreased market share and increased scrutiny by regulatory and accreditation agencies. These outcomes are associated with real costs that a more complete risk assessment should take into account.

Furthermore, traditional risk management fails to take into account the effect of one risk upon another. Understanding the relationship between risks allows for better utilization of resources (people, money, time, ideas), decreases duplication of effort, encourages and supports "out of the box" approaches, and supports the early identification and assessment of risk across the continuum of care. For example, the literature is replete with human resource/human capital issues relating to:

- Workforce fatigue[2,3,4,5]
- Educational levels of hospital nurses and their effect on patient outcomes[6]
- Staff intimidation in the area of safe medication practices[7]
- The decreasing professional labor pool

However, the effect that these issues have on each other has not been easily or readily identified (for example, a decreasing professional labor pool likely creates a demanding and stressful work environment that promotes workplace fatigue), nor their collective effect on matters of patient safety, consumer satisfaction, and medical professional liability. This example makes it clear that relationships among risks need to be identified and analyzed to support core organizational goals, such as providing safe, high-quality patient care.

Finally, it is possible that the greatest risk facing the organization is a risk that does not fall naturally into an area identified or treated by a traditional risk management effort (for example, clinical risk management). Bioterrorism, for example, is a significant risk in health care, even though it does not fall neatly into one domain of hospital risk management. In recent years, hospitals have been forced to identify bioterrorism-related risk throughout their enterprises. For example, although the mailroom was never a focus of traditional risk management activities, the recent anthrax scare has changed the way most health care organizations handle incoming mail. Similarly, the tragedy of 9/11 reinvigorated many health care organizations' efforts in emergency management, and to be successful, those efforts were forced to adopt many of the elements of enterprise risk management. In short, health care institutions are beginning to realize that the risk with the highest potential cost to the institution as a whole might never be considered without an organization-wide risk approach.

···········

HEALTH CARE ENTERPRISE RISK MANAGEMENT

In contrast to traditional risk management, ERM broadly examines multiple categories of risk and estimates how the repercussions arising from a given risk might affect the organization as a whole. The goal of ERM is to spotlight the greatest risks to the entire enterprise, whether those risks are regularly encountered within the hospital or have never before been considered. Once the greatest risks have been identified, organizations are better able to determine an appropriate, integrated response (including prevention, mitigation, management, and financing).

It is difficult for those outside of health care to grasp the uniqueness of health care risk management. Health care risk management includes some elements that are similar to risk management in other industries (manufacturers, service industries, and so on), in addition to common risk management issues and concerns (workers' compensation, fleet safety, workplace safety, hazard identification and mitigation, and so on). However, the potential severity of a catastrophic injury to a patient is distinct. There are not many other industries that function around the clock every day and where poor outcomes result in such dire consequences. As a result, in the past risk managers have placed emphasis on addressing clinical risk. Such a narrow approach can be limiting and might not result in the greatest enhancement of patient safety. ERM provides a broader approach for addressing health care risk. Another challenge faced by health care risk management programs is the effect of continuous advances in medical research and technology. Although these advances support the goal of improved patient care, they come with a price tag: new risk.

ERM and Health Care: Why Now?

Examining risks on an enterprise-wide basis may be particularly important in today's health care environment for several reasons. For example, one of the greatest challenges facing hospitals today is ensuring patient safety. Variability of patient care represents a significant risk that cannot simply be transferred to insurance. Recent emphasis on patient safety initiatives requires providers to focus on prevention through better management of their risks. Furthermore, health care delivery systems are facing increased financial scrutiny and concerns regarding patient safety. Risk management has come to the spotlight with the Sarbanes-Oxley Act of 2002,[8] which increases requirements for accounting oversight and has forced companies to broaden their assessment of their own risks. As investors and regulators demand greater risk transparency, efforts are increasing to assess a health care organization's myriad risks and cover them in a strategic risk management program.

Several other factors have also combined to intensify the importance of ERM throughout the United States. They include:

- Pressure to manage risk more comprehensively and systematically[9]
- Greater accountability and increased scrutiny for boards of directors and senior executives[10]
- Rising frequency and severity of risk[11]
- Negative effect of adverse legal judgment on reputation

- Increasing importance of evolving risks
  - Growing number of doubtful accounts results in increased credit risk
  - Use of variable rate bonds results in increased interest rate risk
  - Vicarious liability assumes increased importance

According to a recent Economist Intelligence Unit survey in April 2005, entitled "The Evolving Role of the CRO," the top three risk management priorities three years from now will be:

- Ensuring that the organization is in full compliance with regulations
- Monitoring and identifying emergent risk
- Extending risk principles into the wider business strategy[12]

Although these predictions were not specifically related to health care, these issues are clearly etched onto the minds of many health care executives for today and the future.

Risk, as described by Jerry Miccolis and Samir Shah in their monograph on "Enterprise Risk Management—An Analytic Approach," is the possibility that something, directly or indirectly, will prevent the achievement of business objectives. Risk factors are the events or conditions that give rise to risk. Risks in health care cannot be eliminated. However, having a thorough understanding of the underlying factors that cause risk will allow for appropriate management and control of those risks. If unmanaged risk prevents the achievement of objectives, well-managed risk may promote the achievement of objectives. Therefore, it stands to reason that understanding and managing risk enterprise-wide can give an organization a competitive advantage.[13]

Health Care ERM: Strategy and Process

A successful ERM program in a health care institution might yield the following results:

1. Identify and prioritize strategically important risks.
2. Assign risk "ownership" to various groups within the organization to promote consistent risk assessments, responses, and accountability across the organization.
3. Provide analytical models for future scenarios to help predict and prepare for potential risk developments.
4. Create an ongoing ERM process within the institution.

RELATIONSHIP OF OBJECTIVES AND COMPONENTS

"Enterprise Risk Management—Integrated Framework," by the Committee of Sponsoring Organizations of the Treadway Commission, states that there is a direct relationship between objectives, which are what an entity strives to achieve, and the enterprise risk management components, which represent what is needed to achieve them. The following exhibit will depict the relationship in a three-dimensional matrix. Refer to Figure 1.1. This matrix has been used as the model for this chapter.

The first step in the process is to ensure that enterprise risk management is a strategic priority for the organization at the board and leadership level. In health care, this also means obtaining "buy-in" from the medical staff and other clinical providers. Education and communication are vital so that the board, medical staff, and leadership all understand the concepts and use common terminology for enterprise risk management.

FIGURE 1.1　　Three-Dimensional Matrix in the Form of a Cube

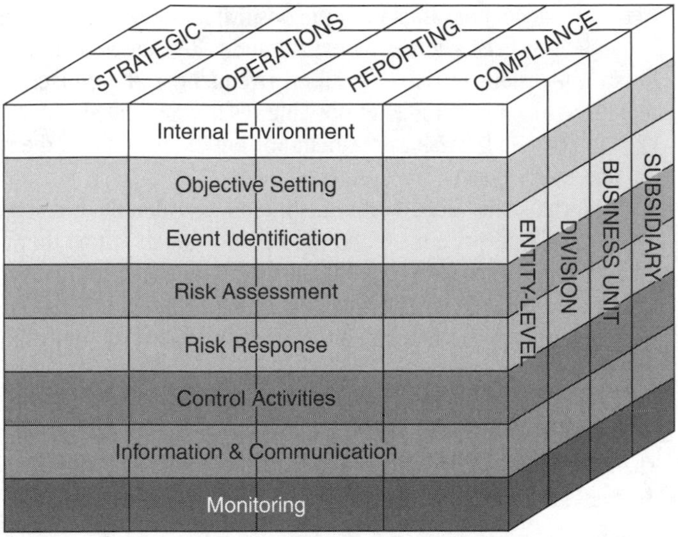

Once buy-in is achieved, it is important to study the internal environment to ascertain the organization's risk management philosophy, risk appetite, ethical values, and management style. Although external factors influence enterprise risk, the internal environment established by the core is the cornerstone for all strategy and objectives.

The next step is to understand how the current risk management program functions, using that knowledge as a baseline or "springboard" from which to restructure the program from one that uses silos to one that is integrated for the total enterprise.

The third step is to identify a core group of individuals (multi-disciplinary) who will function as the enterprise team and be responsible for driving the project forward. This team will define objectives and deliverables and schedule activities accordingly. Because the foundation of any ERM program is information gathering and analysis, much of the core team's work will revolve around data issues.

Event Identification

The enterprise team will need to contemplate the various categories and domains of risk and identify whether any written documents exist that might shed light on the risks resident in each domain. More important, the team will need to develop an interview process that allows key personnel to provide input on potential events that "keep them up at night." Health care has many formal and informal systems by which events, risk, and risk factors are identified. Incident reporting, generic screening, occurrence screening, root cause analysis (RCA), and failure mode effect analysis (FMEA) are all techniques and tools geared to identify events, risk, and risk factors. The identification of non-clinical events, risk, and risk factors is not as robust and requires the coordinated approach of enterprise risk management. The effect of external and internal factors on events also is considered. Increased litigiousness of the public and patient satisfaction are just two examples of external factors to be considered. Examples of internal factors to consider in health care are the increased use of technology and its effect on the workforce and the changing corporate culture.

Risk Assessment

Risk assessment considers both the positive and negative consequences of events underlying identified risks across an organization. Risk assessment takes into account two different dimensions of risk: likelihood (frequency) and impact (severity) and recognizes that there might be a range of possible results associated with a given event.

To conduct the risk assessment portion of the analysis, the risks from both an internal and external standpoint are examined.

Internal risks faced by the institution are identified, discussed, and characterized by both the enterprise team and the key individuals whom they decide to interview. Ideally, these interviews are conducted with employees from several functions in various locations. Interview instruments should be designed to elicit information that will provide insight into current and future risks and into the mitigation techniques currently in use.

The external environment is assessed concurrently. The focus of this assessment is on the effect of external factors on risk management strategy and financial performance. The core team may decide to include additional interviewees in this process. Examples of external factors that affect risk include items such as:

- Professional turnover
- Fixed income and equity market returns
- Changing regulations
- Decreased reimbursement
- Professional liability market trends
- Demographic trends
- Regulatory performance

These sources of information should then be summarized to create a catalogue of potential risks.

Risk Classification

In assessing risk, it is helpful to classify risk factors as manageable or strategic, using a scheme that implies action. Manageable risk factors have the following characteristics:

- Known environment
- Capabilities and resources on hand
- Risks that fell between the cracks.[14] (The risk was somehow missed and is correctable.)

Examples of manageable risk factors might include the risk of wrong-site surgery, the continued inappropriate use of abbreviations, inadequate credentialing, and peer review processes. Health care has the ability and resources on hand to manage these risk factors, and according to Miccolis and Shah at Tillinghast, one might say, "Just get on with it,"[15] meaning fix the problem.

Strategic risk, on the other hand, according to Miccolis[16] et al, requires allocation of capital or a shift in strategic direction. Characteristics of strategic risk factors are:

- Unfamiliar territory
- Capabilities or resources not in place

- Major change in market or business
- Change in reimbursement
- New regulations and requirements

Examples of health care strategic risk factors might include the increased use of technology, such as the implementation of CPOE (computerized physician-provider order entry), bar coding, robotics, use of modeling and simulation, and changes to Medicare reimbursement that affect the products or services offered by the organization. Health care has been ill equipped to deal with these risk factors internally and has forged partnership with outside consultants and vendors for support.

Risk Scoring—Risk Mapping

Once an exhaustive list of risks is assembled, the enterprise team will need to evaluate the importance of one risk versus another. To do so, they must develop a weighting (or scoring) methodology. This methodology may be largely intuitive, but should take into account probability, severity, and time to impact of each of the risks being evaluated. The ultimate score associated with each risk will be (Probability + Time to Impact) × Severity. Refer to Tables 1.1–3 for examples of scoring weights. Remember that these are offered as examples and that each organization needs to personalize them according to its "appetite

TABLE 1.1   Qualitative Measure of Risk Frequency

Level	Descriptor	Example Detail Description
1	Extremely rare	May occur on in exceptional circumstances
2	Rare	Could occur at some time
3	Periodic	Will occur at some time
4	Recurrent	Will probably occur in most circumstances
5	Occurs frequently	Is expected to occur in most circumstances

Reprinted with the Permission of Corey Gooch, IRMG, Aon Limited.

TABLE 1.2   Measure of Time to Impact

Level	Descriptor
1	Warning occurs over a long period of time (**months or years**) providing opportunity to adjust or react
2	Warning occurs over a shorter period of time (**days or weeks**) providing some opportunity to adjust or react
3	No warning, impact is felt immediately (**no warning**)

Reprinted with the Permission of Corey Gooch, IRMG, Aon Limited.

TABLE 1.3   Qualitative and Quantitative Measures of Risk Severity

Level	Descriptor	Descriptor Financial Impact
1	Minor	Less than $50,000
2	Moderate	$50,001–$500,000
3	Major	$500,001–$1,000,000
4	Severe	$1,000,001–$5,000,000
5	Catastrophic	Over $5,000,000

Reprinted with the Permission of Corey Gooch, IRMG, Aon Limited.

FIGURE 1.2   Sample Risk Map

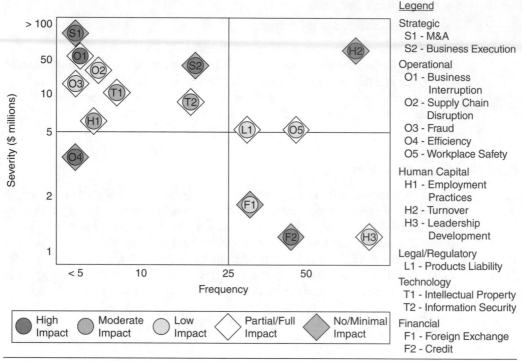

for risk." Once the organization scores each area, the scores are then used to place risks in priority order. The results might then be arrayed graphically for easy viewing. This process is known as risk mapping. It graphically summarizes the potential frequency, severity, and relative time to impact of each risk. Refer to Figure 1.2—Risk Map. Note that risks falling in the upper right-hand corner of the graph are both frequent and severe. These risks are clearly quite important; however, it is likely that many of them have already been identified. Risks in the upper left quadrant, however, are infrequent and severe. This is a particularly important category, as these are risks that might not have been considered in the past, but could have a potentially catastrophic effect on the organization.

Scoring risks one against the other allows the team to create a list of priority items. The team then carefully examines these priority items to determine potential causes (risk factors), impacts, and what techniques are currently being used for risk mitigation. Details about each priority risk might be examined according to the categories or risk domain. Refer to Table 1.4—Risk Categories and Domains.

Risk Response

Once the enterprise team has had the opportunity to consider actions that are currently used to address priority risks, they may begin to consider alternative responses to that risk, including options for avoiding, accepting, reducing, and sharing risk. This part of the process is known as the "risk response" path, during which the team evaluates

TABLE 1.4   Risk Categories and Domains

Financial	Risks such as capital structure, credit and interest rate fluctuations, foreign exchange and accounts receivable. These are risks that affect the profitability, cash position, access to capital, or external financial ratings through business relationships or the timing and recognition of revenue and expenses.
Operational/Clinical	Risks related to the conduct of the business operation that results from inadequate or failed internal processes, people, or systems (medical malpractice) that affect patient safety.
Human Capital	An explosive area of exposure in today's tight labor market including employee selection, retention and turnover, absenteeism, and compensation.
Strategic	Brand, reputation and advertising risks, and risks associated with business strategy. Failure to adapt to changing environment, changing customer priorities, competitive risk, clinical research.
Legal/Regulatory	Incorporates risks arising out of product liability, management liability, failure to comply with statutes, standards, rules and regulations, and issues related to intellectual property.
Technological	An area of tremendous growth in health care including risk associated with the adoption of new systems and processes, (e.g., CPOE, bar coding, EHR, PACS, robotics, simulation, modeling, medical monitoring, telemedicine, cyber-medicine).
Natural Disaster/Hazard	Risks attributable to physical loss of assets or a reduction in their value, including risk arising from earthquakes, windstorms, tornadoes, floods, fires, etc. Traditionally insurable risk related to natural hazards and business interruption.

TABLE 1.5   Fetal Hypoxia

Risk	Cause (Risk Factor)	Impact	Internal Controls	Recommended Actions	Score
• Fetal hypoxic event	• Failure to recognize fetal distress • Failure to interpret fetal monitoring • Inability to perform emergency c-section • Failure to activate chain of command	• Lifetime injury or death • Medical malpractice loss • Increased insurance rates • Loss of reputation • Increased scrutiny by JCAHO, State • Difficulty attracting staff	• Education • Use of technology to facilitate recognition of fetal distress • New policies ensuring emergency c-section readiness • PR advertising new measures	• Bi-annual fetal-monitor training • Identify/purchase new technology • Float obstetricians • Host "mothers-to-be" event	27.5

Carroll RL, Norris GA, Aon Healthcare.

various risk solutions in the context of their organization's risk appetite (the degree of uncertainty an organization is willing to accept to reach its goals) and the cost of capital and competitive position (among other variables), selects appropriate solutions, and assigns implementation responsibility to one or more individuals. For a health care example in the OB area, refer to Table 1.5—Fetal Hypoxia.

Control Activities

Implementation of new risk management techniques must be controlled throughout the organization. In fact, control of risk management activities is increasingly important in the face of HIPAA regulations and electronic health records (EHR). The development of policies and procedures is the core of all control activities. There are policies and procedures in place at all levels throughout the organization. They must be continuously updated and relied upon to ensure that new risk management techniques are properly implemented.

Monitoring

Health care risk is constantly evolving and changing. Continuous monitoring on a real time basis of the internal and external environment is a critical step in enterprise risk management. All risk response components should have a monitoring element built into the activity. Once implemented, solutions should be monitored and evaluated to determine whether:

- The current strategy and tactics achieve their objectives
- The risk owners are properly implementing the strategy
- Information is being appropriately communicated to senior management.

....
INFORMATION AND COMMUNICATION

Communicating the success, failure, and imperfections of new risk management responses is key to ongoing program improvement. High-quality information is needed to identify, assess, manage, and monitor both risk and risk management efforts. Quality information may come in many forms. It may be retrospective (the use of claims loss runs), concurrent or real-time data from systems and record review, or prospective information from trending, forecasting, and modeling. The failure to communicate promptly and appropriately for the situation and the failure to adequately document medical care continue to be the two factors most commonly associated with all medical professional liability claims.

Without information, you have no communication. Understanding data and translating it into meaningful information is a skill set, as are good communication skills. Any organization embarking on establishing an enterprise risk management program needs to assess the availability of relevant information and develop specific methods to communicate across all organizational lines to encompass all employees.

The New Risk Manager: The Chief Risk Officer (CRO)

The advent of enterprise risk management in health care supports the new position of chief risk officer (CRO). James Lam at GE Capital in 1993 was the first person to use the term *chief risk officer* (CRO). Since then, many more CROs have emerged.

The complexities of health care and uncertainty of risk have prompted some health organizations to hire chief risk officers. Some CROs function under the old traditional risk management style and simply carry a new title, whereas other CROs are engaged in enterprise risk management strategy and are charged with the centralization of risk at their organizations. Chief risk officers offer an organization many benefits, not the least of which is the ability to understand the relationship among and between risks across a broad continuum and all business units. An acceptable level of risk for one business unit might have dire consequences for other business units, and therefore might be unacceptable to the organization as a whole.

According to Ross in "The Evolving Role of the CRO," the best CROs tend to have a broad business background, combined with the communication skills required to influence the board, management, and employees responsible for making day-to-day decisions. "CROs are most effective when they provide the board with a clear vision of where enterprise risk lies, help define a policy for distributing and offsetting those risks and work to communicate that vision so that individual managers understand and support it . . . A successful CRO does not command from above. Instead the CRO sets the framework for risk management, while day-to-day decisions on what is or isn't an acceptable risk fall to managers and employees in the frontline of the business."[17]

···········

CONCLUSION

Collaboration, teamwork, trust, willingness to take risk, and open communication are central elements of an ERM program. A common risk framework and common risk taxonomy are necessary to be successful. Enterprise risk management is an organization-wide, ongoing process aimed at identifying, assessing, and minimizing risk to the organization. To be successful, the program requires support from the board and senior leadership of the organization. Enterprise risk management is not a single task, nor can a single person take responsibility for an enterprise risk management program. Although a risk manager or chief risk officer might manage and facilitate the process, it requires the collective power of cross-functional teams throughout the organization. Risk managers and others charged with identifying, assessing, managing, and monitoring risk within the health care organization have a tremendous opportunity to add personal value to the organization by leading this initiative. Those risk management professionals who seize upon this opportunity will be responding to an exciting challenge that is sure to make a difference to their organization.

Endnotes

1. For more information on "Enterprise Risk Management—Integrated Framework" by the Committee of Sponsoring Organizations of the Treadway Commission, visit www.aicpa.org.

2. Rosekind, PhD, Mark, "Managing Fatigue 24/7 in Health Care: Opportunities to Improve Safety"; *APSF Newsletter,* Volume 20, No. 1, Spring 2005.

3. Howard, MD, Steve, "Fatigue & the Practice of Anesthesiology," *APSF Newsletter,* Volume 20, No. I, Spring 2005.

4. ISMP Medication Safety Alert, "An exhausted workforce increases the risk of errors," June 2, 2005.

5. Gaba, MD, David, "The Costs of Clinician Fatigue and Its Prevention," *APSF Newsletter,* Volume 20, No. I, Spring 2005.

6. Aiken et al, "Educational Levels of Hospital Nurses and Surgical Patient Mortality," *JAMA. 2003*; 290: 1617–1623.

7. ISMP Medication Safety Alert, "Intimidation: Practitioners speak up about this unresolved problem" (Part I) March 11, 2004, "Intimidation: Mapping a plan for cultural change in healthcare" (Part II) March 25, 2004 (www.ismp.org/survey0311.asp).

8. On July 30, 2002, President Bush signed into law the Sarbanes-Oxley Act of 2002, which he characterized as "the most far reaching reforms of American business practices since the time of Franklin Delano Roosevelt." The Act mandates several reforms to enhance corporate responsibility, enhance financial disclosures, and combat corporate and accounting fraud, and created the "Public Company Accounting Oversight Board," also known as the PCAOB, to oversee the activities of the auditing profession. The full test of the Act is available at www.sec.gov/about/laws/soa2002.pdf. You can find links to all Commission rulemaking and reports issued under the Sarbanes-Oxley Act at www.sec.gov/spotlight/Sarbanes-oxley.htm.

9. Wason, S., "Enterprise Risk Management, Implementing New Solutions," AFIR Colloquium Toronto, September 7, 2001. Available at www.actuaries.ca/meetings/afir/handouts/s%5fwason.pdf.

10. *Ibid.*

11. *Ibid.*

12. Ross, Alasdair, author; Lofthouse, Gareth, editor; "The Evolving Role of the CRO." A report from the Economist Intelligence Unit's Global Risk Briefing, May 2005.

13. Miccolis, Jerry; Shah, Samir; "Enterprise Risk Management—An Analytic Approach," Tillinghast-Towers Perrin Monograph, 2000, p. 8.

14. *Ibid.,* pp 10–11.

15. *Ibid.,* pp 10–11.

16. *Ibid.*

17. Ross, p. 2.

Suggested Reading

Gooch, C., Kaufman, C., What is Enterprise Risk Management? Risk Management and Claims Management Insights, "An Urgent Call to Action: COSO, ERM and the role of the risk manager," *Risk Financing and Claims Administration Interest Network*, Introductory Issue / Fall 2004.

2

Health Care Legal Concepts

Peter Hoffman

At some time during his professional life, each person who works in the modern world of health care is likely to encounter a variety of legal concepts. These might include, among others, general and professional negligence issues, contract and employment considerations, privacy concerns, and crucial questions such as when life-sustaining treatment may be withheld. The specific issues each person will face depends on her role in the health care field, and also on the type of facility in which she works. Some issues that arise on a regular basis in an acute-care hospital might be less, or even more common in the context of an ambulance service, nursing home, or integrated delivery system. Given the plethora of legal concepts that routinely affect participants in the field of health care, it is useful to have at least some general knowledge about these concepts.

This chapter will provide basic information about several legal concepts and will describe specific issues that occur with frequency in particular settings. The reader is encouraged to read other chapters within this series for more detailed information about the concepts touched on here.

LEGAL ISSUES COMMON TO ALL HEALTH CARE PROVIDERS

There are many levels of liability that affect the health care industry. We will discuss several of them here.

Negligence

Negligence is the primary civil cause of action that health care providers face. A negligence action can involve either a claim of general liability or one of professional liability.

In either circumstance, there are four basic elements in any cause of action that alleges negligence.

1. Duty—One person must be under a duty to another person (or to society) before negligence becomes an issue. In the context of professional liability, duty usually attaches when the provider undertakes to care for the patient.

2. Breach of the duty—The person under the duty must breach the duty in some way (such as allowing a hazard to exist or failing to meet the required standard of care) to allow negligence to attach.

3. Cause of injury—The plaintiff must suffer an injury as a result of the defendant's breach of duty. If the injury did not arise out of the breach of the duty, or the plaintiff cannot prove causation, the cause of action fails.

4. Damages—The plaintiff must be able to show legally cognizable damages as a result of the injury sustained. Damages typically include pain and suffering (sometimes capped by tort reform efforts), medical expenses, lost wages, emotional distress, loss of consortium or companionship, and so on.

General Liability   These issues for health care providers typically include claims that allege negligence for hazards in the environment and nonprofessional judgments and actions.[1] General liability primarily involves premises liability, as many claims entail injuries arising out of the maintenance of premises, including slips and falls, but it can also involve causes of action alleging defamation, employment issues, and slander, to name a few. Claimants asserting general liability causes of action may include patients, physicians and other providers, family members, visitors, or even trespassers.

All four of the above mentioned elements apply in any claim for negligence. The only real difference between medical professional and general liability (negligence) is in the manner of proof. A claim for general negligence does not normally require that an expert witness testify as to the duty that a reasonably prudent person owes to another person, or to show that a breach in that duty occurred (unless the matter is unduly technical).

Medical Professional Liability   Also referred to as malpractice liability, medical professional liability involves claims that allege professional negligence for patient care activities. Typically, these causes of action involve allegations of negligent acts or omissions of health care providers or employees that result in injury to the patient. Patients, or their legal representatives, may allege separate theories of negligence against treating physicians, health care entities, nurses, and other employees.

To state a successful cause of action for medical negligence, a plaintiff must demonstrate all of the elements of negligence discussed previously. In the context of professional negligence, the duty is often referred to as the standard of care. Most arguments during litigation surround the proper standard of care and whether the standard was breached. Another focus is often whether the alleged substandard care was the cause of the plaintiff's injuries. Expert testimony is required to show the appropriate standard of care, whether it was breached, and to show that the plaintiff's injuries were caused by the breach of the standard of care.

Concept of Standard of Care   A physician owes a duty of care to his or her patients to conform to certain standards of reasonable medical care.[2] Generally, a physician's standard of care is measured by the degree of care and skill possessed by other physicians within the same or similar circumstances.[3] The standard of care requires that—among other things—a physician is to remain up to date regarding medical developments and advancements, secure a careful history, perform a comprehensive examination, arrive at an appropriate diagnosis, recommend and implement appropriate therapies, and refer for consultation when indicated.[4]

Historically, the standard for the adequate level of care rendered by a physician was determined by the prevailing standard of care practiced by physicians within the physician's community.[5] This is known as the "locality" rule.[6] Because physicians were reluctant to give expert testimony against a fellow physician in the same community, many states have modified this rule.[7] As a result, some states have implemented either the "similar locality" standard or the "national" standard.[8] Note that physicians who specialize in a particular area of medicine and who hold themselves out as specialists have been required to possess a greater level of skill within that specialty than would a general practitioner.[9]

To prevail in a medical negligence action, a plaintiff must affirmatively prove both the relevant recognized standard of medical care exercised by other physicians, and that the defendant physician departed from that standard when treating the plaintiff, causing the plaintiff to sustain injury or damage. Generally, it is necessary for the plaintiff to have expert witness testimony concerning the standard of care applicable to the defendant.

Expert Testimony   Some states require that specific qualifications and credentials be met before a party can testify as an expert witness in medical malpractice cases. Generally, a person shall not give expert medical testimony unless licensed as a health professional. To determine if a witness is qualified to be an expert, the court typically will consider the witness's education and professional training, the witness's area of specialization, and the length of time the witness has been engaged in the active clinical practice or instruction of the health profession or specialty. Additionally, there are two general standards, or tests, that the court will apply to consider whether an expert witness's testimony will be admissible in court—the Daubert standard and the Frye standard. In federal and many state cases, Daubert defines the standard for admitting expert scientific testimony. According to Daubert, the proposed testimony must be supported by appropriate validation.[10] In other states, Frye is the standard that applies. Under the Frye test, an expert's opinion is admissible if the principle or method underlying that opinion is generally accepted by scientists active in the relevant field.[11] State laws should be reviewed to determine the applicable qualifications and standard applied in the specific jurisdiction.

In any medical negligence case, the physician experts must testify that their expert opinions are based on a reasonable degree of medical certainty. Expert testimony fails to meet this "reasonable certainty" requirement when the plaintiff's expert testifies that the alleged negligence "possibly" caused or "could have" caused the plaintiff's injury, that such negligence "could very properly account for the injury," or even that it is "very highly probable" that defendant's negligence caused the poor result.[12]

Negligence per se   The court may adopt a statute as defining the standard of care in a negligence action if the court determines that the purpose of the statute was to protect the class of persons to which the plaintiff belongs from the type of risk that has ensued.[13] The violation of a statute can be treated as negligence per se if it is unexcused.[14] This allows the plaintiff to handily prove the existence of a duty and the breach of the duty, but the plaintiff still must prove injury and damages.

Privity   Generally, "privity" means a derivative interest founded on a contract or connection between two parties. It also can be thought of as a mutuality of interest. In the context of potential liability of a health care provider stemming from the care of a patient, the concept of "privity" usually applies when a party other than that patient—or that patient's spouse or parent (of a minor patient)—claims that the health care provider also caused that other party injury and seeks to recover for this claimed injury.

Duty of Health Care Providers to Third Parties (Non-Patients)

To sustain a professional negligence cause of action against a physician, the plaintiff normally must be a patient. A patient is defined as a natural person who receives, or should have received, health care from a licensed health care provider under a contract, express or implied.[15] Most states have implemented the general rule that a physician does not owe a professional duty to a non-patient or a third party. Several jurisdictions have held that a hospital does not owe a duty to protect a non-patient who is present in the emergency room from fainting,[16] and that a physician does not owe a duty to a third-party non-patient for injuries arising from the use of prescription medication by the physician's patient.[17] Some states have limited this "no duty" rule by recognizing a duty to non-patient bystanders when the patient poses a danger of harm to an identifiable third party;[18] when the patient's behavior must be controlled to prevent a danger to a third party;[19] or when the bystander becomes a participant in the treatment of a patient, for example, being used by the medical staff to hold the patient down.[20]

In contrast, a limited number of states have held that medical professionals have a duty to third parties in two circumstances: when doctors exert control over a patient and when a doctor is aware of threats against specific, identifiable third parties. Many courts have even concluded that physicians owe a duty to injured third parties and the general public to warn their patients about side effects of prescription medication (such as drowsiness).[21]

Due to the different approaches taken by various states, it is important to review state laws to determine the approach followed by the specific jurisdiction.

Contractual Liability of Doctor to Patient

An agreement to provide medical care to a patient can be expressed or implied. When a patient seeks the assistance and treatment of a physician, and the physician accepts the patient, they enter into an implied contract that the physician will treat the patient. Such a contract can only be terminated by the physician when the physician gives proper notice to the patient. The patient, of course, may terminate the agreement at any time. When an implied contract is formed, the physician does not guarantee the success of treatment, or that beneficial results will occur, but only that the physician possesses, and will carefully apply, professional skills, which are ordinarily possessed by the general practitioner in the physician's locality.[22] General reassurances by the physician to the patient are considered to be an expression of opinion or hope, and do not amount to an expressed contract.[23] These reassurances are considered therapeutic and do not constitute a basis for an express contract.

To be enforceable, an expressed contract must be expressed and must be supported by consideration. Physicians and patients can enter into express written contracts regarding the care provided. Such contracts are not usual but can include various treatment plans, the likelihood of success, and even the physician's promise to cure. Traditionally, courts have respected a physician's freedom to contract as the physician chooses.[24] However, once a contract is formed, a plaintiff might have a cause of action for breach of contract, in addition to other potential claims (such as medical malpractice) if the outcome of the treatment is not what was promised.

Informed Consent   The physician-patient relationship is a consensual one. For more than a century, courts have required the patient's consent prior to any touching, examination, or medical procedure. Consent is traditionally defined as a voluntary agreement to do something proposed by another. There are two kinds of consent: general consent (to allow touching, examination, and non-invasive procedures) and informed consent (to allow the performance of an invasive procedure). If the procedure is an invasive procedure that carries a material risk of harm, the patient's informed consent will probably be required. If the touching is without consent at all, the provider might be liable for battery. Generally, if the patient appropriately consents to a procedure, the patient cannot hold the physician liable unless the physician fails to perform the surgery according to the applicable medical standards (malpractice). Therefore, a physician must obtain full, knowing, and voluntary general and informed consent from the patient concerning any non-emergency surgical procedure.

Informed consent requires more from a physician than simply having the patient sign a form. Health care providers must ensure that patients are aware of the diagnosis, the benefits of the proposed treatment, the material risks of the treatment, alternative options to the proposed treatment, and possible consequences of declining the treatment. This information must be communicated to the patient so that the patient clearly understands it.[25] Once properly informed, the patient can make an intelligent decision regarding the course of treatment, regardless of whether the patient chooses rationally.

Failure to obtain adequate informed consent can give rise to a claim, even if the procedure is performed appropriately.[26] In most states a patient's legal cause of action in a lack of consent case is premised on the plaintiff's ability to prove that the defendant failed to reveal a significant risk that materialized and caused the plaintiff to suffer adverse consequences,[27] and that had the potential risk been disclosed, a reasonable person would not have consented to the treatment or procedure.[28] Although a physician does not generally have a duty to disclose remote risks,[29] a duty may arise if the plaintiff expressly requests that all known complications be revealed.[30]

There are three generally accepted exceptions to the rule that informed consent is required. First, health care providers may assume that informed consent would be obtained in emergency situations if the emergency did not exist.[31] This, of course, does not give the provider the right to assume consent in the face of a prior refusal. Also, traditionally it is the treating physician, not the hospital, who has the duty to obtain informed consent.[32] However, courts have held that a hospital may be held liable when members of its staff neglect to inform the physician that the patient has withdrawn consent prior to treatment.[33] Additionally, hospitals that sponsor or permit experimental procedures may be liable when they fail to ensure that informed consent according to the research protocol is obtained.[34]

Some parties are unable to consent. As a general rule, minors are deemed incapable of providing effective consent to medical treatment. Accordingly, the physician must obtain consent from the parent or guardian before proceeding with any examination or treatment of the minor. There are exceptions to the requirements of consent by a parent or guardian. In certain emergency situations, no consent is required prior to treatment of the minor. Medical, dental, and health services may be rendered to minors of any age without the consent of the parent or legal guardian when, in the physician's judgment, an attempt to secure consent would result in delay of treatment, which would increase the risk to the minor's life or health, or when the minor is emancipated. Minors may consent to the examination or treatment of their minor children in most states. [For further information on informed consent refer to Chapter 4 in Volume II.]

Contractual Negotiation and Approval

Entering into a successful contract requires both parties to think about what the transaction is really about. It involves addressing many details beyond the price of a product or service. The particulars in any specific instance or facility will differ, but the material described here gives a general picture of the negotiation and approval process. As a starting point, it is helpful to ask several questions, such as:

- Who will provide the goods or services and who will provide payment?
- What exactly is each party required to do?
- When will each party be providing the goods or services and when will payment be made?
- Where will the services be performed or where will the goods be delivered?
- Why is each party performing these obligations and why is the deal important to each party?
- How will satisfactory performance or delivery be measured?

As you begin to determine the terms of the proposed arrangement, it is often helpful to consult with your corporate counsel. Generally, most corporate counsels have developed several standard contracts that can help expedite the negotiating process while ensuring that the health care facilities' interests are effectively protected.

Typically, each party will have a starting position and an idea about what it wants to get out of the agreement. Certain points might be very important to one party and less important to the other. It is essential to negotiate a contract that clearly defines the relationship between the parties; characterizes each party's expectations, rights, and responsibilities (including payments terms, warranties, limitations on advertising, and confidentiality); and describes what should happen if something were to go wrong (for example, termination for breach, indemnification [hold harmless] clause, insurance). These clear designations allow both parties to have an adequate understanding regarding each party's intentions, thereby allowing the parties to predict what to anticipate. This is an important element regardless of whether the contract is performed in a few hours or a few years.

Health care providers and administrators should work together with corporate counsel and professional staff to draft and negotiate the agreement. Negotiating a successful contract often involves discussions within the health care facility and consultation with other health care facility departments and committees. It is essential for every member of the health care facility who negotiates a proposed contract to consider the relationship of the product to the overall strategic goal of the health care facility. In drafting or negotiating a contract, corporate counsel should work with the health care facility management to ensure that the contractual obligations are consistent with the legal obligations of the health care facility, and that the risk of liability and other legal consequences are fully understood by the key players and ultimate decision makers. In the contracting process, it is important that the anticipated benefits of the contractual relationship outweigh both the financial and legal risks to the health care facility.

All health care facilities should have an approval process, which must be followed when entering into any contractual agreement. For major contracts (in which the dollar amount is greater than $100,000), both corporate counsel and the financial department should be contacted before negotiations begin to guarantee a coordinated and prompt approach to contract review and approval.

For all purchasing contracts and agreements, the health care facility's purchasing department should be contacted before the acquisition process begins, to ensure that subsequent negotiations conform with the competitive bid process and do not conflict with any new or existing agreements, contracts, or understandings. The purchasing department will also ensure that the process is consistent with the health care facility's commitment to group purchasing memberships and the health care facility's strategy.

The purpose of legal review is to provide advice and counsel concerning the proposed contract: (1) to ensure that the proposed terms and conditions comply with the applicable law; and (2) to identify and minimize significant legal risks.

The legal department should help negotiate and draft the contract and should identify legal issues so that the business decision makers can evaluate the risks or benefits of the arrangement, to finalize the contract. Approval of a contract should be withheld only if there is a significant issue as to whether the terms and conditions of agreement comply with the law.

Most proposed contracts should also be reviewed by the health care facility's finance and administrative departments so that they, respectively, can evaluate issues relating to financial liability, cash flow, and operational matters, whether a contract makes good business sense, and whether it is consistent with the facility's objectives and policies.

The finance department generally would withhold approval of the contract only if there were a significant concern about its financial liability. The purpose of an administrative review is to ensure that contracts make good business sense and are consistent with the health care facility's objectives and policies.

Once a contract has been reviewed by the appropriate departments and offices, and once all necessary changes and revisions have been made based upon that review, the contract is ready for final approval and execution. Each of the departments and offices required to review and approve the contract should indicate final approval of the contract by signing the contract approval form. All copies of the contract should be signed and dated by the authorized health care facility representative.

Once the copies have been signed by the other party, copies of the contract should be forwarded by the originator to the appropriate authorized health care facilities' representatives for signature. Note that if the other party makes additional changes, the contract must be re-reviewed by everyone who previously had signed off. In certain cases it may be preferable that the copies of the contract first be executed by the authorized health care facility representative, and then executed by the other parties.

Once a contract has been fully executed, a copy should be forwarded by the originator to:

- Other parties (as appropriate)
- Health care facilities contract originator (or that person's department)
- Office of legal affairs or contract administrator (if applicable)
- Finance department
- Purchasing department

Fully executed contracts need to be safeguarded and maintained in accordance with the state's or the facility's records retention requirements.

When a contract comes up for renewal, the originator should contact the administrator and the purchasing department (where appropriate) at least ninety days before the expiration date, particularly if any automatic renewal rights or options are involved. In all cases the specific contract language for renewal or termination should be reviewed to ensure compliance. All amendments, modifications, or renewals of the contract should go through the same approval process that was followed for the original contract.

If serious performance problems arise at any time during the contract term, the health care facility employees involved should immediately communicate concerns regarding performance or termination to the contract administrator or the legal department. All performance problems and efforts to resolve these problems should be carefully documented by the health care facility employees. (Please refer to Chapter 12 for further detail on contract review.)

Information Release: Privilege and Privacy Issues

There are several levels of information release that need to be carefully examined.

Peer Review Information   Many state legislatures have agreed, at least to some extent, with the view that because the practice of medicine requires a level of expertise that can be reviewed only by other medical professionals, the medical profession should police its own activities through peer review organizations. Peer review involves the review of physicians' performances by other physicians for quality of care and appropriateness of decision making. Review committees are established by hospitals and used to investigate candidates for clinical privileges and to monitor the existing medical staff.

Many states have enacted statutes designed to protect the peer review process and those individuals on the peer review committee. The legislature has recognized that patients need protection from physicians who deviate from an appropriate professional standard of care. Simultaneously, the legislature has acknowledged that health care providers want limited involvement with peer review committees due to concerns that they will be held liable for the ultimate decision rendered by the board. As a result, many states have implemented peer review protection that grants immunity to members of the peer review committee and grants protective status to documents prepared during the peer review process. This type of legislation ensures that members of peer review organizations are at liberty to speak without restraint about controversial matters such as quality assurance, medical staff credentials, and qualifications. Review your state laws to determine the content of the statute and the extent of its protections in your specific jurisdiction.

Typically, individuals who supply information to peer review committees are protected from criminal and civil liability. This immunity, however, is not absolute. An individual will not be granted immunity if the information reported is unrelated or irrelevant to the peer review committee's purpose and scope. The individual is also not protected if the information reported was false and the individual knew or had reason to believe it was false, or if the individual's appearance before the peer review board was motivated by malice.

Documents used and information recorded by peer review committees are not subject to discovery or admissible as evidence in a civil action against the health care provider, if the civil action stems from a matter that is the subject of the committee's review. This protection also is not absolute. Peer review protection does not apply and the document may be disclosed in accordance with applicable law if the document used by the peer review committee can be obtained from its original source.

In addition, those testifying before a peer review committee cannot be compelled to testify at civil hearings regarding:

1. Evidence that was produced or relied upon at the proceedings
2. Conversations, opinions, or evaluations discussed during the proceedings

3. Testimony before a peer review protection committee or opinions formed as a result of committee hearings. However, a person in attendance is not immune from testifying at other civil proceedings as to information within personal knowledge and learned outside the peer review proceeding

Generally, peer review protection is granted to the following licensed health care providers: physicians, dentists, podiatrists, chiropractors, optometrists, physiologists, pharmacists, registered nurses, practical nurses, and physical therapists. In addition, health care facility administrators, corporations, or organizations acting as health care facilities and committees evaluating the quality of health care and credentialing are also covered.

Patient Confidentiality Communications between a physician and that physician's patients are private and confidential. Those in need of medical attention greatly benefit from being able to discuss their medical situations with health care professionals without the concern that such information might be disclosed to others. A patient's disclosure of pertinent information pertaining to that patient's illness will help the physician provide appropriate medical treatment. Due to this benefit, most states have implemented legislation that provides protections for confidential medical information obtained by the physician.[35] This protection is generally found in the form of the physician-patient privilege. This privilege creates a confidential atmosphere intended to prevent the embarrassment that patients might face upon the disclosure of their illnesses, and encourages patients to disclose all possible information pertaining to their illnesses, thereby enabling the physician to render effective diagnoses and treatments for their patients.[36]

The improper disclosure of information by physicians violates state confidentiality statutes, which generally provide criminal or civil penalties, or civil causes of action for the inappropriate release of a patient's confidential information. Additionally, for hospitals and physicians, the improper disclosure of medical information may subject them to civil liability, including breach of contract, invasion of privacy, intentional infliction of emotional distress, breach of confidential relationship, defamation, and negligence.[37,38]

Under federal law, wrongful disclosure of one's protected health information is a federal crime.[39] Any person who knowingly and in violation of federal law uses or causes to be used a unique health identifier, or obtains individually identifiable health information relating to an individual, or discloses individually identifiable health information to another person, shall be punished depending upon the nature and the scope of the offense.[40] Individually identifiable information includes any information created or received by a health care provider that relates to an individual's physical or mental health, health care, or payment for health care, and identifies or could reasonably be used to identify the individual.[41] The penalties begin with an initial penalty of a $50,000 fine and imprisonment of not more than one year, or both.[42] If the offense is committed under false pretenses, the fine is increased to $100,000 and imprisonment is increased to five years.[43] If the offense is committed with the intent to sell or transfer or use the individually identifiable health information for commercial advantage, personal gain, or malicious harm, then the fine is increased to not more than $250,000 and imprisonment of not more than ten years.[44]

It should be noted that exceptions to the physician-patient relationship arise in personal injury cases and criminal cases. Where the patient is the plaintiff in a personal injury case, defense counsel is entitled to obtain the plaintiff patient's medical records and depose the patient's physicians. In criminal matters, no physician-patient privilege exists.

AIDS- and HIV-Related Issues   The testing and confidentiality issues related to AIDS and HIV are numerous. Strict adherence is necessary for patient safety and to decrease an organization's exposure to liability.

HIV Testing   Generally, a human immunodeficiency virus (HIV) test cannot be performed without the patient's informed written consent. Before consent can be given, a health care provider must explain the nature of the test, including its purpose, potential uses, limitations, and meaning of the results. Pre-test counseling must be made available regarding HIV prevention, exposure, and transmission.

Once results have been obtained, the physician or physician's designee must make a good faith effort to inform the patient of the test results. Medical standards may require that positive test results be confirmed before they are revealed to the patient. Upon receiving the results, the patient must be afforded the opportunity for immediate, individual, face-to-face counseling regarding the significance of the test results and measures for preventing HIV transmission. Counseling should also include the benefits of locating and counseling individuals who might have exposed the patient to HIV.

Partial waivers of the voluntary HIV testing requirements are granted in limited circumstances. In medical emergencies, when the patient is unable to grant consent or if the patient withholds consent and the HIV-related test result is medically necessary to provide appropriate emergency care, the patient must be provided only with notice of the test results and post-test counseling. In addition, individuals who donate organs, body parts, tissues, or semen for use in medical research, therapy, transfusion, or transplantation and test negative for HIV do not need to receive notice of their test results or be given post-test counseling. However, the donor must give written consent to the test and have the opportunity to receive pre-test counseling. Notice of a negative test result also must be given to any individual who asks to be provided with such results.

To protect the welfare of health care providers and those who have rendered assistance to an HIV-positive patient, various exceptions to voluntary HIV testing have been implemented. A patient's existing blood sample can be subjected to involuntary HIV-related testing to protect the welfare of health care providers and emergency medical personnel. However, health care providers who rendered care must obtain certification from a physician, other than from themselves or their employers, that they have had a significant exposure to HIV. A significant exposure is defined as the direct contact with blood or bodily fluids in a manner that, according to the most current guidelines of the Centers for Disease Control and Prevention, is capable of transmitting HIV. This certification must be obtained within seventy-two hours of the exposure. The certifying physician must also provide the health care provider with an opportunity to undergo voluntary HIV-related testing as outlined previously.

A copy of the written certification must be provided to the physician of the individual whose HIV test is sought or to the institutional health care provider in possession of the individual's available blood. The physician or institutional health care provider must make a good faith effort to notify the individual, or that individual's substituted decision maker, of the certification, and request consent to an HIV test within twenty-four hours of the request for HIV testing. If the individual agrees to the test, written consent must be obtained and the individual must be afforded the opportunity for pre-test counseling. If the individual does not agree to an HIV test or cannot be located, an entry must be made on the individual's medical records to that effect. If the individual's blood has already been obtained, that blood may be tested, provided the person was given the opportunity to consent or refuse to consent to the HIV test. Involuntary HIV testing will not proceed unless the health care provider requests the testing and submits to baseline testing.

The patient must be given notice of the test result and the same opportunity for appropriate post-test counseling as afforded in voluntary HIV-related testing. The health care provider may be notified of the patient's test results only if the provider's own baseline HIV test is negative.

Confidentiality of HIV-Related Information   Medical records and other tests, which reveal whether an individual has contracted acquired immunodeficiency syndrome (AIDS) or human immunodeficiency virus (HIV), have been the basis of considerable litigation and legislation. Many of the confidentiality issues discussed previously have arisen in the context of AIDS. Generally, physicians, their employees, and agents are required to maintain the confidentiality of all HIV-related information. This rule applies whether the information is disclosed voluntarily, involuntarily, or pursuant to a court order. Patients whose HIV/AIDS status has been improperly disclosed by health care providers have causes of action under the common law theories of breach of contract, invasion of privacy, intentional infliction of emotional distress, breach of confidential relationship, defamation, and negligence.[45]

Generally, this duty of confidentiality protects only the patient and not the treating physician. The right of privacy regarding one's HIV status has not been extended to treating physicians who are HIV-positive. Courts have permitted hospitals to notify patients who participated in invasive procedures that the physician involved in their care was HIV-positive.[46] This disclosure however, is limited, as the hospital is not permitted to release the physician's name to the patients.[47] The hospital is, however, entitled to release the physician's name and HIV status to certain colleagues with whom the infected physician might have performed surgery and to those who were in that physician's training program.[48] It should be noted that physicians who are patients are protected by the duty of confidentiality. Courts have concluded that hospitals owe a duty of confidentiality to physicians who are patients,[49] so hospitals must take reasonable precautions with physicians' medical records when they are being treated in the hospital.[50] Physicians who are being treated for AIDS have an expectation of privacy that their AIDS diagnoses will not become a matter of public knowledge.[51] This changes, however, once the physician becomes a treating physician and is performing invasive procedures on a patient.[52]

States approach confidentiality as it relates to AIDS in different ways. Some states have strict confidentiality laws to protect the privacy of HIV-infected individuals.[53] HIV status is a private matter, and there are enforceable civil penalties for disclosure of another individual's HIV status.[54] Other states take a less rigid approach regarding confidentiality. Some require reporting of HIV status to public health authorities.[55] This reporting includes the revelation of all new HIV diagnoses, including diagnoses involving the status of physicians.[56] Review your state laws to determine the approach taken in your jurisdiction. (Also refer to Chapter 18, Volume III, in this series for further information on the Health Insurance Portability and Accountability Act [HIPAA] or on the release or disclosure of protected health information.)

Attorney-Client Privilege   This privilege is an essential component of our legal system. It promotes full communication between an attorney and a client. This assures clients that conversations with their attorneys will not be disclosed to others. The privilege belongs to the client, and the attorney must hold client communications in the strictest of confidence.

The elements of the attorney-client privilege are:

- The party seeking the protection of the privilege must be an actual or prospective client.

- The communication must be between a client and an attorney acting as counsel for the client.

- The communication must be made in confidence, outside the presence of third parties.

- The purpose of the communication must be to secure or provide an opinion of law or legal assistance.

- The privilege must be asserted by one holding the privilege. The privilege does not automatically attach.

- The privilege is easily lost or "waived" by improper disclosures to third parties.

The privilege does not attach to communications in furtherance of an ongoing or prospective illegal activity. In addition, the privilege does apply when attorneys defend themselves against charges of wrongful misconduct brought by clients.

Health care providers should be mindful of maintaining the attorney-client privilege in varying circumstances, including:

- In anticipation of potential litigation

- During the investigation of past conduct that may raise legal concerns

- Seeking advice on structuring new ventures (for example, a proposed merger)

- Peer review and risk management (such as quality improvement or malpractice defense)

- Any other sensitive issue where legal input might be helpful and confidentiality is critical

For the attorney-client privilege to protect oral communications, it is best to have an attorney participate directly in the discussion. Therefore, counsel should be present when the purpose of any meeting is to obtain or discuss legal advice or to gather information needed to obtain legal advice or assistance. Only employees who have a "need to know" should attend such meetings and non-client third parties should not attend. Be careful not to divulge privileged communications in meeting minutes or other memoranda. Do not discuss attorney-client information on mobile telephones or in public places (such as elevators) where you might be overheard.

The attorney-client privilege may be invoked in memoranda, correspondence, and other written communications by adhering to the following guidelines:

- Identify and assert the privilege on the document—that is, mark the document "Attorney-Client Privileged Communication."

- Send the document to or from your attorney and limit distribution to a need-to-know basis. Identify all recipients on the document, with no blind copies.

- Avoid the attachment of unprivileged material or written notes on the document.

- Treat the document in a confidential manner and maintain the document in a secure place.

- Information contained on computer disks, hard drives, and back-up systems may also be protected by the attorney-client privilege.

Executives may communicate legal advice received from counsel to other executives or employees who have a need to know without destroying the privilege by identifying the communication as legal advice, limiting communication to counsel's advice, not including underlying facts, and segregating legal discussions from other topics.

When there are disclosures, take immediate action by consulting counsel, telling the recipient that disclosure was inadvertent, requesting return of any written materials, and confirming these steps in writing, if appropriate.

The attorney-client privilege can and should be invoked to safeguard the health care provider's interest whenever legal questions arise. Contact an attorney with any questions regarding the attorney-client privilege.

Employment Issues

Respondeat Superior Liability   In Latin, *respondeat superior* means "let the master answer." In the context of an acute-care facility or hospital, it is a legal doctrine under which an employer may be liable for wrongful acts of its employee that are done within the scope of that employee's job. Under this theory, the hospital is vicariously liable for the actions of its employees who the hospital had a duty to supervise. Essentially, to bring an action under this theory, the plaintiff must establish that:

- the health care provider was a servant or agent of the hospital;
- the act or omission of the health care provider occurred in the scope of employment. If, however, the health care provider is an independent contractor, the theory of respondeat superior is not applicable.[57]

Contracted employees

Non-Discrimination Laws   Laws exist at the federal, state, and local levels that prohibit discrimination against employees on the basis of race, sex, age, disability, sexual orientation, national origin, and religion. The ultimate goal of these laws is to prevent discrimination by providing equal opportunities throughout all facets of employment relationships. These non-discrimination laws require that employers do not take any actions that might infringe on an employee's terms of employment based on that person's status as a member of a protected class.

Federal laws have been implemented in an attempt to rectify past discrimination and prevent future discrimination. These laws include Title VII of the Civil Rights Act of 1964, the Age Discrimination in Employment Act (ADEA), and the Americans with Disabilities Act (ADA). All health care facilities are bound by the terms of these federal laws.

credentialing

Title VII of the Civil Rights Act of 1964 is the heart of anti-discrimination legislation. It prohibits harassment and discrimination of an employee based on that employee's race, gender, and national origin. Prohibitions against sexual harassment also fall within this act. Title VII applies to employers, employment agencies, and labor organizations that employ fifteen or more employees during twenty or more calendar weeks in either the current or previous calendar year. It should be noted that in limited situations, Title VII allows employers to make employment decisions that are based on religion, sex, and national origin when there is a legitimate work-related requirement that is reasonably necessary for the operation of that specific industry (for example, hiring only women for the position of a women's bathroom attendant).[58]

To assert a Title VII claim, plaintiffs must show that they are members of a protected class and were treated differently than similarly situated people from another class. The burden then shifts to the employer to convey a justifiable, non-discriminatory basis for the decision that has been viewed as discriminatory. If the employer is able to articulate such grounds, the burden shifts back to the employees to establish that the employer's discriminatory reason was the primary basis for the decision made. In cases where plaintiffs assert that a particular employer engaged in the practice of discrimination against members of a protected class, the plaintiffs must prove that they were deterred from applying for a job or were not hired for a job because of the employer's discriminatory practices. Most federal courts have determined that supervisors may not be held individually liable under Title VII.[59] However, individual liability for supervisors is allowed under many states' discrimination laws. Review state laws to determine the liability laws applicable to supervisors in the specific jurisdiction.

It is an employer's legal obligation to take prompt and appropriate action in response to a complaint alleging a violation of Title VII. Managers confronted with a complaint based on race, gender, or national origin discrimination should contact human resources departments for assistance. The complaint should be investigated in a timely and thorough fashion. Every health care facility has implemented various policies regarding non-discrimination. All individuals should familiarize themselves with the reporting and investigatory structures set forth in each policy.

The Age Discrimination in Employment Act (ADEA)[60] forbids the discrimination of employees in hiring, discharging, and denying employment on the basis of an individual's age.[61] The act provides that employers who retain twenty or more employees for twenty or more work weeks are prohibited from discrimination against employees who are forty years of age or older.

Employees, applicants, and former employees may file a charge of age discrimination with one of several administrative agencies that investigate and attempt to mediate these claims. After the relevant commission has been given an opportunity to investigate the claim, the claimants may initiate legal action in either state or federal court. An employer may not defend a discrimination claim by asserting that it hired another individual in the protected age category.

Those concerned about issues of age discrimination due to the discipline or termination of an employee should contact the human resources department during the decision-making process. In addition, complaints received regarding discriminatory conduct from an employee or applicant should also be referred to the human resources department.

The Americans with Disabilities Act (ADA) prohibits employment discrimination against qualified individuals on the basis of disability.[62] It requires that employers provide reasonable accommodations to qualified individuals with disabilities (QIWD) to help them perform the essential functions of their jobs. Although most states have laws that forbid discriminating against people with disabilities, the ADA provides uniform national protection.

Many state and local laws extend employment discrimination protection to people outside federally protected categories. Employers should consult specific state and local laws to ensure compliance. Additionally, many employers have voluntarily chosen to extend protection to certain employee groups and have added marital status and sexual orientation to their anti-discrimination policies. To be effective, any equal employment program must have support from top management and supervisors. Such policies should be distributed to all employees and should be clearly understood and implemented by supervisors.

Sexual Harassment   Sexual harassment is prohibited by Title VII of the Civil Rights Act of 1964. Sexual harassment so severe or pervasive as to alter the conditions of the victim's employment can create an abusive working environment. This violates Title VII.[63]

To be actionable under the statute, a sexually objectionable environment must be one that a reasonable person would find to be hostile or abusive, and one that the victim, in fact, did perceive to be hostile or abusive.[64] Sporadic use of abusive language, gender-related jokes, and occasional teasing are not considered severe enough to violate Title VII.[65]

Federal courts have acknowledged two types of sexual harassment claims based upon two different legal theories: quid pro quo harassment and hostile environment harassment. Quid pro quo harassment occurs when a superior demands sexual favors from a subordinate in exchange for continued employment or job benefits. Hostile environment harassment is a situation in which an employee's terms and conditions of employment are altered as a result of pervasive sexual conduct. This includes unwanted sexual advances, demands for sexual favors, and any conduct of a sexual nature that unreasonably interferes with an individual's work performance or creates an intimidating, hostile, or offensive working environment. In both quid pro quo and hostile environment harassment, employers can be held strictly liable for harassment by supervisors that results in tangible job actions, even if they have no knowledge of the conduct. Employees can even recover damages when no tangible job action occurs without showing that the employer was negligent or at fault for the supervisor's conduct.[66] An employer may avoid liability where no tangible job action occurs by establishing an affirmative defense showing that the employer exercised reasonable care to prevent and promptly correct sexual harassment, and that the employee unreasonably failed to take advantage of any preventative or corrective opportunity provided by the employer.[67] For employers to limit potential exposure to sexual harassment claims, an employer must disseminate and enforce an effective sexual harassment policy that incorporates effective procedures for report, investigation, and discipline of sexual harassment in the workplace.[68]

It is an employer's legal obligation to take prompt and appropriate action in response to a complaint of sexual harassment. It is important for a manager confronted with a sexual harassment complaint to investigate the complaint in a timely and thorough fashion, with the assistance of human resources and according to facility policy. Every health care facility must implement anti-sexual harassment policies. All individuals should familiarize themselves with the reporting and investigatory structures set forth in each policy. (Refer to Chapter 6 in Volume III of this series for further information on employment practices liability.)

Staff Credentialing   Credentialing involves the careful selection, review, and evaluation of health care providers. It is a process whereby health care entities select, review, and periodically evaluate the competency of the physicians and other licensed health care practitioners within their facility. Courts have held health care institutions vicariously liable for the negligent acts of independent physicians through the doctrine of apparent agency or ostensible agency and have imposed liability on health care entities through respondeat superior, for the acts of employees committed within the scope of employment.

The Joint Commission on Accreditation of Healthcare Organization (JCAHO) accredits and sets standards for hospitals, health systems, and home care programs to follow regarding the selection of its medical staff. The JCAHO recommends, at a minimum, that a hospital require its medical staff to:

1. Adopt bylaws and rules and regulations, subject to approval by the governing body, that establish a framework for the conduct of the medical staff.

2. Make recommendations to the governing body regarding the structure of the medical staff.

3. Organize itself to accomplish its required function.

4. Describe and implement a process for appointment and reappointment to the medical staff.

5. Describe and implement a process for delineating clinical privileges and determining the appropriate qualifications required to perform these privileges.

6. Monitor and evaluate the quality and appropriateness of patient care.

7. Require members of the medical staff to participate in continuing education.

Individual hospitals should be queried as to their specific requirements for their medical staff.

Impaired Professionals   The American Medical Association (AMA) defines the impaired physician as one who is unable to practice medicine with reasonable skill and safety to patients because of physical or mental illness, including deterioration through the aging process or loss of motor skills, or excessive use or abuse of drugs or alcohol. An institution's primary responsibility is to provide quality medical care to its patients. An impaired physician significantly deviates from this responsibility. Therefore, once the hospital becomes aware of, or has reason to be aware of, an impaired physician, it has a duty to investigate immediately and take appropriate measures in an effort to protect its patients. Efforts to rehabilitate impaired providers must be structured in such a manner that does not compromise the hospital's primary obligation.

Every institution should establish a written policy regarding how impaired physicians should be handled, and it should be properly enforced. This benefits the patients by ensuring high-quality care, identifying the physician who requires assistance, and ultimately protecting the hospital from potential liability. Although hospitals implement different policies, typically a health care facility's guidelines will require that impairment be reported to the institution's in-house impairment program or to an external impaired physician's program. This report is intended to get needed help to the physician. If these reports do not assist the impaired physician into entering an impairment program, then according to state law, the health care facility, hospital peer, or colleague must report the physician to the medical board. Depending on the specifics of applicable state law, a facility, peer, or colleague that fails to report an impaired physician to the medical board in such a circumstance could be fined. Upon recording suspected impairment, the medical board will assess the situation and conduct its own investigation deemed appropriate. Any person who makes a report in good faith is immune from liability. Additionally, some states have mandatory reporting statutes. Therefore, individual state requirements should be built into the institution's policies.

Generally, once an impaired physician has satisfactorily undergone treatment, that physician is likely to return to practice. Certain types of accommodations might be required to assist the physician returning to work, as impairments may constitute a disability under the Americans with Disabilities Act (ADA). Additionally, hospital administration and medical staff members involved in the credentialing process should be aware of the impaired practitioner's problem so they can impose controls designed to prevent injury to patients that are consistent with the ADA and applicable state laws. There may be specific state-imposed requirements that affect when and under what circumstances the physician can return to practice. Generally, it is suggested that before affected practitioners are permitted to return to work, they should be required to produce satisfactory evidence of completion of a rehabilitation program; required to continue in an organized program of ongoing monitoring for a period of two to four years; agree to arrange with other physicians who will assume responsibility for the care of the affected physicians' patients should the need arise; agree to submit to random substance abuse screening tests at the request of the hospital or medical staff leadership; and agree to abstain from addictive substances as a condition of continued medical staff membership and clinical privileges. These precautions are highly recommended measures designed to protect patients and reduce hospital liability. Those aware that a medical professional is impaired should follow the health care institution's guidelines and should contact the risk management department or the legal department within the institution. Precautions should be taken by all parties to guarantee confidentiality concerning the practitioner's condition.

············

LEGAL ISSUES RELATED TO SPECIFIC HEALTH CARE PROVIDERS

The numbers of actors involved in providing health care, and the intricate relationship among those actors and patients, create a maze of liability for specific health care providers.

Acute-Care Hospitals

Throughout a lifetime, a patient may deal with different types of specific health care providers in various settings, including but not limited to: acute or hospital care, long-term care, hospice care, mental and behavioral health care, and integrated delivery systems. It is critical to appreciate the relationships among these providers as, typically, several health care providers might be subject to suit under varying negligence theories when a patient sustains injury during the course of care or treatment.

Ostensible or Apparent Agency   As noted previously, a hospital can be held vicariously liable for the actions of its employees under a theory of *respondeat superior,* as can any employer. A hospital may also be held vicariously liable for the acts or omissions of independent contractors who are not its employees under a theory of ostensible or apparent agency. Under this theory, a hospital may be subjected to liability if the patient looked to the institution rather than the individual physician for care, and the hospital's actions led the patient to reasonably believe that the physician was one of the hospital's employees. This theory is often used to hold the hospital liable for the acts of non-employed physicians and other health care providers with hospital-based practices. The origin of this theory is set forth in the Restatement Second of Torts as follows:

> One who employs an independent contractor to perform services for another which are accepted under reasonable belief that the services are being rendered by the employer or by his servants, is subject to liability for physical harm caused by the negligence of the contractor in supplying such services, to the same extent as though the employer was supplying them himself or by his servants.[69]

This theory of liability is most often applied when a patient is admitted into the emergency department of a hospital and, instead of choosing a particular physician, the hospital has provided the patient with a physician. Subsequently, the patient alleges that the emergency department physician provided negligent care or treatment and, under a theory of ostensible agency, the patient asserts that the hospital is liable for the alleged negligent conduct. Courts have also applied ostensible agency where the conduct of hospital-based health care providers other than emergency department physicians is at issue. For example, this theory has been applied to pathologists, anesthesiologists, and radiologists.[70] Notably, some states have even permitted an ostensible agency cause of action to be asserted against an HMO.[71] To minimize the possibility of any misconceptions that patients might have related to the legal status of independent health care providers providing care and treatment within a particular facility, many hospitals have implemented procedures to inform patients and clearly identify individuals as independent from the hospital. For example, some hospitals began noting on all literature including admission forms, letterheads, advertisements, and billing statements that the physicians within the facility were independent from the hospital itself. Additionally, if the hospital provided uniforms or hospital clothing for the independent contractors, the name of the hospital did not appear on these garments. Further, upon presentation to the emergency department, all patients were given the opportunity to select their own physician or be informed by hospital that the emergency department was staffed with independent contractors.[72]

Corporate Negligence   Under the theory of corporate negligence, a hospital has a non-delegable duty to the patient to ensure the patient's safety and well-being while the patient is in the hospital. The hospital is not vicariously liable for the health care provider's negligent act; rather, the hospital is liable for its own negligence in failing to ensure that a proper standard of care is upheld. To prevail under this theory, the plaintiff must prove:

1. That the hospital knew or had reason to know of a defect in its procedures; and
2. That the defect was a substantial factor in bringing about injury to the patient.[73]

Long-Term Care Liability

The aging of the "Baby Boom" generation, in the next few years, will make senior citizens the largest-growing segment in our society.[74] It is projected that by the year 2030 there will be approximately ten million Americans eighty-five years and older.[75] As the population ages, it is likely that many more people will be living in long-term care facilites.

Types of Long-Term Care Facilities   As the population ages, the services related to the senior population will expand.

Continuing Care Retirement Community   Continuing Care Retirement Communities (CCRC) offer a long-term contract with residents to provide housing, food, and graduated services, including nursing care for the remainder of the resident's life. Usually, the CCRC campus consists of independent housing, personal home care services, and ultimately a nursing facility. Generally, as a resident's needs increase, the need for care increases and the appropriate level of care is provided. Liability issues as to standard of care may vary depending on the level of care that is provided, meaning, whether it is independent, personal home care services, or skilled nursing services.

Personal Care Homes   A licensed personal care home (PCH), commonly referred to as an assisted living facility (ALF), is a facility that provides food, shelter, personal assistance, and supervision for individuals who do not require the services of a licensed nursing facility, but do require some assistance with activities of daily living. PCHs and ALFs are not medical facilities, although they may hire individuals with nursing backgrounds. They are often regulated by state agency, but the level of regulation is usually far less than for a nursing home. Liability issues again depend on the level of care being administered to the patient. A common liability issue arises when the facility keeps residents who require a higher level of care than they can provide.

Nursing Homes   Nursing homes are licensed nursing facilities that provide food, shelter, nursing care, and assistance to individuals who have special needs or need assistance with multiple activities of daily living. Nursing homes are medical facilities. They employ individuals with medical or nursing training. They are either for-profit or not-for-profit. There is no practical difference between the standard of care in a for-profit and a not-for-profit facility. However, many governmentally operated nursing facilities enjoy governmental immunity for common law negligence claims, for which immunity depends entirely on state law.[76]

Regulations   The Omnibus Budget Reconciliation Act of 1987[77] (OBRA) is the basis for the uniform regulations that govern the care and assessment of nursing home residents. The statute established the requirements relating to the provision of care, such as assessing residents, training for nurse's aides, physician supervision, and level of nursing care. Also included in the statute are provisions for various residents' rights, such as the right to be free from physical and chemical restraints, the right to choose one's physician, and the right to confidentiality and privacy.

Included in OBRA is the Federal Nursing Home Reform Act. This establishes the standards of care for facilities receiving Medicare and Medicaid payments. The vast majority of facilities seek reimbursement through Medicare or Medicaid and are therefore subject to these requirements. Facilities that fail to comply with the regulations are subject to sanctions, the withholding of payments, and, under extreme cases, termination of participation in the Medicare and Medicaid system. This statute makes it the individual state's responsibility to establish, monitor, and enforce the state's requirements for licensing and for the federal regulations.[78]

To participate in the Medicare and Medicaid program, a nursing home must go through a survey and certification process every nine to fifteen months. Standard surveys are designed to assess whether the nursing home is in compliance with federal and state regulations. They are typically conducted without any prior notice to the facility. They cover four factors:

1. A survey of the quality of care furnished (as measured by indicators of medical, nursing, and rehabilitative care), dietary and nutrition services, activities and social participation, sanitation, infection control, and the physical environment
2. Review for adequacy of written plans of care
3. An audit for accuracy of the residents' assessments
4. A review of compliance with residents' rights

The survey typically consists of a team of investigators, from a local field office, that examine records, observe care provided by the staff, interview the staff, and interview residents or families.[79] If a facility is found to be out of compliance, a Statement of Deficiencies is reported. Once this is reported, the facility must submit an acceptable plan of Correction, which is then followed by a post-survey revisit to ensure that the plan of correction is implemented.[80] These regulations vary by state and should be reviewed accordingly.

Types of Liability   The liability issues related to health care continue to expand.

Vicarious Liability   Like hospitals and other care providers, nursing homes and long-term care facilities can be held vicariously responsible for the actions or omissions of their employees. For example, in *Bryant v. Hunt*,[81] the Court of Appeals of Michigan found that a nursing home has a responsibility to provide its residents with an "accident-free environment." In this case, the patient died of asphyxiation when she became wedged between the mattress and the bed rail due to the alleged negligence of the nursing home's employees. The Court of Appeals of Michigan found that this was an ordinary negligence claim for which the defendant nursing home could be found to be vicariously liable. The case was remanded to the trial court to be tried on vicarious liability.

An extension of vicarious liability was created through the theory of ostensible agency. The ostensible agency theory holds that a nursing home could be held vicariously liable under an agency theory for the acts of an independent physician, if the patient looks to the institution rather than the individual physician for care, and the nursing home "holds out" the physician as its employee.[82] The key is whether the facility acts or fails to act in some way, which might lead the patient to a reasonable belief that the facility or one of its employees is responsible for treatment. Although not particularly common, this issue can become relevant in the case of physicians employed by, or under contract to, the nursing home, or outsourced contractors such as occupational or physical therapists.

Corporate Liability   This theory holds that a defendant facility owes certain non-delegable duties to the resident, which, if breached, may subject it to liability for damages. Most recently, in *Aptekman v. City of Philadelphia*,[83] the District Court for the Eastern District of Pennsylvania declined to dismiss the suit against the defendant nursing home on the theory of corporate liability. The District Court reasoned that although corporate liability has not yet been extended to include nursing homes, it has been expanded to include HMOs and, given the right set of circumstances, a state court may extend corporate liability to include health care organizations other than hospitals, such as nursing homes and long-term care facilities.

Claims   As in other medical malpractice and medical negligence cases, plaintiffs must present an expert report or an expert witness to establish their case. In *Perdieu v. Blackstone Family Practice Center, Inc.*,[84] the Supreme Court of Virginia determined that the issues surrounding treatment in a nursing home are beyond the ordinary scope of a jury's understanding; therefore, expert testimony is required. The court further stated that the experts employed must be engaged in the actual performance of the procedures at issue in the case. The court therefore excluded testimony of experts who had not treated nursing home patients for more than thirty years, did not have experience in the field of nursing home care, or did not have an active clinical practice within a year of the alleged incident.

Claims against nursing homes include those for negligent hiring or firing[85] and failure to enforce policies and procedures.[86] Statutory claims may also be brought against a nursing home or long-term care facility such as a claim under the Unfair Trade Practices Act[87] or Consumer Protection Law.[88] Claims for care issues can range from discrete events such as a fall or an assault and battery, to a course of treatment, such as wound care.

Elder Abuse   One issue that has been gaining more attention recently is elder abuse. Nearly one out of every three nursing homes in the United States has been cited for an abuse violation in the past few years.[89] To facilitate risk management in nursing homes, many have implemented procedures that require them to report instances of abuse to local authorities and state agencies quickly, to fully prosecute those involved if need be, and to establish safeguards to protect residents from further abuse.[90] Despite these efforts, the physical and sexual abuse of nursing home residents continues to be a rampant problem with large consequences.[91] In response to this, many states have adopted measures for reporting and dealing with allegations of abuse, including registries of employees who have been guilty of abusing residents.

For example, Pennsylvania law protects adults over the age of sixty who cannot perform tasks necessary for their physical or mental health. A majority of those who reside in nursing homes or long-term care facilities fall into this category. Reporting is mandatory in assisted living facilities such as nursing homes and long-term care facilities. In *Delaney v. Baker*,[92] the Supreme Court of California affirmed the judgment of a lower court that awarded the plaintiff with "heightened attorney's fees" and pain and suffering damages. The plaintiff sued the defendant nursing home and two administrators for damages under a theory of elder abuse, willful misconduct, negligence, neglect of an elder, and wrongful death, after the plaintiff's mother died while a resident at the home. At the time of death, the plaintiff's decedent had bed sores down to the bone.

Penalties for elder abuse are different in every state. Some states might even begin to hold long-term care facilities and nursing homes criminally responsible for elder abuse.

Hospice Care

Hospice care differs from traditional health care treatment in its emphasis on palliative treatment for persons who are in the process of dying. In other words, unlike hospitals where curative or restorative treatment is sought, a hospice focuses on pain management for patients facing impending death. Generally, hospice care addresses the physical, psychological, and spiritual needs of the patient. Because hospice patients are suffering from a terminal illness or disease, health care providers operating within the context of a hospice routinely encounter issues related to the Patient Self-Determination Act of 1990, advance directives, and withholding and withdrawing life-sustaining treatment.

Patient Self-Determination Act of 1990   It is imperative that all health care providers, including hospice providers, are knowledgeable regarding the statutory requirements of the Patient Self-Determination Act (PSDA) of 1990.[93] This federal statute prescribes that all providers subject to the act must provide each patient with written information on the patient's right under state law to: (1) accept or refuse life-sustaining treatment, and (2) to formulate advance directives (or living wills). The provider is also required to outline its written policies regarding the implementation of a patient's right to refuse such treatment. The provider is further required to document in each patient's medical record whether the patient has executed an advance directive and to ensure compliance with the requirements of state law regarding advance directives. Additionally, the provider is prohibited from conditioning the provision of care based upon whether or not the patient has executed an advance directive. Finally, the act requires the provider to educate its staff and the community on issues regarding advance directives.

Advance Directives   An advance directive is a legal document that communicates an individual's medical decisions or appoints someone else to make decisions on that person's behalf should the individual become incapacitated and either permanently unconscious or terminally ill. There are two basic kinds of advance directives. Living wills are typically effective to communicate the patient's wishes within a period of time prior to the patient's anticipated death. Durable powers of attorney, on the other hand, usually allow a surrogate to make decisions on the patient's behalf whenever the patient is incapable of making such decisions, regardless of the imminence of death. To be effective, advance directives must comply with state statutes. State and federal governments are currently required to disseminate information about advance directives. In fact, states that fail to comply with the mandates of the Patient Self-Determination Act of 1990 risk losing Medicare and Medicaid funding.

Withholding and Withdrawing Life-Sustaining Treatment

In the absence of an advance directive, health care providers will likely encounter various legal, ethical, and moral issues related to the propriety of withholding or withdrawing of life-sustaining treatment from a patient suffering from an incurable or irreversible medical condition, which might lead to death, regardless of continued life-sustaining treatment. These issues can greatly complicate the decision as to whether treatment should be witheld or withdrawn, particularly when the patient can no longer communicate.

When a patient has an incurable and irreversible medical condition, the classes of treatment involved in sustaining life are typically: (1) surgery, (2) cardiopulmonary resuscitation, (3) antibiotic therapy, (4) respiratory support, (5) renal dialysis, and (6) artificial nutrition and hydration.

Because the essence of the physician-patient relationship is consensual, continuing treatment of the type necessary to sustain life under these circumstances is nearly always invasive and therefore would constitute a technical "battery" if continued over the objection of a competent individual. The law is well settled that such an individual has a legal right to refuse life-sustaining procedures even though refusal might shorten or terminate life. The patient's right in these circumstances is founded upon a common law right to self-determination and a constitutional right to privacy. In the case of a terminally ill patient, the courts have generally held that the patient's right to self-determination and privacy outweigh the countervailing interest of the state in: (1) preserving life, (2) preventing suicide, (3) safeguarding the integrity of the medical profession, and (4) protecting innocent third parties (such as minor dependents or unborn children of the patient). In general, courts considering the "right to die" issue conclude that the state's interest weakens and the individual's right grows as the prognosis dims and the intrusiveness of the treatment increases.

The situation presented by the permanently unconscious or otherwise incompetent patient, however, is greatly complicated because the individual is not in a position to consent to or refuse continued life-sustaining treatment, even if refusal might have been the patient's preference. Under such circumstances, courts, attending physicians, and members of the patient's family usually attempt to achieve the appropriate balance among the various interests involved.

As a practical matter, in the case of the incompetent patient receiving life-sustaining treatment, the attending physician who favors withdrawal of such treatment must balance the probable but often unstated wishes of the patient against the potential of: (1) civil liability for medical malpractice, (2) criminal liability for homicide, and (3) professional censure for unprofessional and unethical conduct. On the other hand, continuing such treatment over the objection of the next of kin might lead ultimately to a civil lawsuit on behalf of the patient or the estate for the tort of battery (nonconsensual bodily invasion). Some courts have held that the surrogate decision maker who wishes to discontinue treatment, in which the patient is incapable of consenting or refusing treatment, may be required to prove what the patient would wish, if the patient were competent, by clear and convincing evidence.[94] This decision is very difficult in the case of a patient in a persistent vegetative state and even more difficult in the case of a conscious, but incompetent, patient. The decision can be further complicated when a patient's family members do not agree about what should be done.

The American Medical Association (AMA) takes the position that in deciding whether potentially life-prolonging medical treatment is in the best interest of the incompetent patient, the physician and the surrogate decision maker should consider several factors, including: (1) the patient's values about life and the way it should be lived; (2) the patient's attitudes toward sickness, medical procedures, and death; and (3) the possibility for extending life under humane conditions.

The AMA maintains that it is not unethical to discontinue all means of life-prolonging treatment to a patient who is beyond doubt permanently unconscious. It is the AMA's position that medication, artificially supplied respiration, nutrition, and hydration constitute life-prolonging medical treatment. Of course not everyone agress with this position, and it can be difficult to achieve consensus even within the medical community as to whether a particular patient is beyond doubt permanently unconscious.

Mental and Behavioral Health Care

The unique circumstances surrounding the relationships among mental and behavioral health care providers, their patients, and third parties requires the imposition of exceptional duties on providers while simultaneously affording them immunities. It is imperative that health care providers know the law in their respective states, as these duties and immunities vary by jurisdiction.

Duty To Warn   A psychiatrist or licensed psychologist cannot disclose information acquired while rendering professional services to a patient without the written consent of the patient. The protection against disclosure applies to both civil and criminal matters. However, individuals may waive this privilege by placing their psychiatric state at issue in a lawsuit. A court then has discretion to permit disclosure of the information.

Since the landmark case of *Tarasoff v. Regents of University of California*, a majority of states have imposed some form of the Tarasoff duty to warn by statute or case law, thereby creating an exception to the physician-patient privilege.[95] In Tarasoff, the court held that "a psychotherapist treating a mentally ill patient has a duty to use reasonable care to give threatened persons such warnings as are essential to avert foreseeable danger arising from his patient's condition or treatment."[96] Significantly, in Tarasoff, the psychotherapist's efforts to contact law enforcement regarding his patient's violent threats did not satisfy his duty to warn.

In most jurisdictions, when a psychotherapist determines that a patient presents a serious danger of violence to another individual, the psychotherapist has a "duty to warn" or an obligation to use reasonable care to protect the intended victim against such danger. The psychotherapist does not violate the psychotherapist-patient privilege when disclosing such patient communications. However, in most jurisdictions, for this duty to warn to come into play, there must be a specific, identifiable victim and a clear means of carrying out the threat to the intended victim. In preventing the threatened danger, the psychotherapist should act in a manner that best preserves the privacy of the patient. Notably, some states have expanded the duty to warn beyond merely psychotherapists. In fact, the law in some states has imposed a duty to warn of an actual threat of violence upon a broad range of mental health providers, including professional counselors, licensed psychiatrists, marriage and family therapists, social workers, and psychiatric and mental health nurse specialists.[97] Therefore, in an effort to avoid third-party liability, it is crucial to know the law of the state in which your particular health care facility is located.

Ambulance Services

An ambulance is defined as a vehicle that is specifically designed for transporting the sick or injured, contains certain specified equipment, and is staffed by trained personnel.[98] Ambulances must be equipped with emergency warning lights, sirens, and telecommunication equipment, including at a minimum, one two-way radio or wireless telephone as prescribed by state and local law. Further, an ambulance must also contain standard patient care equipment, including a stretcher, clean linens, first aid supplies, oxygen equipment, and such other safety and lifesaving equipment as is required by state and local authorities.[99] Generally, there are two types of ambulance vehicles, which are subject to different regulations. A basic ambulance is one that provides transportation, equipment, and staff needed for basic services, including controlling bleeding, splinting fractures, treating shock, delivering babies, or performing cardio-pulmonary resuscitation.[100] The ambulance crew of a basic life support (BLS) vehicle must consist of at least two members. One of these members must be legally authorized to operate all life-sustaining equipment and be certified as an emergency medical technician by the state or local authority. By contrast, an advanced life support (ALS) vehicle is equipped with complex specialized life-sustaining equipment, and, ordinarily, equipment for radio-telephone contact with a physician or hospital. An ALS vehicle must contain two members, with at least one crew member certified as a paramedic or an emergency technician by state and local authority.[101]

Further, an understanding of the distinctions between these ambulance services is important for purposes of Medicare reimbursement. Medicare requires the ambulance supplier to provide documentation that the ambulance service provider is in compliance with emergency and staff licensure and certification requirements.[102] (Refer to Chapter 9 in Volume II of this series for information on Pre-Hospital Medical Services.)

Integrated Delivery Systems

During the last dozen years, the spiraling cost of health care and health insurance premiums has contributed to the development of various types of health care delivery systems, otherwise known as integrated delivery systems (IDS). The Clinton Health Care Reform Plan proposed in 1993 hastened this development and prompted many states to adopt their own health care reform plans.

Thus, in a relatively short period of time, numerous questions have been raised concerning the liability of operating and administering an IDS.

Profile of an IDS   The perceived advantage of an IDS is its economic and administrative efficiency. An IDS consolidates a variety of professional, laboratory, and technical services to control costs. For example, most IDSs contain the following cost containment features:

1. Preadmission review: Requires hospital admissions to be approved in advance
2. Discharge planning: Establishes general guidelines for length of hospitalizations and post-discharge case management

3. Utilization review: Controls the allocation of HMO resources

4. Individual case management

5. Second opinions

6. An appeal process: A mechanism to contest case management decisions

Further, an IDS may be set up to enter into "capitation" agreements with managed care organizations or employers. Capitation generally means that the physician or group receives a fixed monthly or annual payment for each member enrolled in the plan. The pool of proceeds available to each physician or provider diminishes with each patient referral to a nonmember physician or provider. Virtually all theories of liability asserted against an IDS stem from the competing goals of containing health care costs while maximizing health benefits.

There are several theories of liability that may be asserted against a particular IDS:

1. Vicarious liability: Liability imposed upon an IDS by a patient subscriber for the negligent acts of its employees

2. Direct liability: Liability brought by a subscriber directly against an IDS for negligently selecting health care providers or managing resources; most often arises in the case of a refusal to allow services

3. Breach of contract or warranty: Failing to honor or fulfill terms of the patient subscriber or member-physician's contract

4. Intentional misrepresentation or fraud: Nondisclosure of material facts regarding the operation of the IDS

It is helpful to keep in mind the source of each type of liability when studying these theories. Allegations of vicarious and direct liability are vertically imposed theories that can be made only by a patient-subscriber (including parents of a minor or an estate), whereas breach of contract actions are horizontal and may be brought by the subscriber to the HMO, or by the member-physician and provider.

Likewise, it is also important to consider which type of IDS is involved, because application of these theories of liability depends largely on the particular type of IDS model present. The different IDS structures are discussed here.

Structuring an IDS The structure of an IDS is particularly important, as each IDS provides different mechanisms for balancing the competing goals of health care cost containment and maximum health care service. Each IDS creates different incentives for providers and determines the treatment available to patients.

The Health Maintenance Organization (HMO) An HMO is an IDS that provides for the financing and delivery of comprehensive health care services to participants for a prepaid fee. This is in contrast to traditional health care insurance, which reimburses the policyholder or provider for the cost of services ("fee-for-service basis"). HMOs provide services to their members through a system of prepaid physician-providers.

Common to the HMO is the primary care physician who acts as a "gatekeeper." It has been observed by some critics of the traditional health care insurance model that there is an incentive by the provider to perform unnecessary services, and thereby generate fees. The HMO model, on the other hand, has no such incentive and theoretically should be more economical. However, because there is no fee for service, critics of managed care argue that there is also a disincentive to treat.

As established previously, many IDSs and HMOs have a system of capitation in which the participants' premiums are pooled. This pool is used to pay the health care providers. Typically, HMO participants are bound by the HMO to seek treatment from approved physicians. The HMO's limitation on the member's choice of physician, the right to see a specialist, and the system of capitation are the major criticisms of the HMO delivery system.

There are generally four different types of HMOs, which are categorized on the basis of their relationship with the medical providers. As demonstrated below, an HMO's exposure to liability depends largely upon its organizations.

- Staff Model—HMO directly employs staff physicians and other providers who render services only to members. This model is characterized by the employer-employee relationship, which is formed between the physician and the HMO. Staff models also occasionally own or lease their own health care facilities.

- Group Model—HMO contracts with independent medical groups or physician corporations that provide medical care to the HMO members at the group's own offices. Generally speaking, a group model pays its contract physicians a set fee per month, per covered individual. However, unlike staff model physicians, group model physicians are not restricted to treating only HMO participants.

- Network—HMO contracts with different groups of physicians who are permitted to continue to treat non-HMO patients.

- Individual Practice Associations—IPA Model HMO contracts on a capitation basis with independent practice associations, which in turn contract with individual private practice physicians to provide medical care to HMO members in their own offices. IPA physicians, like network physicians, may treat non-HMO patients.

The Preferred Provider Organization (PPO)   A PPO consists of physicians, hospitals, and other medical providers who contract to provide medical care to a defined group of patients on a negotiated, discounted fee-for-service basis.

In contrast to the HMO, a PPO member may seek treatment from a non-approved physician. Further, unlike an HMO member, the PPO member is usually not required to see a gatekeeper before seeking treatment with a specialist.

Insurance Features   A patient's insurance coverage determines the amount of flexibility in choosing health care coverage. Recently there has been an increased effort to expand the patient's choice in this area even if it is at the expense of less covered benefits.

Point of Service (POS)   This is a plan that combines the basic features of an HMO and PPO. Under a POS plan, the covered person may treat with a non-network provider, but at a reduced level of benefits. There is a primary care physician-gatekeeper who approves specialty and hospital services. POS organizations have been set up because HMOs are under both legal and marketing attack because of the lack of freedom of choice in selecting providers.

Exclusive Provider Organization (EPO)   Similar to a PPO, an EPO consists of a group of participating providers with contractual arrangements to an insurer or other sponsoring group to provide services. Like an HMO, EPOs generally have a primary care gatekeeper, and the covered person must seek services exclusively from the participating EPO provider.

Physician Hospital Linkages   Traditional arrangements between hospitals and physicians, like those between physician and patient, are also rapidly changing throughout the country. This has produced a confusing variety of organizational alliances between physicians and hospitals. Whether this is being driven by hopes of economic survival for the hospitals, the physicians, insurance companies, or large employers is unclear. It is clear, however, that the terrain is shifting and will continue to do so. Accordingly, it is important to understand the emerging relationships between hospitals, physicians, and insurers.

The most familiar, and perhaps most interesting organization, the physician-hospital organization (PHO) is a venture between a hospital(s) and a group(s) of physicians, generally the hospital's medical staff and other ancillary providers, who have streamlined their services to act as an integrated whole. The benefits of these systems are the reduction in administrative costs and greater bargaining power in the marketplace to negotiate contracts with an IDS employer or insurance company. There are four basic models:

1. ***Traditional PHO***   A traditional PHO is a joint venture between one or more hospitals and physicians. The physicians may participate in the joint venture as individuals or as an organization such as an IPA or professional corporation. The advantage of a PHO is that it serves as the contracting agent for multiple HMOs and PPOs, and for employers who fund their own benefit plans. Thus, the PHO can exert greater leverage in the marketplace with health care payers. In some situations, the PHO may actually own an HMO or PPO (or vice versa). Within the PHO, the financial and reimbursement interests of the hospital and physicians are aligned. As physicians and hospitals cooperate to achieve their common goals, they deliver care more efficiently, generating greater profitability.

2. ***Management Services Organization (MSO)***   An MSO is an organization that provides management services to one or more medical practices, such as a large group, physician practice, or hospital. MSOs may assume the financial risk associated with health care management by purchasing the assets of a professional corporation and then leasing the assets back to the group. In return, they provide physicians with a full range of administrative services. The MSO can also serve to transfer hospital capital to physicians in exchange for assets, expanded clinical services, more affordable administrative systems, and comprehensive ambulatory and inpatient services.

3. ***Foundation Model***   A foundation is a corporation that is organized by a hospital, a group of hospitals, or a group of non-profit doctors with a common parent organization. The foundation thus provides the physical plant, administrative and marketing services, and non-medical personnel, and negotiates with managed care plans, insurers, and so on. For the most part, physicians have little control in a foundation model. Foundations grew out of the strong prohibition on hospital employment of physicians in California and other states.

4. ***Integrated Health Organization (IHO)***   An IHO is an organization that requires a separate legal entity, such as a parent corporation, with at least two subsidiaries (such as a hospital and a management services organization), and often a third

subsidiary, such as an educational or research foundation. The physicians are employed by the management services corporation, which provides coverage, the physical plant, and so on. An IHO generally sponsors its own managed care activities such as an HMO or PPO.

This is the most integrated of any of the PHO models. It is thought to embrace a comprehensive, community-based system of health care services, which would avoid duplication, minimize competition, and be more cost-effective.

Liability Issues   Essential features common to all integrated delivery systems include strong utilization review and case management procedures, and the exercise of significant control over the panel of providers. Many of the models also include some form of capitation.

As noted previously, capitation generally means that the physician or group receives a fixed monthly or annual payment for each member. This payment goes to compensate the physician or group, but can also pay for referrals to specialists or entities outside of the group. The press is replete with horror stories of physicians or insurers who refused to allow such referrals, even when conventional wisdom supports their medical necessity. For this reason, the capitation issue has strong emotional appeal in claims against a health care provider or an IDS.

Under traditional theories of medical malpractice, liability for negligent treatment rests with the provider. An HMO or PPO does not technically provide medical care directly to its members. During recent years, however, liability for medical malpractice has been extended to IDSs as a result of their restrictions on their members' choice of physician, right to receive certain types of medical care, and the perceived economic disincentive to treat created by capitation.

Thus, while claimants continue to pursue garden-variety professional liability claims of negligent treatment by a participating IDS physician, they may also pursue claims against an IDS on the grounds that: (1) no medical negligence would have occurred if they had had the right to seek treatment from other providers; (2) no medical negligence would have occurred if their right to seek treatment from other providers were not restricted; or (3) that the treatment they requested was arbitrarily denied or delayed, resulting in personal injury.

These new avenues of recovery expose IDSs to significant operating risks.

Respondeat Superior   As previously discussed, *respondeat superior* is a doctrine by which an employer may be held vicariously liable for the negligent acts of its employee performed in the course and scope of employment. In the context of the IDS, the master-servant or employer-employee relationship is most readily apparent in the staff model. In the staff model, an HMO's physician's negligence may be imputed to the physician's employer, the HMO, if it is established that the HMO directly controlled the physician's activities. Because staff-model HMOs place tight restrictions on the scope of their physicians' practices and pay them directly, evidence of control sufficient to impose *respondeat superior* liability is relatively easy to establish.[103] Liability imputed to an IDS is not limited to the staff model. In fact, courts have extended the *respondeat superior* theory of liability to group-model HMOs and even to HMOs who hire non-member physicians to provide independent consultations.[104] Nevertheless, not all jurisdictions are uniform in their approach, and many have held that where the HMO does not directly employ its own physicians, the master-servant relationship might not exist, and therefore, no liability may be assessed against the HMO under the doctrine of *respondeat superior*.

Ostensible Agency   As noted, the theory of ostensible agency is an exception to the general rule of contract law that an employer cannot be held liable for the negligent acts of an independent contractor. Under the theory of ostensible agency, an HMO can be held vicariously liable for the medical malpractice of a contracting physician in which: (1) the patient looked to the institution (the HMO) rather than the individual physician for care; and (2) the HMO "held out" the physician as its employee, thereby creating a reasonable perception in the eyes of the patient that the physician was the apparent agent or employee of the HMO. Ostensible agency is applied almost exclusively to group- and IPA-model HMOs. However, recent developments in federal law, particularly in the interpretation of the Employee Retirement Income Security Act[105] (ERISA), have questioned its continued application. Increasingly, federal courts have ruled that ERISA, a federal regulatory scheme devised by Congress to control disputes related to employee benefits, may preempt state law claims against HMOs on theories of vicarious liability. The ERISA preemption is addressed later in this chapter.

Courts often look to marketing materials to see if they contain statements that imply that, despite the independent contractor status of the physician, the doctor was "held out" as competent by the HMO or IDS. For this reason, marketing directors of health maintenance organizations need to be aware that their statements might ultimately be used to support theories of liability against HMOs. Indeed, if these and other materials suggest that the HMO held out a physician as its employee, and that subscribers relied on these representations to their detriment, courts may ignore the legal distinction of "independent contractor" and impose liability against the HMO. A subscriber may prove reliance on the representations of an IDS by producing marketing materials that hold out the physician or provider as an employee.

Advertisements by some IDSs describing a "total care" program, which not only provides payment for medical services, but also "guarantees quality and service," might haunt an IDS in subsequent litigation. In many plans, the subscriber-plaintiff may not see a specialist or obtain a procedure or test without prior approval or referral from the gatekeeper. This too may create an inference that the patient looked to the IDS for care, and not to a specific physician.

Direct Liability or Corporate Negligence   In addition to being found liable on a vicarious liability basis for the negligent acts of a third-party physician, an IDS may also be directly liable to a patient-subscriber under theories of:

1. Corporate negligence
2. Breach of contract or breach of warranty
3. Intentional misrepresentation or fraud

As applied in the managed care context, courts have upheld theories of corporate negligence against an IDS on the grounds that: (1) the IDS negligently selected its member physicians; or (2) failed to properly allocate its available resources.

Credentialing by a managed care organization of the physicians who will provide care to its participants has become an area of increasing direct liability for an IDS. Because the patient's freedom to choose a physician or specialist is generally limited by the IDS, individuals who are harmed by one of a plan's physicians may plausibly argue that they never would have been subjected to the physician's malpractice, if the IDS had more carefully screened the health care providers for whose services it provides payment under the member's benefit plan.

One of the more hotly contested areas of managed care liability, and also responsible for producing some of the most extraordinary verdicts against health care organizations, is an IDS's system of comprehensive utilization review. In accordance with this system, decisions are made regarding to whom and on what basis treatment will be given. Liability may attach if it is determined that an IDS arbitrarily denied coverage for a given procedure, or that it delayed approving a procedure, resulting in personal injury to a patient-subscriber.[106]

Employee Retirement Income Security Act (ERISA) of 1974[107]

ERISA was designed by Congress to serve as a comprehensive regulatory system for resolving employee benefit disputes. To place ERISA in its proper context, it is helpful to understand the political climate that prompted its passage.

ERISA was passed in reaction to widespread concern regarding the integrity of nationwide employee benefit or pension plans. Throughout the 1960s and early 1970s, as the United States fell into recession and became less competitive in the world market, manufacturing and industrial plants started closing. One of the reasons cited for their failure was the increasingly high cost of maintaining employee benefit plans.

As a result of plant failures, senior "vested" employees, on the verge of retirement, discovered that many of their pension plans were underfunded or insolvent. Simultaneously, Congress began to question whether the Social Security system would be able to meet the demands of these future retirees. These public policy concerns prompted Congress to pass ERISA. In so doing, Congress intended to simplify the administration of pension plans by administering them under a single, cohesive federal body of law. Further, Congress sought to limit an employee's right to sue a plan for mismanagement and thereby protect the financial integrity of employee benefit plans.

As set forth more fully here, by routing litigation to the federal courts, Congress effectively nullified traditional state law causes of action for negligence and breach of contract for mismanagement of employee benefit plans, and required litigants to pursue their claims under ERISA, which permits only the recovery of benefits, not monetary damages, and attorneys' fees. This is the essence of the ERISA preemption.

Without a doubt, ERISA is the most effective tool in defending managed care liability cases. ERISA states:

> Except as provided in subsection (b) of this section [the savings clause], the provisions of this subchapter and subchapter 3 of this chapter shall supersede any and all state laws insofar as they may now or hereafter relate to any employee benefit plan.[108]

This is referred to as the ERISA "preemption clause."

There are only three narrow exceptions to the general rule of ERISA preemption for claims "relating to" an employee benefit plan. They include: (1) any state law that "regulates insurance, banking, or securities,"[109] otherwise known as the "savings clause;" (2) any state cause of action that relates only tangentially to an employee benefit plan; and (3) "run-of-the-mill-type lawsuits," such as collection fee cases for unpaid rent or attorneys' fees, libel, and slander. [110]

Federal court decisions regarding the scope of ERISA preemption have varied somewhat over the years. However, most jurisdictions across the country, and in particular federal courts in Pennsylvania and New Jersey, have until recently applied ERISA preemption broadly to prevent state lawsuits against HMOs under theories of vicarious liability, breach of contract, loss of consortium, and intentional infliction of emotional distress.

Since the Third Circuit case *Dukes v. U.S. Healthcare, Inc.*,[111] courts have generally divided derivative claims into two categories: (1) quality of care, or (2) quantity of care.

Generally, courts have held that quantity of care claims are preempted by ERISA. In contrast, a plaintiff's claim that challenges the quality of care will not be preempted by ERISA. "In other words, if the claim involves a denial of treatment or payment pursuant to the terms of the employee benefit plan, the claim 'relates to' an ERISA plan and will be preempted."[112] Alternatively, "if the claim relates to the quality of care received, such as a claim for physician malpractice, courts often hold that these claims do not relate to an ERISA plan and are not preempted."[113] The Third Circuit acknowledged in *Dukes* that a determination as to whether a cause of action is based on the managed care organization's quality of care or the quantity of care may at times be inextricably intertwined. Consequently, courts are apt to struggle in determining whether ERISA is triggered by a plaintiff's claim where both quality of care and quantity of treatment may arguably be at issue.

········

CONCLUSION

The study of health care potential liability and regulation is a dynamic and expanding endeavor. Plaintiffs continue to try new theories of liability, and courts continue to recognize them. Potential liabilities and regulations relate directly to the nature of health care organizations and operations. Careful selection and management of the corporate form and operation are keys to reducing some of the liabilities inherent in health care. Understanding the legal environment in which organizations exist, once the corporate form has been selected, is the next key to controlling liability.

Although the amount of liability and regulation can be extremely frustrating at times, it is helpful to remember that people's health is typically the number one determinant of their quality of life. All the laws and regulations are merely intended to help protect this precious gift.

Endnotes

1. *Osborne v. Montgomery*, 203 Wis. 223, 234 N.W. 372 (1930).
2. *Young v. Cerniak*, 467 N.E.2d 1045 (Ill. App. Ct. 1984).
3. *Cline v. William H. Friedman & Assoc.*, 882 S.W.2d 754 (Mo. Ct. App. 1994).
4. *Young v. Cerniak*, 467 N.E.2d 1045 (Ill. App. Ct. 1984).
5. *Logan v. Greenwich Hosp. Assoc.*, 191 Conn. 282, 302, 465 A.2d 294, 305 (1983); *Shilkret v. Annapolis Emergency Hosp. Association.*, 349 A.2d 245 (Md. 1975).
6. *Ibid.*
7. *Shilkret v. Annapolis Emergency Hosp. Association*, 276 Md. 187, 349 A.2d 245 (1975); *Pederson v. Dumouchel*, 72 Wash. 2d 73, 431 P.2d 973 (1967).
8. *Sheeley v. Memorial Hosp.*, 710 A.2d 161, 167 (Rhode Island, 1998); *Vergara v. Doan*, 593 N.E.2d 185 (Ind. 1992).
9. *Williams v. Hotel Dieu Hosp.*, 593 So.2d 783 (La. Ct. App. 1992); *Jordan v. Bogner*, 844 P.2d 664 (Colo. 1993).
10. *Daubert v. Merrell Dow Pharmaceuticals, Inc.*, 509 U.S. 579, 590 (1993).
11. *Frye v. United States*, 293 F. 1013 (1923)
12. *Hreha v. Benscoter*, 381 Pa. Super. 556, 554 A.2d 525 (1989).
13. Restatement (Second) of Torts, Section 286 and 288.
14. Restatement (Second) of Torts, Section 288A and 288B.

15. Del. Code Ann., tit. 18, §6801(8).

16. *Kananen v. Alfred Dupont Institute of the Nemours Foundation*, 796 A.2d 1,- (Del. Super. 2000); *Sacks v. Thomas Jefferson University Hospital*, 684 F. Supp. 858 (E.D.Pa. 1988); *Walters v. St. Francis Hospital*, 932 P.2d 1041 (Kan. Ct. App. 1997).

17. *Webb v. Jarvis*, 575 N.E. 2d 992, 995 (Ind. 1991); *Conboy v. Mogeloff*, 567 N.Y.S.2d 960, 961 (App. Div. 1991); *Kirk v. Michael Reese Hosp. & Med. Ctr.*, 513 N.E. 2d 387, 395 (Ill. 1987); *Rebollal v. Payne*, 536 N.Y.S. 2d 147, 148 (App. Div. 1988).

18. *McElwain v. Van Beek*, 447 N.W.2d 442 (Minn. Ct. App. 1989).

19. *McElwain v. Van Beek*, 447 N.W.2d 442 (Minn. Ct. App. 1989).

20. *O'Hara v. Holy Cross Hospital*, 561 N.E.2d 18 (Ill. Supr. 1990).

21. *Watkins v. U.S.*, 589 F.2d 214, 219 (5th Cir. 1979); *Zavalas v. State Dep't of Corrections*, 861 P.2d 1026, 1027 (Or. Ct. App. 1993); *Kasier v. Suburban Transp. Sys. Corp.* 398 P. 2d 14, 16 (Wash 1965); *Schuster v. Altenberg*, 424 N.W.2d 159, 161 (Wis. 1988).

22. 61 Am Jur 2d, Physicians, Surgeons, and Other Healers §186.

23. *Rogala v. Silva*, 305 N.E.2d 571 (Ill. App. 1973).

24. *Noel v. Proud*, 367 P.2d 61 (Kan. 1961); *Colvin v. Smith*, 92 N.Y.S. 2d 794 (1949); *Brooks v. Herd*, 257 P. 238 (Wash. 1927).

25. *Hudson v. Parvin*, 582 So.2D 403 (Miss. 1991).

26. *Gouse v. Casse*, 615 A.2d 331 (Pa. 1992).

27. *Corrigan v. Methodist Hospital*, 869 F. Supp. 1202, 1206 (E.D. Pa. 1994).

28. *Craig v. Borcicky*, 557 So.2d 1253 (Ala 1990); *Tappe v. Iowa Methodist Medical Center*, 477 N.W.2d 396 (Iowa 1991); *Hudson v. Parvin*, 582 So.2d 403 (Miss. 1991); *Roybal v. Bell*, 778 P.2d 108 (Wyo. 1989).

29. *Craig v. Borcicky*, 557 So.2d 1253; *Smith v. Cotter*, 810 P.2d 1204 (Nev. 1991).

30. *Distefano v. Bell*, 544 So.2d 567 (La. Ct. app.), writ denied, 550 So.2d 650 (La. 1989).

31. *Douget v. Touro Infirmary*, 537 So.2d 251 (La. Ct. App. 1988).

32. *Kelley v. Kitabama*, 675 So.2d 1181 (La. Ct. App.), writ denied, 679 So.2d 1352 (La. 1996); *Petriello v. Kalman*, 576 A.2d 474 (Conn. 1990); *Kershaw v. Reichert*, 445 N.W.2d 16 (N.D. 1989); *Johnson v. Sears, Roebuck & Co.*, 832 P.2d 797 (N.M. App.); *Johnson v. St. Joseph Hospital*, 832 P.2d 1223 (N.M. 1992); *Friter v. Iolab Corp.*, 607 A.2d 1111 (Pa. Super. 1992).

33. *Urban v. Spohn Hospital*, 869 S.W.2d 450 (Tex. App.-Corpus Christi 1993, writ denied).

34. *Friter v. Iolab Corp.*, 607 A.2d 1111 (Pa. Super. 1992).

35. 81 Am. Jur. 2d Witnesses §436 (1992).

36. *Ibid.* at §441.

37. *Hammonds v. Aetna Cas. & Surety Co.*, 243 F. Supp. 793, 797 (N.D. Ohio 1965).

38. Va. Code Ann §32.1–36.1 (some statutes provide the negligence standard as a basis for bringing an action for improper disclosure).

39. Health Insurance Portability and Accountability Act of 1996 (HIPAA), Public Law 104–191, at §1177(a).

40. *Ibid.*

41. HIPAA, at §1171(6).

42. HIPAA, at §1177(a).

43. *Ibid.*

44. *Ibid.*

45. *Doe v. Shady Grove*, 598 A.2d 507 (Md. App. 1991) (Patient brought an invasion of privacy action against the hospital where he was treated because employees of the hospital allegedly disclosed that he was being treated for AIDS. The patient also sought an injunction barring the hospital from publicly identifying him in court proceedings. The court held that the failure to uphold such a request would undermine the state statutes that established a presumption of confidentiality for medical records.); *Estate of Behringer v. Medical Ctr.*, 592 A.2d 1251, 1272 (N.J. Super. 1991) (Physician was treated for AIDS at the hospital where he had staff privileges. Word of his condition spread to other physicians within the hospital who were not involved in his treatment. The court found the hospital negligent for failing to protect the plaintiff's medical information from other hospital employees.)

46. *In re Milton S. Hershey Med. Ctr.*, 407 Pa. Super. 565, 595 A.2d 1290 (1991), appeal granted, Application of Milton S. Hershey Med. Ctr., 531 Pa. 640, 611 A.2d 712 (1992), and aff'd, In re Milton S. Hershey Med. Ctr., 535 Pa. 9, 634 A.2d 159 (1992).

47. *Ibid.*

48. *Ibid.*

49. *Estate of Behringer v. Medical Ctr.*, 592 A.2d 1251 (N.J. Super. 1991).

50. *Ibid.*

51. *Ibid.*

52. *Estate of Behringer v. Medical Ctr.*, 592 A.2d 1251 (N.J. Super. 1991).

53. Cal. Health & Safety Code §120980.

54. *Ibid.*

55. An Overview of 1992 State HIV/AIDS Laws (George Washington Intergovernmental Health Policy Project, June 1992). Maryland requires the Department of Health and Mental Hygiene to report HIV and CD4k counts of less than 200 mm^3.

56. 45 N.Y. Pub. Health Law §2130(1).

57. See *Hale v. Sheikholeslam*, 724 F.2d 1205 (5th Cir. 1984); *Townsend v. Kiracoff*, 545 F. Supp. 465 (D.Colo. 1982); *Ruane v. Niagara Falls Memorial Medical Ctr.*, 458 N.E.2d 1253 (N.Y. 1983); *Schloendorff v. Society of N.Y. Hosp.*, 133 N.Y.S. 1143 (App. Div. 1912), aff'd, 105 N.E. 92 (1914); *Tabor v. Doctors Memorial Hosp.*, 563 So. 2d 233 (La. 1990); *Berel v. HCA Health Servs.*, 881 S.W.2d 21, 23 (Tex. App.-Houston [1st Dist.] 1994, writ denied).

58. 29 U.S.C.A §623(f)(1).

59. *Sheridan v. E.I. DuPont de Nemours & Co.*, 100 F.3d 1061, 1077–1078 (3d Cir. 1996).

60. 29 U.S.C.A. 621.

61. 29 U.S.C.A. §623(a)(1).

62. 42 U.S.C.A. §12101.

63. *Meritor Savings Bank, FSB v. Vinson*, 477 U.S. 57, 67 (1986).

64. *Harris v. Forklift Systems, Inc.*, 510 U.S. 17, 21 (1993).

65. *Faragher v. City of Boca Raton*, 524 U.S. 775, 777 (1998).

66. *Faragher v. City of Boca Raton*, 524 U.S. 775 (1998); *Burlington Indus. Inc., v. Ellerth*, 524 U.S. 742 (1998).

67. *Ibid.* at 807.

68. *Faragher v. City of Boca Raton*, 524 U.S. 775 (1998).

69. Restatement of Torts, Sec. 429 (1965).

70. See e.g., *Mitchell v. Shepperd Memorial Hospital*, 797 S.W.2d 144 (Tex.App.—Austin 1990, writ denied); *Pamerin v. Trinity Memorial Hosp.*, 423 N.W.2d 848 (Wis 1988).

71. *Boyd*, 547 A.2d at 1229.

72. See 1 Health L. Prac. Guide § 2:30 (2002).

73. *Thompson v. Nason Hosp.*, 527 Pa. 330, 591 A.2d 703 (1991).

74. See statistics on the Administration on Aging Web site at www.aoa.gov, last updated March 22, 2005.

75. *Ibid.*

76. Mundy, W. J. "Nursing Home Litigation: Defense Considerations from Initial Assessment to Discovery." In Nursing Home Negligence Conference iv. Mundy-z (Prof. Educ. Sys. Ins.), 2002.

77. 42 U.S.C. §1395, §1396.

78. *Ibid.*

79. See 1 Health L. Prac. Guide §2.37 (2002).

80. *Ibid.*

81. 2002 Mich. App. LEXIS 725 (May 21, 2002).

82. See generally, *Adamski v. Tacoma General Hospital*, 579 P.2d 970 (Wash. App. 1978), *Capan v. Divine Providence Hospital*, 430 A.2d. 647 (Pa. 1980), *Rodebush v. Oklahoma Nursing Homes, Ltd.*, 867 P.2d 1241 (Okla. 1993).

83. 2001 U.S. Dist. LEXIS 19120 (E.D. Pa. November 21, 2001).

84. 2002 WL 61048324 (Va. September 13, 2002).

85. Barry by and through *Cornell v. Manor Care Nursing Home*, 1999 U.S. Dist. LEXIS 5928 (E.D. Pa. 1999).

86. *Ex parte McCollough*, 747 So.2d 887 (Ala. 1999) (where plaintiff sued defendant nursing home for a "systematic failure to enforce policies which minimize the risk of wrongdoing").

87. *Schenck v. Living Centers-East*, 917 F. Supp 432 (E.D. La. 1996).

88. *White v. Moses Taylor Hosp.*, 763 F. Supp. 776 (M.D. Pa. 1991).

89. www.aoa.gov (last updated 2005).

90. United States General Accounting Office Report to Congressional Requesters: "Nursing Homes, More Can Be Done to Protect Residents from Abuse," found at www.gao.gov (last updated 2002).

91. *Ibid.*

92. *Delaney v. Baker*, 971 P.2d 986 (Cal. 1999).

93. 42 U.S.C. §1395ccc(f)(1).

94. Conservatorship of Wendland,___ Cal. 4th___, No. S087265 (Cal. August 9, 2001).

95. *Tarasoff v. Regents of University of California*, 529 P.2d 553 (Cal. 1974). See also, George C. Harris, The Dangerous Patient Exception to the Psychotherapist-Patient Privilege: The Tarasoff Duty and the Jaffe Footnote, 74 Wash. L. Rev. 33, 47–48 (1999).

96. *Tarasoff*, 529 P.2d at 559.

97. 25 MPHYDLR 495, Mental and Physical Disability Law Reporter, (May–June 2001).

98. 42 C.F.R. §410.40(e).

99. 42 C.F.R. §410.41(a)(4).

100. Irwin Cohen, 2 Health L. Prac. Guide §19:2 (2002).

101. 42 C.F.R. §410.41 (b)(1)-(2).

102. 2 Health L. Prac. Guide §19:2.

103. *Sloan v. Metropolitan Health Counsel of Indianapolis, Inc.*, 516 N.E. 2d 1104 (Ind. App. 1987) (holding that where an employer-employee relationship exists, a corporation may be held vicariously liable for the malpractice of its employee-physicians).

104. See *Dunn v. Praiss*, 256 N.J. Super. 180, 606 A.2d 862, appeal denied, 611 A.2d 657 (1992) (holding that an HMO was liable under respondeat superior for medical malpractice committed by a urologist who was a member of a group of urologists that contracted to treat HMO subscribers. Significant to the court's finding that an employer-employee relationship existed was the fact that the group urologists were paid on a per capita, as opposed to a fee-for-service basis, and that they were not free to accept or reject a particular patient).

105. 29 U.S.C. §1001 et seq.

106. See *Fox v. Health Net*, 219692 (Cal. Super. Ct. Riverside County, December 29, 1993) (verdict entered against an IDS awarding $12 million in compensatory damages and $77 million in punitives).

107. 29 U.S.C. §1001 et seq.

108. *Pilot Life Ins. Co. v. Dedeaux*, 481 U.S. 41, 44–45 (1987) (quoting § 514(a), 29 U.S.C. § 1144 (a)) (emphasis supplied).

109. ERISA §514 (b)(2) (A). See *Kentucky Assn of Health Plans, Inc. v. Miller*, 538 U.S. 329 (2003).

110. *Settles v. Golden Rule Ins. Co.*, 927 F.2d 505 (10th Cir. 1991); *Nealy v. U.S. Heathcare HMO*, 844 F. Supp. 966, 971 (S.D.N.Y. 1994).

111. *Dukes v. U.S. Healthcare, Inc.*, 57 F.3d 350 (3rd Cir.), cert. denied, 516 U.S. 1009 (1995).

112. Bondurant, E. J., Cataland, A. K., Dean, R. Update on ERISA Litigation Developments. American Law Institute, American Bar Association Continuing Legal Education, SG092 ALI-ABA 249, (May 2–3, 2002).

113. *Ibid.*

Appendix 2.1

ESSENTIALS OF AMERICAN LAW

John C. West

In many respects, American law has grown in the absence of a grand design or consistent vision. It has grown by the accretion of statutes, constitutions, and court decisions in individual cases. New statutes are passed by new generations of legislators; new cases are decided by new generations of judges. American law, to some extent, has evolved to meet the needs and expectations of society as it evolves. There has been, of necessity and invariably, some lag time built into the process. Sometimes all of this has meshed well; at other times, and perhaps more frequently, needs and expectations have conflicted with each other. It is something of a misnomer to refer to something as "American law," because there really is no single American law. It is a complex mixture of fifty different state and federal laws and it varies from location to location. However, there are enough basic similarities between all of the various jurisdictions that certain observations can be made regarding "American law."

American law is based on, or was a reaction to, the Common Law tradition that was received from England during the Colonial period. Many of the most revered institutions of American law, such as trial by jury, can be traced back to medieval England. One of the chief characteristics of the Common Law is that the law is largely built upon court decisions, rather than statutes. A great deal of the Common Law has never been codified, and a court is not dependent upon a statutory enactment to determine whether one party might be liable to another. Where statutes have been enacted in a particular area, court decisions tend to elucidate and clarify what the statutes mean, and courts are free to interpret statutes in ways that might not have been envisioned by the legislature. The Civil Law system, which predominates in most of continental Europe, by contrast, is heavily dependent upon statutory enactments. In Civil Law systems, courts are only allowed to put a "gloss" on statutes when deciding cases; they are not allowed to make new law.

A particularly interesting aspect of American law is the preeminence of the court system. Shortly after independence was secured, the court system secured for itself the right to be the ultimate arbiter of the constitutionality of statutes or governmental regulations. In many, if not most other countries, the legislature determines whether statutes or regulations are constitutional. The reservation of this right by the court system is uniquely American.

What follows is not intended to be an expansive treatise on American law. That is not possible within this context. However, this should give readers who work in a health care setting a good introduction to the vagaries of American law, and should help them understand some of the bases for actions taken during litigation.

....

THE COURT SYSTEM

The United States does not have a single court system, rather it has fifty-one distinct court systems. There is a federal court system, that can draw upon state or federal law, and there are fifty different state court systems. Although each is different, there are certain similarities inherent in each system.

All courts must have jurisdiction over the parties and the subject matter of the dispute to render a competent judgment in any particular case. (Although "jurisdiction" is often used as a shorthand term for the geographic area over which a particular court may have the power to hear cases, the term actually refers to a court's power to hear and decide cases.) Some courts are courts of general jurisdiction, which means that they can hear a wide range of cases, or they may be courts of limited jurisdiction, which means that there are certain types of cases that they are prohibited from hearing and deciding. Jurisdiction over a person or entity usually requires that the person or entity be found within the area over which the court may exercise jurisdiction. This means that the person or entity must either reside or have a place of business within the jurisdiction, transact business within the jurisdiction, or submit to the jurisdiction of the court. Jurisdiction is normally conferred upon a court by statute and may not normally be conferred upon a court by the parties (except in the case of a non-resident defendant who submits to the jurisdiction of the court). If a court does not have jurisdiction over a matter, it must dismiss the action or, if permitted, transfer the action to a court of competent jurisdiction.

All potential plaintiffs must have standing to bring a lawsuit. This generally means that they must have suffered an injury that may be redressed by the law, or they may be threatened by or in fear of an injury that could be prevented by legal means. In this context, "injury" is very broad. It can mean a physical injury to a person, illness, damage to reputation, loss of income or revenue, damage to property, diminution of the value of property, loss of property, loss of business opportunity, loss of or damage to intangible rights, or damage to several other matters recognized by the law.

All actions should be brought in the proper venue. Venue is normally determined by statute and generally is concerned with issues of fairness, efficiency, and judicial economy. Issues concerning proper venue often involve the locations of the residences of the parties, the location of the defendant's principal place of business, or the location where the dispute arose. Venue and jurisdiction are completely separate concepts: a court may have jurisdiction to hear a case, but the venue may not be proper if it would be more appropriate for another court to hear the case. A doctrine related to venue is that of *forum non conveniens*. This, however, is a common law, rather than statutory, doctrine. It is usually the case that *forum non conveniens* issues should be considered to be in conformity with statutory construction relating to venue, but *forum non conveniens* gives the trial court greater discretion. This doctrine usually requires that, if there is a location in which the litigation would clearly be more efficient and convenient for the parties and witnesses, the court should dismiss or transfer the action.

Virtually all jurisdictions have some form of statute of limitations for virtually all civil causes of action or criminal actions (usually with the exception of murder or other particularly serious or heinous crimes). The statute of limitations normally operates to preclude a claimant from bringing a cause of action after a specified period of time (often in the range of one to six years). Statutes of limitation vary by jurisdiction and by cause of action. However, most jurisdictions also have tolling provisions that operate to suspend the running of the statute for certain periods of time. Most statutes will be tolled during periods of legal incompetence, including infancy (to age eighteen in most states). In addition, most jurisdictions will not consider that the statute of limitations has begun to run until the claimant knows or, in the exercise of reasonable judgment, should have known that he may have a cause of action against another person. This is generally referred to as the "late discovery" exception. This exception is frequently used in health care when foreign bodies are left in the patient after surgery, when the patient is unable to have children after damage to a reproductive organ, or anytime a patient discovers a material fact or that a misrepresentation occurred after the procedure or treatment was performed. There may also be an exception in the case of continuing or ongoing treatments. For example, a physician may commit malpractice, but continue to treat the patient for several years. The period of the statute of limitations may not start to run until the course of treatment has ended. A variant of, or complementary to, the statute of limitations is the statute of repose. A statute of repose tends to place a final limit on the time period in which a lawsuit may be brought. Not all jurisdictions have a statute of repose. Unfortunately, as well-meaning as legislatures often are in enacting a statute of repose, they also are often riddled with exceptions that tend to diminish their effectiveness.

All courts, in all court systems, are at least in theory bound to follow cases that have value as precedent. While this is a commonly understood concept, it is difficult, if not impossible, to put into actual practice. In actual practice, the only courts that are absolutely bound to follow precedent are courts of inferior jurisdiction within a given jurisdiction with regard to the cases decided by a court of superior jurisdiction within that jurisdiction. Thus, trial courts and intermediate courts of appeal within a given state are bound to follow the precedent set by the supreme court of that state. However, the state supreme court is not required to follow its own precedent, although overruling previously established precedent is not a step that most supreme courts take lightly. The precedents set by other jurisdictions can be considered to be persuasive authority in any given case, but the court will not normally be required to follow it. Within the federal system, all federal courts must follow the precedent set by the Supreme Court of the United States, but federal circuit courts of appeal are not required to follow precedent set by other circuit courts of appeal, nor are district courts required to follow any precedent set by a circuit court of appeal other than the one for the circuit within which the district court resides. While state courts have concurrent jurisdiction with federal courts with respect to federal statutes, many state supreme courts take the position that they are not bound by any precedent set under federal statutes other than that set by the Supreme Court.

At one time there was a distinction between law courts and courts of equity (chancery). Although this distinction no longer exists in the federal and most state court systems, there are some remnants of the system of which one should be aware. The courts of equity were less concerned with precedent and standardization of the law than they were with dispensing justice in a particular case. The courts were given far more discretion to fashion an appropriate remedy for the parties in equity than they were in law. Equity, by and large, grants relief in the form of personal decrees, rather than money damages. Equity actions were always tried to the court without a jury. Actions that to this day still sound in equity include injunctive relief or specific performance of an agreement.

The Federal Court System

Federal courts are courts of limited jurisdiction. They may hear only cases between certain classes of disputants or certain types of cases. They may hear cases involving disputes between the residents of different states, but only if the matter in controversy exceeds $75,000 (at present). They may hear cases arising out of rights secured by federal statute or by the Constitution of the United States. They may exercise jurisdiction over claims arising under state law that are associated with claims otherwise recognized by federal law. The jurisdiction of federal courts is also limited to hearing only "cases and controversies." This prevents them from deciding matters that are not truly presently in dispute, hence they are incapable of rendering advisory opinions.

Federal District Courts   The federal district courts are the trial level courts in the federal system. As a general rule, entry into the federal court system is through the district court.

United States Circuit Courts of Appeal   Appeals taken from one of the federal district courts will be to a U.S. circuit court of appeal. There are currently thirteen circuit courts of appeal, including the Federal Circuit and the District of Columbia Circuit. Whereas many decisions of the district courts are appealed to the circuit courts of appeal, but few decisions of the circuit courts of appeal are accepted for review by the U.S. Supreme Court, the decisions of the circuit courts of appeal are a source of a great deal of federal case law.

United States Supreme Court   The U.S. Supreme Court is the ultimate appellate court in the nation. It hears appeals from the U.S. circuit courts of appeal, but it does so only upon a grant of certiorari, which is akin to leave of court to file the appeal. It only hears cases that it believes are significant and which will generate clarifications of legal issues. The U.S. Supreme Court also has jurisdiction to resolve disputes between states. It may also hear appeals from the highest court of any state.

State Court Systems

State court systems are highly variable, and there may be no typical state court system. As a general rule, each court system will have at least one court that functions as a trial court (various jurisdictions may have more than one level of trial court, with the amount of damages sought or the amount in controversy as the distinction between them. These are often called district, circuit, common pleas, county, or municipal courts.) All states have a court that functions as an appellate court of ultimate jurisdiction (often called a "supreme court," although, for example, New York calls its supreme court the Court of Appeals, and its Supreme Court is a lower level appellate court).

Many jurisdictions also have an intermediate appellate court, to which appeals are made from the trial court(s) and from which appeals are taken to the supreme court. These are typically called the "court of appeals," but may be called "Superior" or "Supreme" courts.

FEDERAL, STATE, AND LOCAL LAWS AND REGULATIONS

The various laws passed by various governmental units in the United States might appear to be an intertwining, overlapping, and incestuous potpourri of regulations and, to some extent, all of this is true. There are, however, some rules that can be applied to make sense of all of this. There is a certain taxonomy that must be learned. All states and the United States have constitutions. A constitution is a relatively short and very broadly worded instrument that reflects the vision of the governmental entity. Constitutions are by their very nature extremely imprecise. The language is invariably subject to interpretation, which may change over time. Although constitutions are not wholly immutable, they are very difficult to amend or replace.

As a general rule, a statute is a law passed by the supreme legislature of a governmental entity, usually either the federal or a state legislature. It has the force of law upon its passage and may be retroactive in application if so designated by the legislature. All statutes, whether federal or state, must not violate any provision of the Constitution of the United States, which is the supreme law of the land. If they do violate the Constitution, they will be held to be invalid and unenforceable, in whole or in part. The federal government's power to pass and enforce any particular piece of legislation must arise out of a provision in the U.S. Constitution. The federal courts are the ultimate arbiters of the constitutionality of any federal or state statute. In addition, state statutes must not violate provisions within the constitution of that state.

A federal court may render a decision involving a controversy arising out of a state statute, but only if the court has jurisdiction to hear the matter, as discussed previously. This is usually referred to as the pendent jurisdiction of the court. Similarly, a state court may decide a matter involving a federal statute, if the issue is properly before it.

Although an ordinance can be the enactment of any governmental body, it is generally regarded as an enactment of a county or a municipality. County and municipal ordinances must be in conformity with the powers delegated to the entity by the state government.

A regulation is usually considered to be an enactment of an administrative or regulatory agency. Agencies are usually populated with career bureaucrats who are not elected, although the titular head of certain agencies may be appointed by elected governmental officials or the legislature. This idiosyncrasy of agencies may sometimes place them beyond the power of public opinion. Although regulations must be adopted by the agency pursuant to particular procedures, they are not passed by the legislature. Any regulation must be adopted pursuant to a statute or legislation that enables the agency to adopt such a regulation. Regulations frequently add precision to, and assist in the interpretation of, statutes. Regulations generally have the force of law, and, in many cases, their enforcement is by the same agency that enacted them. In many cases, states are entitled to adopt regulations in areas already governed by federal regulations (for example, occupational safety and health or environmental protection). In this event, it is generally the case that the state regulations may be as stringent as, or more stringent than, the federal regulations, but they may not be less stringent.

. . . .

CRIMINAL LAW

American law can be divided into two basic components: criminal law and civil law. There might be some gray areas at the peripheries of the two, or the distinction between the two can be blurred, but they are, by and large, distinct.

The most obvious characteristics of criminal law are that a criminal action is brought by the state or federal government, and that the object of the action is to punish the wrongdoer for transgressions. While a crime might very well injure a particular individual, the wrong that is redressed is an injury to society. Punishment, under criminal law, generally consists of incarceration or the imposition of fines or monetary penalties. It is noteworthy that, as a general rule, it is not possible to obtain insurance for criminal misdeeds or to cover criminal fines or penalties.

Because liberty is one of the fundamental rights secured to all persons by the U.S. Constitution, the burden of proof required to prove that a crime was committed, which might result in the loss of liberty for the convicted individual, is very high. In typical civil litigation, the plaintiff normally is required only to show that the wrong occurred by a preponderance of the evidence (essentially that it is more probable than not that it occurred the way the plaintiff claims). In a criminal proceeding, however, the government is required to prove that a crime occurred beyond a reasonable doubt. If the jurors, collectively, have reasonable doubts that the crime occurred the way that the government claims, they should not convict the defendant.

There are other protections for defendants in criminal cases. The government is foreclosed by the Double Jeopardy Clause, U.S. Constitution Amendment V, from pursuing a second criminal prosecution for the same offense. Also pursuant to the Fifth Amendment, persons may not be compelled to be witnesses against themselves, nor may they be convicted without due process of law. All persons are protected by the Fourth Amendment to the U.S. Constitution from unreasonable searches and seizures. If a search or seizure was unreasonable, the fruits of the search or seizure may not be admitted at trial, which makes it difficult, if not impossible, for the government to prove its case. The Sixth Amendment guarantees trial by jury, a speedy trial, the assistance of counsel, and the right to confront witnesses. The Eighth Amendment prohibits excessive fines and cruel and unusual punishments.

Implications for Health Care Providers

Although there has always been a certain amount of prosecution of health care providers for various offenses, it seems that the level of criminal prosecution is escalating. This is true when one considers the panoply of new regulations to which health care providers can be subjected, many of which carry criminal sanctions, in addition to prosecutions for quality of care decisions. Whether this trend will continue is not known at present, but health care providers should be aware of and attempt to guard against potential criminal sanctions.

....

CIVIL LAW

As opposed to criminal actions, civil actions are usually brought by private individuals (or corporations, rarely by the government) to seek reimbursement or compensation for a wrongful act committed by the defendant(s). The aim of the action is usually not to punish the defendant(s) per se, but rather to redress the wrong. As a general rule, most civil actions seek money damages. Following is a brief introduction to some of the more important aspects of the civil law system, especially as it affects health care organizations.

Negligence

Negligence is perhaps the most common cause of action among the civil law claims. It is undoubtedly the most common allegation against health care providers in civil litigation. It is a far-reaching allegation that can be applied to almost any form of human interaction. The various forms of negligence are addressed here.

There are four elements required in any negligence cause of action. To prevail, the plaintiff will be required to show: (1) the existence of a duty running from the defendant to the plaintiff; (2) a breach of that duty; (3) an injury caused by the breach of the duty; and (4) damages as a result of the injury. If the plaintiff cannot prove any of these elements, he will not prevail.

Ordinary Negligence   An "ordinary" negligence cause of action requires all four of the elements recited, none of which will automatically be assumed in any given case. The existence of a duty is usually present as a simple duty to exercise reasonable care under the circumstances (meaning, the care that a "reasonably prudent" person would exercise under the same or similar circumstances). However, there are certain circumstances in which no duty may be present: there is usually no duty on the part of a landowner to protect a trespasser from hazards on the property, and there is usually no duty to rescue another person who might be in danger. Because the duty is that of an ordinarily prudent person, the plaintiff does not need an expert to show the existence of the duty.

If there is a duty running from the defendant to the plaintiff, the plaintiff will be required to show that the defendant's actions were in some way a breach of that duty. The plaintiff does not need an expert to show that the duty was breached.

The plaintiff must also show that he was injured as a result of the breach of the defendant's duty. Because any action will set into motion another event, or a series of events, it is important to note that the injury must have been proximately caused by the allegedly negligent act. This means, in essence, that the injury must have been reasonably foreseeable. For example, where the defendant pushes another person, who as a result drops a package containing fireworks, which causes the fireworks to go off and injure a third party (the plaintiff), can it be said that the act of pushing the person caused the plaintiff's injury?

Finally, the plaintiff must be able to show damages as a result of injury. Damages must be something that the law can remedy. For example, if the plaintiff alleges a loss of prestige or status, but no lost wages or pain and suffering, there may be no remedy at law available. Damages will be discussed in greater detail further on. Professional Negligence The same elements apply in a "professional" negligence action as in an "ordinary" negligence action, but the methods of proof are different. Whenever a professional, such as a health care provider, undertakes to provide professional services to the plaintiff, a duty arises to provide those services in the same manner as any other competent professional would provide them. The nature of the duty must be established by expert testimony.

Similarly, the plaintiff must show that the defendant's actions deviated from what a competent professional would have done under the same or similar circumstances. The breach of the duty must also be shown by expert testimony.

The element of injury as a result of the negligent action is again required, and causation usually must be shown by expert testimony. Damages may be proven in the same manner as in an action for ordinary negligence.

Negligence per se   Negligence per se is usually reserved for causes of action that are based on a violation of a statute. In this case the statute normally must be of the type that is designed to protect a class of persons, of which the plaintiff is one. For example, if a state has a statute that prohibits a motorist from following another car too closely, it may be considered negligence per se if an accident is caused by a motorist failing to stop in time to avoid hitting another car.

Res ipsa Loquitur   Literally translated, *res ipsa loquitur* means "the thing speaks for itself." In other words, the event or outcome is one that does not normally occur in the absence of negligence. There are three elements involved in a *res ipsa loquitur* case: (1) the accident must be of a type that does not normally occur in the absence of negligence; (2) the instrumentality must have been entirely within the control of the defendant(s); and (3) the plaintiff must not have had any responsibility, through voluntary action or contribution, for the event. The best and most typical example of a *res ipsa loquitur* claim in health care is the case of the retained foreign body following surgery.

Strict Liability

Strict liability attaches when society will not permit a defendant to mount a defense against the allegations of liability made by the plaintiff. Strict liability usually attaches when the defendant undertakes ultrahazardous activities, such as blasting explosives or allowing dangerous animals to run free.

Intentional Torts

As a general rule, allegations of negligence are founded upon actions that the defendant might have taken intentionally, but did not take with the intention of causing harm (for example, a surgeon might intentionally place a sponge inside a patient's abdomen, but not with the intention of causing harm). Intentional torts, on the other hand, arise out of actions taken by the defendant with the intention of causing the outcome that resulted.

Assault   In the context of civil litigation, an assault occurs when one places another in a position in which the other fears that a battery will occur. Thus, lunging at another person with a knife, even if the knife does not contact the person's body, is an assault. There has not been a great deal of civil litigation arising out of assaults that occur in the absence of battery and actual physical injury.

In the context of criminal law, assault has been subsumed into the crime of battery to the point where the two words have become virtually a single term. One rarely hears one word without the other.

Battery   This is a very simple tort. It merely requires the touching of another person's body without that person's consent. In this as in all torts, one must show injury or damage of some sort if one wishes to prevail in a lawsuit. However, it is often possible to make a showing of damages based upon a psychological or emotional injury, such as emotional distress or mental anguish, and succeed in getting one's case heard by a jury.

Consent   In the health care setting, any touching of the body of another is a potential battery. The only defense to an allegation of battery is the defense of consent. If one has the consent of the person to be touched, and if that consent is lawfully obtained and appropriately encompasses the intended scope of the touching, the touching does not constitute a battery. There are two types of consent that are operative in this context. One is a general consent and the other is informed consent. The general consent will suffice for non-invasive, relatively low-risk procedures. Informed consent will be required in any situation where the proposed procedure or treatment carries a material risk of harm.

Informed consent comes in two general varieties. The difference between the varieties lies primarily in the determination of what constitutes a "material risk" of the procedure. For example, should a physician be required to disclose a risk that manifests itself (in the absence of negligence) in one in every million cases? What if the risk manifests itself once in every thousand or hundred cases? When does a risk become material? In the more traditional variety, the physician must disclose the risks that a "reasonable physician," under the same or similar circumstances, would have disclosed. This variety is typically codified in state statutes. In the "reasonable patient" variety, the risks of the procedure that must be disclosed to the patient include those that a reasonable patient would wish to know about before consenting. The patient typically must show that he, as a reasonable patient, would not have undergone the procedure had he been informed of this risk. This variety is often imposed by court decisions.

There have also been several cases involving affirmative misrepresentation of the nature of the procedure. For example, the patient might have expressly consented to the performance of an appendectomy, after which the surgeon performed a hysterectomy. As one might expect, these cases are invariably difficult to defend.

Intentional Infliction of Emotional Distress   The tort of intentional infliction of emotional distress is a somewhat but not terribly uncommon cause of action. It is somewhat unusual in tort law, because the traditional view of emotional distress required a concurrent physical injury, or the placement of the claimant within a zone of danger, for the claimant to prevail. The tort of intentional infliction of emotional distress does not require a concurrent physical injury. It does, however, normally require that the defendant's behavior had been extreme and outrageous, which would normally place it beyond the bounds of ordinarily decent behavior.

Forms of Liability

Liability for damages must be founded upon some legal principle. These legal principles may be separate and distinct from merely being a consequence of a person's actions, as was discussed above. Most of these principles can be traced back to little more than an attempt to get at "deep pockets" to make the injured plaintiff whole.

Direct Liability   Direct liability is imposed upon defendants as a consequence of their actions or failure to act when action might have been legally required.

Joint and Several Liability   Certain states (but not all) allow for the imposition of joint and several liability on multiple tortfeasors (negligent parties). This form of liability, in its simplest form, allows for the imposition of total liability for all of the plaintiff's injuries upon any of the persons potentially responsible for the injuries. For example, A, B, and C each committed negligent acts that ultimately led, it is alleged, to the plaintiff's injuries. However, A and B are bankrupt or have no assets that can be attached (this is only for the purposes of this example—the plaintiff is not required to pursue any particular defendant or avenue of recovery). The plaintiff may seek to recover the full amount of damages from C, even though A and B may have been as responsible, or even more responsible, for the plaintiff's injuries. If the plaintiff obtains complete relief for all of his damages from C, he then has no claim against A or B. However, C may have the right to seek contribution from either A or B, or both, to recover a proportionate share of the damages paid on their behalf (for all the good that it may do him).

Vicarious Liability (Agency)   This is a generic term for liability for the acts or omissions of others. Although liability predicated upon *respondeat superior* principles, as discussed further on, is a form of vicarious liability, this discussion of vicarious liability will focus on liability for the acts or omissions of agents. As a general matter of agency law, the duly authorized agent is permitted to transact any business authorized by the principal, and the agent may be authorized to enter into transactions which obligate the principal to perform certain tasks. In the health care setting, there are two principal types of agency relationships.

Agency by Estoppel (Ostensible Agency)   This arises when the actions of the principal, either implicit or overt, lead the third party to reasonably believe that the putative agent was an agent or employee of the principal. In this instance, as in all estoppel cases, the plaintiff must justifiably rely upon the representations and must change position accordingly. If all of these elements have been met, the defendant will be estopped (not permitted) to deny that the agency relationship exists.

Apparent Agency   This arises when a third party reasonably believes that the putative agent is an agent or employee of the principal and is authorized to transact the business at hand and to legally obligate the principal. In this case, the belief must be generated by the principal affirmatively holding out the putative agent as its agent or employee, or knowingly permitting the putative agent to represent as the agent or employee of the principal. In addition, the third party must justifiably rely on the representation that the agent is authorized to transact the business.

General Comments   In actual practice, the aforementioned distinctions are not germane to the outcome of the case, especially from the lay perspective. They are often used interchangeably by the courts. If an agency relationship can be established, the defendant may become liable for the actions of the agent. In the health care setting, this can mean that a hospital can frequently be liable for the actions of its emergency department physicians. Less commonly, but also possibly, the hospital may be held liable for the actions of its pathologists, radiologists, anesthesiologists, and anesthetists. Some states extend the agency relationship to any physician to whom the hospital, through its recognized agents, refers the patient, as, for example, the on-call roster in the emergency department.

Respondeat Superior   This liability arises out of an employer and employee (master and servant) relationship. As a general rule, the employer will be vicariously liable for the actions of its employee, as long as those actions were taken in the course of the employee's employment and were within the scope of employment. In the health care setting, this defense may be applied in situations where a hospital employee is accused of sexually assaulting a patient: the hospital might argue that it employed the employee to care for patients, not to sexually assault them (this defense might get around *respondeat superior* liability, but will be unavailing against allegations of negligent hiring or negligent supervision).

Respondeat superior liability does not normally attach to actions of an independent contractor. However, in the absence of an employment agreement (whether express or implied) or a clearly recognizable employer and employee relationship, it is not always easy to determine the relationship between the parties (especially when the employer might wish to characterize all persons acting on its behalf as independent contractors). Certain elements might help determine whether a person is an employee. These are: (1) the extent of control exercised by the "employer;" (2) whether the one "employed" is engaged in a distinct business or occupation; (3) the kind of occupation engaged in (and whether it is normally exercised under supervision); (4) the skill required in the occupation; (5) whether the "employer" provides the workplace and the instrumentalities necessary to perform the tasks; (6) the length of time for which the person is "employed" (for a project or for the foreseeable future); (7) the method of payment, if any (by the job or by time period); (8) whether the work is the regular business of the "employer;" (9) whether the parties believe they are creating an employer and employee relationship; and (10) whether the "employer" is in business. None of these elements are determinative. Rather, the court will employ a weighing process to determine whether it is more probable than not that an employer and employee relationship exists. Courts frequently hold that independent medical staff members are independent contractors, rather than employees.

Defenses to Liability

There are certain complete or partial defenses to liability that may be employed to prevent or mitigate an award of damages. Unfortunately, most of these have little application in health care.

Assumption of the Risk   This defense requires that the plaintiff was aware of a known risk and elected to take his chances of injury. There are three basic types of assumption of the risk defenses. In the simplest case, the plaintiff may consent to face the risk and may relieve the defendant of liability for what the defendant may or may not do. Alternatively, the plaintiff may enter into a relationship with the defendant with the knowledge that the defendant will not protect him from the risk. In the third case, the plaintiff may be aware of the defendant's negligence, but nonetheless chooses to encounter the risk. While this defense may serve in some situations (as where the plaintiff has been warned and is aware that a floor is wet but still chooses to walk across it), it will not serve in others (as where a physician warns the patient that he is incompetent or is not properly trained to perform a procedure and the patient still elects to have him perform it). One cannot employ the assumption of the risk defense to defend against negligence that has yet to occur. Like contributory negligence, assumption of the risk has been largely replaced by the doctrine of comparative negligence. Assumption of the risk may be applicable to show the comparative negligence of the plaintiff, but it will rarely be a complete defense.

Contributory Negligence   Also called "contrib" in the jargon, this negligence can be asserted when the plaintiff's own negligent act or omission contributed to the injury that he ultimately suffered. This defense is complete: if the defendant can show that the plaintiff was negligent in any respect, and the negligence was a cause of the injury, no matter how small, the plaintiff will take nothing. This defense has been statutorily abrogated in most jurisdictions.

Comparative Negligence   Unlike contributory negligence, the defense of comparative negligence is not a complete defense to liability. Rather, it can serve to reduce the amount of damages that the plaintiff can receive. The reduction is usually based on the total amount of the award that the plaintiff would have received in the absence of his own negligent act, reduced by a certain percentage of the fault that is allocated to the plaintiff. There are generally two types of comparative negligence defenses. The first, and by far the most common, allows for an award of damages only in the event that the defendant's negligence was greater than the plaintiff's. The second allows for an award of damages to the plaintiff even if the plaintiff's negligence was greater than the defendant's. The defense of comparative negligence can be used in medical malpractice where, for example, the patient failed to adhere to the treatment regimen or to seek follow-up care as directed, and this failure resulted in the harm that he experienced.

Fellow Servant Rule   This rule was most frequently used in defending claims of occupational injury before the advent of workers' compensation laws. It allowed an employer to assert that the plaintiff's injury was caused by the negligent or intentional act of another employee, rather than by any act of the employer. It has been statutorily abrogated in virtually all jurisdictions, at least with regard to injuries that fall under the coverage of workers' compensation.

Last Clear Chance   This defense may be available in the situation where both the plaintiff and the defendant were negligent, but the defendant had the last opportunity to avoid the harm. This is an antiquated and obsolete defense that is not in use, to any great extent, at present.

Damages

There are two basic types of damages: compensatory and punitive. These, and the implications of each, will be addressed in turn.

Compensatory Damages   These damages are intended to compensate the victim for the victim's loss and nothing more. In many jurisdictions, these damages may be divided into two types: economic and non-economic damages. The distinction between the two becomes important when one considers the effect of tort reform measures or the taxability of settlement amounts.

Economic Damages   They may include virtually any compensation that the claimant would have received had it not been for the injury suffered, or expenses that the claimant was or will be required to pay as a result of the injury received. Thus, economic damages may include: lost wages, loss of future wages or earning power, medical expenses, future medical expenses, or such other damages as may be relatively quantifiable. Economic damages may or may not be taxable, depending upon the underlying nature of the claim (they are not taxable if the claim is for an actual physical bodily injury or illness).

Non-Economic Damages   These damages can normally be defined as those that are difficult to quantify, but which are a part of the loss suffered by the plaintiff. These typically include: pain and suffering, emotional distress or mental anguish, loss of companionship or consortium, and loss of enjoyment of life. Clearly, it is extremely difficult to place a monetary value on any of these things. Non-economic damages may or may not be taxable, depending upon the underlying nature of the claim (they are not taxable if the claim is for an actual physical bodily injury or illness).

Punitive or Exemplary Damages   These damages are not designed to make the plaintiff whole following the loss. Rather, they are designed to punish the defendant and to deter future conduct of a similar nature. In most jurisdictions, to award punitive damages, the jury would be required to find that the defendant acted in a willful, wanton, or malicious manner, or that the defendant acted with reckless disregard for the plaintiff's life or health.

Punitive damages may not usually be awarded for simple negligence. Punitive damages are taxable. The availability of insurance for punitive damages varies by jurisdiction. It is against public policy to allow insurers to cover them in some jurisdictions.

TORT REFORM

Tort reform has taken many forms over the past few years, but an assessment of its effectiveness, or the effectiveness of the various forms that it has taken, would yield decidedly mixed results. Various measures taken in the name of tort reform have been struck down by the courts as unconstitutional, under either the federal or state constitutions. Many other measures have simply not been workable, and many appear to have injected additional delay into the litigation process.

Caps on Damages — Michigan has caps

Many jurisdictions have implemented maximum limits on the amount of certain damages that claimants may recover. These "caps" normally cover only non-economic damages, such as pain and suffering or loss of consortium. They do not normally cover economic damages. While many statutory caps have withstood scrutiny by the courts, others have been struck down as unconstitutional under either the federal or a state constitution. The usual ground for finding them unconstitutional has been that they may violate an equal protection clause (for example, why should a person injured by the negligence of a physician be treated differently than a person injured through the negligence of a motorist?). If the cap withstands a challenge, it can be an effective tool in reducing liability in medical malpractice actions.

Elimination of Joint and Several Liability

As noted previously, joint and several liability can pose enormous consequences for the "deep pocket" in a case. If one party has sufficient assets to satisfy a judgment, regardless of its level of culpability, it might find itself liable for the entire judgment. Some states (such as Colorado) have abolished joint and several liability, which leaves all parties potentially liable for only their allocated share of the liability. This is a tremendous improvement over the current state of affairs in most jurisdictions, especially for hospitals, which often find themselves with a disproportionately small share of direct liability.

Comparative Negligence

Most states currently recognize the doctrine of comparative negligence, rather than the more obsolete doctrine of contributory negligence (which bars recovery for a plaintiff who was negligent, regardless of the magnitude or insignificance of the plaintiff's negligence). However, the states that recognize "pure" comparative negligence may allow a recovery for a plaintiff whose negligence greatly exceeded that of the defendant. This is a distinct problem in cases with catastrophic damages (for example, in a case where the plaintiff can show damages of $10 million, but the plaintiff's negligence was responsible for 90 percent of the problem, the defendant can still be liable for $1 million). It is recommended that statutes be amended to allow recovery only in cases where the degree of fault allocated to the defendant's negligence was greater than that allocated to the plaintiff.

Statutes of Limitations or Repose

The relevant statute of limitations tends to place a limit on the time period in which a claim can be brought. A statute of repose tends to bring an absolute close on the time period during which a claim can be brought. Tort reforms that shorten the period of the statute of limitations can help to reduce the number of lawsuits that are brought.

Some states have reformed their statutes of limitations by shortening the time period, but then allowing for an extension of the time period by giving notice of the claimant's intention to sue. This mechanism can be effective if the defendant is actually put on notice of the allegations that the claimant will raise in the lawsuit. Unfortunately, the notice is too often a brief recitation of the party's intention, without actually giving notice of the nature of the claim. This mechanism should require that the claimant specify the nature of the claim.

Affidavit or Certificate of Merit

Some states require that the claimant obtain a certificate or affidavit of merit from an expert before bringing suit. The certificate or affidavit is merely a recitation that the expert believes, to a reasonable degree of medical certainty, that the applicable standard of care was breached and that this breach was a proximate cause of the plaintiff's injury. This mechanism can be an effective method of weeding out frivolous suits. However, these are seldom shared with the defendant and are, in many cases, never actually obtained. These documents should be required, and they should be filed (under seal, if necessary) with the court or shared with the defendant. If a claim is filed without a proper certificate or affidavit, and the court determines that the suit was frivolous, sanctions should be imposed upon the plaintiff or plaintiff's counsel (for example, payment of defendant's legal fees and expenses).

Contingent Fee Arrangements

Contingent fee arrangements usually require the payment of a specified percentage of the recovery to plaintiff's counsel. These sometimes vary according to the mode of recovery (less in the case of a pre-suit settlement, more if the case goes to trial). The amount paid to the plaintiff's attorney might often be greatly in excess of the amount of work done in the case or the difficulty in prosecuting the case. Legislation requiring oversight by the court of all contingent fee arrangements to ensure that they are fair and equitable would be a tremendous improvement. Although some contracts are unenforceable because they might impose obligations on parties that are unlawful, contingent fee agreements are not per se unlawful. Unfortunately, efforts in the past to control contingent fee awards have been struck down as unconstitutional because the U.S. Constitution prohibits laws that might impair the obligations of contracts.

············

CASE CITATION AND LEGAL RESEARCH TERMS

It is recognized that non-lawyers are frequently required to perform some level of legal research. This is often more easily said than done. Legal research employs its own jargon and taxonomy that can often be, at best, inscrutable. Although this brief introduction will not make a non-lawyer into an accomplished researcher, it should give the non-lawyer the tools necessary to perform some legal research functions. The two most commonly retrieved items of interest for the non-lawyer are cases and statutes.

Cases

Cases are cited in legal materials using the following taxonomy. The case name (usually either underlined or italicized) usually includes only the last name of the first plaintiff and the last name of the first defendant. The first number in the citation is the volume number in the case reporter series in which the case may be found. The middle part of the citation is an abbreviation for the reporter in which the case appears (cases often appear in more than one reporter series). The last number is the number of the page on which the first page of the case appears. If there is a second number in the citation, this indicates the page in the reporter where the quotation or concept appears in the case. If the volume numbers and page numbers are blank, this means that the decision has not been published. The parenthetical at the end of the citation indicates the name of the court that rendered the opinion and the date (usually just the year) on which the decision was rendered. This order may be somewhat variable between jurisdictions (some jurisdictions put the parenthetical immediately after the case name). An example of a citation for a published decision is as follows:

Rossi v. Oxley, 269 Ga. 82, 495 S.E. 2d 39 (Ga. 1998)

The plaintiff is Rossi; the defendant is Oxley. This case could be found in Volume 269 of the Georgia Reports at page 82, or in Volume 495 of the Southeastern Reporter (2nd series) at page 39. The decision was handed down by the Georgia Supreme Court in 1998. An example of an unpublished decision is as follows:

United States Fidelity and Guaranty Co. v. St. Elizabeth Medical Center,_____ Ohio App. 3d_____, N.E. 2d_____, No. 16518 (Ct. App. Ohio July 10, 1998)

In this case, the blanks before and after the reporter indicate that the case is unpublished. No. 16518 is the docket number. Citations to unpublished decisions often give the actual date of the decision to assist finding the decision in the court records. Only the year in which the decision was handed down is given for published decisions.

Statutes

Virtually all compilations of state and federal statutes have some form of indexing system to allow people to find relevant statutes. Some indexing systems are, unfortunately, more difficult than others. To find anything in a statutory index, one must know some legal terminology. Such a discussion is far beyond the capabilities of this treatise. Suffice it to say, one must be persistent in attempting to find a statute, sometimes employing numerous key words or phrases, before deciding that there is no statute on point.

State Statutes   These are cited in a manner similar to that employed for cases. There may or may not be a number appearing at the beginning of the citation. If there is, it normally indicates the title or volume of the reporter series in which the statute appears. If there is not, the volume number might appear as the first portion of the statute number.

The state code will be given as an abbreviation. This is followed by the statute number, and possibly the section number of the statute. A parenthetical on the end of the citation will usually give the version of the statute being cited (by year) and possibly the reporter in which the statute appears. An example follows:

Oh. Rev. Code §2317.54 (Page 1995)

In this case, the statute is found in Title 23 of the Ohio Revised Code, in which each statute (and subsections of statutes) are numbered sequentially. "Page" is the name of the reporter. The version of the statute that is being referenced was as it appeared in the 1995 version of the code.

Federal Statutes   These are often cited with the name of the statute. All federal statutes can be found in the United States Code (U.S.C. [sometimes U.S.C.A. or U.S.C.S.]). An example would be:

Health Care Quality Improvement Act, 42 U.S.C. §11101, *et seq.*

This act is found in Title 42 of the United States Code at section 11101. The *"et seq."* Indicates that the statute has more than one section.

Federal Regulations   These typically appear in the Code of Federal Regulations (C.F.R.). These are usually cited by volume number, reporter and regulation number. An example would be:

42 C.F.R. §2.1

Before federal regulations are published in the Code of Federal Regulations, they are published in the Federal Register. In this case, the regulation may be cited as it appears in the Federal Register. An example is as follows:

54 Fed. Reg. 23134 (May 30, 1989)

Again, the material is found in Volume 54 of the Federal Register at page 23134, which was published on May 30, 1989.

Table 2.1 gives a set of standard, and generally accepted, legal abbreviations, although courts and lawyers in a particular state frequently use different abbreviations.

APPENDIX 2.1 TABLE 2.1   Standard Legal Abbreviations[1,2]

Abbreviation	Name of Reporter/Code	Court
A.	Atlantic Reports	
A. 2d	Atlantic Reports, 2nd Series	
A.D.	Appellate Division Reports	New York Supreme Court, Appellate Division
A.D. 2d	Appellate Division Reports, 2nd Series	New York Supreme Court, Appellate Division
Ala. Code	Code of Alabama	
Alaska Stat.	Alaska Statutes	
Ariz.	Arizona Reports	Supreme Court of Arizona
Ariz.	Arizona Reports	Arizona Court of Appeals
Ariz. Rev. Stat. Ann.	Arizona Revised Statutes, Annotated	
Ark.	Arkansas Reports	Supreme Court of Arkansas
Ark. App.	Arkansas Appellate Reports	Arkansas Court of Appeals
Ark. Code	Arkansas Code, Annotated	
Cal.	California Reports	Supreme Court of California
Cal. 2d	California Reports, 2nd Series	Supreme Court of California
Cal. 3d	California Reports, 3rd Series	Supreme Court of California
Cal. 4th	California Reports, 4th Series	Supreme Court of California
Cal. App.	California Appellate Reports	California Court of Appeals
Cal. App. 2d	California Appellate Reports, 2nd Series	California Court of Appeals
Cal. App. 3d	California Appellate Reports, 3rd Series	California Court of Appeals
Cal. App. 4th	California Appellate Reports, 4th Series	California Court of Appeals
Cal. [subject] Code	California Code	

(Continued)

APPENDIX 2.1 TABLE 2.1   Standard Legal Abbreviations[1,2] *(Continued)*

Abbreviation	Name of Reporter/Code	Court
C.F.R.	Code of Federal Regulations	
Colo. Rev. Stat.	Colorado Revised Code	
Conn.	Connecticut Reports	Supreme Court of Connecticut
Conn. App.	Connecticut Appellate Reports	Connecticut Court of Appeals
Conn. Supp.	Connecticut Supplement	Connecticut Superior Court
Conn. Cir. Ct.	Connecticut Circuit Court Reporter	Connecticut Circuit Court
Conn. Gen. Stat.	Connecticut General Statutes	
D.C. Code Ann.	District of Columbia Code, Annotated	
Del. Code Ann.	Delaware Code, Annotated	
F.	Federal Reporter	U. S. Circuit Courts of Appeal
F. 2d	Federal Reporter, 2nd Series	U. S. Circuit Courts of Appeal
F. 3d	Federal Reporter, 3rd Series	U. S. Circuit Courts of Appeal
Fed. Reg.	Federal Register	
Fla. L. Weekly	Florida Law Weekly	Supreme Court of Florida
Fla. Supp.	Florida Supplement	Florida Circuit and County Courts
Fla. Supp. 2d	Florida Supplement	Florida Circuit and County Courts
Fla. Stat.	Florida Statutes	
Fla. Stat. Ann.	Florida Statutes, Annotated	
F. Supp.	Federal Supplement	U.S. District Courts
F. Supp. 2d	Federal Supplement, 2nd Series	U.S. District Courts
Ga.	Georgia Reports	Supreme Court of Georgia
Ga. App.	Georgia Appellate Reports	Georgia Court of Appeals
Ga. Code Ann.	Official Code of Georgia, Annotated	
Haw.	Hawaii Reports	Supreme Court of Hawaii
Haw. App.	Hawaii Appellate Reports	Hawaii Court of Appeals
Haw. Rev. Stat.	Hawaii Revised Statutes	
Idaho	Idaho Reports	Supreme Court of Idaho and Idaho Court of Appeals
Idaho Code	Idaho Code	
Ill.	Illinois Reports	Supreme Court of Illinois
Ill. 2d	Illinois Reports, 2nd Series	Supreme Court of Illinois
Ill. App.	Illinois Appellate Reports	Illinois Court of Appeals
Ill. App. 2d	Illinois Appellate Reports, 2nd Series	Illinois Court of Appeals
Ill. App. 3d	Illinois Appellate Reports, 3rd Series	Illinois Court of Appeals
Ill. Ct. Cl.	Illinois Court of Claims Reporter	Illinois Court of Claims
Ill. Ann. Stat.	Smith-Hunt Illinois Annotated Statutes	
Ill. Rev. Stat.	Illinois Revised Statutes	
Ind. Code	Indiana Code	
Iowa Code	Code of Iowa	
Kan.	Kansas Reports	Supreme Court of Kansas
Kan. App.	Kansas Appellate Reports	Kansas Court of Appeals
Kan. 2d	Kansas Appellate Reports, 2nd Series	Kansas Court of Appeals
Kan. Stat. Ann.	Kansas Statutes, Annotated	
Ky. Rev. Stat. Ann.	Kentucky Revised Statutes, Annotated	
La. Rev. Stat. Ann.	Louisiana Revised Statutes, Annotated	
La. [subj] Code Ann.	Louisiana [subject] Code, Annotated	
L. Ed.	Lawyers' Edition	U.S. Supreme Court
Me. Rev. Stat. Ann.	Maine Revised Statutes, Annotated	
Md.	Maryland Reports	Court of Appeals of Maryland
Md. App.	Maryland Appellate Reports	Maryland Court of Special Appeals
Md. Code Ann.	Annotated Code of Maryland	
Mass.	Massachusetts Reports	Supreme Judicial Court of Massachusetts
Mass. App. Ct.	Massachusetts Appeals Court Reports	Massachusetts Court of Appeals
Mass. App. Div.	Massachusetts Appellate Reports	Massachusetts District Court Division

(Continued)

APPENDIX 2.1 TABLE 2.1   Standard Legal Abbreviations[1,2] (*Continued*)

Abbreviation	Name of Reporter/Code	Court
Mass. Gen. Laws	General Laws of the Commonwealth of Massachusetts	
Mich.	Michigan Reports	Supreme Court of Michigan
Mich. App.	Michigan Appeals Reports	Michigan Court of Appeals
Mich. Comp. Laws	Michigan Compiled Laws	
Minn. Stat.	Minnesota Statutes	
Minn. Stat. Ann.	Minnesota Statutes, Annotated	
Miss. Code Ann.	Mississippi Code, Annotated	
Mo. Ann. Stat.	Vernon's Annotated Missouri Statutes	
Mo. Rev. Stat.	Missouri Revised Statutes	
Mont.	Montana Reports	Montana Supreme Court
Mont. Code Ann.	Montana Code, Annotated	
N.C.	North Carolina Reports	Supreme Court of North Carolina
N.C. App.	North Carolina Appellate Reports	North Carolina Court of Appeals
N.C. Gen. Stat.	North Carolina General Statutes	
N.D. Cent. Code	North Dakota Century Code	
N.E.	Northeast Reporter	
N.E. 2d	Northeast Reporter, 2nd Series	
Neb.	Nebraska Reports	Supreme Court of Nebraska
Neb. Rev. Stat.	Nebraska Revised Statutes	
Nev.	Nevada Reports	Supreme Court of Nevada
Nev. Rev. Stat.	Nevada Revised Statutes	
Nev. Rev. Stat. Ann.	Nevada Revised Statutes, Annotated	
N.H.	New Hampshire Reports	Supreme Court of New Hampshire
N.H. Rev. Stat. Ann.	New Hampshire Revised Statutes, Annotated	
N.J.	New Jersey Reports	Supreme Court of New Jersey
N.J. Super.	New Jersey Superior Court Reports	New Jersey Superior Court
N.J. Rev. Stat.	New Jersey Revised Statutes	
N.M.	New Mexico Reports	Supreme Court of New Mexico; New Mexico Court of Appeals
N.M. Stat. Ann.	New Mexico Statutes, Annotated	
N.Y.	New York Reports	Court of Appeals of New York
N.Y. 2d	New York Reports, 2nd Series	Court of Appeals of New York
N.Y.S.	West's New York Supplement	New York Supreme Court, Appellate Division
N.Y.S. 2d	West's New York Supplement, 2nd Series	New York Supreme Court, Appellate Division
N.W.	Northwestern Reporter	
N.W. 2d	Northwestern Reporter, 2nd Series	
Ohio St.	Ohio State Reports	Supreme Court of Ohio
Ohio St. 2d	Ohio State Reports, 2nd Series	Supreme Court of Ohio
Ohio St. 3d	Ohio State Reports, 3rd Series	Supreme Court of Ohio
Ohio App.	Ohio Appellate Reports	Ohio Courts of Appeal
Ohio App. 2d	Ohio Appellate Reports, 2nd Series	Ohio Courts of Appeal
Ohio App. 3d	Ohio Appellate Reports, 3rd Series	Ohio Courts of Appeal
Ohio Misc.	Ohio Miscellaneous Reports	Ohio lower courts
Ohio Misc. 2d	Ohio Miscellaneous Reports, 2nd Series	Ohio lower courts
Oh. Rev. Code	Ohio Revised Code	
Okla. Stat.	Oklahoma Statutes	
Or.	Oregon Reports	Supreme Court of Oregon
Or. App.	Oregon Reports, Court of Appeals	Oregon Court of Appeals
Or. Rev. Stat.	Oregon Revised Statutes	
P.	Pacific Reporter	
P. 2d	Pacific Reporter, 2nd Series	

(*Continued*)

APPENDIX 2.1 TABLE 2.1   Standard Legal Abbreviations[1,2] (*Continued*)

Abbreviation	Name of Reporter/Code	Court
Pa.	Pennsylvania State Reports	Supreme Court of Pennsylvania
Pa. Super.	Pennsylvania Superior Court Reports	Pennsylvania Superior Court
Pa. Commw.	Pennsylvania Commonwealth Court Reports	Pennsylvania Commonwealth Courts
Pa. Cons. Stat.	Pennsylvania Consolidated Statutes	
Pa. D&C	Pennsylvania District and County Reports	Pennsylvania lower courts
R.I.	Rhode Island Reports	Rhode Island state courts
R.I. Gen. Laws	Rhode Island General Laws	
S.C.	South Carolina Reports	Supreme Court of South Carolina
S.C. Code	South Carolina Code	
S. Ct.	Supreme Court Reporter	U. S. Supreme Court
S.D. Codified Laws	South Dakota Codified Laws	
So.	Southern Reporter	
So. 2d	Southern Reporter, 2nd Series	
S.E.	South Eastern Reporter	
S.E. 2d	South Eastern Reporter, 2nd Series	
S.W.	South Western Reporter	
S.W. 2d	South Western Reporter, 2nd Series	
Tenn. Code Ann.	Tennessee Code, Annotated	
Tex. Sup. Ct. J.	Texas Supreme Court Journal	Supreme Court of Texas
Tex. [subj] Code	Texas [subject] Code	
U.S.	United States Reporter	U.S. Supreme Court
U.S. App. D.C.	U.S. Court of Appeals Reports	District of Columbia Circuit Court of Appeals
U.S.C.	United States Code	
U.S.L.W.	U.S. Law Week	U.S. Supreme Court
Utah Code Ann.	Utah Code, Annotated	
Va.	Virginia Reports	Supreme Court of Virginia
Va. App.	Virginia Appellate Reporter	Virginia Court of Appeals
Va. Code Ann.	Virginia Code Annotated	
Vt. Reports	Vermont Reports	Supreme Court of Vermont
Vt. Stat. Ann.	Vermont Statutes, Annotated	
Wash.	Washington Reports	Supreme Court of Washington
Wash. 2d	Washington Reports, 2nd Series	Supreme Court of Washington
Wash. App.	Washington Appellate Reports	Washington Courts of Appeal
Wash. Rev. Code	Revised Code of Washington	
W. Va.	West Virginia Reports	West Virginia Supreme Court of Appeals
W. Va. Code	West Virginia Code	
Wis.	Wisconsin Reports	Supreme Court of Wisconsin
Wis. 2d	Wisconsin Reports, 2nd Series	Supreme Court of Wisconsin
Wis. Stat.	Wisconsin Statutes	
Wyo.	Wyoming Reports	Supreme Court of Wyoming
Wyo. Stat.	Wyoming Statutes	

1. Only the reporters in which decisions of the named courts are currently published are given. One may encounter older decisions that are cited to discontinued reporters.
2. These abbreviations are in the format given in The Bluebook: A Uniform System of Citation (17th ed.), Brockton, MA: Star Printing (2003). Lawyers and courts within a given jurisdiction, especially to statutory compilations, may routinely abbreviate citations in different, frequently shorter formats.

3

Governance of the Health Care Organization

John Horty
Monica Hanslovan

The mark of a good health care corporation, like that of any corporation, is the way it is governed. Governance determines how any organization is centered. Governance in health care is particularly important because of the responsibility of the organization to patients and to the community. Governance is the art and skill, developed over many years, of making important corporate decisions. Making decisions is the ultimate legal authority of the corporation.

The board is not passive. It makes decisions. In most instances, the corporation board should confine itself to important decisions and let management manage. However, in some situations, decisions that appear to be small or limited are (or become) important. The decisions of the board, along with the culture and values of board and management, forge the culture and values of the corporation. The culture and values of the corporation are the essence and the result of leadership—good or bad. There is no other way to govern.

The principles of corporate governance do not change. The problems that an organization faces and the decisions that it must make do change. All those who support the governance of the corporation, the CEO and top management personnel, including the risk management professional, must understand the essentials of governance.

Obviously, different health care organizations face different degrees of risk. Medical groups, health care systems, long-term care organizations, insurance companies, surgical centers and hospitals—all have boards. All have the same governance responsibilities, yet the need for risk management in each type of organization is different. All have significant responsibilities for the care of patients. Even insurance companies (who by their actions may sometimes effectively deny care by refusing to pay for it under the terms of their policy) shoulder this responsibility.

There are several types of corporate structures, particularly in health care. Some are organized as for-profit corporations, but the majority are not-for-profit corporations. All of the health care corporations previously stated may be organized either as for-profit or not-for-profit in every state in America.

The crux of the difference between for-profit and not-for-profit corporations is in two areas. For-profit corporations have shareholders who own the corporation and hope to profit from its business. Not-for-profit corporations have no shareholders, and those who govern do not own the company or profit. Any profits must be applied to the non-profit purpose of the corporation.

Not-for-profit boards have a duty to those they serve. It is their only duty. Keeping the organization fiscally and organizationally strong is the means to that purpose. The mission of a not-for-profit corporation in the health care field is to provide quality care. In contrast, the board of a for-profit corporation (in addition to its duty to patients) owes a duty to the owners of the corporation—the shareholders—to make the business a success and to pass the profits along to the shareholders.

Although, as stated previously, there are many different kinds of organizations in health care, the greatest liability and risks are in hospitals. Hospitals have the largest number of employees, physicians, and other independent practitioners, the greatest interaction with patients (by far the greatest number of interactions that carry risk and potential liability), and are where procedures with the greatest risk and complexity are performed.

ESSENTIAL RESPONSIBILITIES OF THE HOSPITAL BOARD

The essential responsibilities of the hospital board are, first and foremost, patient safety; second, that the hospital is fiscally prudent to ensure that sufficient funds are available to accomplish its mission; and third, improvements to the hospital and what it does.

Patient Safety

The foremost responsibility of any hospital board is to see that patients are safe. This is such an overriding responsibility that it almost needs no discussion. It is what every patient who enters the hospital expects and takes for granted. A board that does not see to patient safety is not doing its job. Anyone who cares for patients (physicians and others alike) must be competent and must act responsibly. The hospital must be adequately staffed, and equipment must be appropriately maintained and available as needed. The entire operation must put the patient first.

Finances

Hospitals (including for-profit hospitals) are in business to serve the patients who come to them for care. They must make enough money to do this job well, and the board is responsible to the community that it serves to ensure that the hospital has the financial resources to accomplish its mission—now and in the future. Almost all boards wisely take this financial responsibility seriously. Patient safety must come first and be before profit.

Improvements

The third major responsibility of the hospital or health care board is to improve the hospital's ability to serve those who come to it as medicine changes. This responsibility has three segments:

(handwritten note: "would board say this?")

New Services   Health care is a dynamic part of our society. Advances in technology are continuous. They allow hospitals to provide new services and new methods for the delivery of care. Other advances such as the exploration of our genetic code will revolutionize health care in ways yet to be fully understood. A hospital board's responsibility is to weigh finances, safety, and community needs as it decides how these advances and new technology will affect the services to provide and equipment to purchase.

Better Patient Outcomes   Every hospital must strive to deliver quality care and to continuously improve patient outcomes. Patient safety must always come first. By improving patient outcomes, the quality of care is enhanced and patient safety is maintained. Improved outcomes are the result of better equipment, better training of staff, and the understanding of new and better modalities of care. But, equally important is the ability to measure and quantify continuing improvement of outcomes and the changes in care that make them possible. Again, the board must see that this continuous measurement and improvement is a priority. Management, the medical staff, and the hospital must make it happen, but the board makes it a continuing priority and responsibility.

A Patient-Friendly Hospital   Finally, it is the responsibility of the board to set the goal of a patient-friendly hospital. This is easy to say, but sometimes hard to do. Putting the hospital's patients first is a cliché, but one with real meaning. If the board does not think that this is a major goal, it won't be!

The hospital or health care board must continually strive to improve the ability to serve those who come to the hospital as medicine changes. By breaking board responsibilities into three segments, the understanding of the word "quality" is separated into three distinct and different parts: patient safety, better outcomes, and a patient-friendly environment. Clearly, the board should put patient safety first, with outcomes an important second, and a friendly environment third. "Quality" has become a buzzword in this field. It often seems to be in the eye of the beholder, seen to mean whatever is being emphasized at the time. Safety, outcomes, and a friendly atmosphere are concrete and can be measured. Thus, the board has a yardstick to measure that its responsibilities in all these areas are being met.

. . . .

BASIC LEGAL DUTIES OF HEALTH CARE TRUSTEES

Two terms describe the individuals who serve on boards of corporations. For-profit corporations almost uniformly use the term *director.* Many not-for-profit corporations use the term *trustee* because many early not-for-profit corporations began as charitable trusts. The term *trustee* emphasizes the duty of trust to patients and the community. In this chapter, the term *trustee* also is used to encompass directors.

Management personnel who support the governance of a health care organization must understand the two basic duties of trustees: the duty of care and the duty of loyalty. These two duties are shared by all board members of all corporations, but are particularly important in the governance of a hospital or health care organization because the "business" of a health care corporation has immediate effects on the lives and well-being of patients.

Duty of Care

The duty of care imposed on health care board members means the duty to act in good faith, with the care that an ordinarily prudent person in a similar position would use under those circumstances, and in the reasonable belief that actions taken are in the best interest of the corporation. Courts call this the *reasonable person standard* because the action or any failure to act by the board is judged by what a reasonable person would do. Health care and hospital board members have the duty to act reasonably under the circumstances—to exercise good business judgment and to use ordinary care and prudence in fulfilling their duties. Trustees can be held liable for negligent acts or omissions in the performance of their duties and actions taken on behalf of the hospital.

Good Faith   This means that hospital and health care trustees must act honestly and faithfully, observing reasonable commercial standards of fair dealing. It means acting without intent to defraud or to take advantage of others. It's easy to see the importance of good faith actions for any trustee, health care or otherwise. Recent examples of the breach of this duty by some for-profit directors and executives make this painfully obvious.

Acting in the Best Interest of the Corporation   This translates into a duty of reasonable care, meaning that board members have the duty to explore all options before they make an important decision—to "do their homework," so to speak. In a for-profit corporation, the duty to act in the best interest of the corporation generally means maximizing the return on the shareholders' investment. In contrast, in a non-profit hospital or health system where no shareholders or owners exist, the board members' fiduciary duty is to act in the best interest of the people served by the organization.

Duty of Loyalty

The duty of loyalty imposed on health care board members establishes the duty not to compete with the corporation, not to disclose confidential information obtained in the performance of one's duties as a board member, not to usurp corporate opportunity, and not to gain personal enrichment at the corporation's expense.

non-compete clause

No Competing with the Corporation   Board members have a duty not to compete with the corporation they serve. A hospital or health system board would be wise to define "significant competition" in an official board policy so that it's clear to all involved exactly what this term means. Such a policy would give the board an objective template by which to measure any future situation that occurs. Significant competition might mean dealings with another organization that create a net job loss for the hospital or cost the hospital 1 percent of its market share.

No Disclosure of Confidential Information   The reasons for this duty are obvious. Any trustee (health care or otherwise) inevitably will obtain confidential, privileged information while performing as a board member. Such information must remain confidential in all respects, which prohibits idle chatter and gossip and the deliberate release of information.

No Usurping Corporate Opportunity   In legal terms, this is known as the *corporate opportunity doctrine*. It means that a board member's fiduciary duty of loyalty prohibits the trustee from profiting from any business that properly belongs to the corporation. A hospital or health care trustee must first give the corporation ample opportunity to act before taking personal advantage of an opportunity that the corporation itself might have taken.

No Personal Enrichment at Corporate Expense   Board members should not participate in any decision involving a transaction between the health care corporation and an organization in which the board members have a personal interest without disclosure and board approval. Personal interest might mean that the board member would profit from the transaction; that a close family member of the board member would profit from the transaction; or that the board member serves on the boards of two corporations that might be transacting business with each other.

Every hospital or health system should have a conflict of interest policy in place to address these situations. The board chair should see that the policy is followed when a conflict arises. Adoption of such a policy eliminates the need for the organization to have a separate "non-compete" policy.

From time to time, all board members have conflicts of interest. In almost every case, board members need not resign if they declare the conflict to the board chair and do not participate in decisions concerning these transactions.

Care and loyalty are the two basic duties shared by all trustees. Because of the nature of health care today, and because non-profit hospital trustees ultimately are responsible for the quality of patient care, health care trustees must take these duties very seriously. Health care governance is not an easy task.

∙∙∙∙∙∙∙∙∙∙∙∙
LESSONS FROM THE PANEL ON THE NON-PROFIT SECTOR REPORT TO CONGRESS

It became apparent that health care governance is not an easy task when, in June 2005, the Panel on the Nonprofit Sector issued a report to Congress and the non-profit sector entitled *Strengthening Transparency, Governance and Accountability of Charitable Organizations.* The report made fifteen major recommendations about how non-profit organizations should be regulated and governed. When discussing the structure, size, composition, and independence of governing boards, the report noted that, "A knowledgeable, committed board of directors is the strongest protector of a charitable organization's accountability to the law, its donors, consumers of its products and services, and the public."[1] This is certainly true for those who serve on the boards of non-profit hospitals and health care organizations. Directors of non-profit hospitals are strong protectors of the very people the hospital serves—its patients.

Major policymakers are sitting up and taking notice of the recommendations in the report. Senator Charles Grassley, Chair of the Senate Finance Committee, said: "This report . . . will be of great use as the Finance Committee . . . now begins drafting legislation. My goal is legislation that will seek to encourage more checks to charities while also ensuring that the dollars are being spent appropriately to help the community and those in need. The panel report will inform the committee and its work, particularly in the important areas of governance and transparency."[2]

Some of the report's recommendations will make it into law. And other provisions, while not becoming legislation, may well become "best practices" that boards and management of non-profit organizations ignore at their peril. Although the report is wide-ranging, many of its observations about governance duties and roles are quite succinct.

The following discusses three of the report's more pertinent observations and recommendations for non-profit boards.

"Independent" Board Members

The report defines "independent board members" as those individuals: (1) who have not been compensated by the organization within the past twelve months, including full-time and part-time compensation as an employee or as an independent contractor (except for "reasonable compensation" for board service); (2) whose own compensation, except for board service, is not determined by individuals who are compensated by the organization; (3) who do not receive, directly or indirectly, material financial benefits (such as service contracts, grants, or other payments) from the organization except as a member of the charitable class served by the organization; and (4) who are not related to any individuals described above. The report clarifies that "related to" means related as a spouse, sibling, parent, or child. Non-profit hospitals should also remember that the Sarbanes-Oxley Act of 2002 sets forth standards for the independence of members of board audit committees of publicly traded corporations. Although Sarbanes-Oxley generally does not apply to non-profit corporations, it provides, with regard to director "independence," that companies registered with the New York Stock Exchange must have a *majority* of directors who meet the Exchange's definition of "independence."

With regard to public charities, the report recommends that at least one-third of their board members be free of the conflicts of interest that can arise when they have a personal interest in the financial transactions of the charity. Individuals who receive compensation for services, or who receive material financial benefits from the hospital (and their spouses or family members), would have inherent conflicts of interest and would not be considered to be "independent" board members.

Founders of many non-profit hospitals probably initially turned to family members, business partners, even neighbors and friends to serve on the hospital's board. The authors often hear from hospitals that finding independent board members can be particularly problematic in smaller communities and rural areas. Although it can be difficult at times, hospitals should make every effort to find independent board members. The report even goes so far as to state that this should be a legal requirement for public charities that are eligible to receive tax-deductible contributions on the most favorable terms.

Disqualification from Board Service

The report recommends that Congress amend the regulations to prohibit individuals who are barred from service on boards of publicly traded companies or convicted of crimes directly related to breaches of fiduciary duty in their service as an employee or board member of a charitable organization from serving on the board of a charitable organization for five years following their conviction or removal.

The Sarbanes-Oxley Act (discussed in greater detail later in this chapter) grants the Securities and Exchange Commission (SEC) the authority to bar individuals from serving on the boards of publicly traded companies subject to the approval of a federal judge or an SEC administrative law judge (ALJ). Currently, there is no prohibition on individuals barred by the SEC from serving on the boards of non-profit hospitals or health care organizations. But, obviously, non-profit hospitals and other health care organizations should recognize that, if someone has been barred from service on the board of a publicly traded company or convicted of a crime directly related to a breach of fiduciary duty while serving as an employee or board member of a charitable organization, this should raise serious concerns about the person's perceived ability to fulfill the fiduciary responsibilities of a board member of a non-profit hospital.

Non-profit hospitals should begin to ask and remind current and prospective board members about this prohibition. Ultimately, though, the responsibility for resigning or declining board service should rest with the individual who has been prohibited from such service. The report suggests that individuals who fail to inform the hospital that they are ineligible to serve should be subject to a penalty equivalent to penalties imposed on tax preparers for omission or misrepresentation of information.

Board Compensation

In the authors' experience (and confirmed in the report), the vast majority of board members are not compensated for their services. However, charities and foundations are permitted under current law to pay "reasonable compensation" for services provided by board members. "Reasonable compensation" is defined as "the amount that would ordinarily be paid for like services by like enterprises (whether tax-exempt or taxable) under like circumstances." Federal tax laws prohibit payment of excessive compensation, contracts, and transactions that provide excessive economic benefit to board members and other "disqualified persons." The report defines a "disqualified person" for public charities and also for private foundations. For public charities, a disqualified person is someone who, at any time during the five-year period ending on the date of the transaction in question, was *"in a position to exercise substantial influence over the affairs of the organization."* Any member of a disqualified person's family, and any entity in which one or more disqualified persons together own, directly or indirectly, more than a 35-percent interest, is also considered to be a disqualified person.

The report "strongly encourages" charitable organizations to ask board members to serve on a voluntary basis. In situations where a non-profit hospital or health care organization feels that it is necessary to compensate board members, the report recommends that there be significant disclosure requirements to detail the amount of, and reasons for, the compensation, including the services provided and responsibilities of board members. Compensation for service as a board member must be "reasonable" and must be clearly differentiated from any compensation paid for services in the capacity of the staff of the organization.

In situations where the organization feels that board members should be compensated because of the complexity of the responsibility, the time commitment involved in board service, and the skills required for the particular assignment, the organization should, as a "best practice," review information on compensation provided by organizations comparable in size, grant-making or program practices, geographic scope, location, and with similar board responsibilities, to determine the "reasonableness" of any compensation provided to board members.

....
FEDERAL SENTENCING GUIDELINES FOR ORGANIZATIONS

Establishing and maintaining an effective compliance and ethics program is another responsibility of the health care organization's governing board. On November 1, 2004, the United States Sentencing Commission revised the Federal Sentencing Guidelines for Organizations, which apply to non-profit and for-profit organizations. The Guidelines were created in 1984 to respond to a perception and some evidence (in the case of individual, not corporate, defendants) that judges in the federal circuits were adopting very different sentences for similarly situated defendants found guilty of criminal charges. Chapter 8 in the Guidelines, addressing sentencing of organizations, was added in 1991.

The Guidelines set a baseline range of determinate sentences for different categories of offenses; judges increase or decrease the sentence depending on enumerated circumstances listed in the Guidelines (setting a culpability score from which "upward or downward departures" are made). The November 1, 2004, amendments to Chapter 8 seek to strengthen the importance of the characteristics of an effective corporate compliance program defined in the Guidelines.

The revised Guidelines broadly define the term "organization" to include "corporations, partnerships, associations, joint-stock companies, unions, trusts, pension funds, unincorporated organizations, governments and political subdivisions thereof, and non-profit organizations." Section 8A1.1, Application Note #1. The Guidelines also speak directly to the responsibilities placed on the board. Specifically, the Guidelines provide that "The organization's governing authority shall be knowledgeable about the content and operation of the compliance and ethics program and shall exercise reasonable oversight with respect to the implementation and effectiveness of the compliance and ethics program." Section 8B2.1 (b)(2)(A). Application Note #1 of Section 8B2.1 defines "governing authority" as (a) the Board of Directors; or (b) if the organization does not have a Board of Directors, the highest-level governing body of the organization.

The Guidelines make it very clear that, for an organization to receive a reduction in fines and penalties, oversight of programs designed to prevent and detect criminal activity is the responsibility of an organization's board. The key changes to the Guidelines from a board member's perspective are:

- An explicit recognition of the important role ethics and culture play in ensuring effective compliance programs. The Commission changed the definition of an effective program from one that provides due diligence to prevent and detect criminal violations, to one that also must "promote an organizational culture that encourages ethical conduct and a commitment to compliance with the law." With this revision, the Commission sought to emphasize that, without ethics, compliance becomes about following a minimum set of rules, and reflects the emphasis on ethics and values incorporated into recent legislative and regulatory reforms.

- The placement of responsibility for reasonable oversight of the compliance and ethics program with the board. This means that the board must ensure that management and employees act legally and ethically to protect the company's reputation and the value that derives from that reputation.

- A requirement that senior management "ensure" that the organization has an effective compliance and ethics program (ECEP) by working closely with senior leadership to develop a strong program.

- A risk assessment requirement that demonstrates that the organization has identified risk areas where criminal violations may occur. This may include the use of auditing and monitoring systems to detect criminal conduct, ongoing risk assessment, and periodic evaluation of the effectiveness of the program.

- A requirement that the organization encourage "appropriate incentives to perform in accordance with the compliance and ethics program."

- A requirement that organizations provide employees with a means to seek guidance regarding potential or actual criminal conduct without fear of retribution. Practically, this means that boards should assess employee willingness to use the system in place in the organization.

- Required training in relevant legal standards and obligations. It is no longer an option. The revised Guidelines include a mandatory training requirement for high-level officials and for employees.

- A requirement that compliance officers be given adequate authority and resources to carry out their responsibilities, including a direct reporting responsibility and access to the organizational leadership and the organization's board.[3]

In sum, the amendments have both raised the bar for compliance and ethics and have put responsibility for an effective compliance and ethics program in the hands of the board.

THE SARBANES-OXLEY ACT OF 2002

Even though not legally required to do so, some hospitals and health care organizations are revising their bylaws to be more consistent with the requirements of the Public Company Accounting Reform and Investor Protection Act of 2002 ("Sarbanes-Oxley" or the "Act"). Sarbanes-Oxley established new requirements for the corporate governance of issuers of securities that are regulated by the Securities and Exchange Commission. Because non-profit hospitals and health care organizations do not issue securities that are regulated by the SEC, the Act does not apply directly to these organizations.

At the same time, non-profit boards should recognize that some of the concepts that have been included in the Act are being adopted by the Exempt Organizations Branch of the Internal Revenue Service. Non-profit boards should also be aware that some states are in the process of considering legislation that would impose the requirements of the Act on those states' non-profit corporations. Therefore, the boards of health care organizations are well advised to consider the concepts upon which Sarbanes-Oxley was based. An open question is the extent to which the Act's approach to implementing corporate accountability and other principles of governance may be applied to the non-profit setting either through subsequent legislation or judicial review.

Although the Act generally does not apply to non-profit corporations, it contains certain provisions that reflect principles that directors and CEOs of non-profit organizations have long been expected to follow. At the very least, the Act is educational in that it highlights these principles and expectations. It is also possible that, at some point in the future, a court would look to the Act for guidance when interpreting duties of directors and CEOs of non-profit organizations. Similarly, at some future point, legislatures may impose similar requirements on non-profits. The following discusses the main provisions of the Act that could potentially be applied to non-profit organizations.

Accountability   Just as the Sarbanes-Oxley Act is intended to hold corporate executives and auditors more accountable to the shareholders of public companies and impose new obligations and restrictions on directors and senior executives of such companies, similar accountability could eventually be placed on directors and senior executives of non-profits. For example, certain sections of the Act require senior executive certification of financial reports. The Act holds signing officers responsible for establishing and maintaining internal controls to ensure that material information relating to the company and its consolidated subsidiaries is made known to such officers by others within those entities. It requires the signing officers to have disclosed to the company's auditors and the board's audit committee all significant deficiencies in the design or operation of internal controls which could adversely affect the company's ability to record, process, summarize, and report financial data.

Another section of the Act prohibits directors and officers of public companies from taking any action to "fraudulently influence, coerce, manipulate or mislead" any independent public or certified accountant engaged in the performance of an audit of the company's financial statements for the purpose of rendering such financial statements materially misleading.

It's easy to see how the same technical requirements could be placed on directors and officers of non-profits. Even though there are no shareholders in a non-profit to bring derivative suits against corporate officers for such actions, a state attorney general could decide to look more closely into these matters.

Under Sarbanes-Oxley, the SEC is empowered to prohibit any person who violates federal securities laws, rules, or regulations from acting as an officer or director of any public company. Again, it is not a stretch to imagine that potential bars could be placed on officers and directors of non-profits who violate certain laws, rules, or regulations, prohibiting them from serving in that capacity for any other non-profit organization. In fact, the exclusion from Medicare of individuals convicted of certain crimes is one example of how this principle has already been applied in the non-profit setting.

Audit Process and Oversight   Sarbanes-Oxley establishes an "Accounting Oversight Board" to oversee firms that audit public companies in the United States and abroad. Regulations of that board will affect the same independent auditing firms as they also audit non-profits. Non-profit boards should remember that annual external audits should be conducted and should be reviewed by the health care organization's board of directors. Equally, it is as important for accounting firms and auditors of non-profit health care organizations to avoid conflicts of interest and to have no business relationship with the organization outside of the auditing duties being provided.

Disclosures   One significant aspect of Sarbanes-Oxley is that it requires public companies to disclose material changes in financial condition or operations on a rapid and current basis. The same "real-time disclosure" requirement could likewise be placed on non-profits. It is foreseeable that non-profits will be called upon in the future to disclose (in plain English and on a rapid and current basis) information concerning material changes in financial condition or operations. Such a requirement would lessen (or perhaps completely avoid) deferral of disclosures by non-profits.

The Act similarly requires each public company to disclose in its periodic reports whether the board's audit committee has at least one member who is a "financial expert." This requirement for a "financial expert" on the audit committee of a non-profit health care board where possible is reasonable, and it would not be a surprise if such a requirement were also applied to non-profits in the future.

Sarbanes-Oxley requires public companies to disclose whether their senior financial executives have adopted a "Code of Ethics." Likewise, senior financial executives of non-profit corporations might be expected to follow this same type of code in the future (or at least to profess their allegiance to such a code to some governmental agency).

Finally, the Act requires attorneys to report violations of securities laws and breaches of fiduciary duty by a public company or its agents to the chief legal counsel or CEO of the company. If the counsel or CEO does not respond appropriately, the attorney must report the evidence to the audit committee of the company's board of directors, to a committee composed entirely of outside directors, or to the board as a whole. In our estimation, it is possible that the same reporting obligations could, in the future, be placed on attorneys for non-profit corporations to report breaches of fiduciary duty by senior executives.

....

THE VOLUNTEER PROTECTION ACT OF 1997

One little-known but very important protection afforded to hospital trustees is the federal Volunteer Protection Act of 1997. This statute was passed to protect volunteers active in not-for-profit corporations such as the Boy Scouts, playgroups, Little League, and other community organizations. While not specifically incorporating trustees or hospitals, the language is broad enough to cover them.

The act defines not-for-profit organizations as "any organization which is described in section 501(c)(3) of Title 26 [of the Internal Revenue Code] and exempt from tax under section 501(a) of Title 26 . . . or any not-for-profit organization which is organized and conducted for public benefit and operated primarily for charitable, civic, educational, religious, welfare, or health purposes . . ."[4] Because most hospitals and health systems are tax-exempt organizations under 501(c)(3) of the IRS Code and are conducted for public benefit and operated primarily for health purposes, most hospitals easily fit within the act's definition of a not-for-profit organization.

Furthermore, trustees are specifically identified as "volunteers" under the act. The Volunteer Protection Act defines "volunteer" as "an individual performing services for a non-profit organization or a governmental entity who does not receive compensation . . . or any other thing of value in lieu of compensation . . . and such term includes a volunteer serving as a director, officer, trustee, or direct service volunteer."[5]

The act specifically limits liability for volunteers such as hospital trustees. It states, in part, ". . . no volunteer of a non-profit organization . . . shall be liable for harm caused by an act or omission of the volunteer on behalf of the organization or entity if the volunteer was acting within the scope of the volunteer's responsibilities in the non-profit organization . . . at the time of the act or omission . . . if the harm was not caused by willful or criminal misconduct, gross negligence, reckless misconduct, or a conscious, flagrant indifference to the rights or safety of the individual harmed by the volunteer."[6]

Punitive damages are also limited by this act. The general rule states that "punitive damages may not be awarded against a volunteer in an action brought for harm based on the action of a volunteer acting within the scope of the volunteer's responsibilities to a non-profit organization . . . unless the claimant establishes by clear and convincing evidence that the harm was proximately caused by action of such volunteer which constitutes willful or criminal misconduct, or a conscious, flagrant indifference to the rights or safety of the individual harmed."[7] Although the Act lists exceptions to volunteer liability protection based on certain provisions in state laws that may be applicable in some circumstances, it still takes great strides in limiting liability for trustees of not-for-profit organizations in many circumstances.

The purpose of the Volunteer Protection Act is to sustain the viability of not-for-profit organizations (such as hospitals) that depend on volunteers. This act is an important federal law that, by its very nature, can limit the liability of hospital trustees should a claim be brought against them. Hospital trustees and counsel should be familiar with this

D&O liability offers better protection

protection. It is particularly valuable in this time of medical professional liability insurance crisis. Risk management professionals should be well aware of it.

....

RISK MANAGEMENT AND THE BOARD

A risk management professional's duty is inherent in the title of the position itself—to prevent or minimize corporate loss from legal liability. This may involve developing systems to prevent adverse events and attempting to handle events that do occur in such a manner that the organization's financial and reputation cost are minimized. For example, in the case of a *sentinel event* or other unexpected occurrence that could risk both liability, reputation, and accreditation, the risk management professional may: (1) interview central figures to determine what went wrong; (2) hold personal discussions with the injured party or parties; or (3) attempt to reach a satisfactory settlement without a lawsuit.

Board accountability and responsibility for risk management and quality is nothing new—this has always been the duty of the health care organization governing board. This section discusses what the relationship between the health care organization's risk management professional and governing board should be, to most effectively and efficiently prevent or minimize the organization's losses from legal liability.

Risk Management's Role in Educating the Board

Although it is not common for the risk management professional to report directly to the board (as will be discussed later in this chapter), the CEO and the risk management professional still need to ensure that the board is educated about the overall task of risk management and the crucial part the board itself plays in reducing potential liability by effectively discharging its risk management oversight role.

Board members must understand that they play a key part (along with the risk management professional) in preventing patient injury, preventing medical professional liability, and overseeing the corporation's prevention of loss from legal liability. This means that the board must work closely with the risk management professional and other hospital management staff, with the understanding that ineffective governance might cause harm to patients if it goes uncorrected, and also could generate liability for the corporation. Board education is key, but remember that management of risk is the result of board attention to medical and other errors that harm or could harm patients, and a plan for preventing repeat errors. As previously stated, one of the most important responsibilities of the board is to see that care is taken by the hospital and physicians so that patients are not harmed.

The risk management professional and CEO should play a dual role in educating the board with regard to its risk management and oversight duties. Periodically, and for new board members, the risk management professional and CEO may conduct a "risk management orientation program." In-house counsel and medical staff leadership may also participate in this introduction or orientation to risk management. The risk management professional and hospital management can use this opportunity to ensure that the board is familiar with the following concepts:

- The relationship between the health care organization's quality improvement program and medical staff credentialing function and the risk management program
- The health care organization's definition of risk management and the scope of the hospital or system's risk management program

- The role and job of the risk management professional
- The relationship between the insurance, loss of control and claims functions, and the risk management program
- How the risk management professional gathers data and identifies risks—incident reporting, occurrence reporting, generic screening, patient complaints, or other methods
- The highest-risk areas of patient injury and medical professional liability claims within the hospital and throughout the system and how they compare with national data
- Insurance coverage and costs
- The health care organization's claims history
- The part the board plays in preventing patient injury and malpractice liability and reducing overall liability exposure by effectively discharging its risk management oversight role
- The role of ineffective governance in generating liability losses[8]

Participation in such an "orientation process" can ensure that both new and current board members have a basic understanding of the hospital or health system's organizational structure vis-à-vis risk management, and a basic understanding of the crucial role that they play in accountability and responsibility for patient safety. The implementation of such an orientation program, however, is only the beginning of the larger role that the risk management professional (and hospital management) can play in establishing a comprehensive board orientation program.

While a periodic or "new board member" risk management orientation program is a good idea, it only scratches the surface of the knowledge that board members will need to effectively discharge their duties as corporate fiduciaries. The risk management professional can and should continue this educational process for the board by working with management to create a series of ongoing, well-designed activities for both new and current board members, so that they are continually made aware of any issues of patient safety. Such ongoing activities (as opposed to educational sessions held once or twice a year) ensure that the board's education regarding its oversight duties is not merely a one-time event but, rather, a continuing process.

What are the core competencies that board members should possess to keep themselves and their organizations accountable? From a risk management perspective, at least some board members should possess specific competencies in law, accounting, financial expertise, and clinical care. It is also important for trustees to understand:

- Governance obligations, functions, processes, and best practices
- The health care industry and their individual market and organization
- Key success factors including strategic, financial, operational, and clinical variables
- How to read, analyze, and interpret basic financial statements[9]

A hospital or health system board cannot effectively discharge its oversight role in patient safety until it has been properly educated. The risk management professional can play a pivotal role in ensuring that this education takes place.

Delivery of Information to the Board

Management could ask the risk management professional to report directly to the board, but this is unusual. Risk management professionals generally report to hospital management, either directly to the CEO or through a chief operating officer or senior vice president. It is not unusual for the risk management professional to report to the chief medical officer or vice president of medical affairs. Information generally comes to the board through the hospital's management. How this is accomplished is a matter to be worked out between the CEO and the board chair. Only in an extreme situation (in which the risk management professional believes that management is *creating liability* for the corporation and not telling the board about it) should a risk management professional bypass management and report concerns directly to the board.

Some organizations have the risk management professional report to a board committee, usually the professional affairs committee (PAC) of the board or the equivalent committee responsible for receiving and making recommendations on credentialing and peer review recommendations from the medical staff executive committee. Because the role of the PAC is generally to receive recommendations from the various medical staff committees and to make recommendations to the board regarding such things as initial appointment, reappointment, the delineation of privileges, "disciplinary" actions taken against medical staff appointees, bylaws, and rules and regulations of the medical staff, PAC is an ideal committee for the risk management professional to report to in lieu of a report to the full board. This is especially true when potential liability involves a physician, as it does in almost all major cases.

Medicare and Medicaid Fraud and Abuse

The Medicare definition of fraud is "an intentional representation that an individual knows to be false or does not believe to be true and makes, knowing that the representation could result in some unauthorized benefit to himself/herself or some other person."[10] The most frequent kind of fraud arises from a false statement or misrepresentation made or caused to be made that is material to entitlement or payment under the Medicare program. The violator may be a physician or other practitioner, a hospital or other institutional provider, a clinical laboratory or other supplier, an employee of any provider, a billing service, a beneficiary, a Medicare carrier employee, or any person in a position to file a claim for Medicare benefits.

Fraud schemes that a risk management professional might become aware of could include one or more of the following: offering or acceptance of kickbacks; routine waiver of co-payments; fraudulent diagnosis; billing for services not rendered; unbundling charges; or falsifying certificates of medical necessity, plans of treatment, and medical records to justify payment.

A risk management professional's discovery of Medicare or Medicaid fraud and abuse may sometimes represent the type of extreme situation referenced above that requires a risk management professional to bypass higher authority and go directly to the board. This would, of course, occur only if top management either were implicated or refused to take effective action.

What Should the Board Know?

What information should the hospital trustees have? First, it is very important to keep in mind that the risk management professional should couch all reports to the board in terms that maximize state peer review protection. Risk management professional reports should *always* provide a road map for peer review protection under state law. Also, it is important to strike a proper balance as to how much information to provide to the board. Nothing productive will be accomplished if trustees are overwhelmed with information.

At the same time, it is essential that they be given enough information to enable them to thoroughly understand the issue. There are a few basics, however. The board should *always* know:

- All sentinel events and follow-up
- All lawsuits filed and the nature of claims and what is being done to address any quality questions these raise
- All payments, settlements, and judgments
- Any quality trends
- Any questions raised by the death of a patient

There is little point in having a risk management professional if this kind of information is not given to the board.

Content and Format of Reports to the Board

It is no easy task for hospital management to decide what information the board should be privy to, nor is it easy for risk management professionals to strike the difficult balance between enabling the board to thoroughly understand an issue without overwhelming it with data. Aside from the basic information already discussed that the board should always be provided, risk management reports should strive to provide meaningful information about issues of patient safety to the board in a clear, concise, graphic format.

As opposed to giving board members a three-ring binder filled with stacks of paper, or a large packet of data that overwhelms them, risk management professionals should ensure that the information they provide to the board is broken down into one report, which should be short and easy to read. Any reports given to the board (whether from risk management or hospital management) should tell board members in plain English where the organization stands with respect to incidents that affect patient safety compared with where it strives to be in this regard.

It also may be helpful to include a "consent agenda" to help streamline board meeting procedures. Consent agenda items are considered to be routine and non-controversial, with documentation provided to the board that is adequate and sufficient for approval without discussion unless a board member raises a specific question. For instance, items that may routinely be found on a consent agenda include such things as approval of the minutes from the last board meeting or approval of reports from the Medical Executive Committee. The consent agenda is intended to minimize the time required for the handling of any non-controversial matters, and to permit additional time to be spent on more significant matters. Any item on the consent agenda should be moved to the regular agenda upon request from any board member. Such items also may be held to a subsequent meeting for further consideration.

Recommendations of the Credentials Committee of the Medical Staff for physician appointments and clinical privileges are usually non-controversial and often become part of the consent agenda. We believe this is a bad idea.

The recommendations of the Credentials Committee that deal with appointment and clinical privileges directly go to the most important board responsibility—the safety of patients. These recommendations must be acted on directly by the board after the board asks for and receives the assurance of the Credentials Committee chair that these recommendations are the result of the thoughtful work of the Committee.

Even though the recommendations pass through and are approved by the Medical Staff Executive Committee, they should be presented to the board by the chair of the Committee who did the work. The approval may, in most cases, be *pro forma,* but it should be received from the Committee and be endorsed by the Committee chair before the board acts.

Reports to the board should include a carefully selected group of risk management indicators that show board members at a glance how well their organization is performing in patient safety. Indicators might include such items as analyses of trends identified through incident reports and occurrence screens, and open and closed claims trends and costs of claims, or results of insurance audits and costs—all the while remembering that claims and their costs represent problems that need to be fixed. Board members and risk management professionals alike should not forget that the harm done to patients is important, not the insurance loss.

The report should track the organization's risk management trends over time in a graphic format, and should show how the organization compares with benchmark organizations. By presenting information to boards in this way, risk management professionals and hospital managers will do more than lay out the data for trustees, they will be helping board members to *interpret* such data.

By helping trustees interpret data, risk management professionals and hospital managers will be giving trustees what they really need—the information (risk management or otherwise) to know where their organization stands. Moreover, when assessing the risk management status of an organization, boards will benefit by being provided with a global "big picture" as opposed to being bogged down in data.

Risk management professionals can begin such a process in their organizations by first analyzing the most important five to ten risk management variables that the board needs to know over the course of the next year. The risk management professional, CEO, and board chair should all play a part in answering this question and deciding on the crucial indicators that should be presented to the board. Then, a chart should be prepared for each indicator containing one black line showing the organization's target for each indicator. Before each board meeting, management (with the risk management professional's help) fills in what actually happened so that all board members need do is look at the chart to see if what actually happened is over or under the organization's "target line."[11] Such a format facilitates quick review of the essential indicators and will provide the board with the easily understood, big-picture view of the issues that it needs to effectively govern in the areas of patient safety and risk management.

How the Board Can Help Hospital Management and the Risk Management Professional

It is important for the governing board and the risk management professional of any health care organization to realize that all duties delegated to the risk management professional ultimately flow from the board through the chief executive officer. The governance of the organization should be the source of responsibilities that the risk management professional carries out. From a managerial perspective, this eases the blame or resistance to things that must be done that could potentially fall upon the risk management professional should others in the organization perceive that orders are flowing from one individual alone. It must be clear that the risk management professional is carrying out delegated authority and responsibilities of the chief executive officer of the corporation.

....

THE MEDICAL STAFF, RISK MANAGEMENT, AND THE BOARD

The medical staff, whether of the hospital or other health care organization, is central to risk management. The most serious liability any health care organization (and particularly a hospital) faces is always at the intersection between the organization and the physicians who practice within it.

One of the difficulties in understanding the medical staff is that the term itself has two different meanings: (1) individual physicians who have received from the board an appointment to the hospital medical staff and treat patients in the hospital; and (2) an organization of physicians established by the hospital board with various delegated duties pertaining to quality and the ability to act as a group to influence the hospital, its management and board.

How does the medical staff, both as an organization and as individuals, relate to governance? The purpose of the individual members of the medical staff is to provide good quality medicine, whereas the purpose of the medical staff as an organization is to monitor the care provided.

The medical staff organization acts as a consultant to the hospital board. It is asked to make recommendations on quality, appointments, discipline of medical staff appointees, and hospital needs and procedures. Members of medical staff committees who make such recommendations must act with the same care and loyalty as board members. The medical staff is not organized for political purposes or to protect the economic interests of one or all physicians.

The hospital's relationship with members of the medical staff does not fit easily within ordinary corporate law or organization. That is why it is sometimes difficult for the risk management professional to deal with quality or liability issues that involve members of the medical staff. However, it is essential that this be done. Management, including the risk management professional, is responsible to the board for investigating all potential liability, whether physician-related or not. The medical staff organization does not have exclusive jurisdiction over acts by physicians in the hospital.

The Board Must Step In

The board delegates responsibility for monitoring and overseeing the quality of care to the medical staff. However, if the medical staff fails or is unable to fulfill its responsibilities in monitoring the safety and outcome of care provided by the organization, the board has the legal authority and, more important, the obligation to step in to oversee the safety and outcomes.

Medical Staff Development Plans[12]

A medical staff development plan defines what it means to be a member of the medical staff, including sharing the hospital's vision, mission, and commitment to the community. Many boards have found the development of such plans to be effective. For many hospitals, such plans have become critical to maintaining a good relationship with their medical staffs. Just going through the process of developing a plan has been helpful. Critical steps in the development of a plan follow:

Step 1: Board Adopts Resolution and Statement of Community Service Principles   The board adopts a resolution that authorizes the research and

analysis that lead to the plan. That resolution also establishes a staff development committee or task force composed of board members, management representatives (including the chief executive officer), and physicians. It is important that the physicians selected for this committee not be those who might be economically advantaged by its recommendations. A Statement of Community Service Principles, adopted by the board, provides the foundation for further discussions and possible actions with respect to physicians who have economic conflicts of interest.

Step 2: Communicate   It is critical that physicians, especially those in leadership positions, know and understand how and why a medical staff development plan is being developed, its purpose, and its objectives. The physicians should be kept apprised of the progress of the study and, when appropriate, input from physicians should be sought and considered.

Step 3: Gather Data and Analyze Community Needs   The ultimate purpose of the plan (and of the hospital itself) is to meet the needs of the community. That, obviously, is part of a hospital's charitable purposes as articulated in its Statement of Community Service Principles.

A "community needs assessment" involves collecting data regarding individuals currently practicing in the hospital; information about their practices and referral patterns, including what care is referred outside of the community and why; demographic information regarding the population served by the hospital and that population's health care needs; the study of the existing health resources in the community; and areas underserved from either a geographic, medical specialty, or income level standpoint.

Visits to the emergency department, calls from individuals seeking physicians to provide care, waiting lists for care in physician office practices, or the inability to obtain an appointment can all indicate a community need for specific services.

The task force analyzes the data collected to determine on a specialty-by-specialty basis what is necessary to meet the current and projected needs of the community.

Step 4: Communicate Again   As this information is collected, it should be made available for physicians to review and comment on. Physicians should also be surveyed to gain insight into what services the hospital might offer, what services the hospital could provide better, and where efficiencies or additional progress could be achieved.

Step 5: Analyze Financial Relationships and Their Impact   The task force should also analyze the financial relationships that physicians on the medical staff may have with competing entities, and how each type of financial relationship could compromise physicians' abilities to fulfill their responsibilities as members of the medical staff, or could otherwise impair the hospital's ability to fulfill its charitable mission.

Two types of physician financial relationships should be specifically analyzed: ownership or investment interests in competing facilities or services and compensation arrangements, such as employment contracts or medical directorships with competing facilities, including other hospitals or health systems. The task force's analysis should include: (a) information about competing entities in the market and how those entities affect the hospital both financially and operationally; (b) disclosures from medical staff members and applicants of their financial relationships; and (c) whether the hospital can be made a more attractive location in which to practice.

Step 6: Task Force Recommends   Based on its analysis of community needs and the effect of physicians' conflicting financial relationships, the task force might recommend: (a) adding, expanding, reducing, or eliminating clinical or new services; (b) recruiting new practitioners to meet clinical service needs; (c) identifying specialties which are recruitment priorities; or (d) setting organizational criteria for applicants in specialties in which applications will be accepted. Examples of such criteria may include: (i) potential applicants must indicate an intention to actively use the hospital's facilities to permit reasonable monitoring of their practices and to assure working familiarity with the hospital's technology, regulations, procedures, and personnel; (ii) potential applicants must be willing to work with the medical staff and hospital to develop protocols and best practices in their specialties, to practice in accordance with such protocols or to document the reasons for variance, and to attend meetings at which such practices and protocols are reviewed and improved.

Additional organizational criteria may relate to financial concerns, including whether physicians who have conflicting financial relationships: (i) should be permitted to serve on the board or in medical staff leadership positions; (ii) should be eligible for appointment or reappointment to the medical staff or to categories of the staff that would given them the ability to participate in the governance of the staff or hospital; and (iii) should be eligible for financial relationships with, or assistance from, the hospital, for example, employment agreements, exclusive contracts, and malpractice premium assistance.

Step 7: Board Adopts Plan   The board adopts a plan that is reviewed and revised on a regular basis, at least every three years.

....

CONCLUSION

The ever-expanding responsibilities faced by health care organization governing boards today make it more important than ever that those who support governance, such as risk management professionals, are up to the task. Health care governing boards have always been ultimately responsible for the quality of patient care provided, physician performance, risk management, and appointment and disciplining of physicians. In the future, health care governing board responsibilities will only increase.

As discussed, current media emphasis on medical errors will encourage boards to be proactive in monitoring and improving quality data, and the fallout from the recent corporate accounting scandals is certain to result in greater board responsibility for nonprofit corporate financial statements. The necessity for risk management in organizations other than the hospital is growing as lawyers for plaintiffs look for additional deep pockets to pay claims.

This will only intensify if the medical professional liability insurance crisis becomes more widespread. A strong, cooperative relationship between an organization's risk management professional, hospital management, and, particularly, medical staff committees with quality responsibilities can ensure that the organization's loss from legal liability is prevented at best, and minimized at the very least.

Endnotes

1. Panel on the Nonprofit Sector. Strengthening Transparency, Governance, and Accountability of Charitable Organizations, a Final Report to Congress and the Nonprofit Sector. June 2005, p. 75.

2. Remarks of Sen. Charles Grassley, News Conference of the Panel on the Nonprofit Sector's Final Report, Wednesday, June 22, 2005.

3. Seidman, D. "What Every Board Member Needs To Know About Compliance." *Compliance Today*, July 2005, pp. 6, 9.

4. 42 U.S.C.A. Section 14505 (4)(A)(B).

5. 42 U.S.C.A. Section 14505 (6)(A)(B).

6. 42 U.S.C.A. Section 14503 (a)(1)(3).

7. 42 U.S.C.A. Section 14503 (e)(1).

8. Carroll, RL., Editor., *Risk Management Handbook for Health Care Organizations— 3rd Edition*, Chapter 3: The Health Care Organization Governing Board, Orlikoff, J. E, San Francisco: Jossey-Bass, 2001. pp. 69–70.

9. Mycek, S. "Accountability Stops Here: Educating the Board to Meet Its Responsibilities." *Trustee*, Vol. 55, no. 6, June 2002, p. 13.

10. Centers for Medicare and Medicaid Services. "Medicare Definition of Fraud." http://cms.hhs.gov/providers/fraud/DEFINI2.ASP. Last visited 6/05.

11. Strenger, E. W., "The Data Game." *Trustee*, Vol. 50, No. 4, April 1997, p. 28.

12. "Medical Staff Development Plans." Reprinted from *Action Kit for Hospital Trustees*, by permission, January/February 2004, Copyright 2004, by Horty, Springer & Mattern, P. C.

4

Development of a Risk Management Program

Jane J. McCaffrey
Sheila Hagg-Rickert

Organizations and individuals have always sought ways to identify and reduce the risks that threatened their existence. In primitive agrarian societies, where families and villages produced barely enough to meet their most basic needs, the loss of a year's harvest, whether to forces of nature or to the plunder of warring tribes, surely spelled disaster. The attempts of such cultures to protect their food supplies and other necessities of life from destruction by fire, flood, and theft represent history's earliest risk management efforts. As societies developed into industrialized economies, individuals and organizations continued to seek ways to understand and anticipate the risks associated with such perils in an attempt to protect valuable property from such threats, ultimately establishing mechanisms for transferring the financial consequences of such losses through policies of insurance.

Despite the age-old concern with protecting assets from the risks associated with accidental losses, risk management has existed for only about fifty years.[1] Health care risk management in its present form did not really begin to emerge until the malpractice crisis of the mid-1970s, when hospitals and other health care entities experienced rapid rises in claims costs, and subsequently insurance premiums, and witnessed the exit of several major medical professional liability insurers from the market.[2] This crisis formed the basis for health care entities to develop the first risk management programs. The American Society for Hospital Risk Management (ASHRM) was established in 1980 in response to this developing interest in risk management among health care organizations. Over the years, health care risk management has moved from a discipline focused almost exclusively on medical professional liability issues to a profession concerned with all of the risks associated with accidental losses facing a health care organization.[3] In addition to hospitals, managed care organizations, long-term care, and ambulatory care, other providers of health care have come to realize the value of effective risk management and have developed formalized programs.[4] Increasingly, risk management is moving towards the concept of enterprise risk management and considering the myriad of complex legal, regulatory, political, business, and financial risks facing health care organizations. As risk management moves toward this more strategic orientation and risk management professionals prepare themselves for new roles as chief risk officers, diverse work experience, higher education, and broad-based business, financial, and technical skills will be valued in health care risk management professionals more than ever before.[5] Another recent development in risk management has been the return focus on patient safety.

The patient safety movement was prompted in large part by the 1999 publication of *To Err is Human: Building a Safer Health System,*[6] which articulated the findings of an Institute of Medicine study of the devastating consequences of widespread medical error in the nation's hospitals. Risk management professionals who had long had primary responsibility for investigating, analyzing, and maintaining data regarding adverse patient incidents joined with colleagues from performance improvement, health care administration, and a variety of clinical disciplines in an attempt to systematically identify the underlying causes of medical errors in their organizations, and to design and implement effective interdisciplinary organization-wide patient safety programs.

RISK MANAGEMENT PROGRAM DEVELOPMENT

Whatever the health care setting or the sophistication of the risk management professional, an effective risk management program requires certain elementary building blocks: key structural elements, sufficient scope to cover all applicable categories of risk, appropriate risk strategies, and written policies and procedures. This chapter focuses on these building blocks, giving the novice risk management professional guidance in developing a comprehensive risk management program and providing the experienced risk management professional with a program overview that may be used as a self-assessment guide.

Developing a comprehensive risk management program depends on addressing several specific considerations. An effective risk management effort is built on key structural elements that enable the risk management professional to develop and enforce a risk management plan and enact the necessary changes in organizational policy. The program must include a defined scope of risks to be managed, including an examination of the risks associated with patients, medical staff, employees, governing bodies, property, automobiles, and other risks that subject the health care organization to potential liability or the threat of loss. Risk management strategies represent the mix of techniques employed to prevent or reduce potential losses and preserve the organization's assets. The final building block is a set of written policies and procedures that ensures program uniformity and consistency, and assists in communication of the program to affected parties. This chapter describes how each of these four important considerations contributes to an effective risk management program.

KEY STRUCTURAL ELEMENTS OF THE RISK MANAGEMENT PROGRAM

The exact structure of a health care organization's risk management program depends on the size and complexity of its functions, and the scope of other services that it offers. Several key structural components are necessary for any health care risk management program to succeed. Whether an entity is just beginning to organize its risk management program or is seeking to revamp or expand an existing program, attention to these structural factors will help ensure that the program has a solid foundation.

Authority

The risk management professional in a health care organization must maintain sufficient authority and respect to enact the changes in clinical practice, policy and procedure, and in employee and medical staff behavior that are necessary to fulfill the purpose of the risk management program. The risk manager must deal on a daily basis with highly sensitive and confidential information that directly affects the organization's public image and financial status. The risk management professional is responsible for coordinating risk management activities with members of the medical staff and outside parties, and with managers and employees at all levels of the organization. For these reasons, the risk management professional's position should be relatively high in the organizational hierarchy. Ideally, the risk management professional should report directly to the CEO, or at least to another member of the senior administrative management team. Risk management professionals whose positions rank below the department manager level on the organizational chart will almost certainly face difficulty in dealing authoritatively with medical staff, nursing administration, and department managers. They also may have difficulty gaining access to senior management and representing the organization in its relations with insurers, attorneys, and other outside parties involved in the risk management process. In many non-hospital health care organizations, and in smaller hospital facilities, the designated risk management professional may serve primarily as a senior manager or clinician and devote only a relatively small percentage of work time to risk management activities. Under such a model, risk finance and insurance program administration typically are handled by the organization's finance department; workers' compensation programs are managed by human resources personnel; and safety programs are developed and overseen by a facility or maintenance manager. Although this division of labor might be efficient for apportioning the workload required for a successful risk management effort, it creates special challenges when establishing ownership of the risk management function and creating an identity for those activities that comprise risk management. Such part-time risk management professionals, especially those who view their risk management responsibilities as subordinate to their other job duties, might find it difficult to acquire the wide range of expertise necessary to adequately fulfill their risk management obligations and to stay abreast of rapidly changing and often complex legal and regulatory developments affecting the field.

Visibility

The risk management professional should be highly visible in the health care organization. No one individual can perform every function of a comprehensive risk management program single-handedly, even in the smallest health care facility. Therefore, it is necessary for the organization's risk management professional, through consciousness-raising, education, and communication, to foster an awareness of risk management practices and techniques among senior management and the governing body, medical staff members, and employees at all organizational levels. The risk management professional's position should be structured to enhance opportunities for interaction with others through service on appropriate committees, participation in educational activities such as employee orientation and staff in-service offerings, and access to organization-wide communication mechanisms.

Communication

As health care facilities have merged into alliances and networks and acquired physician practices, clinics, and managed care organizations to form integrated delivery systems (IDSs), additional issues relating to potential liability, insurance coverage, claims management, and loss control have emerged. To anticipate risk management pitfalls and opportunities in this environment, the risk management professional must be an insider who is provided with information on proposed mergers, acquisitions, and joint ventures early in the due diligence process. (Refer to Volume III, Chapters 7 and 8, in this series for more information) Equipped with such information, the risk management professional is in a position to advise senior management on the risk management implications of various new business arrangements, many of which can be substantial, but frequently are overlooked by executives not attuned to risk management issues and specific insurance requirements.

Coordination

Because of the wide range of risk management functions and the diversity of activities necessary for a successful risk management program, the health care organization should establish both formal and informal mechanisms for the coordination of the risk management program with other departments and functions. To adequately integrate and coordinate risk management with other functions, the risk management professional needs to establish reporting and communication relationships with key individuals within the organization:

- The chief executive officer (CEO) provides a vital link to the entity's governing board and medical staff and establishes the necessary support for the risk management program. The CEO serves as the key decision maker for many activities crucial to the risk management program, such as authorizing the settlement of larger claims and establishing insurance limits. Additionally, the CEO often heads the team of senior managers responsible for the development of new business opportunities, mergers, and acquisitions.

- The chief financial officer (CFO) may have multiple risk financing responsibilities and provides valuable information for the risk management program. These functions include establishing limits on self-insured retentions or trusts, monitoring the financial operations of captives, and overseeing the performance of actuarial analyses. In some organizations, the CFO is the primary purchaser of insurance coverages and must therefore rely on information provided by the risk management professional to make appropriate decisions regarding risk-financing activities on behalf of the organization.

- The performance improvement or quality management director serves as an important source of information regarding adverse clinical events occurring within the facility that potentially have serious risk management implications. The risk management standards promulgated by the Joint Commission on Accreditation of Healthcare Organizations (JCAHO) emphasizes the interdependence of risk management and performance improvement activities.[7] Both the development of proactive patient safety initiatives and an effective root cause analysis process for post-occurrence sentinel events depend on the active leadership and close coordination of the risk management professional and performance improvement director. The performance improvement director may also be able to assist a risk management professional who lacks clinical training in interpreting and analyzing information contained in medical records, and in providing clinical loss prevention services.

- The patient safety director has responsibility for systematically analyzing the sources of human error and systems issues that affect patient care. Patient safety directors may report to the risk management professional or performance improvement director, or to senior management in a health care organization. Patient safety directors are very involved in the development of clinical risk management loss prevention initiatives.

- The compliance officer guides the development of policy and staff education efforts related to legislative and regulatory initiatives such as HIPAA, Sarbanes-Oxley, and Medicare fraud and abuse prevention.[8]

- The infection control nurse (or staff epidemiologist) provides information on patient infections that might give rise to liability claims and can assist the risk management professional in understanding infection control protocols aimed at reducing the frequency and severity of nosocomial infections, establishing guidelines for coping with AIDS, tuberculosis, and other communicable diseases.

- The safety officer may have primary responsibility for, or assist the risk management professional in, performing fire safety, hazardous materials management, emergency preparedness, and employee safety activities in compliance with JCAHO standards.[9] The safety officer usually chairs the organization's safety committee, which serves as a vital source of risk management information and organizational problem solving.

- The patient representative (or ombudsman) relays information regarding patient complaints and works with patients and families who have experienced difficulties with the organization or specific staff members to reach satisfactory resolutions of their concerns. Patient representatives, whether employees or volunteers, must be trained to recognize and appropriately manage risk management concerns that arise in the course of their activities and to relay information to the risk management professional.

- The employee health nurse (or workers' compensation coordinator or personnel director) may, in some organizations, manage the daily operational aspects of the facility's workers' compensation program and provide claims and injury information to the risk management professional. Often this individual is instrumental in developing transitional duty return-to-work and other injury management programs. The risk management professional in some health care organizations is personally responsible for the operation of workers' compensation programs, but nonetheless must coordinate activities with the human resources director and various line managers.

- The health information manager (or medical records director) notifies the risk management professional of requests from attorneys for medical records that might signal initiation of legal proceedings or claims. The health information manager also develops policies and procedures relating to the documentation of patient care activities, patient confidentiality, and appropriate release of information, and ensures the organization's compliance with the privacy requirements of HIPAA. (See Volume III, Chapter 18, for more information on HIPAA.)

- The medical director (or chief medical officer) serves as a liaison between the risk management program and the medical staff and assists the risk management professional in "selling" risk management to physicians. The risk management professional must also work with the medical staff services professional to ensure that the organization's medical staff appointment, credentialing, privileging, and disciplinary procedures are conducted in accordance with sound risk management practices.

- The patient accounts representative works with the risk management professional to identify patient complaints and concerns that surface during the billing and collections process. Such concerns may be based on perceived patient care problems. They hold the potential for becoming liability claims if collection efforts are vigorously pursued.

- Nursing and departmental managers offer the risk management professional the technical and clinical expertise necessary to identify and analyze potential patient-care risks and assist with the investigation of liability claims and incidents. Middle management personnel also play a crucial role in building and maintaining support for the risk management program and in educating and raising the risk management consciousness of employees within their areas of responsibility.

- The education director (or in-service program coordinator) assists the risk management professional in identifying staff education needs pertaining to risk management and in planning, organizing, and presenting orientation and in-service education programs.

- The human resources director maintains responsibility for developing effective job descriptions and performance appraisal processes, employee background checks and competency testing, verification of licenses and certifications, and maintenance of a drug-free workplace, all of which are critical to the prevention and defense of medical professional liability actions. In addition, the human resources staff generally takes the lead in preventing and managing claims and complaints related to employment practices issues, such as alleged sexual harassment, discrimination, and wrongful termination.

Accountability

Just as risk management professionals need sufficient authority to perform assigned functions, they should be held accountable for that performance. Every health care organization's risk management professional, including those in small institutions that have job duties in addition to risk management, should have a written job description that outlines key risk management responsibilities. Annual performance appraisals assessing the risk management professional's achievement of specific, measurable risk management goals and objectives should be conducted to gauge and document the individual's effectiveness. The risk management professional should prepare an annual report to senior management and the governing body that summarizes claims, insurance, and risk management program activities, and documents the progress made toward the attainment of established goals.

SCOPE OF THE RISK MANAGEMENT PROGRAM

The purpose of a health care risk management program is to protect the organization against risks associated with accidental losses, regardless of the cause. One of the building blocks of an effective program is sufficient scope to cover all potential sources of risk. Although many risk management professionals focus on the medical professional liability aspects of health care risk management, the discipline extends into many other areas that are equally important to the survival of the modern health care organization. Defined broadly, health care risk management is concerned with a tremendous variety of issues and situations that hold the potential for liability or casualty losses for the organization. To be truly comprehensive, a risk management program must address the full scope of the following categories of risk:

- Patient care-related
- Medical staff-related
- Employee-related
- Property-related
- Financial
- Other

Patient Care-Related Risks

Over the course of the last several years, U.S. health care institutions and practitioners have once again experienced a "malpractice crisis" evidenced by rising jury verdicts, settlement amounts,[10] insurance premiums,[11] dwindling insurance availability due to carrier withdrawals from the medical malpractice market,[12] and the imposition of more stringent underwriting criteria.[13] The reduction in insurers' investment income resulting from the general economic downturn in the early part of the twenty-first century and the huge unanticipated insurance losses associated from the terrorist attacks of September 11, 2001, only served to exacerbate the worsening trends for health care medical professional liability insurers and their insureds.

Given the substantial proportion of total health care risk management costs associated with medical professional liability claims and insurance premiums and the current national focus on patient safety issues, it is not surprising that most health care risk management efforts begin with patient care-related issues. Patient care or clinical risk management, including information gathering, loss control efforts, medical professional liability risk financing, and claims management activities, forms the core of most health care risk management programs. Although most patient-related risk management activity focuses on direct clinical patient-care activities and the consequences of inappropriate or incorrectly performed medical treatments, other important patient-related issues also confront the risk management professional, including:

- Confidentiality and appropriate release of patient medical information, especially in light of HIPAA and other privacy requirements
- Protection of patients from abuse and neglect and from assault by other patients, visitors, or staff
- Securing appropriate informed patient consent to medical treatment
- Nondiscriminatory treatment of patients, regardless of race, religion, national origin, or payment status
- Protection of patient valuables from loss or damage
- Appropriate triage, stabilization, and transfer of patients presenting to dedicated emergency departments (DEDs)
- Patient participation in research studies and the use of experimental drugs and medical procedures
- Utilization review decisions related to the timing of patient discharges and the provision of medically necessary services under various third-party managed care arrangements
- Access to care concerns

Medical Staff-Related Risks

Closely aligned with patient care-related risk management issues are those experienced by medical staff and other clinically privileged practitioners. Many, if not most, of the potentially serious occurrences related to the delivery of clinical patient care involve a facility's medical staff. It is imperative that the health care risk management professional include physicians in clinical loss prevention and claims management programs, and elicit their support for overall risk management activities. Risk management concerns that stem from the unique relationship between a health care organization and its medical staff merit the risk management professional's particular attention. Of special importance are:

- Medical staff peer review and performance improvement activities, and maintaining the confidentiality and protection of the data generated through such peer review processes

- Medical staff credentialing, appointment, and privileging processes

- Medical staff disciplinary proceedings, due process considerations, and potential allegations of antitrust and restraint of trade

- The identification and treatment of impaired physicians and other credentialed providers who pose a threat to patient or employee safety

- Business arrangements and financial incentives to physicians that might have fraud and abuse or other implications under federal Medicare regulations[14]

- Physician gatekeeper obligations and incentives under various managed care plans

In this era of expanding legal theories of corporate liability and vicarious liability, the activities of the medical staff are often deemed the activities of the health care organization. It has become increasingly difficult for defense attorneys to persuade judges and juries to distinguish between the institution and its independent contractor physicians. As physicians become business partners with health care entities and assume ownership interests in new ventures, and as hospitals and other organizations purchase or assume management of physician practices, the distinctions become even more blurred.

Employee-Related Risks

Several issues relating to the employment of personnel deserve the health care risk management professional's attention. Of obvious importance is maintaining a safe work environment for employees, reducing the risk of occupational illness and injury, and providing for the treatment and compensation of workers who suffer on-the-job injuries and work-related illnesses. In this regard, it is important that risk management professionals maintain a working knowledge of relevant state workers' compensation law, and regulations promulgated by the federal Occupational Safety and Health Administration (OSHA). Such understanding allows them to work effectively with human resources departments, employee health nurses, and designated safety officers to establish successful employee injury and management programs.

Posing particularly serious problems for today's health care organization are allegations of discrimination in recruitment, hiring, and promotion based on age, race, sex, national origin, or disability; wrongful termination; and other claims filed with the Equal Employment Opportunity Commission (EEOC). Claims involving alleged sexual harassment are also increasingly common.[15,16,17] The risk management professional must work closely with the facility's human resources director to help minimize such claims exposures, manage the claims that do occur, and finance the costs associated with such losses.

Property-Related Risks

Many complex health care entities have significant property assets, including large hospital and clinic structures, medical office buildings, and valuable medical and data processing equipment. It is incumbent upon the risk management professional to protect these assets from risk of loss due to fires, acts of God, floods, natural disasters, and other perils that might damage or destroy such property. In addition, health care institutions typically maintain a large volume of paper and electronic records that are essential to the ongoing operations of the entity and that must be protected from damage or destruction. Obviously, the costs associated with repairing and replacing damaged assets can be significant, and the revenues lost during the period of business interruption can have disastrous effects on the organization.

Many health care employees routinely handle cash, checks, and credit cards in the course of their job duties. Hospitals and nursing homes often are requested to safeguard cash and other valuables belonging to patients and residents. Home health workers, who function independently and without direct supervision in a client's home, are particularly vulnerable to allegations of theft. Thus, it is important for the risk management professional to evaluate hiring and screening protocols for such workers, to review policies and procedures for handling cash and safeguarding valuables, and to consider various bonding and insurance alternatives to adequately protect the facility from such losses.

Financial Risks

Although the ordinary business risks associated with new ventures or services, and the continued financial viability of the organization's existing operations, are traditionally considered to be outside the sphere of risk management concerns, there are at least two areas of financial risk with which the risk management professional must be concerned.

First, the directors and officers of health care organizations, like those of other corporate entities, may face liability imposed by suits from shareholders or others alleging inappropriate conduct in the fulfillment of the directors' and officers' duties. Corporate charters and bylaws frequently require the entity to defend and indemnify its directors and officers against such claims. Likewise, the entity itself may be named in such actions. It is therefore important for the risk management professional to understand the corporate structure of the organization; any requirements imposed by the charter, bylaws, or other documents; and the opportunities to transfer such risks through policies of insurance, to adequately protect the organization's assets.

Second, risk management professionals who represent the interests of health care providers who contract with managed care organizations (MCOs) on an "at-risk" basis (typically through capitated payment arrangements) need to consider available options for limiting the financial risks inherent in such agreements. These risks may be characterized as either specific, in which the costs associated with providing care to an individual plan subscriber greatly exceed expectations, or aggregate, in which the total costs of providing required health care services under the plan agreement are higher than anticipated. Various options exist for contractual transfer of risks above a certain level back to the MCO or for the purchase of "stop-loss" insurance coverage.

Other Risks

There are, of course, other areas of potential concern for the health care risk management professional. Among these are property and liability losses related to the operation of automobiles, trucks, vans, and ambulances owned or leased by the organization. Many facilities also own or operate helicopters or fixed-wing air transport services, or maintain heliports or helipads that pose additional liability and property risks.

Since September 11, 2001, U.S. health care institutions have become increasingly aware of their vulnerability to terrorist and bioterrorist attack.

Organizations have sought to augment existing disaster and emergency preparedness plans to address scenarios in which the facility itself is the target of such an attack, and those in which the institution plays a key role in triage and treatment response in an attack occurring elsewhere. Planning for such contingencies requires an analysis of patient care, employee-related and property-related risks of potentially staggering proportions, and the coordination of resources on a local, statewide, and national level.[18] (For more information on emergency management, see Chapter 18.) Although typically representing a lesser proportion of the total cost of risk, hospitals and most other health care entities are accessible by the public, and vulnerable to a wide variety of general liability claims stemming from visitor injuries caused by slips, falls, and other mishaps. The risk management professional must therefore be concerned with the overall maintenance of buildings, parking lots, and sidewalks, and with visitor access and supervision.

Hazardous materials management is yet another area of concern for health care risk management. Ensuring that appropriate protocols are in place for the safe storage, use, and disposal of the myriad toxic chemicals and radioactive materials routinely used by health care organizations is a highly regulated[19] and important risk management activity. The implications for patients, employees, and the community at large should such materials find their way into the environment are chief considerations in managing hazardous materials programs. Proper disposal of infectious biological waste generated by hospitals and other health care entities continues to be a significant public health and environmental concern.

Special issues involving auxiliary personnel and other volunteers who may provide services at hospitals, and students involved in clinical training experiences who sustain injury in the course of their duties or may inflict harm on others, also merit the risk management professional's attention. Such individuals may not be routinely covered under the organization's workers' compensation and liability insurance programs, and the risks pertaining to both groups must be specially considered by the risk management professional from both a risk financing and loss prevention perspective. Requirements for training and supervision of volunteers and students, and clearly delineated duties appropriate for such non-employees, must be adequately defined.

For senior-level health care risk management professionals rising within their organizations to the level of chief risk officer (CRO), an even larger universe of potential risks merits attention. The CRO concept was developed initially in banking and financial services industries to describe the role of a broadly experienced executive charged with responsibility for identifying and analyzing risks to an organization, whether or not insurable, developing strategies for handling such risks, and advising the governing board and senior management team. While still rare in health care settings, CROs often address issues ranging from the risk of increased market competition to the risk of regulatory sanctions if a certain course of corporate conduct is pursued, and typically work closely with an organization's internal audit, legal, and finance departments to formulate risk identification, loss prevention, and risk financing strategies.

············

THE RISK MANAGEMENT PROCESS

Viewing risk management as a process helps the risk management professional set priorities and assists in ensuring a comprehensive risk management effort. The risk management process consists of five steps (see Figure 4.1 for a graphic representation):

1. Identify and analyze loss exposures
2. Consider alternative risk techniques
3. Select what appears to be the best risk management technique or combination of techniques
4. Implement the selected technique(s)
5. Monitor and improve the risk management program[20]

The sections that follow describe how each step of the risk management process should be considered in developing a comprehensive risk management program.

Step 1—Identify and Analyze Loss Exposures

Risk identification is the process through which the risk management professional becomes aware of risks in the health care environment that constitute potential loss exposures for the institution. Such exposures can include loss of financial assets through liability judgments and out-of-court settlements, or casualty losses to physical plant and property, human losses through death or injury of employees, and intangible losses to public image and reputation.

The risk management professional uses many information sources to identify potential risks. Incident reporting, in which employees report accidents and occurrences not consistent with normal operating routines or expected outcomes, is the cornerstone of most risk identification systems. Incident reporting systems range from sophisticated point-of-service electronic reporting and analysis packages to simple paper forms. Regardless of the format, incident reporting systems allow caregivers to provide the risk management department with basic early warning information about occurrences that are inconsistent with normal, expected patient care processes and that result (or have the potential to result) in injury to patients, visitors, staff, or property. Other common risk identification processes include:

- **Generic occurrence screening.** Generic occurrence screening is a risk management process often performed as part of a health care organization's performance improvement program. In a generic occurrence screening process, patient records are reviewed retrospectively to determine whether the care provided meets specific pre-determined criteria. Generic screening criteria of interest to the risk management professional might include, "Did the patient sustain a fall during this admission?" or "Were all medications administered as ordered?" Although generic occurrence screening often provides information that duplicates that reported through incident reports, the systematic nature of the process may capture incidents that should have been reported, but were not. The major disadvantages of generic occurrence screening from a risk management perspective are the time lag inherent in reviewing records retrospectively, and the fact that only incidents meeting pre-selected criteria will be identified though the process.

FIGURE 4.1   Steps in Risk Management Decision Making

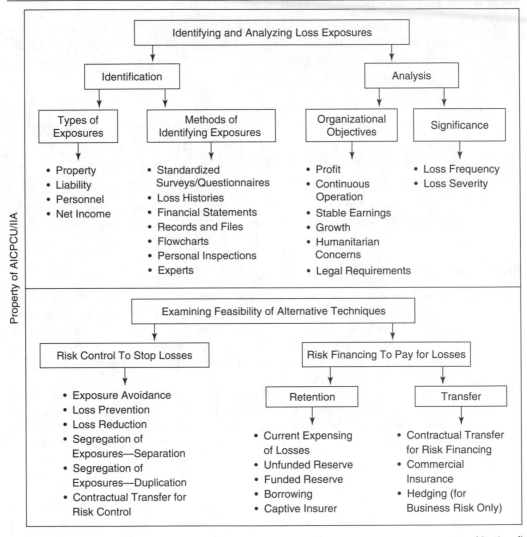

(Continued)

- **Patient complaints and satisfaction survey results.** Survey data tallied by patient representatives (or community relations or marketing departments) is another source of risk management information. Such survey results may provide insight into individual patient issues, and may offer aggregate trend data regarding patient experiences with the health care organization.

- **Prior medical professional liability, property and casualty, and workers' compensation claims data.** The analysis of such claims is a frequently used and valuable risk identification tool. By studying the specific services, procedures, and activities that have resulted in claims against the organization in the past, the risk management

FIGURE 4.1   Steps in Risk Management Decision Making (*Continued*)

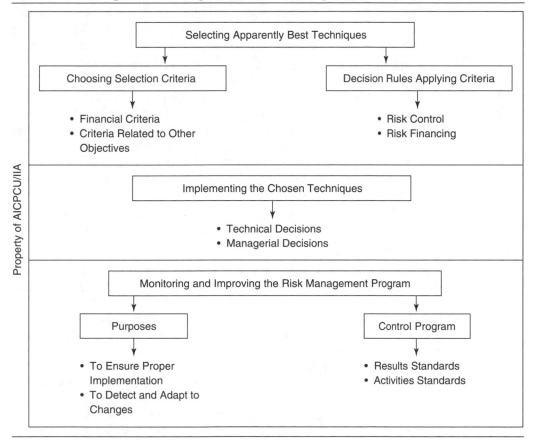

Source: George L. Head and Stephen Horn II, *Essentials of Risk Management*, 3rd ed., vol. 1 (Malvern, PA: Insurance Institute of America, 1997), p. 15. Reprinted with permission.

professional is in a better position to anticipate future areas of concern and take appropriate action to mitigate subsequent losses.

- **Surveys by the JCAHO,[21] the National Committee on Quality Assurance (NCQA),[22] liability or other insurers, and risk management consultants.** Such survey processes help enable the risk management professional to identify sources of potential risk that might have previously been overlooked by the organization. Outside experts and consultants draw on their experience to provide insight into the risk identification process for the organization and compare the organization's performance with national standards, pointing out areas meriting the risk management professional's additional attention.

- **State licensure surveys.** These surveys play an important role in risk identification. Although sometimes less important in hospitals and acute care settings, state surveys are an important part of risk management programs in long-term care facilities and outpatient settings. Findings from such surveys frequently identify areas of concern for risk management and performance improvement staff, and guide loss prevention efforts.

- **Contracts, leases, and other agreements entered into by the health care facility.** The review of salient contract provisions entered into by the organization frequently reveals risk exposures that must be addressed through modification of the contract or agreement, insurance, or enhanced loss prevention activities.

- **Information generated through the facility's infection control and performance improvement functions.** The data generated through such related functions should be routinely reviewed by the risk management professional to the extent permitted by law. (Concerns have been expressed in some jurisdictions that free access to medical staff peer review information by a risk management professional, who might use it in part to prepare for the defense of medical professional liability claims, may waive statutory protections provided under state peer review protection statutes. The reader is advised to seek the counsel of an attorney with expertise in this area when developing a mechanism for reviewing such information.)

- Finally, informal discussions with line managers and other staff members are excellent sources of information about potential risks with which the risk management professional might previously have been unfamiliar.

Risk analysis is the process of determining the potential severity of the loss associated with an identified risk, and the probability that such a loss will occur. Together, those factors establish the seriousness of a risk and guide the risk management professional's selection of an appropriate risk treatment strategy. Risk management professionals need to give priority to the areas of greatest potential risk of financial loss, such as an anesthesia or obstetrical mishap, even though claims in these areas may occur infrequently. Ordinarily, less emphasis is given to small claims that occur frequently, unless the total costs associated with a certain type of incident are especially significant. Although risk analysis is, in part, an "art"—a judgment call based on the training, experience, and instincts of the risk management professional—it also is a "science" in that certain data and objective sources of information are taken into consideration in evaluating a given risk. In particular, closed claims data, which reveal the frequency and severity of prior losses, should be reviewed to gain insight into the analysis of current risks. The organization's legal counsel, insurance brokers, and insurance carriers may be consulted for additional information, or for more information on risk identification and analysis, see Chapter 20, "Early Warning Systems for Identification of Organizational Risk," in this volume.

Step 2—Examine Risk Management Techniques or Treatments

Risk management techniques or treatments refer to the range of choices available to the risk management professionals in handling a given risk. Risk treatment strategies include two general categories: risk control and risk financing. Risk control involves preventing losses or mitigating the magnitude of the loss, while risk financing involves paying for those losses that do occur.

Risk Control Risk control includes the following treatments or techniques:

- Exposure avoidance
- Loss prevention
- Loss reduction
- Segregation of loss exposures (separation or duplication)
- Contractual transfer for risk control

Exposure Avoidance   Exposure avoidance reduces the possibility of a loss to "zero." Whereas other risk control techniques will reduce the frequency or severity of a loss, avoidance is the only risk control technique to eliminate any possibility for the loss to occur. When a given risk poses a particularly serious threat that cannot be effectively reduced or transferred, think about eliminating it. For example, a hospital might elect not to provide obstetrical services, thereby avoiding the risk of a birth trauma claim. Although the strategy might be very effective in terms of controlling risk exposure, it could come at the high cost of a loss of hospital mission effectiveness, market share, revenues, patient satisfaction, and medical staff relations, which could outweigh the risk management benefit of the avoidance technique.

Loss Prevention   Loss prevention as a risk control technique reduces the likelihood of an untoward event occurring and focuses on reducing the frequency of loss. Loss prevention efforts are at the core of most health care risk management programs, are proactive in nature, and include staff education, policy, and procedure review and revision. These interventions aim to control the number of adverse occurrences without unduly eliminating potentially risky activities.

Loss Reduction   Loss reduction or minimization involves various loss control strategies aimed at limiting the potential consequences of a given risk without totally accepting or avoiding them, thus focusing on reducing the severity of losses. Loss reduction or minimization efforts may also include risk management techniques, such as establishing and maintaining a rapport with injured patients and their families, thus limiting the severity of a loss that has already occurred. Other loss reduction treatments include: prompt incident investigation, disaster and business continuity drills, written plans to support emergency management, fire drills, and building structures equipped with sprinkler and alarm systems. Also, a facility offering obstetrical services may develop a protocol to save placentas from births meeting certain criteria for pathological review. Such an examination may encourage an early settlement if the examination is unfavorable and does not support quality care. If the review does support the care rendered, the pathological findings become a defense tool in any subsequent claim against the facility or the practitioner. Although such a process does not prevent poor obstetrical outcome, it tends to reduce the potential financial consequences of such occurrences to the organization.

Accreditation agencies such as the JCAHO have instituted formal requirements for clinical loss prevention efforts, such as prescribed root cause analysis (RCA) and failure mode and effects analysis (FMEA) processes. These analytical methodologies have long been intuitively applied by risk management professionals and are considered key patient safety and risk control activities. RCA represents a systematic approach to identifying the underlying causes of adverse occurrences so that effective steps can be taken to modify processes and prevent future losses. Through the use of FMEA, organizations analyze processes associated with high-risk procedures and clinical services so as to identify weaknesses in systems before a problem actually occurs. The processes examined need not be complex, but typically are those that can have serious consequences if a systems failure occurs. The Universal Protocol, a methodology adopted by health care organizations to reduce the occurrence of wrong-site surgeries, was the result of an FMEA process.[23]

Segregation of Loss Exposures   The fourth risk control technique is segregation of loss exposures. This technique involves arranging an organization's activities and resources so that if a loss occurs, it will not affect the entire organization. Segregation of loss exposures consists of two categories: separation and duplication. Separation, when properly applied, results in the distribution of a particular activity or asset over several locations, thereby confining the extent of the loss to only a portion of the organization should a loss occur at a single location. For example, a medical supply company might distribute its inventory among multiple warehouses or purchase supplies from different vendors to reduce the potential losses associated with a warehouse or manufacturing plant fire. In a medical office, separation may be evidenced by obtaining medications from multiple suppliers, and the practitioner maintaining staff privileges at several hospitals. Duplication results in a reserve, or substitute for a product or service, being available for use even if the primary source or activity is affected by a loss. Keeping duplicate electronic records and computer files is a form of duplication. Although duplication of records is generally a convenient method to mitigate loss, duplicate records and files should be stored off-site to prevent accidental loss.

Risk Financing   Risk financing strategies include many ways to generate funds to pay for losses that risk control techniques do not entirely eliminate. These treatment techniques include both risk retention and risk transfer.

Risk Retention   One strategy for managing an identified risk is risk retention. This treatment strategy involves assuming the potential losses associated with a given risk and making plans to cover the financial consequences of such losses. The retention options open to health care organizations include the current expensing of losses, using an unfunded loss reserve (an accounting entry denoting a potential liability to pay for a loss), using a funded loss reserve (a reserve backed by set-aside funds within the organization), borrowing funds to pay for losses, and providing insurance through an affiliated captive insurer.[24] Another (less thought of) form of risk retention occurs when the risk of exposure to loss is unknown and has not been identified by the organization or risk management professional, and therefore the opportunity to evaluate appropriate risk financing strategies is lost. Failure to identify a risk will result in unwitting risk retention unless insurance coverage is available under an existing policy. Risk retention is most appropriate for managing: (1) those risks that cannot be otherwise reduced, transferred, or avoided; (2) those risks for which the probability of loss is not great and for which the potential consequences are within the institution's ability to self-fund; (3) those losses that are quantifiable and predictable; and (4) those small risks (such as missing dentures and eyeglasses) for which the purchase of cost-effective insurance coverage might not be feasible.

For purposes of illustration, assume that a risk management professional has identified a risk of injuries related to misdiagnosis of patients seen in the facility's emergency department. Because the hospital's governing board and administration might have identified the provision of emergency services as central to both its mission and market-positioning strategy, the hospital is unwilling to forgo providing such services as a means of eliminating the risk. The hospital may then choose to self-insure for losses associated with injuries (retention) or perhaps purchase an insurance policy to cover such losses (a risk transfer strategy). The purchase of insurance combined with a deductible, or a program of primary self-insurance, may be a viable option to help reduce cost. Likewise, a physician's office practice in California may elect (absent any loan covenants, mortgage restrictions, or regulatory requirements to the contrary) not to purchase earthquake insurance coverage on its office building. The risk management professional may determine that the chances of the building being seriously damaged or destroyed in an earthquake are sufficiently remote and the costs of securing such coverage are sufficiently high to merit "going bare" for the exposure. If such a risk retention strategy is selected, it may be appropriate for the risk management professional to increase loss prevention and loss reduction efforts, such as the installation of sway bracing near sprinkler heads to reduce potential water damage in the event of an earthquake. Thus risk retention, like other available risk treatment strategies, should not be viewed in isolation, but rather as part of an overall strategy for managing an identified risk.

Risk Transfer   Contractual transfer techniques for risk financing involve shifting the financial obligation for a loss, but not the ultimate legal responsibilities for losses, to an outside entity, through the purchase of insurance from a third-party, unaffiliated insurer or non-insurance transfer through a contract provision, commonly described as a hold-harmless agreement. Through risk transfer an institution can continue to engage in a risk-producing activity while transferring the financial risk of loss to another party. For example, a hospital may purchase a medical professional liability policy to pay for any losses associated with medical malpractice, thereby transferring the financial obligation for the loss to an insurance company while remaining legally liable for patient injuries caused by the negligence of its staff.

Step 3—Select Best Risk Management Technique(s)

Selecting the best risk management technique or treatment for a specific situation is a two-part activity. The first step requires forecasting the effects that the available risk management options are likely to have on the organization's ability to fulfill its goals. The second is defining and applying criteria that measure how well each alternative risk management technique contributes to the organization's objectives in a cost-effective way.[25] For most identified risks, the health care facility will employ a combination of risk treatment and risk financing techniques to manage a given risk. At a minimum, one risk control technique and one risk financing technique should be combined to address each significant exposure. The risk management professional may elect to employ any available combination of risk control and risk financing techniques to obtain the desired results. Typically, health care organizations accept a certain amount of patient care liability risk through an insurance deductible or self-insured retention; attempt to limit potential risk by not offering some inherently high-risk services; seek to reduce the severity of loss for incidents that have already occurred through prompt incident investigation and claim resolution; prevent future losses through in-service education, appropriate staffing, and credentialing; and transfer the remaining financial risk by purchasing insurance.

Step 4—Implement the Selected Technique

The implementation process involves both the technical risk management decisions that must be made by risk management professionals and the related decisions that are made by other managers within the organization to implement the chosen risk management technique(s). Technical expertise exercised by risk management professionals may include selecting an appropriate insurer and choosing appropriate policy limits and deductibles. In working with managers and other personnel, risk management professionals advise and influences others in implementing selected techniques that are not within their direct areas of responsibility.

Step 5—Monitor, Evaluate, and Improve the Risk Management Program

The final step in the risk management process is to evaluate and monitor the effectiveness of the risk management program by assessing the adequacy and appropriateness of the techniques employed to identify, analyze, and treat risks. Risk management evaluation involves not only the risk management professional, but also senior management, medical staff and governing board, insurers, claims managers, and legal counsel. A multidisciplinary approach to evaluating the risk management program ensures that the impact of risk management activities on various constituencies is measured accurately, and that additional opportunities to improve the risk management function are fully explored. To facilitate the risk management evaluation process, the risk management professional needs to prepare a comprehensive annual report of risk management efforts, highlighting significant claims activity, new program developments, changes in insurance coverage, and contractual modifications having risk management significance. These results should be compared against clearly defined benchmarks that have been identified in advance of the review. Such benchmarks can be internal or external to the organization and may be as simple as comparing the current program results against those from the previous year. The risk management professional can also use data from independent but similar organizations against which to benchmark. Benchmarks frequently include a comparison of claims data. Claims data provide frequency and severity information for losses incurred, including the number of events reported and dollars spent to defend and settle them. For more on benchmarking and program evaluation, refer to Chapter 6 on Risk Management Metrics.

EVOLUTION OF THE RISK MANAGEMENT PROGRAM

As the delivery of health care continues to change, so must the structure of risk management programs. The existing and emerging principles that apply to risk management will need to adapt to ensure safe, cost-effective, and clinically effective care. The health care organization as it is known today will be different in the future, with multiple levels and both horizontal and vertical integration. Interdependency on organizational strategic and financial goals must be integrated into risk management program development and must meet the needs of the changing customer base and payer mix. It is possible that within one organization there will be a need to create different risk management program structures and take different steps in assessing risk management needs in the health organization's different areas.

SELECTING AN APPROPRIATE RISK MANAGEMENT PROGRAM STRUCTURE

A variety of risk management program structures can be considered based on organizational size, scope of services and activities, available resources, and locations. Generally, acute-care hospitals have preexisting systems that introduce and enhance risk management program components, whereas integrated delivery systems (IDSs), long-term care settings, physician's office practices, home health care, and ambulatory care centers are less likely to have formalized risk management efforts.

The overall level of risk management responsibility can vary greatly. It can be any one of the following (or a combination, depending on organizational structure and expectations):

- **All related risk management functions:** In a traditional model, this structure requires an experienced risk management professional and a vast array of resources that can address each type of service provided within the organization. Knowledge of and experience in clinical care delivery, plant engineering, safety, claims, and finance are particularly helpful in large, multi-institutional organizations. The more recent enterprise risk management model encompasses strategic planning, marketing, and even branding components. In many situations, on-site risk management coordinators integrate activities with the corporate or home office. In many smaller organizations, all related risk management activities may be managed by one department or by one person. A physician's office practice is an example where one employee may have responsibility for risk management, quality improvement, safety, medical records, disaster planning, infection control, and so on.

- **Responsibility for a set of defined risk management activities and services:** This structure continues to be the model of choice at community hospitals and hospitals in a system. Responsibility in this structure is spread among multiple departments. The coordination and facilitation of activities that affect risk management activities should still be managed and controlled out of a single office, preferably the risk management department. In this model there are generally separate departments for safety, security, quality improvement, corporate compliance, education and in-service, risk financing, contract review and negotiating, claims administration, and so on. For example, the CFO may have responsibility for the risk financing program, in-house legal administration may have responsibility for the claims administration and contract review, or the director of the emergency department may have responsibility for disaster planning, to give a few examples. The hospital or other health care setting that is part of an organized health system also has a limit to the breadth and depth of risk management responsibility at the local level. In many cases, the corporate office mandates the risk financing program and may also manage all claims. Risk management positions at the local site generally revolve around loss control activities and are far more common than control of all risk management functions. The intent of system-wide programs is to create a general operational structure that encourages consistency and cost control while allowing for flexibility, timeliness, and accountability at the lowest possible levels.

- **Consultative and outsourcing only:** At specific times, an organization may choose to supplement its risk management functions. Consistent with the consulting and outsourcing structure model is a process to internally manage the flow of information and facilitate communication. Consultative and outsourcing structures are commonly used during times of merger, acquisition, and divestiture, when the organization faces severe financial constraints, has a loss of key risk management personnel, is undergoing reengineering efforts, or management change. It is not unusual that in this structure there is still the need for a risk management professional. This individual then becomes the contact point between the outsourced organization or consultant and senior management, and the outsourced organization becomes the risk management "backroom."

Regardless of the health care organization's choice of formal structure, its risk management program should incorporate the basic elements, components, and functions described throughout this chapter. All risk management activities require alignment with the organization's mission and strategic plan.

. . . .

ASSESSING AREAS OF THE ORGANIZATION THAT NEED RISK MANAGEMENT

A critical factor is that an assessment methodology might vary, but consistency in its application should be maintained. Assessment findings, and any improvement strategies, should be presented uniformly so that the organization and individuals maintain a clear understanding of the findings and resulting recommendations.

There are various ways to approach any assessment, but most risk management professionals find that having written guidelines helps avoid overlooking key points. There are many tools from which to choose, one of which is the *Risk Management Self-Assessment Manual* (2000).[26] Other sources can be found through literature searches and in outside organizations such as insurance companies, regulatory agencies, and consulting firms.

Identify the Various Areas for Assessment

Because assessments can take time, after evaluating basic organizational structures, the focus usually should start with high-risk, high-volume, and high-visibility areas. In multi-institutional organizations, assessments should be tailored so that organization-wide processes and institutional specific programs are assessed. This will allow for more comprehensive findings that reflect the organizational status.

In general, profiling the organization's current services and business relationships is important in identifying the various areas for assessment. The assessment process should include the organization on an enterprise-wide basis, assessing it from an operational, clinical, and business perspective. This process could be viewed as "taking inventory" of activities that might have potential risk, and as finding a starting point for developing or renewing the risk management program's focus. This inventory includes a systematic review of the organization's functions, data, budget, and workforce, and a survey of perceptions about the effectiveness of systems and processes already in place. The assessment may reveal findings and needs that differ according to the organization's various areas. An example could be if an organization decides to institute a research department, but lacks a defined and operational institutional review board, which could result in regulatory noncompliance and direct-patient risk.

Analyzing Current Systems

The second phase of the assessment is to analyze those systems that are already in place for minimizing risk and then determine current effectiveness. Profiles should include identification of key contacts and responsibilities, level and types of risk financing, contractual relationships, and risk management activities (including policies, orientation, job and credentialing requirements, integration into current organizational structure, and safety and quality program integration). Areas or topics to be inventoried may include:

- Educational relationships—levels and types of agreements, formal or informal.
- Staff relationships—employed, contracted, independent, network where staff float from one entity of a large organization to another), or consulting (may involve the assessment of staff issues).

- Scope of services—not only types, but also where and to what degree. This also might include reporting relationships.
- Subsidiaries owned, partnered, or otherwise associated with the organization.
- Accreditations, licenses, certifications, or other designations in which any or all parts of the organization participate.
- Human resources issues, with focus on pre-employment screening, ongoing competency evaluation, and staffing.
- Information management methodologies, computerized information and access, and other information issues such as retention and release.
- Clinical technology issues—selection, maintenance, user training, and product and equipment problem-tracking systems, and level of support technology such as bar coding and order entry software.
- Level of consistent application of systems throughout the organization.
- Assessment of the organizational core values, including philosophy and practice with regard to disclosure and non-punitive environment.
- Loss assessment data, loss runs, and results of inspection by regulatory agencies.
- Credentialing and orientation processes for non-employee staff, both initially and at reappointment.
- Contract management protocols.
- The safety and quality management program structure and its integration and effectiveness.
- Emergency preparedness protocols and emergency management relationships external to the organization.

Assessing Compliance

Risk management programs must meet not only organizational needs, but also provide support for meeting the requirements of outside entities that, by either choice or mandate, make demands on the health care organization's operation. The demands in the managed care market may not come with only a list of activities and reporting provisions, but also might require that certain accreditations be maintained. Rules set forth by regulatory agencies must also be factored into the activities and processes as the risk management program develops and expands. One should first review and analyze the most recent findings of all external reviews, inspections, and surveys, and any reports from consultants. These reports and the status of the action taken in response, along with appropriate standards issued by various bodies, can be used to compile assessment tools that can assist in evaluating the risk management program and in planning for improvement. During this review of external demands, attention to the organization's ability to identify, track, and integrate external mandates also should be assessed.

Reviewing the Assessments

Assessments are often performed to identify risk management program strengths and opportunities for improvement. Analysis should include categorizing findings according to severity, frequency, effect on the organization's strategic plan, areas identified for improvement, and best practices identified. Good practice without supporting documentation should be assessed as both a practice strength and an information weakness. For example, even if it is identified that the patient care process might need no immediate attention, the recording or tracking of patient care information well might require integration into a better-defined information process, to substantiate practice patterns.

Setting Priorities for Program Implementation

Established risk management programs should undergo continuous reassessment, particularly as new areas are added or for those previously identified as weak. Regulations and other external mandates, along with areas of severe loss, should command the most immediate attention. Organizational emphasis (what the strategic plan and the mission support) also will need to be factored into the list of areas to be addressed first. One useful tool is to map out a strategy to take advantage of the many activities that are interdependent. Some risk management activities that might seem less important may need to be initiated to lay the groundwork for success in high-impact areas. An example might be the development of user-friendly reporting or early identification tools that are adapted for the organization's various departments and services. Such a project could be multidisciplinary and supported by various areas within the organization, which can lead to an enhanced quality-improvement database. In setting priorities for program implementation, risk management professionals should clearly define the desired outcome. Having done an analysis, the risk management professional should be aware of the organization's strengths and weaknesses, and of improvements or expansions that need to be accomplished. Preliminary work may consist of collecting data and drafting early versions of future measurement tools. An other key item is to identify levels of understanding, not only during the assessment, but also once an analysis is formulated. The result of action or inaction must be clearly defined in relation to the direct effect on the organization.

....

KEY COMPONENTS FOR GETTING STARTED

For any risk management program to achieve its goals, several key components must be in place. Organizational commitment—that is, acceptance of roles and support for program aspects by the various levels of leadership, starting with the board—is a necessity. Commitment is often demonstrated through assignments of responsibility, commitment to accountability systems, approval of the program, and participation in aspects requiring support and action. The ultimate goal is to achieve integration of risk management components, systems, and strategies into the overall organizational culture of safety.

Access to all levels of the organization, with defined accountabilities and identification of resources, also is part of the initial structure formation. No risk management program can function in isolation; its integration with other initiatives, particularly safety, is critical to its success. By relying on already established relationships, risk management professionals can enhance programs with limited resources by strengthening operational linkages and avoiding duplication of efforts. Negative perceptions about the risk management program might damage its credibility before it even gets under way. Physicians often perceive that risk management's involvement after an event has occurred only makes matters worse or that the only motivation is to minimize costs. Frequently, risk management programs are viewed as reactive to crisis rather than proactive in creating a safe culture.

Risk management activities should focus on support and service, using facilitative techniques in guiding the clinicians' understanding of the nonnegotiable forces (regulatory fines, accreditations, citations, and agency requirements) and the alternatives available. Clinical staff should have input into not only the risk management process but also the analysis, redesign, and monitoring stages. Most program elements that affect clinical functions require that the clinical staff members become committed to risk management concepts and understand the desired outcome. Ensuring that duplication of effort is minimized can be a key selling point to staff members in accepting their roles in the risk management effort. Simplification of any process is always welcome. A method for seeking continual staff feedback also should be developed to ensure ownership of the program by all staff.

....

WRITING A RISK MANAGEMENT PROGRAM PLAN

The written risk management program plan includes an overview of the purpose, structure, and process of risk management activities within the organization. Within this framework, organizational performance objectives can be developed in addition to policies and guidelines to support the identified processes that maximize achievement of the program's objectives. It is critical to maintain an integrated approach at this point of development to achieve a consistency of purpose within the organization and to avoid duplication of effort. Rather than create new systems for the risk management process, the risk management professional should evaluate how best to enhance existing systems.

As with all programs that have a data collection and monitoring function, reports, memos, and minutes will be generated as communication tools. To be most effective, these tools must meet the needs of those responsible for the implementation and change of risk management and safety practices. Therefore, it is important that those served by such information have input into its ultimate design and format as a means of maximizing its usefulness. (Refer to Exhibit 4.1 for a sample risk management program plan).

....

ACHIEVING PROGRAM ACCEPTANCE

Often the quickest way to gain support for a program is to provide visibility and education on its related topics. A well-designed risk management program will not be successful unless staff members at all levels understand its purpose and methods. In some cases, the risk management professional may even provide unrelated services simply as a means to gain the acceptance and trust vital to the program's success. Often the support of an interested medical staff member serving as an advocate familiarizes others with the merits of the risk management program. The risk management program achieves visibility through participation in employee orientation and continuing education activities. Focus on prevention aspects of risk management creates a less threatening atmosphere and aligns efforts with the ever-increasing focus on safety. Maintaining a subject file on risk management topics such as consent, information release, falls, medication process, human factors that contribute to error prone behavior, and credentialing allows the risk management professional to have supplemental resources when participating in education and quality and performance improvement projects. Another strategy is to become involved in the organization's efforts in responding to external initiatives or mandates such as JCAHO National Safety Goals, insurance carrier criteria, state licensing requirements, and Conditions of Participation from CMS.

EXHIBIT 4.1   Risk Management Program (Sample)

POLICY

Risk Management Program Plan

PURPOSE

The Risk Management Program is designed to protect the human and financial assets of the organization against the adverse effects of accidental losses, effectively managing losses that may occur, and to enhance continuous improvement of patient care services in a safe healthcare environment.

    Risk Management is the process of creating and implementing strategies directed at minimizing the adverse effects of accidental loss on the (Entity's) human, physical, and financial assets through the identification and assessment of loss potential and selection of appropriate loss assumption, transfer, prevention, and control mechanisms.

AUTHORITY

The governing body has the ultimate responsibility to assure the provision of a safe environment. The governing body delegates authority for the establishment of a comprehensive, organization-wide risk management program to (Entity) administration.

SCOPE

The Risk Management Program is designed to identify, assess, prevent, and control losses that arise from employee work-related injury, liability, property, regulatory compliance and other loss exposures arising from operations.

    The Risk Management Program involves loss prevention, control, and continuous quality improvement activities. Team effort to implement the risk management program will include physicians, administrators, management, supervisors, and line employees to identify, review, evaluate, and control risks that interfere with quality patient care, safety and services rendered in the (Entity) and to take appropriate corrective and preventive action as necessary.

PROGRAM ELEMENTS

The Risk Management Program at (Entity) will utilize a five-step process which includes:

1. Identification of potential loss exposures;
2. Assessing the feasibility of alternative techniques to treat the exposure identified;
3. Selecting the appropriate risk management technique;
4. Implementing the chosen technique; and
5. Monitoring the effectiveness of the action taken.

OBJECTIVES

The objectives of the Risk Management Program are to preserve the assets, reputation, and quality of care of (Entity) by utilizing a process to identify, reduce, or eliminate the risk of loss.

    To meet these objectives, the Risk Management Program will undertake the following activities:

1. Administer all insurance or self-insurance programs so as to maximize coverage and minimize expenses;
2. Inspect all (Entity) premises to discover and correct potentially hazardous conditions which may present unnecessary risk to employees, patients, and others;
3. Review the performance of all persons providing care to patients to identify and correct practices which may present unnecessary risks to patients or deviate from acceptable practices;
4. Review policies and procedures to update, amend, edit, and revise to reflect appropriate care, legislative requirements, and minimize or prevent liability ramifications;
5. Investigate adverse occurrences to assess and determine how similar occurrences might be averted and to control the loss related to the adverse occurrence;
6. Handle complaints and grievances to resolve disputes and improve patient care and associated services;
7. Coordinate the local management of claims against (Entity) in a timely, organized, and cost effective manner as required by coverage documents; and
8. Organize educational programs on risk management topics to promote awareness of risk management issues and safer practices.

(Continued)

EXHIBIT 4.1   Risk Management Program (Sample) (*Continued*)

PROGRAM PLAN

1. GOVERNING BODY

    The Governing Body has the ultimate responsibility to assure that a Risk Management Program is established and implemented. The Governing Body will delegate the responsibility for the Risk Management Program to (Administrative Vice President or President).

    In discharging its responsibilities for the Risk Management Program, the Governing Body will:
    a. Assure that a comprehensive, ongoing and effective Risk Management Program is in place;
    b. Assure that significant deficiencies identified by the risk management process are corrected;
    c. Assure financial and administrative support necessary for the effective implementation of the Risk Management Program;
    d. Receive periodic reports on Risk Management Program activities as described in the plan.

2. ADMINISTRATION

    (Entity) administration actively supports the Risk Management Program. Administration is responsible for the general management of (Entity) and authorized to act on behalf of the Governing Body to assist with the implementation of the Risk Management Program and related activities. Administration/management
    a. Assigns accountability for Risk Management Program components within (Entity) as follows:

    Clinical Risk

    (Title): _____

    Essential functions:
        Quality assurance, utilization review, infection control, pharmacy and therapeutics, medical staff credentialing and committees, and clinical practice guidelines or standards

    Regulatory/Accreditation/Licensing Risks

    (Title): _____

    Essential functions:
        Safety management and loss control, employee accidents, department hazard analysis, equipment management, plant safety and management including fire suppression, Safe Medical Device Act compliance, EMTALA compliance, and OSHA compliance programs

    Business Risk

    (Title): _____

    Essential functions:
        Risk financing and insurance, employee benefits and workers' compensation, employment practices, contract review systems, administration and operational activities, disaster planning and preparedness, and security systems
    b. Support the integration of the Risk Management Program into the overall management control system used to evaluate the delivery of quality care and services;
    c. Participate in the review and evaluation of patient care and safety within (Entity);
    d. Identify, implement, and support corrective action plans for (Entity) related to the Risk Management Program; and
    e. Monitor results for effectiveness of techniques employed to manage risks for (Entity), and make any adjustments necessary to the corrective action plan.

3. PROFESSIONAL STAFF (Physicians, Nurses, and other licensed health care practitioners)

    The professional staff are responsible for providing diagnostic and therapeutic medical care, and:
    a. Actively participating in the functions of the Risk Management Program by monitoring, evaluating, and maintaining applicable standards of care within his/her licensure and position;
    b. Report variances in care to responsible individuals in order to identify and resolve clinical risks;
    c. Identify, recommend, and implement corrective action needed.

INTEGRATION WITH KEY ASPECTS OF OPERATIONS

The Risk Management Program interfaces with other key aspects of operations and shares pertinent information as appropriate with organizational functions/committees such as:

1. Quality Management
2. Medical Staff Services

(Continued)

EXHIBIT 4.1   Risk Management Program (Sample) *(Continued)*

---

3. Human Resources
4. Utilization Management
5. Performance Improvement
6. Safety
7. Infection Control
8. Medical Records
9. Patient Billing Office
10. Security

CONFIDENTIALITY

Risk management documents and records include information which relate to sensitive patient and provider information. It is the intent of this Risk Management Program to apply all existing legal standards and state or federal statutes to provide protection to the documents, proceedings and individuals involved in the program.

Any and all documents and records that are part of the internal Risk Management Program, as well as the proceedings, reports and records from any of the involved committees, shall be maintained in a confidential manner. Disclosure to any judicial or administrative proceeding will occur only under a court order or legal mandate. The Risk Management Program will ensure:

1. Documents/records generated as part of the organizational Risk Management Program, as well as the proceedings, reports/records are to be confidential and subject to the state and federal laws protecting such documents from discovery.
2. Copies of minutes, reports, worksheets, and other data summaries related to risk management are stored in a manner to maintain strict confidentiality.
3. Employees, volunteers, and physicians/medical staff are obligated to maintain complete confidentiality of all pertinent information to protect patient rights, as required by state and federal law.

EVALUATION OF THE RISK MANAGEMENT PROGRAM

The Risk Management Program and (Entity's) progress toward achieving objectives listed in this plan will be reviewed at least annually by the Governing Body of (Entity).

Approval:

_____   _____

Governing Body (Board Chair)   Date

_____   _____

President/CEO   Date

_____   _____

Medical Staff President   Date

Adventist Health, 2005 Reprinted with permission

············

CONCLUSION

Establishing a risk management program is no simple task, particularly in today's complex health care environment. Assessment of the health care organization's internal and external relationships and forces will provide an excellent basis for the issues the risk management program must address. Establishing risk management's role in the overall safety initiatives and safety culture development must also be included in the risk management program. Obtaining commitment to the program from all levels of the organization, top to bottom, can be a slow process, but must be achieved for full integration to occur. Translating a written plan into functional risk management processes requires collaboration and facilitation skills now more than ever. No matter how defined the risk management plan, the program will always be evolving as it adapts to the changes in health care.

Endnotes

1. Kuhn, A. M. "Introduction to Risk Management." In B. J. Youngberg (ed.), *The Risk Manager's Desk Reference.* Gaithersburg, Md.: Aspen Publishers, 1988.

2. *Ibid.*, p. 1.

3. *Ibid.*

4. Taravella, S. "The Rise of Risk Management." *Modern Healthcare,* Oct. 8, 1990.

5. *Ibid.*

6. Kohn, L. T., Corrigan, J. M., and Donaldson, M. S. (eds). *To Err is Human: Building a Safer Health System.* Washington, D.C. National Academy Press, 1999.

7. Joint Commission on Accreditation of Healthcare Organizations. *2005 Comprehensive Accreditation Manual for Hospitals.* Oakbrook Terrace, Ill.: JCAHO, 2004.

8. The Health Insurance Portability and Accountability Act of 1996 (Public Law 104–191); 45 CFR Parts 160 and 164 (August 14, 2002). The Sarbanes-Oxley Reform Act (Public Law 107–204); 116 Stat.746, US Code Title 15, Section 7201 et seq.

9. JCAHO, *op. cit.*

10. *Medical Malpractice: Verdicts, Settlements and Statistical Analysis.* Horsham, Pa.: LRP Publications, 2002.

11. "What's Ahead on the Medical Liability Front in 2002?" *Medical Liability Monitor,* 27(1), January 21, 2002.

12. *Ibid.*

13. *Ibid.*

14. 42 U.S.C. 1320.

15. *Laughinhouse v. Risser,* 786 F. Supp. 920 (Kan. 1992).

16. *Trotta v. Mobil Oil Corp.,* 798 F. Supp. 1336 (DC NY 1992).

17. *Jewell v. Palmer Broadcasting Ltd.,* Iowa District Ct. No. CL94–56040, Dec. 30, 1993.

18. Gamble, R. H. "The Insurance Renewal Marathon," www.BusinessFinancialMag.com. Last visited February 2002.

19. Hazard Communication Standard. Final Rule. Occupational Safety and Health Administration. 29 CFR.1910.1200.

20. Head, G., and Kudk-ske, R. *Risk Management for Public Entities.* Malvern, Pa.: Center for the Advancement of Risk Management Education, 1999, pp. 4–5.

21. JCAHO, *op. cit.*

22. National Committee on Quality Assurance. NCQA Standards for Accreditation (CR 8.0, CR 13.0) Washington, D.C.: NCQA, 1995.

23. Joint Commission on Accreditation of Healthcare Organizations. Universal Protocol for Preventing Wrong Site, Wrong Procedure, Wrong Person Surgery™ (Effective July 1, 2004.)

24. Head, and Kudk-ske, *op.cit,* pp. 4–5.

25. *Ibid.*

26. "ASHRM Risk Management Index Measures Task Force." *Risk Management Self-Assessment Manual.* Chicago: American Hospital Association, 2000.

Suggested Readings

Brown, B. L. *Risk Management for Hospitals: A Practical Approach.* Rockville, Md.: Aspen Publishers, 1979.

Healthcare Risk Control (published monthly by the Emergency Care Research Institute [ECRI], 5200 Butler Pike, Plymouth Meeting, Pa. 19462).

Hospital Peer Review (published monthly by American Health Consultants, Inc., 3525 Piedmont Rd. N.E., Bldg. 6, Ste. 400, Atlanta, Ga. 30305).

Hospital Risk Management (published monthly by American Health Consultants, Inc., 3525 Piedmont Rd. N.E., Bldg. 6, Ste. 400, Atlanta, Ga. 30305).

Jessee, W. F. *Quality of Care Issues for the Hospital Trustee: A Practical Guide to Fulfilling Trustee Responsibilities.* Chicago: Hospital Research and Educational Trust, 1984.

Journal of Healthcare Risk Management (published quarterly by the American Society for Healthcare Risk Management of the American Hospital Association, One North Franklin, Chicago, Ill. 60606).

Hospital Patient Safety Standards: Examples of Compliance. JCAHO Chicago: Joint Commission Resources, 2002.

Kraus, G. P. *Health Care Risk Management: Organization and Claims Administration.* Owings Mills, Md.: National Health Publishing Co., 1986.

Risk Management Pearls Series (published by the American Society for Healthcare Risk Management of the American Hospital Association, One North Franklin, Chicago, Ill. 60606).

Rowland, H., and Rowland, B. *Hospital Risk Management: Forms, Checklists, and Guidelines.* Gaithersburg, Md.: Aspen Publishers, 1993.

5

The Health Care Risk Management Professional

Jeannie Sedwick

Jeannie Sedwick

....

OVERVIEW

Health care has changed dramatically over the past thirty-five years, and this has led to an expansion in the role and responsibilities of health care risk management professionals. In the early years of the profession, health care risk managers focused primarily on exposures that related to general and professional liability. Today, health care risk management professionals must manage not only those exposures, but also exposures that relate to managed care and capitation risks, mergers and acquisitions, employment and workers' compensation risks, and risks related to corporate compliance and organizational ethics. Despite the significant changes in health care over the past three and a half decades, the risk management process has remained virtually unchanged and continues to serve the same purpose: to maintain a safe and effective health care environment for patients, visitors, and employees, thereby preventing or reducing loss to the organization. Many risk management professionals are adopting the enterprise risk management (ERM) approach, described as a comprehensive process that evaluates all risk exposures confronting an organization from the top down. ERM is a discipline broad in scope and reflects an organization-wide, ongoing commitment to risk management principles. To be effective, ERM should be part of the organization's strategic plan and viewed as a *proactive,* and also a *reactive* process.[1] The basics of health care enterprise risk management were discussed in more detail in Chapter 1.

This chapter provides an overview of the role of the health care risk management professional and the skills necessary for performing this function in an ever-changing health care environment. Information is provided about the educational and experiential backgrounds of risk management professionals, and about commonly held designations.

Information about the availability of educational programs for those who wish to enter the field, or for those in the field who wish to further their education, is also discussed.

. . . .

THE RISK MANAGER'S JOB—FUNCTIONAL AREAS OF RESPONSIBILITY

The roles and responsibilities of health care risk management professionals vary widely. Risk management program components—and therefore the role of the risk management professional—are greatly influenced by the size and structure of the organization and by the risk financing strategies it employs. The profession itself has evolved along functional needs and growing regulatory mandates, without benefit of extensive scientific study or a well-defined body of knowledge. Until recently, no attempt had been made to quantify the many activities that have come to make up the health care risk management professional's functional job responsibilities. Thus, it is not possible to describe the "typical" health care risk management professional's job.

The risk management professional often performs specific duties that may result in a variety of titles for the position. It is not unusual to see the risk management professional with a title of risk manager, chief risk officer, or patient safety officer, to encompass the expanding role and responsibilities of the health care risk professional. The evolving role of the chief risk officer (CRO) in the health care setting is gaining more visibility in larger organizations and usually resides at the senior management level. The title "Chief Risk Officer" was first used by James Lam, at GE Capital in 1993, to describe a function to manage "all aspects of risk," including risk management, back-office operations, and business and financial planning.[2] The CRO position is quickly finding a place in health care organizations to respond to increased regulatory pressures and a variety of business risks better known as ERM.

The role of the patient safety officer (PSO) is founded on the growth of the modern patient safety movement and new patient safety regulations and requirements. Restructuring within health care organizations so as to formalize the PSO responsibilities offers risk management professionals and others an opportunity to highlight their current contributions to patient safety, develop additional skills, and expand their profile. The job description for a patient safety officer can vary, but the basic functions are contained in Exhibit 5.1. Risk management professionals assuming the additional responsibilities of the PSO may need to enhance their job descriptions with the responsibilities in the level one, two, or three for the health care risk management professional as contained in Exhibits 5.2, 5.3, and 5.4, respectively. Additional information on the Patient Safety Officer Program can be found in Volume II, Chapter 1.

In 1999, the American Society for Healthcare Risk Management (ASHRM) conducted the first role delineation study in health care risk management.[3] The purpose of this study was to identify those activities that make up a health care risk management professional's job and thereby define health care risk management's body of knowledge. A list of approximately 160 task statements describing various risk management functions and activities was sent to 2,500 health care risk management professionals, who were asked to rate the importance of each task. The findings suggest that the health care risk management professional's job responsibilities can be divided into six major functional areas: loss prevention and reduction, claims management, risk financing, regulatory and accreditation compliance, risk management operations, and bioethics.

EXHIBIT 5.1   Patient Safety Officer Job Description

Position Summary

The Patient Safety Officer will supervise personnel responsible for the delivery of patient safety services and risk management. The Patient Safety Officer incorporates and utilizes methods to improve all aspects of patient safety, risk management, and quality. The PSO will oversee the collection, analysis and dissemination of PS data and information. The PSO will analyze clinical processes, identify potential risks for patients and employees and develop strategies to maximize safety, effectiveness and efficiency. The PSO will oversee the development and implementation of medical error reduction strategies in collaboration with all departments and patient care areas. Additionally, the Patient Safety Officer will be primarily responsible for communication and marketing related to patient safety initiatives.

Reports To: Chief Patient Safety and Quality Officer

PRINCIPAL ACCOUNTABILITIES AND ESSENTIAL DUTIES OF THE JOB

Service Excellence (100% of time)

- Provides excellent service to all customers, meeting or exceeding their needs/expectations, to ensure continuous improvement of customer-focused environment.
- Exemplifies excellent customer service towards physicians, patients, families, staff, visitors, co-workers and other departments. Shows courtesy, compassion, and respect in communication with all customers.
- Contributes to teamwork and harmonious working relationships.
- Partners with healthcare teams, patients and families to continuously solicit feedback and information to improve patient safety and quality. Actively supports patients, families and employees involved in serious PS events.

Provides clinical and operational guidance to all personnel performing patient safety and risk management duties (100% of time)

- Acts as coach and mentor to PS and Risk Management personnel, providing feedback about performance routinely.
- Performs all duties of manager at BJH including: hiring and firing, budget preparation, performance appraisals and other human resource/personnel functions.
- Assists Chief Patient Safety and Quality Officer and Chief Medical Officer with all responsibilities related to PS.

Responsible for Data Management, Analysis and Safety Event Reporting (30% of time)

- Oversees activities related to data collection, data review, analysis and dissemination of patient safety information.
- Reviews safety event data from Safety Event Reporting databases.
- Identifies trends, clusters, and risk factors; establishes benchmarks for comparison.
- Oversees the dissemination of accurate, user-friendly PS reports in a timely fashion to key stakeholders.
- Demonstrates expertise in use of PS software and databases.

Oversee all activities related to: Risk Prevention and Medical Error Reduction (30% of time)

- Uses risk factor data to develop evidence-based PS interventions and process improvement strategies.
- Collaborates with healthcare teams to rapidly identify risk, employ prevention and risk reduction strategies.
- Demonstrates expertise and participates in PI team facilitation, leadership and membership.
- Participates in Root Cause Analysis (RCA), Failure Mode and Effects Analysis (FMEA) and cluster investigation.
- Utilizes systems thinking, human factors and complexity science, principles of epidemiology and PI improvement to prevent and mitigate risk to patients and employees.

Education, Training and Safety Performance Maintenance (10% of time)

- Oversees the development and implementation of basic PS education and training curriculum, on-going training, employee orientation, and competency testing.
- Collaborates with clinical and administrative leaders to identify areas of educational need to enhance PS.
- Provides just-in-time education and routine PS presentations to key stakeholders.
- Actively participates in Patient Safety Council Forums and educational programs.
- Promotes a culture where errors and near-misses are openly discussed and used as learning opportunities.
- Provides education and consultation to patients, families, visitors and healthcare teams on PS issues.
- Conducts patient safety rounds to gather information and educate on routine basis.

(Continued)

EXHIBIT 5.1   Patient Safety Officer Job Description (*Continued*)

Committee and Team Responsibilities:

- Patient Safety and Quality Committee.
- PI, RCA, FMEA teams.
- Patient Safety Council.
- May be member of policy-making committees of hospital or medical staff (e.g., Infection Control Committee, Risk Mgt. & Safety Council, Pharmacy & Therapeutics, Unit Practice Council).

Experience and Position Requirements

- At least 10 years of clinical experience and 5 years of management experience preferred.
- Masters in nursing, public health or other related field required.
- Team building and budget experience required.
- Demonstrates excellent: written and verbal communication skills, computer proficiency, relationship management and conflict negotiation problem-solving skills.
- Use of quality improvement tools and methods preferred.

Reprinted, with permission, Barnes Jewish Hospital, 2005.

EXHIBIT 5.2   Risk Manager Position Description, Level One

Position Summary

The risk manager is responsible for the facility's risk management activities, which includes, but may not be limited to a general knowledge of facility insurance programs, managing claims against the facility, interfacing with defense legal counsel, administering the risk management program on a day-to-day basis, managing and analyzing risk management data, and conducting risk management educational programs, complying with risk management related standards by JCAHO and other accrediting and regulatory agencies with the objective of enhancing patient safety , promoting patient safety ,quality care, and minimizing loss to protect the assets of the facility. This individual participates in formulating policy and/or organizational changes, but must seek advice and approval from higher authority. Risk management may be one of several areas of responsibility for this individual.

OPERATIONS/COMPLIANCE

Overview

The level one risk manager has specific responsibilities regarding gathering and analyzing data and preparing reports to management and outside agencies as required, which may be subject to final approval by facility management. Responsible for keeping management advised of developments in professional liability, entailing ongoing review of applicable literature. May recommend budget items to management.

Specific Activities

- Develops, coordinates, and administers facility-wide systems for risk identification, investigation, and reduction; maintains a network of informational sources and experts; performs risk surveys and inspects patient care areas; reviews facility and to assess loss potential.
- Participates on committees directed towards promoting patient safety issues.
- Maintains risk management statistics and files in compliance with JCAHO and state and federal agencies; promotes maximum confidentiality by limiting access of such information. Also strives to verify that the following information is accurate, available, and secure: includes medical records, patient billing records, policies and procedures, incident reports, medical examiner's reports (if available), as well as any other data pertinent to a particular claim.
- Collects, evaluates, and distributes relevant data concerning patient injuries: aggregate data summaries, monthly trend analyses of incidents, claims profiles, and workers' compensation trends; provides aggregate analysis of risk data; maintains statistical trending of losses and other risk management data.
- Informs directors of service and department heads regarding occurrences, issues, findings, and risk management suggestions; provides feedback to directors at all levels in the effort to eliminate risks; assists clinical chairs and department heads in designing risk management programs within their departments.
- Works with legal counsel to coordinate the investigation, processing, and defense of claims against the facility; records, collects, documents, maintains, and provides to defense attorneys any requested information and documents necessary to prepare testimony in pending litigation.

(Continued)

EXHIBIT 5.2   Risk Manager Position Description, Level One (*Continued*)

- Responds to professional liability and facility liability questions posed by physicians, nurses, and other personnel.
- May have on-call responsibility.
- Advises security on procedures to reduce the frequency and/or minimize the severity of property loss or assets.
- Provides assistance to departments in complying with Joint Commission or other accrediting agencies, regarding risk management related standards.
- Recommends appropriate revisions to new or existing policies and procedures to reduce the frequency of future occurrences; recommends ways to minimize risks through system changes; reviews and revises facility policies as appropriate to maintain adherence to current standards and requirements.

LOSS PREVENTION/PATIENT SAFETY

Overview

The level one risk manager is responsible for development of loss prevention programs that may include but not limited to patient safety issues. Periodic in-services and routine orientation may be conducted for facility employees/ medical staff regarding health care risk management and related subjects. This position may utilize outside speakers and faculty for such programs, subject to the approval of management, and may coordinate such efforts with the facility's education department.

Specific Activities

- Proactive analysis of patient safety and medical errors processes.
- Participates in the process of disclosure for medical errors.
- Participates in root cause analysis investigation and reporting of adverse drug events and sentinel events to the appropriate parties.
- Maintains awareness of legislative and regulatory activities related to health care risk management.
- Complies with various codes, laws, rules, and regulations concerning patient care, including those mandated by state and federal agencies, incident reporting. Includes investigation activities of federal, state and local enforcement authorities.
- Provides in-service training to medical center personnel to enhance their awareness of their role in reducing liability exposures.
- Disseminates information on claim patterns and risk control, as well as legislative and regulatory changes.
- Maintains a risk management education calendar.
- Takes steps to ascertain that risks are minimized through follow-up and actions on all regulatory/insurance survey report recommendations/deficiencies.
- Receives and investigates reports of product problems to determine appropriate response (in-house recalls, independent evaluations, etc.).
- Participates on select committees related to provision of patient care.
- Receives incident reports and other information regarding untoward occurrences in the facility, such as quality assurance outliers or variations, and collates such information systematically to permit analysis pursuant to risk management policy and procedure.
- Reviews collated data to identify trends regarding accidents or occurrences, and recommends corrective action to management, if appropriate.
- Prepares reports to management regarding trends/patterns and findings. Recommends electronic data programming initiation and improvement

CLAIMS MANAGEMENT

Overview

The level 1 risk manager receives complaints/claims related to professional and general liability and transmits that information to the appropriate department manager, administrative representative, patient ombudsman, insurance carrier or legal counsel. At the request of management, legal counsel, or the adjuster, participates in responding to the complaint or claim to obtain information and facilitate settlement at an early stage. Works in coordination with patient ombudsman or acts as same to resolve complaints before they develop into professional/general liability claims.

Specific Activities

Designs, implements, and maintains a direct referral system for staff to report unexpected events and potential claims against the facility through such input sources as medical records, business office, patient advocate, nursing, medical staff, quality improvement, etc.

- Investigates and analyzes actual and potential risks in the institution; assesses liability and probability of legal action for potential notification of insurance carriers.

(*Continued*)

EXHIBIT 5.2   Risk Manager Position Description, Level One (*Continued*)

- Directly refers to administration those incidents with claims potential; reports to higher authority any serious event involving actual or potential injury to patients, visitors, or employees.
- Assists in processing summons and complaints served on present and previous employees; assists defendants in completing necessary documents.
- With director of patient representatives, reviews patient complaints that may be the source of potential legal action; discusses and offers solutions when possible to resolve with patient and/or family any grievances perceived as potential liability claims.
- Participates in evaluation of claims for settlement; negotiates settlement of small claims within administrative authority; advises collection department of appropriate action for unpaid accounts involved in litigation; approves payment for or replacement of lost property after evaluating claim.
- Reviews national and local claims data; analyzes prior claims, lawsuits, and complaints against the facility.

RISK FINANCING

Overview

The level 1 risk manager has general knowledge of, and is familiar with, the facility's insurance coverage against liability and casualty loss, including self-insurance funding and budgeting for payment of deductibles, risk retention, and coinsurance. Usually participates in management reviews of insurance coverage and related issues. May prepare summaries of the facility's insurance program for management and staff.

Specific Activities

- Notifies the liability insurance carrier of all actual and potential claims, including primary and excess carriers as necessary.
- May verify with the Medical Staff Services Coordinator that each independent practitioner provides proof of adequate professional liability insurance at the time of initial credentialing and at reappointment.
- May act as liaison with the insurance carrier; completes insurance applications and responds to surveys; prepares materials necessary for renewal of primary and excess insurance policies.
- Provides insurance information to outside agencies; assists in compliance with state insurance reporting requirements.

SUGGESTED PARAMETERS FOR POSITION

- Experience is entry level, 0-3 years in risk management.
- Position title risk analysis, risk manager, patient safety coordinator, various titles reflecting combined job responsibilities i.e. QA/RM, Medical Staff Coordinator, Human Resources Manager.
- Reports to position of middle to top level management, Director of Risk Management.
- Certification/Education may include associate degree, RN, ARM, pursuing CPHRM.
- Organization Size may be one facility/organization with less than 100 licensed beds.
- Key attributes: Strong written and oral communications skills, presentation skills, team player, ability to influence change without direct authority, and negotiation skills.

Reprinted, with permission, from the American Society for Healthcare Risk Management.

EXHIBIT 5.3   Risk Manager Job Description, Level Two

Position Summary

The risk manager is responsible for the facility's risk management activities, which include, but may not be limited to, coordinating insurance coverage and risk financing, managing claims against the facility, interfacing with defense legal counsel, administering the risk management program on a day-to-day basis, managing and analyzing risk management data conducting risk management educational programs, complying with risk management related standards by JCAHO, all with the objective of maintaining patient safety, enhancing quality care, and minimizing loss to protect the assets of the facility. The level two risk manager performs these functions reporting to management at the vice-president level. This individual is responsible for reviewing and formulating policy or organizational changes and making recommendations for final approval by senior management.

OPERATION/COMPLIANCE

Overview

The level two risk manager performs the functions outlined under level one and, in addition, manages a facility department or office of risk management. Is responsible for data management, claims management, and the education components of the facility's risk management program. Promotes the organizational patient safety initiatives. Develops department budget for management

(*Continued*)

EXHIBIT 5.3   Risk Manager Job Description, Level Two (*Continued*)

approval. Works directly with legal counsel as a team member in the defense of claims. Has ongoing access to facility liability defense counsel to consult regarding both preventive and corrective measures to be taken in situations having legal connotation. On request, may provide information to facility management concerning reasonableness of cost and quality of legal services

Specific Activities

- Has full responsibility for operations of the risk management program that may include an enterprise liability approach to exposures.
- Directs loss control/loss prevention activities and reports results to senior administration.
- Supervises the statistical trending of losses and analyzes patterns.
- Designs and implements risk management surveys and studies; conducts surveys, studies, and special projects to assist in long-term planning and changes to facility policies and systems that reduce risk and losses.
- Responsible for identifying and communicating regulatory requirements.
- Leads development of organization-wide approach on disclosure of medical errors and obtains physician support.
- Designs and/or administers safety systems and procedures to minimize loss from employee casualties, and complies with OSHA regulations.
- Analyzes the risk of loss versus cost of reducing risk.
- Supervises accumulation of risk management cost data for budgetary and historical purposes: prepares budgets for departmental operations.
- Works with Medical Staff Services to develop and maintain risk management profiles on physicians and integrates that information into the credentialing process in compliance with state and federal agencies, Joint Commission and/or other accrediting bodies, and institutional requirements.
- Submits recommendations for changes in the existing risk control and risk-financing procedures based on changes in properties, operations, or activities.
- Evaluates correspondence from attorneys, patients, and other outside sources, and formulates responses, as necessary.
- Records, collects, documents, maintains, and communicates to insurance carrier and/or attorney any information necessary to prepare testimony in pending litigation.
- Directs and coordinates release of records and information in response to subpoenas, court orders, attorney requests, state and federal agency investigations, and other inquiries from outside sources.
- Maintains legal case files and strives to maintain maximum protection from discoverability of such files.
- Approves defense postures or settlement values at lower levels routinely.
- Answers medical/legal inquiries of physicians, nurses, and administrators regarding emergent patient care issues and loss control.
- Resolves treatment issues, including patient decisions made against medical advice (AMA), refusals of treatment, and consent issues; initiates court orders as appropriate via in-house and outside legal counsel.
- Reviews relevant contracts for risk exposure and insurance purposes before approval, including affiliation agreements, leases, construction agreements, and purchase orders, as appropriate.
- Maintains awareness of legislative activities that may affect risk management programs and participates in the legislative process.

LOSS PREVENTION/PATIENT SAFETY

Overview

The level two risk manager performs the functions as outlined under level one and, in addition, organizes and manages facility-wide educational programs on health care risk management and related subjects for health care practitioners. Presents such programs in conjunction with the facility's education department or other organizations. Supports the patient safety initiatives through direct participation on committees/task forces. Develops risk management budget for senior management approval.

Specific Activities

- Plans, develops, and presents educational material to administration, the medical staff, nursing personnel, and other department personnel on topics related to risk management as they affect personnel.
- Develops and implements educational programs designed to minimize the frequency and reduce the severity of actual and potential safety hazards throughout the facility.
- Leads root cause analysis and makes recommendations for improvement.
- Active participation in patient safety goals by providing data to support priorities.
- Active role in FMEA (Failure Mode and Effects Analysis).
- Acts as resource, internal consultant, and educator for patient safety/risk management issues.

(*Continued*)

EXHIBIT 5.3   Risk Manager Job Description, Level Two (*Continued*)

- Complies with various codes, laws, rules and regulations concerning patient care, including those mandated by state and federal agencies, incident reporting, also includes investigative activities with federal, state and local enforcement authorities.
- Leads investigations for adverse drug events and sentinel events.

CLAIMS MANAGEMENT

Overview

The level two risk manager performs the functions outlined under level one and, in addition, works actively with legal counsel or the adjuster in investigating claims, developing defense strategy, and evaluating the monetary value of the claim. Participates as a team member in negotiating settlements for management approval. In litigated claims, assists legal counsel in accessing facility records and personnel and may act as a corporate representative during pretrial and trial. Recommends defense strategies for approval by CEO, governing board, and legal counsel. Provides advice to senior management or the chief financial officer regarding reasonableness of expenses for claims defense.

Specific Activities

- Authority to initiate medical write-offs to mitigate potential claims.
- Oversees investigation of incidents/accidents/events that could lead to financial loss, including professional liability, general liability, and workers' compensation.
- Investigates risks involving actual or potential injury to patients, visitors, and employees; collects information necessary to prepare for the defense of claims.
- Serves as liaison to brokers and insurance company representatives in negotiating and settling specific general liability claims; directs conferences with claimants, attorneys, and insurance carriers, when applicable.
- Interacts with legal counsel, insurance carrier, and patients/families to effect timely settlement.
- Coordination of defense with co-defendants.
- Provides direction and advice to medical staff, as necessary, in connection with malpractice litigation and medicolegal matters.
- Reports patient care-related incidents to the Department of Health if required by law; directs investigation and development of corrective plans; submits required reports to state and federal agencies.

RISK FINANCING

Overview

The level two risk manager performs or coordinates the functions outlined under level one and, in addition, participates in negotiating coverage issues with carriers or trust administrators, including levels of coverage, scope of coverage, and premiums. Participates in formulating recommendations for purchase of coverage or funding of self-insurance for submission to management for final approval. Participates in preparing other financial analyses of facility's insurance program for the information of management and the governing body.

Specific Activities

- Reviews and maintains insurance policies; analyzes existing policies for coverage and exclusions; anticipates and deals with policy expirations.
- Participates in managing the facility's insurance programs and financing by preparing statistical data to support the continuation or reduction of premiums paid or reserves.
- Participates in negotiating policy provisions.
- May assess appropriate reserve funding levels, both insured and self-insured, in conjunction with an actuary.

SUGGESTED PARAMETERS FOR POSITION

- Experience is intermediate level position with 4-8 years in risk management.
- Position title may include Risk Manager, Director RM, Director Patient Safety.
- Reports to VP Risk Management , COO, CFO, or CEO.
- Certification/Education may include Bachelor Degree, RN, single risk management certification, ARM, CPHRM, FASHRM.
- Organization size may include 1-2 facilities, with 100-400 licensed beds.
- Key attributes: All in Level I job description, plus management of insurance portfolio and claims handling.

EXHIBIT 5.4   Risk Manager Position Description, Level Three

Position Summary

The risk manager is responsible for the facility's risk management activities, which include, but may not be limited to, procurement of insurance coverage and risk financing, managing claims against the facility, interfacing with defense legal counsel, administering an enterprise risk management program on a day-to-day basis, managing and analyzing risk management data, conducting risk management educational programs, complying with risk management related standards by JCAHO other accrediting and regulatory agencies with the objective of promoting patient safety, enhancing quality care, and minimizing loss to protect the assets of the facility. While the level 3 position may be responsible for the functions in level one and two job descriptions, this position most often supervises and offers overall program direction to staff performing the task in the first two job description levels. This position reviews, formulates, and implements policy and organizational changes, performing within general programmatic authority delegated by the CEO, chief financial officer, or governing body.

OPERATIONS/COMPLIANCE

Overview

The level three risk manager performs the functions outlined under levels one and two and, in addition, oversees aspects of data management and analysis for the organization's loss control program. Establishes budget for data management and analysis aspects of loss control. Directs risk management program for a large health care system and/or multi-hospital system with facility risk managers. Works within broad guidelines established by the CEO, chief financial officer, or governing body regarding the use and integration of loss control data with other types of organizational data systems for audit and accountability purposes on a facility or system-wide basis. May serve as the organization's compliance officer. Leads patient safety initiatives in the organization. Responds to all regulatory/compliance issues and strives to incorporate processes to address the results of these surveys/requirements.

Specific Activities

- Works with senior leadership in organizational operations, quality, etc.
- May serve on subcommittees of the Board of Directors.
- Authorities to retain, direct, and approve compensation of defense counsel.
- Conducts systems analyses to uncover and identify patterns that could result in compensable events.
- Assists clinical chairs and department heads in designing risk management programs within their departments.
- Develops and implements departmental and facility policies and procedures that affect liability exposures.
- Minimizes risk by responding to all regulatory/insurance survey report recommendations/deficiencies.
- Selects and utilizes services of consulting services, brokers, carriers, etc.
- Provides board summary reports on incidents, claims, reserves, claim payments, etc.
- Works with Medical Staff Services Coordinator to provide risk management information into the credentialing process in compliance with state and federal agencies, accrediting bodies, and institutional requirements.
- Complies with various codes, laws, rules, and regulations concerning patient care/safety, including those mandated by state and federal agencies, incident reporting, also includes the investigation activities of federal, state, and local enforcement authorities.
- Implements relevant statutes and regulations, including mandated mechanisms of physician monitoring with feedback to medical staff office, reappointment process, etc.
- Assumes responsibility for contract compliance within appropriate guidelines and legal concepts; in preparing contracts for board approval, provides advice on contract language necessary to fulfill insurance and risk management requirements; evaluates each contract negotiated by the organization to verify that insurance and liability issues are adequately addressed and that risk is transferred to the other party, if feasible; establishes insurance requirements for all projects and contracts; where appropriate, negotiates changes in contracts with other parties; verifies that affiliated institutions have adequate insurance coverage.
- Reviews and approves plans and specifications for major new construction, alterations, and installation of equipment.

LOSS PREVENTION/PATIENT SAFETY

Overview

The level three risk manager performs the functions outlined under levels one and two and, in addition, develops loss control educational programs for the organization's use. This position establishes education budget, subject to approval of the CEO, chief financial officer, or governing body. May develop educational programs relative to health care risk management utilizing well known experts in the field for national or regional representation. May develop risk management educational programs with broad appeal for marketing to other organizations. May serve as Patient Safety Officer/Advocate or Sponsor.

(Continued)

EXHIBIT 5.4   Risk Manager Position Description, Level Three (*Continued*)

Specific Activities

- Plans and implements a facility-system wide program for both loss prevention and loss control, and a comprehensive orientation program; those programs will be directed to all current and future employees of the board, physicians, and employees to advise them of their responsibilities, obligations, and part in the facility's risk management program.
- Participates in new business development activities by providing due diligence on new ventures/acquisitions.
- Serves as FEMA consultant/process expert.
- Directs and conducts educational sessions on risk management for medical staff and employees.
- Procures outside loss prevention services.

CLAIMS MANAGEMENT

Overview

The level three risk manager performs the functions outlined in levels one and two and, in addition has authority within broad guidelines established by the CEO, chief financial officer, or governing body to approve settlement of claims against the facility or system. Has authority to direct legal counsel and other personnel involved in claims management and to give final approval to defense strategies. Approves payment of fees of defense counsel and payment of other expenses of claims defense.

Specific Activities

- Manages the claims program, which contains the following components: reporting procedures, system maintenance, detailed claim investigations, establishment of reserves, selection and monitoring of legal counsel, conferring directly with claimants, attorneys, physicians, employees, brokers, carriers, and consultants, settlement of claims, selection and utilization of actuarial firms, as needed and/or required.
- Compliance with Medicare/Medicaid regulations as related to claims.
- Recommendations to senior management for funding requirements and necessary limits of coverage.
- Reporting claims information to senior management.
- Directs activities of investigators.
- Directs claims handling and defense preparation activities of the insurance company and defense counsel.
- Is responsible for administering claims initiated in the boiler/machinery, fire, and other loss areas.
- Projects future costs of losses, services, insurance, and other risk management expenses.
- Authority to manage and resolve claims within self-insured programs.

RISK FINANCING

Overview

The level three risk manager performs or coordinates the functions outlined under levels one and two and, in addition, manages the organization's insurance or self-insurance program within broad guidelines established by the CEO, chief financial officer, or governing body. This position has authority to finalize selection and retention of carriers or self-funding mechanisms in conjunction with the chief financial officer. Ensures the preparation of loss experience reports and summaries for the information of the CEO, chief financial officer, and governing body.

Specific Activities

- Evaluates property exposures, including new construction and renovation programs, to provide coverage and minimize risk.
- Develops familiarity with insurance markets through frequent market contact and attendance at meetings and market symposiums.
- Plans, coordinates, and administers a broad, comprehensive insurance program involving such activities as insurance purchasing, insurance consulting, administering self-insured coverage, and coordinating claims handling for all insurance lines.
- Directs and coordinates all aspects of insurance management for the institution, including developing alternatives such as self-insurance, excess insurance, and other risk-financing mechanisms.
- Develops and manages the overall risk management program, involving risks of all types, which may include using deductibles, self-insurance, captive insurance companies, financial plans, commercial insurance, and insurance/reinsurance programs.
- For property insurance, boiler and machinery insurance, crime insurance, student health insurance, automobile insurance, and all other purchased insurance coverage, analyzes values and verifies that exposures are adequately insured; in the event of a loss, prepares data required by brokers and carriers and manages process through to settlement of claim.

(*Continued*)

EXHIBIT 5.4   **Risk Manager Position Description, Level Three** (*Continued*)

- Prepares specifications for competitive bidding; negotiates with brokers, agents, or companies on insurance coverage, premiums, and services.
- Establishes and administers self-insurance trust funds for various types of insurance needs.

SUGGESTED PARAMETERS FOR POSITION

- Experience is senior level position with 8-10 years in risk management
- Position title may include Vice President Risk Management/ Patient Safety, Chief Risk Officer, VP Legal Services Reports to CEO, Board of Trustees/Directors
- Certification/Education may include JD, Masters Degree, multiple certifications such as ARM, CPHRM, DFASHRM, CPCU
- Organization Size may include multiple facilities, IDS, with more than 400 licensed beds
- Key Attributes: Include all of those in Levels I and II, plus advanced business/healthcare management skills.

Reprinted, with permission, from the American Society for Healthcare Risk Management.

Loss Prevention and Reduction

This category encompasses all aspects of risk identification, loss prevention, and loss reduction, and represents the largest functional area.

- Developing formal and informal mechanisms for risk identification, such as incident reporting, staff referrals, medical record reviews, review of patient complaints, and review of pertinent quality-improvement information
- Developing and maintaining collaborative relationships with key departments, such as quality management, nursing, medical staff, safety, security and infection control, to enhance program effectiveness
- Developing statistical and qualitative reports on risk management trends and patterns, and communicating this information effectively to appropriate audiences
- Developing root cause analysis and failure mode and effects analysis (FMEA) for incidents and potential areas of risk
- Developing policies and procedures in key areas of risk management interest, such as informed consent, product recalls, confidentiality, and handling of sentinel events
- Developing educational programs for all levels of staff on a variety of risk management topics
- Developing a program for management of exposures resulting from contracts, such as affiliation agreements, construction agreements, leases, management contracts, and purchase agreements
- Serving as a resource to organizational staff on issues related to professional liability and other risks

Claims Management

This category includes all activities associated with managing actual or potential claims, from reporting and investigation to resolution.

- Notifying carriers of actual or potential claims
- Establishing claim files and coordinating investigation
- Supervising investigators, third-party administrators (TPAs), and defense counsel

- Coordinating the organization's response to discovery requests and interrogatories
- Developing standards for the selection and evaluation of service providers
- Setting expense and indemnity reserves
- Approving and authorizing settlements
- Ensuring that the organization's senior management are kept informed of high-exposure cases and aggregate claims experience, including their effect on the risk financing program

Risk Financing

This category includes many activities associated with financing losses, whether the organization transfers or retains the risk.

- Maintaining and coordinating exposure data for the organization
- Coordinating insurance applications and renewals
- Collaborating with brokers, underwriters, actuaries, and other service providers to determine the risk financing needs of the organization
- Evaluating coverage limits, deductibles, attachment points, and lines of coverage to ensure that all exposures are adequately covered
- Evaluating risk financing options such as commercial insurance, retention, captives, and risk retention groups, and selecting the best option based on the organization's needs
- Monitoring and evaluating the organization's risk financing program

Regulatory and Accreditation Compliance

This category includes all activities associated with compliance with accreditation standards and with major health care regulations.

- Promoting compliance with requirements to report specific incidents to state and federal agencies
- Promoting compliance with regulations such as Americans with Disabilities Act (ADA), Occupational Safety and Health Administration (OSHA), Patient Self-Determination Act (PSDA), Safe Medical Devices Act (SMDA), Emergency Medical Treatment and Active Labor Act (EMTALA), Health Care Quality Improvement Act (HCQIA), Health Insurance Portability and Accountability Act (HIPAA), and the Patient Safety Initiatives prompted by the Institute of Medicine (IOM) report
- Promoting compliance with Joint Commission on Accreditation of Healthcare Organizations (JCAHO) requirements, including those pertaining to sentinel events and National Patient Safety Goals and Standards
- Promoting compliance with requirements to report deaths to the medical examiner or coroner
- Collaborating with key departments to ensure compliance with life safety codes and emergency management
- Promoting compliance with specific regulatory initiatives such as Project Lookback programs

Risk Management Operations

This category covers activities associated with managing a risk management department.

- Developing an organizational risk management policy statement and plan
- Training and supervising risk management staff
- Coordinating and administering risk management and patient safety committees
- Developing annual goals for the risk management department
- Evaluating the effectiveness of risk management activities

Bioethics

This category includes all activities related to issues such as do not resuscitate (DNR) orders, brain death criteria, advance directives, withdrawal of life support, and human subjects research.

- Reviewing policies and procedures related to end-of-life issues for conformance with ethical principles and adherence to applicable regulation
- Reviewing policies and procedures relating to human subjects research for adherence to applicable regulation and organizational policy
- Providing risk management consultation for specific ethical dilemmas
- Providing education for staff, patients, families, and communities on patients' rights

....

HEALTH CARE RISK MANAGEMENT ACROSS A SPECTRUM OF SETTINGS

As mentioned earlier in the chapter, the roles and job responsibilities of health care risk management professionals are determined by the characteristics of the organizations in which they work. The size and structure of the organization determine the needs of the organization, and this in turn influences the size, structure, and function of the risk management program. The risk financing strategies of the organization are also important determinants of risk management program structure and function.

The following sections examine the role of the risk management professional in several health care settings—the acute care hospital or medical center, the academic medical center, the integrated delivery system (IDS), multi-hospital system, ambulatory care setting, long-term care facility, and physician practices and clinics. For each setting, the relative importance of each of the six major functional areas of responsibility are examined, as are other unique characteristics of risk management programs in these settings.

The Acute Care Hospital or Medical Center

According to ASHRM's 2005 member survey,[4] 37 percent of respondents are employed in an acute care hospital or medical center, by far the largest category. Refer to Table 5.1 for an inventory of the type of organizations represented by respondents in the ASHRM Member Survey 2005. Acute care hospitals or medical centers can range in size from fewer than 100 licensed beds to more than 500 licensed beds. They can be classified as

TABLE 5.1   Type of Organizations

Organization	Percentage
Acute Care Medical Center	32%
Academic Medical Center	7%
Free-Standing Community Hospital	6%
Integrated Delivery System	12%
Multi-Hospital System	9%
Pediatric Hospital	1%
Specialty Hospital	1%
Tertiary Care Facility	1%
Insurance Brokerage	2%
Insurance Company	9%
Law Firm	1%
Long-Term Care Facility	1%
Managed Care Provider	1%
Physician Office	1%
Behavioral/Psychology Healthcare Facility	1%
Rehabilitation Facility	1%
Risk Management Consulting Firm	2%
Self Employed	1%
Other	11%

Base: 911 respondents

Reprinted with permission from the American Society for Healthcare Risk Management, ASHRM Membership Survey 2005.

community hospitals, which tend to be smaller and typically do not have their own residency programs, and teaching hospitals, which tend to be larger and often have multiple residency programs.

Acute care hospitals or medical centers offer a range of services, although not all hospitals offer every type of service. Patient care services typically offered in acute care hospitals or medical centers include general medicine and surgery, medical and surgical subspecialties such as cardiology and orthopedic surgery, and primary care services such as family medicine, pediatrics, and obstetrics. Most have intensive care units of some type and also have emergency departments. More complex services, such as transplant surgery and advanced trauma care, are typically found in academic medical centers, which are discussed later in this section. The types of services a hospital offers are typically controlled through the state's certificate of need program.

Even within this category, risk management program structure and function varies widely. At a small- to medium-sized community hospital, it is common practice for the risk management professional to assume responsibilities for several related areas, such as quality improvement, safety and patient safety, or infection control. The limitations of the hospital's resources, together with a smaller workload, make this arrangement an attractive one for these organizations. More recently, risk management professionals in such settings have also been called upon to assume the role of the corporate compliance officer, patient safety officer, or chief risk officer.

Small- to medium-sized hospitals are usually commercially insured, thereby decreasing the administrative burden for the risk financing and claims management functions on the risk management department itself. Responsibilities for workers' compensation programs often rest with the human resources department. Thus, the risk management professional's role in such settings often focuses on the activities associated with loss prevention and reduction: risk identification and analysis, management of serious adverse events, staff education, and policy and procedure review and development. Risk management professionals in these hospitals also often have responsibility for ensuring compliance with major health care regulations and requirements and for accreditation activities. Smaller hospitals often face risks associated with access to care, specifically access to specialized or intensive care, not faced by larger hospitals. The risk management professional also may be quite involved in clinical ethics consultations, because smaller organizations typically do not have the resources to employ an ethicist or in-house counsel.

The risk management professional's role in risk financing at smaller hospitals is often limited to collecting and coordinating exposure data and managing the insurance renewal process. The chief financial officer typically assumes the burden for evaluation of carriers and insurance options, selection of new carriers, and decisions regarding risk-financing options. The risk management professional's interaction with brokers and underwriters may be limited.

When risk is transferred, responsibilities for claims management also decrease. In a smaller, commercially insured hospital, the risk management professional's role in claims management is limited to coordinating the investigation and defense activities of the investigators, adjustors, and attorneys employed or retained by the insurance carrier. In this setting, the risk management professional is not responsible for setting reserves or authorizing settlements, as this is usually the exclusive right and responsibility of the insurance carrier.

Risk management professionals in small- to medium-sized community hospitals often enjoy high visibility. They are often viewed as the primary resource on a wide range of topics because the organization cannot afford to employ experts in a variety of disciplines. They very often function as the hospital's liaison to outside counsel, and as such become involved in a variety of interesting legal issues. Risk management professionals in such settings have the opportunity to work and interact with nearly every health care discipline. Thus, these positions offer excellent opportunities for learning and collaboration, and also opportunities for advancement by assuming responsibility for related areas.

In medium to large community hospitals or medical centers, risk management professionals typically have somewhat greater and better-defined responsibilities than in smaller hospitals. They generally retain responsibility for all loss prevention and control functions, but may be assisted by one or more staff members. Such staff assistants often have clinical experience or expertise that enables them to interact very effectively with patient care providers. The nature of loss prevention and reduction activities at such hospitals is essentially the same, though the volume tends to be greater than at smaller facilities. An enterprise risk management program is desirable, as it encourages risk management professionals to act in concert with other managers to fully evaluate the organization's exposures and promotes thinking "outside the box" for solutions. Potential partners with the risk management professional may be internal audit, treasury, security, institutional research, quality and performance improvement teams, or even individuals outside the corporate family that have a direct effect on risk such as credit agencies, regulatory and licensing agencies, fire and rescue, and police.

Credentialing and informed consent issues assume greater significance in these settings because of the greater number of specialists on staff and the riskier nature of treatments and procedures offered.

Medium to large hospitals and medical centers usually employ a greater number of professionals specializing in a variety of disciplines, so that risk management professionals in such hospitals are less likely to assume multiple job responsibilities. Usually, safety and infection control professionals are employed, and often the quality improvement function is separate from risk management. Thus, the risk management professional in such settings focuses almost exclusively on risk management functions, and there is little confusion among the staff as to who the risk management professional is or what the function comprises.

Although many are commercially insured, medium to large hospitals and medical centers are often in the position to use alternative risk financing strategies. It is common for such organizations to have in place self-insured trusts, large deductibles, or captive insurance companies to finance primary liability risks. If that is the case, the risk management professional has a greater role in risk financing and claims management. The risk management professional typically works collaboratively with the chief financial officer and other executives in the development of loss exposure data, setting reserves, monitoring of program results, and evaluating existing and alternative arrangements. Claims management also becomes a higher risk management priority in such circumstances, and the risk management professional is often responsible for directing the activities of an in-house claims staff or of third-party claims administrators, investigators, and attorneys. Risk management professionals in such settings typically have a great deal of interaction with brokers, underwriters, and actuaries, and may also have responsibility for self-funded workers' compensation programs.

Risk management professionals in medium to large hospitals and medical centers are often quite involved in regulatory compliance, but in many cases, there is a designated compliance officer with responsibility for the corporate compliance program. Thus, the risk management professional's role becomes more advisory in nature, serving as a content expert in those areas that relate to risk management. Most often, risk management professionals in these settings continue to play a significant role in accreditation, but this is usually a collaborative role with other administrators. They are involved in ethics consultations, as are their counterparts in smaller hospitals, but their role may be more advisory in nature because larger hospitals typically have more resources devoted to their ethics programs. As the risk management department tends to be larger, the risk management professional in such a setting typically devotes more time to department administration.

Risk management professionals in medium to large hospitals and medical centers require the same skill set as those in smaller hospitals. Effective communication skills and the ability to work collaboratively in other disciplines are critical success factors in either setting. In addition, risk management professionals who work in larger and more complex settings need to develop a better understanding of more complex risks, and of risk financing and claims management.

The risk management professional job descriptions for level one and level two found in Exhibit 5.2 and Exhibit 5.3 are most consistent with the functions of the risk management professional in the acute care hospital or medical center.

Academic Medical Centers

Academic medical centers pose unique risk management challenges. They tend to be large and complex organizations, and the care they provide is equally complicated. Risk management professionals and chief risk officers (CROs) in these settings must deal with risks ranging from simple clinical misadventures to complicated issues involving clinical research, affiliation agreements, and academic freedom.

Academic medical centers tend to have risk management departments with several professional staff members. Some organizations may have their risk management staff or program segmented into areas of clinical risk of the medical center and the affiliated university or school risk. Most often, the risk management staff for the medical center will include staff with clinical training. This is a great advantage given the complex nature of the clinical risks encountered in these settings.

Risk prevention and reduction activities in academic medical centers are made more difficult because of the many individuals involved in patient care. Unlike other hospitals, patients in academic medical centers are often cared for by students, residents, fellows, and specialists not commonly found in other settings. Because of the involvement of so many individuals in patients' care, there is a greater potential for error; thus, risk is increased. In addition, staff rotations and turnover tend to be higher in academic medical centers, and there is a constant need for education and reinforcement of risk management policies and procedures, including reporting requirements.

Risk management professionals in academic medical centers often spend a great deal of time educating the staff about risk management principles and practices. They also devote a great deal of time to the investigation of incidents, because facts and circumstances tend to be more complicated and harder to discern. Credentialing and human subject research also pose special risks in academic medical centers with which the risk management professional is involved. Refer to Chapter 9 in this text, on Physician and Allied Health Professional Credentialing, for more information.

Academic medical centers often face unique risks that make commercial insurance vehicles unattractive options. As a result, academic medical centers are often involved in alternative risk financing arrangements such as captives. The risk management professional in an academic medical center is likely to have some involvement in risk financing arrangements, and therefore must have expertise and knowledge in this area. The level of the risk management professional's involvement will depend on many factors, including whether or not the organization is involved in a group risk financing arrangement, and on the culture of the organization. Often, academic medical centers' risk financing functions are administered at high administrative levels, and the risk management professional's role in these functions may be limited.

Claims management in an academic medical center is usually handled within the organization rather than outsourced. Therefore the responsible manager must have the ability to effectively investigate claims, manage the activities of defense counsel, and establish appropriate reserves. The volume of claims in an academic medical center is such that several dedicated claims professionals may be required. It is especially true if the department is expected to manage other types of claims, such as general liability, directors' and officers' liability, and property claims. Refer to Volume III, Chapter 10 on Claims and Litigation Management, for information.

Regulatory and corporate compliance and accreditation activities in academic medical centers are complicated and time-consuming activities usually handled by professional staff dedicated to those functions; however, the risk management professional typically serves as an advisor. Refer to Volume III, Chapters 16, 17, and 19 in this series for more information on regulations, accreditation, and compliance issues, respectively.

Bioethics consultation in an academic medical center is usually a collaborative effort in which the risk management professional plays an important role. Because of the strong research orientation of academic medical centers, they often have strong clinical ethics programs with dedicated staff. Risk management professionals are often members of the ethics committee and institutional review board (IRB). Refer to Chapter 7, Ethics in Patient Care, in this volume and in Volume II, Chapter 5 as Clinical Research and the IRS, for more information.

Risk management department operations consume a great deal of time because the department tends to be larger in an academic medical center. Also, the risk management professional in an academic medical center may be expected to support the organization's teaching and research mission by accepting interns, teaching in the medical school, and assisting in risk management-related research. All of these activities increase the administrative burden of the risk management department.

The level three risk management job description found in Exhibit 5.4 is most representative of the scope of responsibilities in an academic medical center. Depending upon the organizational structure, a chief risk officer may be better suited for this position. The CRO job description in Exhibit 5.5 provides some suggestions for job responsibilities.

EXHIBIT 5.5   Chief Risk Officer Position Description

Position Summary

The Chief Risk Officer (CRO) has broad responsibility for the protection of the institution and its staff from fortuitous loss. The Chief Risk Officer advises and consults with senior leadership and the Board on potential sources of loss and makes decisions on how to eliminate or minimize loss.

Major Responsibilities

The following are the major areas of responsibility for the chief risk officer. These responsibilities include oversight, facilitation, coordination, supervision and technical competence in the following areas:

RISK FINANCING

Coordinates, advises and facilitates risk-financing strategy with the CFO on issues that could financially put the organization at risk.

Specific Activities

- Reviews documents and issues that impact the availability of risk financing options such as: changes to bond covenants, materials presented to bond rating agencies, all fines and sanctions levied through the OIG, FBI, CMS, and other issues of similar impact.
- Finalize the selection and retention of insurance carriers or self-funding mechanisms in conjunction with the CFO, and corporate office.
- Administer self-insurance trust funds.
- Evaluate property exposures, including new construction and renovation programs.
- Develop familiarity with insurance markets through frequent market contact and attendance at meetings and market symposiums.
- Plan, coordinate, and administer a comprehensive insurance program involving such activities as insurance purchasing, insurance consulting, claims coordination, and administration of self-insured program.
- Directs and coordinates all aspects of insurance management, including developing alternative insurance programs such as self-insurance, risk retention groups, captives, deductible programs, financial plans, reinsurance, commercial insurance and excess insurance.
- Analyze values and ensure that exposures for property insurance, boiler and machinery insurance, crime insurance, automobile insurance and all other purchased insurance are adequately insured; in the event of loss, prepare data required by brokers and carriers and manage the process through to the settlement of claim.
- Develop familiarity with insurance markets through frequent market contact.
- Prepare specifications for competitive bidding; negotiate with brokers, agents or companies.

CLAIMS ADMINISTRATION / EVENT REPORTING

Specific Activities

- Approve settlement of all claims against the facility within broad guidelines established by the CEO, CFO, and/or governing body.
- Direct legal counsel and other personnel involved in claims management and give final approval to defense strategies.
- Approve payment of fees for defense counsel and payment of other claims defense expenses.

(Continued)

EXHIBIT 5.5   Chief Risk Officer Position Description (*Continued*)

- Develop and implement an "early intervention program." Include disclosure of unanticipated events, use of apology, alternate dispute resolution mechanisms, early payments strategy, lessons learned /prevention activities and the use of employee assistance programs.
- Ensure appropriate reporting to all required outside agencies including the NPDB and/or HIPDB.
- Manage the claims program, which contains the following components:
  - Reporting procedures
  - System maintenance
  - Detailed claims investigations
  - Establishment of reserves
  - Use of alternative dispute resolution mechanisms
  - Monitoring of legal counsel
  - Conferring directly with claimants, attorneys, physicians, employees, brokers and consultants
  - Settlement of claims
  - Selection and utilization of actuarial firms as needed or requested

- Comply with Medicare/Medicaid regulations.
- Make recommendations to senior management regarding funding levels and coverage limits.
- Report claims to senior management and board of directors.
- Direct investigative activities.
- Procure outside loss prevention services if necessary to supplement in-house activities.
- Project future cost of losses, services, insurance and other risk financial vehicles.

PATIENT SAFETY

Specific Activities

- Develop, implement and monitor the Patient Safety Plan.
- Coordinate all patient safety activities with other clinical loss control, quality management, performance improvement, and infection control initiatives.
- Coordinate and facilitate all initiatives to comply with the JCAHO Patient Safety Initiatives.
- Plan for creative ways to enhance patient safety by the use and support of technological advances including, CPOE, bar coding, EMR and the like.
- Monitor the Internet and professional journals and publications to remain abreast of current projects and initiatives regarding patient safety.

LOSS CONTROL (CLINICAL AND NON-CLINICAL)

Specific Activities

- Plan and implement an institution-wide program of clinical and non-clinical loss control, including a comprehensive orientation program.
- Direct and conduct educational sessions on risk management for medical staff and employees.
- Develop, implement and manage the event reporting system.
- Conduct systems analyses to uncover and identify patterns that could result in compensable events.
- Assist clinical chiefs, and department heads in the design of risk management program specific to their department and unique risk.
- Research, write and implement departmental and facility policies and procedures that affect liability exposures and assist in regulatory compliance.
- Oversee patient relations/advocate programs.
- Ensure that risks are minimized by following-up and acting on all regulatory/insurance survey report recommendations/ deficiencies.
- Select and utilize all necessary outside consulting services offered insurance carriers, independent risk management consultants, and third-party administrators.
- Provide senior management and board of directors with summary reports of incidents, claims, reserves, claims payments, sentinel events and near misses highlighting "lessons learned" and risk control initiatives implemented.
- Develop and maintain risk management profiles on individual physicians and ensure the integration of that information into the credentialing process in compliance with state and federal agencies, NCQA, JCAHO, and institutional requirements.
- Ensure compliance with various codes, laws, rules and regulations concerning patient care, including those mandated by state and federal agencies, incident reporting and investigation activities.
- Review and approve all plans and specifications for new construction, alterations and installation of new equipment. Ensure that outside insurance carrier has signed off on plans as appropriate.

(*Continued*)

EXHIBIT 5.5   Chief Risk Officer Position Description (*Continued*)

CORPORATE COUNSEL

The CRO will offer assistance to the organizations General Counsel with those legal, regulatory issues that can impact the organization from a patient safety, public relations, marketing, and risk financing standpoint. Those issues might include:

- Fraud/abuse allegations.
- Reporting to outside federal and state agencies.
- Reporting to the NPDDB, state licensing boards, CDC.
- The levying of any sanctions or fines.
- Recommendations that affect licensing and accreditation.
- Review of new and existing legislation to determine appropriate risk response.

HUMAN RESOURCES

The CRO will work with the human resource executive to identify, analyze, and manage through risk control and risk financing techniques those risks related to the workforce.

Specific Activities

- Review all employee related surveys, questionnaires, etc. that address employee morale, turnover, and the climate/culture of the organization.
- Coordinate strategy to reduce turnover, improve morale and to promote an organizational culture that support patient and employee safety.
- Identify and develop with Human Resources initiatives to improve the organizations ability to recruit all positions within the work force including physicians, and to enhance the work experience and educational level of all staff.
- Identify and develop with Human Resource methods to reduce:
  Employee fatigue
  Absenteeism/presenteeism

STRATEGIC PLANNING & MARKETING

The CRO advises senior leadership on mitigation strategy for risk inherent in the following activities:

- Advertising campaigns including all print, TV, and mixed media materials.
- Physician recruitment activities.
- Mergers, acquisitions and divestitures.
- Joint ventures.
- New clinical programs.
- New facilities/construction.
- Clinical research.

INTERNAL AUDIT

The CRO and Internal Auditor are in a unique position to assist each other. Internal audit is charged with the identification and mitigation of the organizations exposure to loss, much like the CRO. Area of assistance and communication can be:

- Investigation of employee related crime issues, e.g., embezzlement.
- Implementation of educational initiatives for the Board of Directors on issues related to the Sarbanes Oxley Act.
- Corporate Compliance Program.

CONTRACT ADMINISTRATION

Assume responsibility for contract administration to include the following components:

- Assist with the development of appropriate working guideline and legal concepts for contract review.
- Work with senior management to develop contract language to protect the institution from liability and financial loss.
- Review all contracts prior to administrative approval for compliance with written guidelines.
- Negotiate necessary changes to bring the contract into compliance with written guidelines.
- Maintain a database (or purchase software) for contract tracking.
- Assume responsibility as the central repository for all contracts.

(*Continued*)

EXHIBIT 5.5   Chief Risk Officer Position Description (*Continued*)

POSITION QUALIFICATIONS

Experience

- A minimum of 10 years of progressive experience in healthcare administration with specific experience in healthcare risk management.

Education

- Bachelor degree required; master's degree preferred.
- Clinical background helpful RN/MD.
- JD, CPCU, and/or MBA desired.
- Associate in Risk Management (ARM) desired.
- Certified Professional in Healthcare Quality (CPHQ) desired.
- Certified Professional in Healthcare Risk Management (CPHRM) desired

KNOWLEDGE AND ABILITIES

- Knowledge of NCQA, HEDIS, and JCAHO, ISMP, NPSF, Leapfrog, IHI initiative, regulations and other patient care related initiatives to improve outcomes.
- Knowledge of regulatory codes, legal requirements and healthcare law.
- Effective presentation skills, articulate, persuasive, and eloquent communicator both verbally and in writing.
- Self-motivated with the ability to work independently. Requires little supervision.
- Ability to manage/handle stress while under pressure from many involved parties
- Ability to interface with a variety of professionals including members of the Board of Directors, medical staff and senior leadership, attorneys, accountants, actuaries, brokers, and the like.
- Knowledge of alternate risk financing/insurance programs.
- Demonstrated skills in strategic planning, implementing and evaluating programs.
- Knowledge of clinical and non-clinical loss control and claims administration.
- Ability to prioritize tasks and see the "big picture."
- Ability to delegate and know when to ask for assistance.
- Demonstrated ability to offer creative, innovative solutions to prevent/reduce difficult risk issues.
- Ability to manage information in a confidential manner.
- Reputation and ethical conduct must be of the highest standard and beyond reproach.

POSITION RELATIONSHIPS

Member of a comprehensive healthcare team, including other healthcare providers, the patient, the patient's family and significant others. Position has managerial responsibilities within the Enterprise Risk Management Unit. The chief risk officer, if not directly responsible the following areas with interface with them to minimize the potential for loss:

- Emergency Management
- Process/Quality Improvement
- Medical Staff Credentialing
- Infection Control
- Workers' Compensation/Employee Health
- Environmental Health
- Patient Safety
- Risk Financing
- Claims and Litigation Management
- Risk Control (clinical and non-clinical)
- Internal Audit
- Human Resources

COMMITTEE RESPONSIBILITY

The Chief Risk Officer will actively participate on the enterprise risk management committee and be a permanent member on the following committees:

- Quality/Performance Improvement
- Patient Safety

(*Continued*)

EXHIBIT 5.5   Chief Risk Officer Position Description (*Continued*)

- Emergency Management
- Customer Relations

The Chief Risk Officer should periodically attend or review the meeting materials / minutes of other committees such as:

- Pharmacy and Therapeutics
- Blood Utilization
- Utilization Review/Case Review
- Morbidity & Mortality
- Medical Products/Purchasing
- Credentialing Committee
- Infection Control Committee
- Surgical Case Review
- Nursing Executive Committee
- Medical Staff Departmental meetings
- Marketing and Strategy
- Human Resource

COMMUNICATION STANDARDS

Frequent contact is made with members of the senior leadership team, board of directors, medical staff leadership and a variety of outside professionals. Position requires the ability to articulately communicate a wide variety of legal, medical, and business subjects as they relate to enterprise risk management. Promote and provide courteous and effective communication with internal and external customers. May be spokesperson for the organization in time of a crisis/disaster.

WORKING CONDITIONS

Working conditions are almost exclusively indoors in a warm, well-lit environment.

- Motor coordination and manual dexterity are frequently necessary for the coordination of eye-hand and motor function in computer and telephone use.
- Occasional inter-office or inter-campus traveling with frequent sitting.
- Requirement for periodic on-call coverage.
- Scheduling flexibility is necessary to meet early morning and evening schedules.
- Ability to handle multiple projects simultaneously some with tight deadlines and minimal staff.

Reprinted, with the permission of Roberta Carroll, Senior Vice President, Aon Healthcare.

Integrated Delivery Systems

An integrated delivery system (IDS) is an organization that encompasses many different types of providers under one corporate structure. An IDS often includes acute care facilities, physician group practices, multi-specialty clinics, post-acute care facilities, and home care services. Providers may be employees or independent contractors, or they may be loosely affiliated with the organization. IDSs often cover broad geographical areas and can be very large and complex organizations in terms of corporate structure. In many cases, an IDS comprises facilities across several states. For all of these reasons, IDSs are particularly challenging for risk management professionals who seek to develop coordinated and consistent risk management plans and strategies.

Within the IDS, there is usually a corporate risk management professional who assumes responsibility for the IDS's overall risk management program. The corporate risk management professional is responsible for risk financing activities and has oversight responsibilities for claims management. This position typically is responsible for risk management activities only and does not assume other related responsibilities. Risk prevention and reduction activities are carried out by risk management staff at the facility level who may report to the corporate risk management professional or to the facility administrator. In many instances, the risk management function is assumed by a clinician or other facility staff member with no formal risk management training. This requires that the corporate risk management professional be an effective teacher and mentor.

The degree of integration and standardization of risk management practices, and of clinical practice, across the IDS is often quite variable and produces significant risk that must be managed. The corporate risk management professional establishes broad goals and objectives for the risk management program, thus providing the framework for the individual facilities to follow. These general guidelines allow individual facilities to adopt policies and practices that address issues unique to their setting. It might take time before all elements of the IDS can be successfully incorporated into a coordinated risk management program within the IDS. Very often, individual facilities are permitted to remain in existing risk financing arrangements because standardization and change across the IDS is too difficult to manage. Thus, the corporate risk management professional may be required to manage and oversee a complex program with many different and varied components.

In addition to the risks noted above, IDSs are particularly vulnerable to the risks associated with merger and acquisition activity. Thus, the corporate risk management professional's role in pre-merger due diligence takes on added significance within the IDS. Establishing strong relationships and being perceived as a valuable resource is essential to influence decisions, and eliminate or mitigate risk, before these organizational changes. More specific information may be found in Volume III, Chapter 8, Mergers, Acquisitions and Divestitures, in this series.

Risk identification can be accomplished in several ways in the IDS. Health plan utilization decisions that limit or deny services require a consistent approach based on currently accepted medical practices and on insuring agreements. Close study of contracts, credentialing practices, marketing and sales initiatives, capitation agreements, health benefit claims and denials, and member and patient satisfaction data are other mechanisms for identifying potential risks.

The risk management professional may oversee or be directly responsible for claims administration, including investigating, analyzing, reporting, and establishing reserves.

The corporate risk management professional within an IDS must be well versed in all aspects of risk financing and must have excellent skills in contract management. This individual must work well with other people to achieve corporate objectives, although the risk management professional exercises no control over these individuals. The level three risk management professional job description in Exhibit 5.4 most closely corresponds with this role in an IDS. The chief risk officer job description in Exhibit 5.5 also might fit this type of organization.

Multi-facility Health Care Systems

Health care systems are composed of multiple facilities providing similar services owned by a single corporation or parent organization. In many ways, health care system risk management programs are similar to IDS programs. They both manage risks across discrete organizations that may have entirely different cultures and identities. However, systems do not face the same challenges that IDSs face, in that their practices and procedures tend to be standardized across the system. Thus, the corporate risk management professional in a system is unlikely to be faced with a broad array of risk financing arrangements or facility-based practices within the system because the risk management program in a system is usually well-coordinated and fairly standardized across the system.

The risk management professional in a health care system most often functions as a senior executive in the organization. Risk prevention and reduction activities are usually carried out at the facility level under the direction of the corporate office. As in the IDS, the corporate risk management professional in a system will likely be responsible for risk financing activities while using alternative risk financing strategies to control costs. Claims management activities are often centralized and handled internally by dedicated claims staff.

System risk managers usually work collaboratively with others in the organization in regulatory and accreditation compliance and bioethics, and are likely to serve in a consultative capacity, or the responsibility may be delegated within the department.

The level three risk management professional or the chief risk officer job description most closely approximates the duties of the health care system risk management professional. The position requires significant risk management knowledge and experience, and the ability to stay ahead of the complexities involved in a changing health care environment.

Ambulatory Care Organizations

Ambulatory care organizations (ACOs) include multi-specialty clinics, freestanding surgical centers, urgent care or walk-in medical clinics, and community health or public health facilities. Physician practices may also be considered in the ACO. The organizational structure of outpatient care can be as varied as the facility itself. Some organizations may have an office manager whose job responsibilities include risk management. It is not unusual to have a physician functioning as the senior administrator to whom the office manager or risk management professional reports. Larger facilities more often have a governing body to guide the organization. As in a small hospital setting, the individual responsible for the risk management function may be responsible for several functions. Refer to Volume II, Chapter 8, Managing Primary Care Risk in the Ambulatory Environment, for more information.

ACOs pose unique risks because of the large number of patient encounters, which increases the risk of exposure to loss. In addition, because patients generally control the progress of their health care in the ACO setting, there is a greater chance that care may be fragmented or prolonged, and a provider might not recognize changes or deterioration in a patient's condition. Finally, ACOs often do not have access, as hospitals do, to other departments that support critical risk management functions, such as safety, infection control, and biomedical engineering.

Risks in ACOs vary with the type of setting. In most ambulatory settings, the risk of "failure to follow up," either from the patient's perspective or the provider's perspective, can be a risk management concern. Also, the use and maintenance of equipment pose risk management concerns, as do concerns regarding adherence to safety standards, universal precautions, and regulatory compliance.

Outpatient surgery centers have risk issues related to appropriate discharge criteria for their patients and in maintaining practice parameters and standards of care for the many different procedures performed. Emerging risks include the performance of an expanding number and complexity of procedures, including surgery, in outpatient and office settings. Credentialing is of particular concern because of the lack of formal procedures in this area.

Incident reports and occurrence screening often provide the mechanisms for risk identification. Patient complaints also provide excellent sources of information about potential risks.

Risk financing strategies used by ACOs may vary, but rarely will an ACO be involved in a self-managed alternative risk financing arrangement. Most ACOs are commercially insured or are part of the risk financing program of a larger organization, often an IDS or system. In that case, the parent organization assumes most of the responsibility, and the ACO risk management professional plays a minor role in risk financing, usually limited to coordinating exposure data and renewals. The administrator or office manager for the stand-alone physician practice(s) is typically more involved with risk finance decisions, claims management, quality improvement, and patient safety issues.

Most ACOs do not manage liability claims internally. Instead, this function is handled by the insurance carrier or a third party administrator (TPA) employed by the parent organization. The ACO may be called upon to assist in the coordination of investigation and defense of claims, but usually will not have any direct responsibility for claims management.

Risk management professionals and office managers in some ACOs do not have significant responsibilities for regulatory or accreditation issues, whereas others have complete responsibility, depending upon the resources available to the organization.

The level one risk management professional job description in Exhibit 5.2 most closely corresponds to this scope of responsibility.

Physician Practices and Groups

The physician risk management professional has emerged as organizations with employed physicians, hospital-owned physician practices, and private physician groups and clinics recognize the need for a person to take responsibility for the risk management functions. Managing physician risks, similar to ACOs, include loss prevention and patient safety, claims management, and risk financing as core job functions. Among the loss exposures for physician practices are high patient visit numbers, unexpected patient outcomes, patient privacy, practice standards, federal and state regulatory requirements, and patient safety issues. The physician risk management professional, like the level one position, may have multiple responsibilities for the practice such as being charged with handling of human resource issues, contract review, education for staff, and management of the office finances. The risk management professional is usually located in the office of the practice for stand-alone physician groups, or may be located in the corporate risk management office of the health care organization for employed physician practices.

Loss prevention activities in this setting include implementing and coordinating continuing education for the staff, coordinating insurer risk assessments, or performing risk surveys for the practice. The risk management professional establishes systems for risk identification, investigation, and reductions and provides analysis of data for management review.

The risk management professional is often responsible for the development of operating standards and procedures to promote quality of care, establishing clinical workflow, procedures, quality improvement initiatives, ongoing evaluation and monitoring of clinical staff credentials, and handling patient complaints. Responsibility for claims management includes reporting claims to the insurers, to the parent organization's risk management office, or to a third-party administrator. This position supports the internal investigation of incidents and claims and may interact with legal counsel.

Risk financing responsibilities may include the coordination of medical professional liability coverage in concert with the governing board of the practice. Contract review may include negotiation of managed care contracts, employment contracts, and vendor contracts. Exhibit 5.6 provides an example of a job description for a physician risk management professional.

EXHIBIT 5.6   Physician Risk Manager Job Description

Position Summary

The Physician Risk Manager leads the risk management/quality programs for the practice. The core job functions include operations/compliance, loss prevention, claims management and risk financing. This position develops and administers various programs that include, but are not limited to, risk-management, quality improvement, patient safety, loss-prevention, and regulatory requirements. The PRM employed in a smaller physician practice may also serve as the administrative director and will often assume additional responsibilities, such as human resources, vendor relationships and managed care contracts.

Loss prevention activities include identification of risks, practice issues, quality of care and the development and implementation of employee educational programs to reduce the exposures to loss. The PRM may spend a significant amount of time developing and implementing policies and procedures/guidelines to meet regulatory and compliance issues. This position typically provides educational programs to the staff and physicians.

The risk manager ensures the reporting of incidents and claims from the staff by developing systems for gathering and tracking data. Analysis of this data is reported to upper management and with recommendations for correcting or improving services.

The PRM is also responsible for the management/investigation of claims and risk financing. This position investigates claims and may be the initial contact for patient complaints while also serving as the liaison to attorneys, third-party administrators (TPAs), or departments who may be supervising the investigation. Claims handling may be delegated to a TPA. The PRM working with larger physician groups may be significantly involved with risk financing issues. Responsibilities include coordination with a broker to obtain insurance coverage for medical professional liability, general liability, director's and officer's liability, and property insurance. Assigned projects may include research on cost effective programs to minimize asset liability. The experienced PRM may participate in the development of major strategic initiatives such as a self-administered professional liability program that may encompass the integration of multiple practices/clinics.

Reports to: Executive Practice Director or Administration

Major Responsibilities

OPERATIONS/COMPLIANCE

- Maintains strictest confidentiality in all responsibilities and accountabilities.
- Establishes clinical work flow, procedures, and improvements for the practices.
- Facilitates communications with clinical staff.
- Manages projects, either self-initiated or assigned by upper administration Develops and maintains RM Intranet site content.
- Supportive of and insures compliance with applicable organizational medical group policies.
- Interpretations and communicates current and future regulatory requirements to achieve accreditation by organizations such as OSHA, CLIA, NCQA, JCAHO, HIPPA and other regulatory bodies.
- Presents a professional role model, exhibiting a team attitude, utilizing a positive problem solving approach with patients, physicians and staff. Works to develop and maintain positive morale of staff.

LOSS PREVENTION

- Communicates with administration and or Executive Practice Director to inform them of practice issues.
- Identify system concerns and make recommendations for reducing loss exposure.
- Development of operating standards and procedures to promote the quality of care, achieve licensure or accreditation with such agencies, as required and operate within the cost constraints of the organizational budget.
- Development and implementation of required employee-training programs required to maintain compliance with regulatory or credentialing organizations; i.e., OSHA annual in-services, ABN education, Clinical Assistant training, etc.
- Ongoing evaluation and monitoring of clinical staff credentials and skills to assure utilization of appropriate staff.
- Participation in care model development.
- Serve as a resource regarding appropriateness of services being rendered by clinical support staff to patients.
- Provides risk management training to physicians and staff.
- Maintains meaningful risk management data.

CLAIMS

- Investigates and manages professional and general liability incidents and minor claims in consultation with legal counsel.
- Responsible for all aspects of claims management, including communication with patients.
- Initiates settlements within authority level and reports to Board upon conclusion.

(Continued)

EXHIBIT 5.6   Physician Risk Manager Job Description (*Continued*)

- Using data from claims annually identifies key areas of exposure and works with Risk Management committee to develop action plans regarding Loss Control and seeks to incorporate meaningful benchmarks where available.
- Within a hospital based practice, may coordinates interface with organizational Risk Management by setting policy, establishing pathways for report investigation, authorizing payment subject to limit determined by the organization.

RISK FINANCING

- Participate in the budgeting process and expense management of the practice.
- Works with broker to obtain medical professional liability insurance or with organizational risk manager to ensure appropriate coverage is provided for the practice and/or the healthcare system.

KNOWLEDGE, SKILLS & ABILITIES

- Maintains current proficiency with Risk Management best practices.
- Strong communication and interpersonal skills to deal effectively with physicians, patients and employees.
- Ability to manage and motivate employees within the environment.
- Strong clinical background, and understanding of medical records.
- Able to inspire confidence in physicians.
- Knowledge of risk management functions, including claims management, investigation, and resolution.
- Knowledge of management practices to direct assigned staff.
- Knowledge of Clinic's strategic business objectives and employee performance objectives.
- Skilled in exercising initiative, judgment, discretion and decision-making to achieve organizational objectives.
- Skilled in establishing and maintaining effective working relationships with Clinic leadership, medical staffs, and supports staff.
- Skilled in identifying and resolving problems. Ability to delegate responsibility and authority to staff. Ability to work creatively with management and department staff to achieve objectives.
- Ability to analyze problems and consistently follow through on solution or delegation.
- Strong analytical skills and interest in interpretation of regulatory requirements.
- Ability to generate quality management reports and documents which clearly and concisely communicates information to management.
- Detailed knowledge of regulatory requirements for clinical support staff.

SUGGESTED PARAMETERS FOR POSITION

- Bachelor's degree in a related area; MBA, MHA, JD preferred.
- Nursing degree may be preferred for smaller stand-alone practices.
- Certifications may include ARM, CPHRM, and FASHRM.
- Ten years experience as risk manager with significant management responsibility.
- One to three years practice management experience with clinical background preferred.
- Position titles may include practice administrator, risk manager, director risk management, or a combined job title with quality/peer review or patient safety.
- Organizational size may range from one physician practice, to multiple clinics/offices or may include a number of employed physicians of a healthcare organization.

The Everett Clinic (Everett, Washington, July 2005) and Carilion Health System, Carilion Medical Group (Roanoke, Virginia, July 2005).

Long-Term Care Facilities

The organizational structure for a long-term care facility (LTC) may be as simple as a standalone privately owned facility, or as complex as a multi-facility, multi-state system. Some hospital-affiliated LTC units may be housed within the acute care hospital, and others may be located separately from the hospital. LTC centers located in the hospital usually use the hospital risk management professional to manage the risk for this area, just as they would other patient care units. Some LTC facilities are independent from the affiliated organizations' management and operations, and will have a separate risk management function. Risk financing most often occurs through the health care facility insurance program. Single, privately held LTC organizations use the facility administrator to develop and oversee the risk management functions, and sometimes have some owner involvement in claims management. Within the smaller setting, the quality and risk responsibilities may be combined and performed by a clinical person with direct oversight by the facility administrator.

A more complex LTC organization with multiple facilities in several states most often employs a corporate position responsible for the development of a system-wide risk management program. As in the multi-hospital system, the challenge is to develop standard policies and procedures, and to maintain consistency in the management of claims. Loss prevention and reduction activities are usually carried out at the facility level under the direction of the system risk management professional.

LTCs pose unique risks because of the patient's length of stay at the facility. The nature of allegations most often identified are administrative (for example, employee-related); clinical (for example, patient care-related); environmental (for example, emergency-related); provider (for example, vendor-related); and regulatory (for example, OBRA). Proactive risk management and quality improvement are essential to the reduction of risk exposures to the LTC facility. Facilities specializing in the care of patients with Alzheimer's disease have specific risk exposures for wandering and elopement of residents. Employee education and training is a significant part of the risk management professional's job responsibilities and is an effective loss prevention strategy for employee turnover in the LTC setting. Refer to Volume II, Chapter 19, in this series for more information on long-term care risk.

Risk financing strategies may include a commercially insured or self-insured alternative risk financing arrangement. In larger systems, the responsibility for insurance placement falls to the corporate risk management professional or senior management at the parent organization. The LTC risk management professional at each facility in the system plays a minor role in risk financing, often limited to coordinating exposure data. In a single facility, the responsibility for risk financing is most often assumed by the LTC administrator, and may include the owner in this process. Currently, LTC facilities have been faced with a limited number of markets for professional liability coverage, which has placed much more emphasis on risk financing alternatives at the corporate level.

Risk identification occurs through incident reporting, occurrence screening, and on-site visits of licensing organizations at the state and federal levels. Patient and family complaints are often a source of information regarding potential risk exposures and claims.

Like the ACO, smaller LTC facilities do not manage their own liability claims. This function may be handled by the insurer or a third party administrator (TPA). Larger LTC systems with self-managed programs may choose to self-administer their claims.

Bioethics issues include end-of-life decisions, such as advance directives and DNR orders. Coordinating the patient's desires and keeping the family involved are challenges in this long term care environment, and can become more complicated if the patient is taken to the acute care setting. Patient records and documents from the LTC facility are significant to the decision making process for the patient during an unexpected hospitalization.

The level one and two risk management professional job descriptions found in Exhibits 5.2 and 5.3 are most consistent with the functions of the corporate risk management professional for a multi-facility LTC system.

....

REQUIRED SKILLS FOR THE SUCCESSFUL
HEALTH CARE RISK MANAGEMENT PROFESSIONAL

To be successful, health care risk management professionals must develop a variety of skills necessary for performing a difficult job in a complex environment. They are called upon to interact with all levels of authority within the organization, and with patients and other customers. They often act as the organization's "official" representative in very sensitive circumstances. This means that they must have communication skills necessary to interact effectively with many different individuals and personalities, and must do so under stressful circumstances. Of primary importance is effective communication, which includes writing, listening, and speaking. Health care risk management professionals are often called upon to conduct educational sessions for other health care workers, including professional and nonprofessional providers and employees. They must also frequently deliver formal presentations to management, board members, or trustees. For this reason, excellent verbal communication skills and a thorough understanding and application of effective presentation styles are of critical importance.

In addition to verbal communication, successful health care risk management professionals also must be able to communicate well in writing. They often must prepare detailed reports of individual cases, reports of trends and patterns, and develop policies, procedures, and other guidance documents that will be used by others at all levels of the organization. For this reason, the health care risk management professional must have the ability to communicate clearly, accurately, and succinctly in writing.

Finally, the ability to listen well is another essential component of excellent communication skills. An essential function is fact-gathering following a serious event and interviewing those involved, carefully listening to their stories, and reconstructing the events that occurred. The health care risk management professional must also be able to glean information about risks and exposures from several sources, including committee reports and informal discussions. The successful health care risk management professional must be able to listen carefully to all information without passing judgment, and to carefully and objectively process information and communicate it to others. Thus, the ability to listen well is a complex and critical skill.

Another important skill is the ability to negotiate. The health care risk management professional often serves as negotiator in different situations, such as the resolution of claims or patient complaints, securing broker services or insurance coverage, or in developing indemnification agreements or contract language. Negotiation skills are desirable and may be developed through education offerings.

Another critical skill is the ability to remain objective despite being in an emotionally charged situation: The risk management professional is often called upon to provide support and direction to those most closely associated with these events and also must assume responsibility for discovering the facts and determining the best course of action. To do this effectively, the health care risk management professional must have the ability to maintain objectivity and professional detachment, even in emotionally difficult situations, and to pursue the best course of action for the organization regardless of personal feelings.

Finally, another critically important skill for the health care risk management professional is the ability to maintain confidentiality. Because of the nature of their work, health care risk management professionals often encounter situations and fact patterns that might seriously damage or destroy the organization and the individuals who work there. The health care risk management professional must be able to perform those activities necessary to protect the organizations and individuals, while also refraining from sharing information needlessly, regardless of how tempting or trying the situation might be. Maintaining confidentiality is critical, not only to protect those involved in an adverse event or potentially damaging circumstance, but also to gain and maintain the trust of those who might provide important information in the future.

········

RISK MANAGEMENT ETHICS

One hallmark of a true profession is a code of ethical conduct to which its practitioners must adhere. This is a familiar concept in health care, as medicine's own code of ethics dates back to the Hippocratic Oath. Nursing, law, and other disciplines related to health care risk management likewise have codes of ethical behaviors that guide practitioners in those fields.

ASHRM's Code of Professional Responsibility articulates the standards of conduct to which its members must adhere. This code is included in Exhibit 5.7. It provides a useful road map for health care risk management professionals who wish to maintain the highest level of professional conduct.

EXHIBIT 5.7　　ASHRM Code of Professional Ethics and Conduct

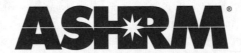

American Society for Healthcare Risk Management

Code of Professional Ethics and Conduct

Preamble

The American Society for Healthcare Risk Management (ASHRM) issues this Code of Professional Ethics and Conduct to assist its members in determining ethically appropriate professional conduct and to recognize conduct which does not meet this standard.

While there are diverse professional disciplines represented by the membership of ASHRM, at the heart of each is the responsibility to serve the public trust in the delivery of healthcare. The Healthcare Risk Management Professional must work to safeguard and foster the rights, interests, and prerogatives of patients or others served. The Healthcare Risk Management professional must maintain standards of professional conduct that will serve to withstand the scrutiny of all constituencies served.

The Responsibility to the Profession

- Practicing the profession with honesty, fairness, integrity, respect and good faith, avoiding conduct which would result in harm to others and promoting conduct which reflects well on the profession;
- Identifying, acknowledging, and disclosing potential conflict of interest;
- Complying with all federal, state, and local laws, regulations, and accrediting standards that impact the delivery of healthcare;
- Conducting oneself as a leader in professional behavior that will merit the trust, confidence, and respect of patients, healthcare professionals and the general public;
- Maintaining and improving professional skills, knowledge and competence;
- Advancing professional standards by supporting risk management research for the evolution of best practices;
- Participating in activities that support and enhance the credibility and dignity of the healthcare risk management profession;
- Maintaining and respecting professional confidences;

(Continued)

EXHIBIT 5.7   ASHRM Code of Professional Ethics and Conduct (*Continued*)

- Upholding the mission of the American Society for Healthcare Risk Management; and
- Upholding the integrity of this Code of Professional Ethics and Conduct by agreeing to abide by all rules of conduct prescribed by this Code and by ASHRM's Bylaws.

The Responsibility to Those We Serve

The fundamental objectives of the Healthcare Risk Management Professional are to enhance the overall quality of life, dignity, safety, and well being of every individual needing healthcare services. The Healthcare Risk Management Professional will support these objectives by:

- Respecting the dignity of all individuals by practicing in a non-discriminatory manner;
- Promoting an environment that supports a non-punitive approach to systems improvement;
- Investigating event factors with due diligence so that steps can be taken to reduce the likelihood of similar injury to other patients and to protect the next patient;
- Communicating and disclosing information to patients and, when appropriate, others, honestly and factually;
- Advising employing organizations and/or colleagues when existing policies, procedures or behaviors are inconsistent with this Code;
- Advocating on behalf of patients' rights;
- Using our knowledge and position in ways that enhance fair and honest communication, avoid manipulation, and not take undue advantage of those with whom we have professional interactions other than patients;
- Respecting that patients and their families are equal partners in the healthcare delivery process and entitled to fair, respectful, and equitable treatment and should not be taken advantage of; and
- Disclosing confidential information only when such disclosure is appropriately authorized or when law requires such disclosure.

Conflict of Interest

A conflict of interest exists when the Healthcare Risk Management Professional is called upon to serve competing interests. Some conflicts of interest, such as transactions with a former employer or dealings with past business associates, may be acceptable as long as disclosure of the conflict is made to all involved parties. Other conflicts, such as business transactions which inure to benefit of the Healthcare Risk Management Professional or his/her family members at the expense of others, are unacceptable even if disclosure to all involved parties is made. In order to avoid conflict of interest, the Healthcare Risk Management Professional must:

- Exercise good faith in all transactions;
- Avoid any interests, investments or activities which conflict or appear to conflict with the interests of the employer or client;
- Make full disclosure of all facts of any transaction which involves the possible conflict of interest to all parties involved; and
- Avoid accepting gifts or other considerations, which might influence the Healthcare Risk Management Professional's judgment.

Reprinted with the permission of the American Society for Healthcare Risk Management.

············

A PROFILE OF THE HEALTH CARE RISK MANAGEMENT PROFESSIONAL

Because of the way in which the health care risk management profession has evolved, health care risk management professionals come from many professional and educational backgrounds, including nursing, law, administration, quality assurance, and insurance. According to the results of ASHRM's Member Survey 2005 and represented in Table 5.2, 82 percent of respondents were identified as having a minimum of a bachelor's degree, and of those, 49 percent had an advanced degree.

Health care risk management professionals hold several professional designations. According to the ASHRM 2004 Compensation Survey,[5] three of the top four most common professional designations were Certified Professional in Healthcare Risk Management (CPHRM) at 26.6 percent, Associate in Risk Management at 20.6 percent, and a Certified Professional in Healthcare Quality (CPHQ) at 11.9 percent. The highest educational level was a bachelor's degree with 35.1 percent, and those having an advanced degree totaled 44.1 percent. These results approximate the subsequent ASHRM Member Survey in 2005. Table 5.3 illustrates the results of the survey's findings regarding highest educational level held by health care risk management professionals.

Table 5.4 identifies the job titles as related to their job function of respondents to the ASHRM Member Survey 2005. The survey classifies the respondent's job functions from senior level to entry level positions, and includes roles dedicated to financial and claims management, compliance, legal, nursing, physician or medical director, and patient safety officer. The majority of the responses centered on some variations of the risk management professional job title.

TABLE 5.2   Level of Education

Education	*Percentage*
High School Graduate	1%
Associate's Degree	7%
Nursing Diploma	4%
Bachelor's Degree	33%
Master's Degree	35%
Doctoral Degree	2%
JD	11%
MD	1%
Other	6%

Base: 911 respondents

Reprinted, with permission, from the American Society for Healthcare Risk Management, ASHRM Membership Survey 2005.

TABLE 5.3   Highest Level of Educational Training by Title

Designation	*Percentage*
Bachelor's Degree	35.1
Master's Degree	25.5
MBA	7.4
JD	9.9
Associate's Degree	7.9
Doctorate	1.3
Other	10.7
None of the above	2.2

Base: n=944

Reprinted, with permission, from the American Society for Healthcare Risk Management, 2004 Compensation Survey of Healthcare Risk Management Professionals.

TABLE 5.4   Job Function/Titles

Job Function/Titles	Percentage
Top Risk Management Officer	19%
Sr. Risk Manager	3%
Risk Manager	16%
Middle Manager Risk Management	12%
Entry-Level Risk Manager	2%
Top Finance/Claims Management	1%
Middle Finance/Claims Management	1%
Top Patient Safety Officer	2%
Middle Manager Patient Safety	>1%
Compliance Officer	1%
Legal/Regulatory	2%
Nurse Executive	1%
Physician/Medical Director	>1%
Third-Party Administrator	1%
Consultant	6%
Insurance Broker	1%
Other	14%
No Response	18%

Base: 911respondents

Reprinted, with permission, from the American Society for Healthcare Risk Management, ASHRM Member Survey, 2005.

• • • • • • • • • • • •

EDUCATION AND PROFESSIONAL RECOGNITION PROGRAMS

An important characteristic that distinguishes a true professional is the desire to further develop and refine mastery of the chosen profession. One of the ways professionals pursue growth and development is by continuing their education through both formal and informal means. In turn, the profession recognizes the efforts of these professionals by bestowing designations extolling their achievements. Thus, continuing education and professional recognition of achievement are important components of a continuously evolving profession, and important milestones for the health care risk management professional.

Academic Training

A growing number of colleges and universities either currently offer or are developing programs leading to a baccalaureate or master's degree in health care risk management. (Information about such programs is available at www.ashrm.org.) This trend signifies the increasing recognition of health care risk management as a discipline worthy of academic attention. As the profession continues to evolve, more entrants into the field will come equipped with formal academic training rather than experiential training, as has been the case in the past. If the trend continues, it is possible that formal academic training in health care risk management will be a requirement for entry into the field. This requirement would also help to provide a steady stream of new and qualified candidates for health care risk management positions, however, such programs are not yet widely available.

Continuing Professional Education

While academic programs fulfill an important role for the profession, they might not meet the needs of those that already hold academic degrees but seek further professional education in the field of health care risk management. Thus, it is important that other means exist for health care professionals to obtain continuing education in the field of health care risk management. Fortunately, in addition to academic programs, several other avenues exist for health care risk management professionals to further their education and professional development.

The major source of professional education programs for health care risk management professionals is the American Society for Healthcare Risk Management (ASHRM), which has developed several educational programs that are available to both members and nonmembers. The Barton Certificate in Healthcare Risk Management Program, which covers key aspects of risk management, is designed with three modules for the risk management professional. The program includes the Essentials Module, which provides the educational foundation for new management professionals, the Application Module, with relevant topics for those with one to five years in health care risk management, and the Advanced Forum, for more experienced risk management individuals facing special risk management challenges. Upon completion of all three modules, attendees are issued a certificate of completion by ASHRM. Participants may also earn undergraduate and graduate college credits and receive credit towards the ASHRM risk management certification program.

ASHRM also presents programs on more advanced topics, such as risk financing, regulatory developments, and other critical issues throughout the year. At its annual conference, ASHRM presents programs on a wide variety of topics both within the field of health care risk management and more broadly within health care. As with other offerings, attendees earn continuing education credits.

In addition to ASHRM, major health care liability insurance carriers and brokers also offer educational programs specifically designed for health care risk management professionals. Although these programs are often limited to clients or insureds, they often cover timely topics and feature nationally known speakers.

Certification

Certification provides evidence of mastery of a defined body of knowledge by requiring certificants to successfully complete an objective test, such as a written examination. It helps to set professional standards by identifying a minimum level of knowledge, which all certificants must possess. It also helps to ensure continued growth and development of the profession, and of individuals practicing the profession by requiring recertification at predetermined intervals.

Currently, there is only one certification program specifically for health care risk management professionals in the United States. This program, administered by the American Hospital Association Certification Center (AHACC), in cooperation with ASHRM, offers the designation of Certified Professional in Healthcare Risk Management (CPHRM). An individual who meets eligibility criteria and successfully completes a qualifying examination becomes certified. Eligibility standards include prior work experience in addition to certain educational requirements. The CPHRM examination tests the applicant's knowledge in each of the six domain areas identified by ASHRM's role delineation study: loss prevention and reduction, claims management, risk financing, regulatory and accreditation compliance, operations, and bioethics. Certificants are required to become re-certified every three years.

The Insurance Institute of America (IIA)[6] also offers risk management education in the form of its Associate in Risk Management (ARM) program. This is a designation program consisting of three courses and accompanying examinations that focus on risk assessment (designated as ARM 54), risk control (ARM 55), and risk financing (ARM 56). Upon successful completion of the examinations, the student earns the designation Associate in Risk Management, or ARM, which is recognized throughout the health care and insurance industry. Although the ARM program does not focus specifically on health care risk management, it offers significant educational benefits to the individual interested in furthering education beyond the borders of health care.

Other designation programs are also offered through the Insurance Institute of America and the American Institute for Chartered Property and Casualty Underwriters, such as the Associate in Claims (AIC) and the Chartered Property and Casualty Underwriter (CPCU). Many equate a CPCU designation[7] to a graduate degree in insurance.

Licensure

Health care risk management professionals should know and understand the specific state statutes and regulations that govern their work environment, and under which their position as risk manager may be managed and controlled. For example, by Florida statute, every licensed hospital, ambulatory surgical center,[8] nursing home,[9] and HMO[10] shall establish as part of its administrative function an internal risk management program. Every hospital, ambulatory surgical center, and HMO[11] shall hire a licensed risk manager[12] for implementation and oversight of the facilities internal risk management program. Within the Florida nursing home environment, the internal risk management and quality assurance program is the responsibility of the facility administrator. The hiring of licensed risk managers is not required.

Professional Recognition Programs

Professional recognition programs serve a valuable function for a profession and the individuals practicing the profession by encouraging continued growth and development of individuals, in turn elevating standards in the profession. Such programs are typically administered by professional societies and membership organizations.

ASHRM offers the highest achievement designations for distinguished fellow (DFASHRM), which is awarded for superior achievement in the profession. The designation of fellow (FASHRM) is awarded for outstanding achievement. Criteria for both designations include a combination of education, leadership, and publication experience and achievement, and designations are awarded to members who meet the criteria.

ASHRM's highest award, the Distinguished Service Award (DSA), recognizes a health care risk management professional whose efforts have advanced the profession and practice of risk management and who has made an outstanding contribution to ASHRM. The award is given only to those whom the ASHRM board of directors feels merits the award.

Other organizations sometimes also offer awards in recognition of superior achievement. *Business Insurance,* a nationally recognized insurance publication, offers recognition to the Risk Manager of the Year, and to members of the Risk Management Honor Roll. These awards are given to winners from all industries, and health care risk management professionals have been so honored.

············
CONCLUSION

The growth and evolution of the health care risk management profession has mirrored that of the health care industry as a whole, although its basic components and processes have not changed. The goal of an effective health care risk management program continues to be to maintain a safe and effective health care environment for patients, visitors, and employees, thereby preventing or reducing loss to the organization. Risk management continues to compose an important part of the delivery of health care, and it has become even more important because of the greater emphasis on patient safety.

The role of the health care risk management professional continues to evolve. Loss prevention and reduction, claims management, risk financing, regulatory and accreditation compliance, risk management operations, and bioethics are the major functional areas that together compose the job description of the health care risk management professional, the chief risk officer, and the patient safety officer. The depth and breadth of these functions, and their vital importance to an organization's survival have been amply demonstrated by this study.

Health care risk management professionals, chief risk officers, physician risk management professionals, and patient safety officers are a diverse group of professionals from several backgrounds. Most are highly educated and have a variety of clinical backgrounds. They value continuing education and professional achievement as demonstrated by the demographic data obtained in the ASHRM studies.

Successful health care risk management professionals must possess certain critical skills. The ability to communicate well, negotiate effectively, remain objective, and maintain confidentiality are the keys to success.

Opportunities for health care risk management professionals to enhance their professional growth and development abound. Academic training programs in health care risk management are increasingly common, and continuing education opportunities have always been plentiful. An opportunity to enhance professional development and recognition comes with the health care risk management certification program developed by ASHRM, in conjunction with the American Hospital Association.

The continuing challenge for health care risk management professionals will be to stay abreast of developments in health care that leads to new exposures, and to develop new risk financing and loss control techniques to manage those exposures. Enterprise risk management (ERM) provides the tools for embedding the discussion of risk into the way an organization does business. The risk management professional who adds value to the organization by aligning risk management strategies in support of business success will not only survive, but thrive in this constantly changing environment.

Endnotes

1. Carroll, R. C., Ed., Preface p. xxxvii, *Risk Management Handbook for Health Care Organizations*, Jossey Bass Publishing, 2004.

2. Kloman, F. H., *Risk Management Milestones 1900–1999*, International Risk Management Institute (IRMI), March 2001 available at www.irmi.com.

3. ASHRM Healthcare Risk Management National Role Delineation Study, 1999, conducted by Applied Measurement Professionals, Inc. Lenexa, KS.

4. ASHRM Membership Survey 2005, Analysis provided by Organizational Research Forum, Inc., Vernon Hills, IL 2005.

5. 2004 Compensation Survey of Healthcare Risk Management Professionals, American Society for Healthcare Risk Management, Chicago, IL.

6. American Institute for CPCU and Insurance Institute of America, Malvern, PA at www.aicpcu.org/.

7. *Ibid.* The CPCU program consists of eleven courses. You must pass eight courses to earn the CPCU designation. All candidates must complete the five foundation courses. In addition, you select either the commercial or personal insurance concentration and complete the three courses in the concentration of your choosing. You may not combine courses from both concentrations. Five foundation courses are:

    CPCU 510
    Foundations of Risk Management, Insurance, and Professionalism
    CPCU 520
    Insurance Operations, Regulation, and Statutory Accounting
    CPCU 530
    The Legal Environment of Insurance
    CPCU 540
    Business and Financial Analysis for Risk Management and Insurance Professionals
    CPCU 560
    Financial Services Institutions
    Three courses in either the personal or commercial concentration:
    Commercial Concentration (with personal survey)
    CPCU 551
    Commercial Property Risk Management and Insurance
    CPCU 552
    Commercial Liability Risk Management and Insurance
    CPCU 553
    Survey of Personal Risk Management, Insurance, and Financial Planning
    Personal Concentration (with commercial survey)
    CPCU 555
    Personal Risk Management and Property-Liability Insurance
    CPCU 556
    Personal Financial Planning
    CPCU 557
    Survey of Commercial Risk Management and Insurance

8. Florida Statute §395.0197

9. Florida Statute §400.147

10. Florida Statute §631.55

11. Only organizations that have an annual premium volume of $10 million or more and that directly provide health care in a building owned or leased by the organization shall hire a risk manager certified under ss.395.10971.

12. 395.10974 Health care risk managers; qualifications, licensure, fees.

    (1) Any person desiring to be licensed as a health care risk manager shall submit an application on a form provided by the agency. In order to qualify, the applicant shall submit evidence satisfactory to the agency which demonstrates the applicant's competence, by education or experience, in the following areas:

        (a) Applicable standards of health care risk management.

        (b) Applicable federal, state, and local health and safety laws and rules.

        (c) General risk management administration.

        (d) Patient care.

(e) Medical care.

(f) Personal and social care.

(g) Accident prevention.

(h) Departmental organization and management.

(i) Community interrelationships.

(j) Medical terminology.

The agency may require such additional information, from the applicant or any other person, as may be reasonably required to verify the information contained in the application.

(2) The agency shall not grant or issue a license as a health care risk manager to any individual unless from the application it affirmatively appears that the applicant:

(a) Is 18 years of age or over;

(b) Is a high school graduate or equivalent; and

(c) 1. Has fulfilled the requirements of a 1-year program or its equivalent in health care risk management training which may be developed or approved by the agency;

2. Has completed 2 years of college-level studies which would prepare the applicant for health care risk management, to be further defined by rule; or

3. Has obtained 1 year of practical experience in health care risk management.

(3) The agency shall issue a [1]license to practice health care risk management to any applicant who qualifies under this section and submits an application fee of not more than $75, a fingerprinting fee of not more than $75, and a license fee of not more than $100. The agency shall by rule establish fees and procedures for the issuance and cancellation of licenses.

(4) The agency shall renew a health care risk manager [2]license upon receipt of a biennial renewal application and fees. The agency shall by rule establish a procedure for the biennial renewal of licenses.

History.—ss. 38, 53, ch. 85-175; s. 4, ch. 86-287; s. 33, ch. 88-166; s. 184, ch. 90-363; s. 4, ch. 91-429; s. 29, ch. 98-89; s. 75, ch. 98-199.

[1]Note.—As amended and transferred to its present location by s. 29, ch. 98-89. The amendment by s. 75, ch. 98-199, added the words "and an appointment" following the word "license."

[2]Note.—As amended and transferred to its present location by s. 29, ch. 98-89. The amendment by s. 75, ch. 98-199, substituted the word "appointment" for the word "license."

Note.—Former s. 626.944.

Suggested Readings

American Society for Healthcare Risk Management, The Growing Role of the Patient Safety Officer: Implications for Risk Managers, Monograph contributors Marva West Tan, Paul Gutting, Julie Gorczyca, June 2004.

Economist Intelligence Unit's Global Risk Briefing, The Evolving Role of the CRO, New York, NY, May 2005.

Business Insurance, Apr. 22, 1996, p. 135.

American Hospital Association, Pearls for Skilled Nursing/Long-Term Care Facilities. Chicago, IL: AHA American Hospital Publishing, Inc., 2002.

American Hospital Association. Mapping Your Risk Management Course in Integrated Delivery Networks. Chicago, IL: AHA American Hospital Publishing, Inc., 1995.

American Hospital Association. Mapping Your Risk Management Course in Stand-Alone Hospitals. Chicago, IL: AHA American Hospital Publishing, Inc., 1995.

American Hospital Association. Mapping Your Risk Management Course in Ambulatory Care. Chicago, IL: American Hospital Publishing, Inc., 1995.

Youngberg, B. J. *The Risk Manager's Desk Reference*. Rockville, MD: Aspen, 1994.

Berkowitz, S. L. Journal of Healthcare Risk Management, Enterprise Risk Management and the Healthcare Risk Manager, Chicago, IL: AHA American Hospital Publishing, Inc., 2001.

6

Risk Management Metrics

Judith Napier
Trista Johnson

This chapter will define metrics that are useful to measure success in a risk management program. Risk management professionals need to determine how risk management is defined in the organization, the essential components to be measured, to whom the measurements will be provided, and how success will be determined. This chapter will focus on traditional measurements and will provide information to assist organizations that are linking patient safety and risk management processes.

BACKGROUND

Risk management is defined in several ways. It has been described as "the system designed to prevent and control patient injury, enhance quality, promote safety, and minimize the losses associated with medical malpractice claims."[1] It is sometimes considered in processes related to adverse outcomes and claims handling when litigation occurs. Unless the risk management process is clearly defined within an organization, it is difficult to determine the appropriate measurements to apply. Also, consideration should be given as to whether one is describing risk prevention or risk mitigation after an event has occurred. Each would have different descriptions, expectations, and processes.

Risk analysis is also a process described in multiple ways. Risk analysis may involve the review of data, a process, or a situation to learn and apply the information for trends or patterns. Risk analysis is sometimes used to quantify risk frequency or severity or to describe the magnitude of potential risk. This would suggest that there is some sort of screening process or severity rating applicable to the events, to establish priorities of actions. A more typical definition of risk analysis, however, equates to liability

*good definition

assessment used to determine the legal liability exposure of a specific event and to subsequently assign a value to the potential financial loss.

These terms often are used interchangeably, yet they have very different meanings. Before measuring a facility's risk management program, the risk management professional needs to establish what the terms mean to the various stakeholders in the organization.

....

BENCHMARKING DEFINED

The American Productivity and Quality Center (APQC) defines benchmarking as "the process of improving performance by continuously identifying, understanding, and adapting outstanding practices and processes found inside and outside the organization."[2] Another well known expert in the area of benchmarking, Robert C. Camp, has described benchmarking "as the search for industry best practices that lead to superior performances."[3]

Background

The Xerox Corporation was one of the first companies in America to develop and use benchmarking as a method to understand its competition. In 1976, after the Japanese excelled in the office copier market, Xerox recognized the need to do things differently. In 1979, Xerox introduced benchmarking methods as a means to study and understand its competitors' products, to compare to and contrast its own products and processes.

When Xerox first applied benchmarking principles to the manufacturing of its products, significant changes were made to the processes that led to incorporating the best features of the competitors' products. Success in manufacturing led to implementation of benchmarking principles in other parts of the organization such as maintenance, warehousing, distribution, billing, and so on. Xerox quickly found that the principles applied to all aspects of the company.

There are many tools now available to assist organizations in benchmarking. In 1994, the U.S. Department of Defense produced a document that establishes a framework for managing process improvement using benchmarking as a process. The tool introduces specific steps for successful performance improvement.[4]

- Establishing a strong foundation by selecting, analyzing the process, and calculating metrics and gaps in performance
- Selecting benchmark partners with "best in class" processes with a benchmark team
- Planning for productive sessions with tight agendas, trained personnel, and defined responsibilities
- Conducting a thorough benchmark with site visits, data gathering, interviews, and questionnaires
- Analyzing the results and planning to create changes for a best in class model

The key process measures are defined in this tool in the following categories:

- *Fitness for Purpose* (FFP): These measures record how well the process is satisfying the stakeholders' interests, requirements, and desires. They define effectiveness measures.
- *Conformance to Standard* (CTS): These measures record how well the process is conforming to rules, regulations, standards, requirements, and specifications. These are quality measures.

- *Cycle Time* (CT): These measures record how responsive the process is. They are considered efficiency measures.

- *Process Cost* (PC): These measures record the fixed or investment costs associated with the process. They are overhead measures.

Currently, benchmarking in risk management relies on national data such as average cost of claims, average verdict data, and number of staff in risk management departments, so as to compare results to other health care risk management departments. The Risk and Insurance Management Society (RIMS) [www.rims.org] produces an annual "benchmark survey" that reviews the overall cost of risk for many different types of organizations. Health care has been adapting these tools for the past fifteen years to measure the effectiveness of risk management programs in the hospital and health care settings. The information compares an organization's cost of risk against industry competitors to gauge the cost of effectiveness of risk management departments.

However, *"benchmarking involves uncovering best practices where ever they exist."*[5] Thus, it is important not only to compare data, but also processes. Benchmarking suggests that the risk management professional look at the processes that are used to achieve results and then modify internal processes to gain same or better results with the benchmark. Instead, the data are often used as a gauge to establish what is an acceptable range of results, and therefore, the organization is able to stay the course. However, an organization should evaluate internal processes affecting the numbers and define, measure, and monitor the processes that affect the data.

True benchmarking through the sharing of lessons learned in system changes and system failures is a new direction. Using process improvement measures in risk management raises the issues of linkages between patient safety, quality, and risk management efforts. Deciding whether these disciplines fit together suggests that the information collected in each of these disciplines has connectivity. The health care industry is trying to understand what the data mean across the enterprise, rather than in each distinct discipline.

With the advent of the IOM report, *To Err Is Human: Building a Safer Health System* (1999),[6] and the follow-up report, *Crossing the Quality Chasm: A New Health Care System for the 21st Century* (2001),[7] the bar was raised for health care to look at its systems in a new way. The industry shifted focus to the patient and asked whether this is the best that health care has to offer our communities. In many cases, the answer was a resounding no, and so began the patient safety movement.

The late Dr. Avedis Donabedian, father of health systems research, introduced a model in which he identified the seven pillars of quality in health care:[8]

1. Efficacy—improving a patient's well-being
2. Efficiency—obtaining the greatest improvement at the lowest cost
3. Optimality—balancing costs and benefits
4. Acceptability—adapting care to the wishes, expectations, and values of the patient
5. Legitimacy—proving care acceptable to society at large
6. Equity—distributing care fairly
7. Cost—providing the greatest benefit at the lowest cost while optimizing the cost/benefit ratio.

Dr. Donabedian built his premises on these pillars—that health problems are not a collection of unrelated events, but rather a complex process that follows general principles. This breakthrough thinking in his initial work is accepted today as a fundamental principle. The patient safety movement and the body of work that has begun to reflect the science of safety clearly recognizes the complexity in health care systems. High-reliability research has focused on the fundamental principles that need to be in place for an organization to develop predictable processes that produce dependable outcomes. Such principles include a just culture, open reporting systems, and teamwork and communication across multiple disciplines.

In a just culture, everyone speaks up. The current model of reporting incidents, which risk management has relied on for several years, is based on a voluntary system. Unfortunately, the feedback loop has often involved disciplining the individual who was involved in the event. To break that cycle, risk management needs to team with patient safety to create a just culture for reporting events, to streamline the reporting process, to decrease the time needed to complete reports, and to develop essential feedback loops to the caregivers when they report the system failures. If the health care facility considers these principles and begins to shape its efforts around these foundations, then the work focuses on the patient rather than on the organization. This moves the risk management program to a multidimensional aspect in the health care organization, rather than one-dimensional in managing post-event investigations and litigation.

Traditional risk management measures continue to be important cornerstones in program evaluation, but they are not the only focus for an organization interested in making significant improvements in safety. Traditional measures will be described, along with how they are typically collected and analyzed.

CLAIMS

Total Number of Claims Most health care risk management professionals track the number of claims that the organization is involved with at any given time. The total number of claims represents, arguably, high-level results of the safety and risk program at a facility. The measurement is created by counting the total number of claims for a given time period and can be tracked in a line graph plotting the monthly, quarterly, or annual number of claims. The advantage of this measure is that it provides a baseline of the volume of claims against the organization in several areas. The disadvantage is that the numbers are often too small to be statistically significant, and the claims that are currently active in an organization reflect events that occurred months and often years before the report.

Just as the organization has to define risk management and risk analysis it also has to define claim. Many organizations identify a claim as any event that the risk management professional thinks could give rise to compensation, or a formal demand for compensation, be it a letter or filed lawsuit. Other organizations define a claim as a filed lawsuit. It is important that the organization define how it will use the term and then consistently apply that definition.

Total Number of Potential Claims Many health care risk management programs track potential claims, such as those events that involve identifiable patient harm, or events where there is no legal activity or demand for compensation, but the risk management professional determines that there is potential for an assertion. These potential claims provide a sense of the volume of potentially compensable events that the organization is experiencing, allowing for early intervention and disposition.

Cost to the Organization for Claims   The total claims costs, along with the claims volume, are good foundational measurements of a traditional risk management program. Total claims costs include expense and indemnity dollars, both reserved and paid. Expense dollars generally include the cost to defend or settle a claim, along with the cost of investigation, medical record copying fees, deposition cost, expert witness fees, attorney fees, and the like. Indemnity costs include those dollars necessary to settle the case with the plaintiff, and can represent medical cost (past, present, and future), lost wages, pain and suffering, and so on. The advantage of this cost measurement is that it provides a direct measure of financial obligation, but the disadvantage is that the values are quite variable.

Potential Claims by Event Type or Cause   Risk management professionals can isolate, per specialty, the number and severity of cases, to implement specific risk prevention strategies. However, the breakdown of claims into sub-groups by event type or cause often results in such small numbers in the sub-groups that they cannot be used effectively for tracking purposes.

Total Cost of Risk   The total cost of risk report is a means of capturing multiple data sets to describe the risk management structure and services so as to focus on the issues relative to the financial measurement of risk. Taking a snapshot in time allows the organization to look at the insurance program structure (limits, coverage, and premium costs), expenses to run the program including salaries of risk and claims staff, funding of the self-insured retention or deductible, claims adjusting costs if an outside TPA is used, medical bill writeoffs, and costs to defend or manage claims. The administrative expenses, including the costs related to risk management and loss control, audit fees, actuary fees, and so on, should be factored into the total cost of risk report.

A total cost of risk report provides a financial snapshot of the cost to the organization of the risk management program across all lines of insurance and operating business units. An example is provided in Exhibit 6.1.

Qualitative Measurements of Risk Management Programs   Many organizations track broad process measures that indicate that the structure of a risk management program has been implemented. These measures are most important in an organization where the risk management program is relatively new. They include the creation of policies and procedures to document the risk management program or the communication of risk management issues to senior leadership or the board of directors. Although these measurements indicate whether a basic risk management infrastructure has been established, it does not indicate the success of the organization in reducing risk exposures to the organization.

The disadvantage of traditional measurements for risk management is they do not provide data which can be acted upon in any meaningful way; rather, the data provide a snapshot of financial risk to the organization for events that occurred in the distant past.

A method often used in the past is to "benchmark" the number (frequency) of claims in a particular area with the cost or severity of those cases. For instance, tracking the number of neonatal injury cases and the average cost of those cases in various parts of the country is one method risk management has used to provide a focus to one clinical area. Defense costs, and the average cost to defend certain claims, are calculated and tracked over time. This might be relevant information; however, it only identifies a potential problem. To address the problem and move toward resolution, it is necessary to apply

EXHIBIT 6.1   Total Cost of Risk Report

Provides a snapshot in time used to summarize, inform, and improve the health care system's total cost of risk by using data to identify risk trends for the health system and individual business units.

YEARS FOR COMPARISONS

	2005	2004	2003	2003

Premium Expense
- Gross Premiums
- Broker Fees
- State Fees
- Bonds/Securities
- Other
- Excess (state-related)

Subtotal

Loss Expenses
- Funded Losses
- Claims Adjusting—TPA
        In sourced
- Medical/Rehab (in sourced)
- Deductible retained
- Investigation (business unit claims and litigation)

Subtotal

Administrative Expenses
- Department Costs related to risk
- Loss control: System
                Local
                Outsourced
- Audit Fees
- Actuary Fees

Subtotal

GRAND TOTAL

process improvement in a quantifiable way to compare a facility's processes against other facilities that might have better results.

Other measurement tools for performance and process improvements include work by W. Edwards Deming and Joseph Juran. Together, their work is viewed as foundational for quality improvement principles and tools for industry and health care.[9]

Deming focused on the theoretical aspects for managing organizations and emphasized systems effect on outcomes. His work to define systems and understand variation in practice supported much of the early work in health care quality.

On the other hand, Juran had a more practical approach to managing quality in organizations. He used principles to implement strategic quality processes to manage quality functions in organizations. Quality improvement, quality planning, and quality controls were touted as the means to affect the strategic quality planning for organizations.

Together, these two giants established the premise that top management needs to be the driver for long-term commitment and change to be effective. Further, systems were more at the root of problems in organizations than the failure of individuals operating within the faulty systems. They began to question the incentives that had been built to motivate practices that were based on faulty premises. Great importance was placed on planning upstream, which would ultimately affect the output downstream. Finally, they recognized the need to understand process variation and the effect this was having on overall improvement.[10]

Tools for Measurement

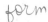

The "Plan, Do, Check, Act" (PDCA) cycle offers health care systems a simple yet effective way to measure and modify change based on the effect on the quality outcome of the change they are attempting to achieve. Sometimes it is referred to as the Deming Cycle, after Deming introduced the concept in Japan in the 1950s. The PDCA is an improvement cycle based on a scientific method of proposing a change in process, implementing the change, measuring the results, and taking appropriate action. The four stages are:[11]

- Plan: Determine goals for a process and changes needed to achieve them.
- Do: Implement the changes.
- Check: Evaluate the results in terms of performance.
- Act: Standardize and stabilize the change or begin the cycle again, depending on the results.

Metrics

A metric is a standard to measure and assess performance or process. The new prospective patient safety measurements provide a robust set of measurements to assess the safety of an organization and guide improvement efforts.

Measurements typically used as part of patient safety work often embrace reactive and proactive measurements. Patient falls data is a key example. A patient falls rate (number of inpatients falling in a given time period divided by the total number of inpatient days) is often a retrospective measurement used to track the outcome of patient safety efforts. The patient falls rate tells leadership, risk management, and the patient safety staff whether process improvements are making a difference in reducing patient falls. Other types of measures often tracked in a patient falls prevention initiative include concurrent data, such as the percent of patients that receive a falls risk assessment, or the number of patients scored as high risk with an intervention in place to reduce the fall risk. These process measures indicate how well the nursing staff is addressing the issue of patient fall risk for the patient population, and implementing appropriate care plans to reduce the risk of falls based on patients' risk profiles.

Another type of measure, called a balancing measure, is also used in prospective patient safety work. A balancing measure for the "patient falls" work would be the number of patients who receive a 1:1 attendant. This measure would help provide an assessment of whether the fall risk is decreasing because of the increased use of 1:1 attendants, rather than the more robust and less resource-draining prevention methods.

Good Catches and Near Misses

Beyond the typically reported safety events in hospitals, hospitals have begun reporting events called "near misses" or "good catches." These events are not truly "events" in the traditional risk management definition, but rather are occurrences that are identified before they become events. The Joint Commission on Accreditation of HealthCare Organizations (JCAHO) has used the term "near miss" in its sentinel event program to mean events that did not have a significant outcome but might have if the situation had been repeated. Similarly, "good catches" is a synonymous term used to describe events caught before they harmed the patient. An example might be a nurse who prepared medications for two patients in separate rooms, walking into the first patient's room to administer the medication and almost giving the patient the wrong medications, but catching the mistake before administering the medication in error.

Tracking these events and reporting on a monthly basis will do little for an organization except to demonstrate how staff members are reporting situations that could be acted upon to prevent events before they happen. The underlying data on the events is most useful to guide organizational improvement efforts aimed at preventing significant events, rather than waiting until a major event occurs before action is taken. The best way to analyze such data is first to organize them into categories and then analyze the details to understand the processes leading to the near misses. Process review and improvement, using tools such as the PDCA model, enable the organization to monitor improvements and continually alter processes and measure results.

Accidents Waiting to Happen

In most health care organizations, potential accidents are rarely reported through traditional safety event or incident reporting systems. The "accident waiting to happen" is an event that most likely does not involve any specific patient, but has the potential to cause harm to patients. For example, this might include the manner in which a medication is stored in a cabinet next to another medication with a similar name, potentially leading to error when the wrong medication is chosen. This type of situation is useful in guiding a health care organization to create process improvements before adverse events occur. This information is important in leadership rounding programs, as an extra or external pair of eyes can pick up potential safety situations more easily than staff routinely working within the environment.

Comparative Data on Patient Safety

Many health care organizations have created patient safety data collection processes, following the IOM report in 1999.[12] So many separate systems were created that the National Quality Forum assigned a council to decide on a standard national patient safety taxonomy that will serve as the foundational data collection taxonomy for future measurements. This taxonomy will be a guide for health care organizations in standardizing the data elements collected. This will allow for comparison of data across hospitals to determine trends of significant events and identify areas for improvement on a larger scale. Alignment with this taxonomy will be a key task for health care organizations over the next several years to enable the creation of comparative data.

The most useful metrics support strategic goals of the health care organization and the risk management program, and produce actionable information for use by the governing body, medical staff, risk management professional, or other stakeholders. Developing meaningful metrics that measure the factor desired requires time and thought. Sometimes, mentally working backwards from desired outcomes or the data needed to support decision making will lead to the needed process or outcome measure.

Small-group brainstorming about the service or program that is being measured may also provide a focus for measurement and potential measures. Typically, developing good outcome measures poses the most difficult challenge, as outcomes may be delayed or under the influence of multiple factors outside of the risk management program's control. Relying solely on process measures may be a prudent first step when devising a new measurement system, or it might be possible to identify some measurable short-term or partial outcomes. It is more desirable to develop a few robust measures than to count multiple items for vague purposes.

DEVELOPING NEW METRICS

The following characteristics are associated with good measures:

- Objective or measurable—Although this is an obvious characteristic, it is also a challenging one, as the broad goal in program evaluation is often to measure the "success" of a specific effort. The subjective term "success" must be operationalized in measurable terms such as fewer claims, reduced legal fees, or increased physician reporting so that the data that must be collected can be identified. Qualitative information, such as comments from clinical staff, might provide some useful data when you cannot identify an objective quantifiable measure.

- Sensitive or responsive—The item to be measured is believed to change over time and to be responsive to risk management activities. The metric can capture or record these changes.

- Meaningful—The metric addresses a key aspect of program operation or desired outcomes and is likely to be important as a basis for decision making. A meaningful measure will be understood both inside and outside the risk management department.

- Unique—The metric measures one item or factor, or if it measures more than one factor, the measure is divided into subcomponents. For example, a metric regarding the number of adverse events and near misses reported in a quarter should have a separate indicator for counting adverse events and another for counting near misses.

- Realm of control—Is the item being measured under the direct control of the risk management program or thought to be influenced by organization-wide risk management activities? If there are other internal or external factors affecting this measure, they need to be identified to factor them into data analysis and reporting. Considering realm of control is particularly important when developing and reporting outcome measures. Jurisdiction, new state medical professional liability legislation, relative number, and expertise of the plaintiffs' bar are external factors that might affect the risk management program's ability to reduce aggregate claims settlement amounts.

- Feasibility—Are the data needed for the measure readily available or easily derived from existing health information management systems? How often will data be needed: quarterly, monthly, weekly, or at some other frequency? Will data need to be pulled from various data sources within the health system, such as from the medical record, incident reports, or audits? If the measure involves new data collection, how would this be accomplished and what resources would be needed? Could data collection be piggy-backed on an existing effort? Could the data collection process be automated through an electronic medical record system, where available? If possible, do a rough cost–benefit analysis of implementing this measure. Reducing the burden of ongoing data collection should be a factor in the design of any new metric.

- Validity—Does the metric actually measure what it is supposed to measure? Few risk management professionals routinely perform any statistical tests of validity of a measure. Most rely on "face" validity, which involves consensus by experts in the field that this is a reasonable measure of "X" or some dimension of "X." Seek some internal or external review of draft measures by professional colleagues or others knowledgeable in risk management and try to improve the validity of new measures. If more assurance is needed regarding validity, get assistance from a statistician or health services researcher. One particular area of concern with relation to validity in risk and safety work is the underreporting associated with voluntarily reported safety events or incidents. When using trends or rates of voluntarily reported safety events, validity of the data is a concern if underreporting of events is present.

- Reliability—Will the measure produce similar data results in the hands of different users over time? If the measure involves considerable additional data collection, a simple test of interrater reliability (reliability among multiple raters) might be worthwhile before proceeding to full implementation. Interrater reliability indicates the consistency of data collection between separate individuals collecting the same data. For example, if two individuals are abstracting the same data elements and end up with the same results, there is high interrater reliability.

- Baseline—It is important when selecting a metric to look for one that has a baseline period available to use as a comparison to the follow-up data once improvements have been put into place. A baseline is a measurement during a period of time before an intervention. It is collected to provide this comparison. Without a baseline measure, it is difficult to ascertain whether the current data indicate a change from the previous environment or if any improvement has been made.

- Multidimensional—Consider measuring different dimensions of the risk management program by using several structure, process, and outcome measures to develop a better picture of program functioning. In addition to these three standbys of measurement, many national evaluation programs such as the Eighth Scope of Work of Quality Improvement Organizations[13] include other types of measurements, such as patients' experience of care, infrastructure enhancements, such as use of health information technology, or cultural readiness for patient safety.

Using the right metrics helps create a dashboard or scorecard for risk management that directs leaders and board members to answer the question: Is the risk management program successful in its efforts?

A *scorecard* is an evaluation tool that specifies the criteria the health care facility's key stakeholders will use to rate risk management performance in relation to the requirements.

On the other hand, a *dashboard* is a tool used for collecting and reporting information about vital customer requirements or your business's performance for key customers. Dashboards provide a quick summary of process or performance outcomes.[14]

An effective performance metrics system:[15]

- Defines what is important from the customer's perspective.
- Builds measures that support the desired performance.
- Creates an environment of trust where real issues can be discussed openly; progress is celebrated.

- Is routinely reviewed and analyzed.

  Effective metrics will have the following attributes:[16]

- They drive better decision making.
- They are objective and easily measured.
- They always result in action.
- Over time, they are predictive in nature, not simply reactive.
- They are easily understood by multiple stakeholders.
- They drive improvements in efficiency, effectiveness, customer satisfaction, and employee satisfaction in an environment of mutual respect.
- They are owned and regularly reviewed by management and employees alike.

Performance metrics can be extremely useful to assess the effectiveness of a risk management program. Using predetermined goals that are measured against performance standards takes the subjectivity out of the effectiveness question. Further, by creating a team of people at the inception of the process to help define the measures, and by monitoring the suitability and effectiveness of the measures, using predetermined goals permits the organization to stay focused on the risk management goals.

The Institute for Healthcare Improvement (IHI)[17] has defined measures for improvement as different from measures for research. It is important to differentiate the two. Measures for research have a purpose to discover new knowledge. The purpose of measurement for process improvement is to bring new knowledge into daily practice.

Research typically relies on one large "blind" test, whereas process improvement uses many sequential and observable tests of change. Volumes of data are gathered in research to ensure that all bases are covered. Just enough data is gathered in PI work to learn and complete another cycle of improvement, and research usually takes long periods of time to report on the results. PI relies on small tests of change to accelerate improvement.

· · · · · · · · · · ·

CONCLUSION

Connecting financial information with the clinical risk information begins to paint a picture for the organization's leadership of the importance of risk management and patient safety to the viability of the health care organization. It is important to represent both components to relate the true picture of risk prevention and management in the organization.

Clinical risk issues that are measures in today's health care structures look at issues such as clinical and environmental risk assessments, identifying gaps from regulatory standards to practice issues with strong linkages to patient outcomes and claims. Integrating the quality data and the risk management data not only provides the organization with a sense of continuity and teamwork between the disciplines, but also begins to describe the various components of the issue from a quality viewpoint, a patient safety vantage, or a risk management and prevention perspective.

Risk management, patient safety, and quality improvement are all vehicles currently used in health care to build a safe and reliable system of patient care. Past work has involved individual departments separately collecting data and analyzing that information to draw conclusions and direct the organization in setting plans and goals independent of each other. As risk management professionals continue to define and expand their professional discipline and assess their organizations' readiness to change, it is incumbent that past models be reevaluated. The disciplines of risk management, patient safety, and quality improvement need to integrate their approach to patient care. This integration will ultimately support the efficient use of organizational resources to improve outcomes.

The authors would like to thank Marva West Tan, Associate Director, Quality Initiative, State of Maryland, Department of Health and Mental Hygiene, for her research assistance in developing this chapter.

Endnotes

1. Carroll, R. L., Editor, *Risk Management Handbook for Health Care Organizations*. 4th Edition, 2004, Jossey- Bass, Inc., San Francisco, CA.

2. "Benchmarking: Leveraging Best-Practice Strategies," an APQC White Paper for Senior Management based on the internationally acclaimed study *Organizing and Managing Benchmarking* | Copyright ©1995, 1999 APQC, all rights reserved. [www.apqc.org].

3. Camp, R. C., Quoted in PSA online, "Benchmarking," Copyright © 2001 Productive Solutions Australia Pty Ltd. All rights reserved. *Available at* www.productivesolutions. com.au/Benchmarking.html. Site, accessed 01.09.06.

4. Davis R. I., R. A. Davis, "How to Prepare For and Conduct a Benchmark Project," Electronic College of Process Innovation, Framework for Managing Process Improvement Benchmark Tutorial, Department of Defense, 7/15/94.

5. Camp, *op. cit.*

6. Kohn, L. T., J. M. Corrigan, and M. S. Donaldson (eds.), *To Err is Human: Building a Safer Health System*; Institute of Medicine, Committee on Quality of Health Care in America, Washington, D.C., National Academy Press, 1999.

7. *Crossing the Quality Chasm: A New Health Care System for the 21st Century*, Committee on Quality of Health Care in America Institute of Medicine, March 2001, National Academy Press, Washington, DC.

8. Best, M., D. Neuhauser. *Avedis Donabedian: Father of Quality Assurance and Poet*; Quality and Safety in Health Care 2004;13;472–473. Available at qhc.bmjjournals. com/cgi/reprint/13/6/472. Accessed 12/30/05.

9. Landesberg, P. "In the Beginning, There were Deming and Juran." *The Journal For Quality & Participation*, November/December 1999.pp. 59–61. [www.aqp.org]

10. *Ibid.*

11. "Capsule Summaries of Key Lean Concepts." Lean Enterprise Institute, Source: *Lean Lexicon,* Brookline, MA [www.lean.org].

12. Kohn, *op. cit.*

13. Centers for Medicare and Medicaid Services; Medicare News April 7, 2005, available at www.cms.hhs.gov/apps/media/press/release.asp?Counter=1421.

14. Copyright © 2000–2005 iSixSigma LLC—All rights reserved reproduction without permission is strictly prohibited. [www. Six Sigma http://health care.isixsigma.com].

15. Romeu M., *Developing a Performance Metrics System; An Introduction to Performance Management Tools*, p. 1, Copyrights MR Group, Inc. 2003 For more information: info@mrgroup-inc.com.

16. *Ibid.*, pp 1–2.

17. Institute for Healthcare Improvement. Online information available at: www.IHI. org/IHI/Topics/Improvement/ImprovementMethods/Measures.

Suggested Readings

Guidelines for managing risk in the health care sector HB 228:2001Standards Australia ASNZ4360.

Juran, J. M. A *history of managing for quality: The evolution, trends, and future directions of managing for quality.* J. M. Juran, editor-in-chief. Milwaukee, Wis.: ASQC Quality Press, 1995.

Juran, J. M. *Juran on leadership for quality: An executive handbook.* New York: Free Press; Toronto: Maxwell Macmillan Canada, 1989.

Donabedian, A. "Evaluating the quality of medical care." *Milbank Memorial Fund Quarterly* 1966;44:166–206.

7

Ethics in Patient Care

Sheila Cohen Zimmet

This chapter is intended to provide the reader with an understanding of the ethics and law affecting everyday patient care issues, particularly those that are the most difficult to resolve—decisions to withhold or withdraw medical treatment, and experimentation on human subjects. It is hoped that an understanding of the relevant bioethical and legal principles will assist the risk management professional in reducing legal exposures by promoting communication among health care providers, patients, and their families as to available treatment options and the benefits and burdens of each. All too often risk management issues arise because patients, their family members, or surrogates[1] are uncomfortable about treatment decisions that have been made either with or without their participation. They feel they have been the subject of experimentation without their knowledge, or they simply are not comfortable deciding to forgo further treatment because they think it might not be the "right" thing to do.

If the families or surrogates of patients with terminal, incurable illnesses were counseled, understood the benefits and burdens of treatment, and understood that it is ethically permissible, or perhaps preferable, to withhold futile care when the burdens of treatment outweighed the benefits of that treatment, there would be far less suspicion and even hostility in intensive care units. It is important that patients and their families understand and believe that treatment recommendations are made on the basis of burdens and benefits to the patient, not to the managed care system. It is the rare family dispute, or stalemate over a terminally ill patient's treatment options, that cannot be resolved by having health care providers, family members or other surrogates, and religious and ethics consultants together in one room, openly discussing the ethically permissible options, including the option of no further treatment.

The suggested readings and Web sites at the end of this chapter contain basic ethics and regulatory documents that are useful reference tools for the risk management professional. The emphasis is on ethics because ethical principles, along with constitutional interpretation, are the source of the law that has developed in this area. The legal concept of patient self-determination that is recognized in judicial opinions and codified into law derives from the ethical principle of respect for autonomy (defined further on), as does the law applicable to research on human subjects.

....

ETHICAL PRINCIPLES AND MORAL OBLIGATIONS

The relationships between health care providers and their patients and families are guided by certain basic ethical principles and the morally binding obligations that are derived from those principles. The basic ethical principles that are most relevant to clinical bioethics are:

1. Beneficence, which creates an obligation to benefit patients and other people, and to further their welfare and interests

2. A principle of respect for patients' autonomy[2]

3. Nonmaleficence, which asserts an obligation to prevent harm or, if risks of harm must be taken, to minimize those risks

4. Justice, which is relevant to fairness of access to health care and to issues of rationing at the bedside

The morally binding obligations between patient and clinician, or other health care provider, that derive from these principles are:

- To respect the patient's privacy and maintain a process that protects confidentiality

- To communicate honestly about all aspects of the patient's diagnosis, treatment, and prognosis

- To determine whether the patient is capable of sharing in decision-making

- To conduct an ethically valid process of informed consent throughout the relationship

The concepts of doing good (beneficence), avoiding harm (nonmaleficence), privacy, confidentiality, and justice that are central to these ethical principles and moral obligations are recognized in the Oath of Hippocrates set forth in Appendix 7.1.

....

RESEARCH

In 1990, *New England Journal of Medicine* Executive Editor Dr. Marcia Angell reiterated the journal's position that only research conducted in accordance with the rights of human subjects would be published. The results of unethical research would not be published, regardless of scientific merit.

> There are three reasons for our position. First, the policy of publishing only ethical research, if generally applied, would deter unethical work. . . . Furthermore, any other policy would tend to lead to more unethical work. . . . Second, denying publication even when the ethical violations are minor protects the principle of the primacy of the research subject. If small lapses were permitted we would become inured to them, and this would lead to larger violations. And finally, refusal to publish unethical work serves notice to society at large that even scientists do not consider

science the primary measure of a civilization. Knowledge, although important, may be less important to a decent society than the way it is obtained.[3]

The primacy of the human subject of which Dr. Angell wrote is the central concept of the modern system of human subject protection in biomedical research. It has its roots in the basic ethical principles of respect for people, beneficence, and justice, the hallmarks of the National Commission for the Protection of Human Subjects in Biomedical and Behavioral Research's Belmont Report (1979). The Belmont Report described the basic ethical principles upon which all biomedical and behavioral research should be based. (See Appendix 7.2 at the end of this chapter for more information on the Belmont Report.)

The Belmont Report was not the first to address these important concepts in the context of human research. In developing its report, the National Commission looked to the principles enunciated in the Nuremberg Code, developed during the Nuremberg War Crime Trials. These principles were used as a set of standards to judge the conduct of those physicians and scientists who had conducted biomedical research on imprisoned populations, and for whom the results of that research took priority over the human subjects themselves. (See Appendix 7.3 for more on the Nuremberg Code.) The commission also looked to the Declaration of Helsinki, first adopted by the World Medical Assembly in 1964, as recommendations to guide medical doctors in biomedical research involving human subjects. The Declaration of Helsinki provides the accepted ethical standards for international human subject research. (See www.wma.net/e/policy/b3.htm for the Declaration of Helsinki.)

The three basic ethical concepts of the Belmont Report, in addition to the current regulations governing research on human subjects, are defined in the report as follows:

- *Respect for persons* means a recognition of the personal dignity and autonomy of individuals, and special protection of those persons with diminished autonomy . . . an affirmative obligation to protect vulnerable populations.

- *Beneficence* involves an obligation to maximize benefits and minimize risks of harm (nonmaleficence).

- *Justice* requires a fair distribution of the benefits and burdens of research.

Adherence to these basic ethical concepts ensures that the disadvantaged are not used as research subjects for the benefit of the advantaged, and that social progress resulting from human research does not justify overriding the rights of the individual subject.[4]

The Belmont Report distinguished between research and practice in discussing which activities require special review. Practice includes interventions designed to enhance the well-being of a patient through either diagnosis or treatment and which have a reasonable expectation of success. Per the Belmont Report, research was defined as an activity designed to test a hypothesis, permit conclusions to be drawn, and thereby to develop or contribute to generalizable knowledge (expressed, for example, in theories, principles, and statements of relationships). A departure from standard practice or the institution of a new treatment was not viewed as research. However, the commission recommended that new procedures should first be made part of formal research protocols, to evaluate safety and efficacy.

Following publication of the Belmont Report, both the Department of Health, Education and Welfare (formerly the DHEW, now the Department of Health and Human Services [DHHS]) and the Food and Drug Administration (FDA) strengthened their human subject protections, increasing but not altering the role of the Institutional Review Boards (IRBs). The DHHS human research regulations, including IRB requirements, are codified at Code of Federal Regulations Title 45, Part 46 (including the Federal Policy or

"Common Rule," followed by all federal agencies that sponsor research). FDA regulations on human research are codified at CFR Title 21 Parts 50 (Informed Consent), 56 (Institutional Review Boards), 312 (Investigational New Drug Application), 812 (Investigational Device Exemptions), and 860 (Medical Device Classification Procedures).

Each health care institution that receives federal funding for human research from a department or agency covered by the Federal Policy or "Common Rule," or that is subject to FDA regulation, must have one or more IRBs with authority to prospectively review, require modification of, approve, or disapprove the research. The IRB may be established by the institution or, less often, may be an independent IRB under contract to the institution to provide IRB services. A document assuring compliance with human subject protections must be negotiated between the institution and DHHS before DHHS-funded research may be conducted. The document, known as an assurance, may be for a single project or, more often, may be a Federalwide Assurance (FWA).

Applicable regulations are codified at 45 C.F.R. 46.103. The DHHS and FDA have the authority to conduct compliance inspections of institutions engaged in research, including the activities of IRBs, and to halt or restrict federally funded research if institutions are found out of compliance with human subject protections. For example, an institution found to be out of compliance may have its assurance restricted or revoked.

FDA and Office of Human Research Protection (OHRP) inspections may be routine, not-for-cause inspections, or may be performed in response to a complaint. In an "Open Letter to the Human Research Community," dated April 17, 2002, Dr. Greg Koski, then Director of OHRP, announced a new quality improvement program that focuses on institutional self-assessment with follow-up "collegial and constructive" on-site consultation visits by OHRP staff. OHRP's Division of Assurances and Quality Improvement (DAQI) would not "ordinarily" share information obtained by OHRP pursuant to voluntary QI evaluations with its Division of Compliance Oversight. (For more information, see the Open Letter, program description, and self-assessment tool on the OHRP Web site at [www.hhs.gov/ohrp/qi/]).

In another open letter, dated September 12, 2002, Dr. Koski renewed OHRP's invitation for institutions to participate in the QI program and noted that OHRP will defer not-for-cause evaluations of an institution that has participated in or is scheduling a QI consultation. In other words, health care organizations are more likely to be subject to a not-for-cause inspection if they do not voluntarily participate in the QI program.

The federal research requirements are founded on respect for the autonomy of the research subject, evidenced by stringent informed consent requirements; the protection of vulnerable populations; the absence of coercion; and the reasonable balance of benefits and burdens of the proposed research for the individual subject, not for society at large. An individual's decision not to participate in research may not in any way affect the ability of the individual to receive medical care or other benefits to which the individual otherwise would be entitled. It is the role of the IRBs to review and monitor the conduct of research and to educate the the research community about the proper conduct of research. A discussion of the role of the IRBs and recent regulatory activity in this area follows.

●●●●●●●●●●●●
INSTITUTIONAL REVIEW BOARDS

For Dr. Gary B. Ellis, former director of the Office for Protection from Research Risks (OPRR),[5] the relationship between subject and researcher is one based on trust, and that trust must be respected:

In the final analysis, research investigators, research institutions, and federal regulators are stewards of a trust agreement with the people who are research subjects. For research subjects who are safeguarded by the federal regulations, we have a system in place that (1) minimizes the potential for harm, (2) enables and protects individual, autonomous choice, and (3) promotes the pursuit of new knowledge. By doing so, we protect the rights and welfare of our fellow citizens who make a remarkable contribution to the common good by participating in research studies. We owe them our best effort.[6]

To Dr. Jordan Cohen of the Association of American Medical Colleges, the successful conduct of medical research in a free society depends on trust between the scientific enterprise and the public, trust in the integrity of the discovery process, and epecially trust in the safety of patients and healthy volunteers who participate in the process. (Cohen, Jordan J., Siegel, Elisa K., "Academic Medical Centers and Medical Research," JAMA, 294, Sept 21, 2005, 1367–1372, 1369).

It is the role of the IRBs to safeguard that trust and to assess research in terms of risks and benefits, the adequacy of informed consent, the adequacy of safeguards to protect the privacy and confidentiality of subjects,[7] and the equitable selection of subjects (for example, is inclusion of vulnerable populations appropriate? Are minorities and women of childbearing potential adequately represented, or is a clear and compelling reason for their exclusion provided?). The IRB must (1) identify risks of the research, (2) determine that the risks will be minimized to the extent possible, (3) identify probable benefits of the research, (4) determine that the risks are reasonable in relation to the benefits to the subject and the knowledge to be gained, (5) ensure that research subjects are provided with an accurate and fair description of the risks, discomforts, and anticipated benefits, (6) ensure that research subjects are offered the opportunity to voluntarily accept or reject participation in the research, or discontinue participation, without coercion or fear of reprisal or deprivation of treatment to which the patient is otherwise entitled,[8] and (7) determine intervals of periodic review and, when necessary, determine the adequacy of mechanisms for monitoring data collection.

Maintaining strong safeguards for the safety of human subjects in medical research is a paramount obligation of clinical investigators and their institutions. Institutional review boards (IRBs) are the heart of the protection regime; they are responsible for reviewing all clinical and translational research conducted at their respective institutions and for making ethical determinations that risks to human subjects have been minimized to the greatest extent possible; that risks are reasonable in relation to anticipated benefits, if any; and that the risks, benefits, and alternative options are clearly communicated to the potential participants in the informed consent process.

In a time of declining clinical revenue, there may be increased pressure from principal investigators and administrators to cut corners and speed up the approval process for sponsored research. Such an approach places the welfare of the researcher and the research institution ahead of the welfare of the subject, and is inconsistent with the ethical foundation of biomedical research and the derivative regulatory framework. The results of research, whether in terms of scientific recognition or of financial reward, may never take priority over the research subject. Furthermore, compliance activities of federal regulatory bodies have shown that an approach to research that minimizes protection of the subject can ultimately prove to be very costly, both in revenue and reputation.

At the 2002 Fraud and Compliance Forum sponsored by the American Health Lawyers Association and the Health Care Compliance Association, Dr. Melody Lin of the OHRP Office of Research Compliance identified common findings and deficiencies associated with compliance oversight activities. These included:

- Initial and continuing review issues
  - Inadequate IRB review, particularly with respect to issues affecting vulnerable populations
  - IRB review without sufficient information
  - Contingent approval with no system for follow-up
  - Inadequate continuing annual review, including failure to review at least once per year
- Informed consent and informed consent documentation issues
  - Language too complex
  - Use of impermissible exculpatory language
  - Standard consent forms inadequate for certain procedures
  - Reliance on standard surgical consent form to collect tissue samples
  - Inappropriate boilerplates
  - Failure to minimize possibility of coercion or undue influence
- IRB membership and expertise issues
  - Lack of researcher diversity
  - Lack of IRB expertise for research
  - Lack of IRB expertise for research involving children and prisoners
  - Lack of sufficient understanding of regulations
  - Designation of an additional IRB without OHRP approval
- Documentation of IRB activities
  - Inappropriate application of exemption (not in six categories)
  - Inappropriate use of expedited approvals
  - Failure to document consideration of additional safeguards
  - Inadequate minutes (meaning votes not recorded, no summary of important issues, inability to reconstruct what was approved)
  - Poorly maintained files
- IRB convened without a quorum
  - Non-scientist absent
  - Majority not present
- Conflict of interest issues
  - IRB members
  - Office of sponsored research
  - Institutional officials
  - Inappropriate waiver of informed consent
- Lack of written standard operating procedures
- Failure to report unanticipated problems to OHRP
- Inadequate IRB resources and overburdened IRBs, which is considered the primary problem

Government oversight compliance activities have increased significantly since 1999 and are expected to continue at increased intensity, signaling an increase in public interest in the ethical and procedural propriety of biomedical research. OHRP posts its compliance activities on its Web site, including the text of determination letters sent to research institutions operating under OHRP assurances. It is useful for risk management professionals to review the posted letters at (ohrp.osophs.dhhs.gov/detrm_letrs/lindex.htm) to determine OHRP compliance priorities.

A review of the 2005 OHRP Determination Letters posted on its Web site reveals a similar pattern of common deficiences: (1) Consent form deficiencies such as language not understandable to the public, inadequate explanation of potential risks, failure to address all required elements of informed consent, failure to describe all research procedures; (2) IRB procedural and process deficiencies, such as inadequate written policies and procedures; improper use of expedited review for research not within permissible categories; inadequate information considered by the IRB to make required risk and benefit determinations, particulary with respect to research involving pediatric subjects for which specific documented findings are required; substantive changes to protocols and consent forms without full Board re-review; failure of documentation of IRB actions, including attendance, specific votes on actions taken, and summary of IRB discussions; (3) Lapsed IRB approval-IRB approval is valid for no greater than one year-study approval expires after one year and the study administratively terminates; all research activity must stop, unless the IRB specifically finds that it is in the best interest of subjects already enrolled to continue research activities, 4) Failure to report to OHRP unanticipated problems involving risks to subjects, serious or continuing noncompliance, suspensions and terminatinons.

The risk management professional should review the OHRP Determination Letters, Informed Consent Checklist, Guidance documents,and Decision Charts, and on the OHRP Web site (www.hhs.gov/ohrp/) for a more detailed analysis of and useful tools for compliance with the IRB's obligations in each of these areas. Comprehensive, mistake-proof IRB application forms, consent form templates, and IRB reviewer forms that elicit all required information, address all necessary informed consent elements, and contain required IRB findings, are important tools for maximizing the safety of human subjects and minimizing institutional liability.

The failure of some IRBs to consider whether the investigator has a potential conflict of interest and to determine how to manage or eliminate that conflict, along with the failure to inform the subject of potential conflicts of interest of the investigator or the institution, has resulted in significant public condemnation and increased regulatory scrutiny. It is essential that each research institution establish its own policies and procedures for the reporting and managing of investigator and institutional conflicts of interest. Does an investigator, for example, have an impermissible financial conflict of interest because of a paid consultancy or an equity interest in the sponsor? Can the conflict be managed with an independent oversight committee to verify the integrity of the data? (For more information, see [grants1.nih.gov/grants/policy/coi/index.htm and www.aamc.org/members/coitf/].

It also is the responsibility of each research institution and its IRB to educate investigators to monitor the conduct of research and to ensure that the IRB members themselves are adequately and continually trained in human research protection. Ultimately, the expectation is for increasing institutional support for the research compliance infrastructure, including adequate staff resources that incorporate a research compliance officer function for implementation and monitoring of research activities and for management of research funds.

Gene or Recombinant DNA Research

Research involving recombinant DNA or gene therapy that has any federal funding requires additional levels of review and approval at the institutional level (Institutional Biosafety Committee) and at the federal level (Recombinant DNA Advisory Committee [RAC] of the Office of Biotechnology Activities [OBA]). The RAC was established to respond to public concerns about the safety of research that involves gene manipulation. See "Frequently Asked Questions" on the OBA Web site at (www4.od.nih.gov/oba/RAC/RAC_FAQs.htm).

Summary

Each research institution should review its own policies and procedures and its IRB records for compliance with federal regulations to determine whether it is vulnerable to an adverse action on the basis of the mentioned criteria. For example, does the institution have an internal for-cause and random monitoring/audit system to verify that investigators are complying with research protocols? Do all subjects sign consent forms? Do IRB policies and procedures satisfy federal requirements? Are minutes of IRB meetings adequate? Does training of IRB members and investigators meet the regulatory compliance emphasis on education? The risk management professional should assess whether and how to assist the institution in meeting its obligations in the area of human biomedical research, or how a research compliance officer or similar official, could do it. The risk management professional should also assess coordination of the activities of its research regulatory bodies—the IRB, the Institutional Biosafety Committee (for recombinant DNA and biohazards), and the Radiation Safety Committee (for radiologic safety; radiation safety review and approval is required by the institution's Nuclear Regulatory Commission license).

If compliance is not adequate, the loss to the institution, in terms of funding and reputation, could be enormous. Institutions must be vigilant in their review and monitoring of the activities of the IRB and investigators and mindful of their own institutional financial conflicts of interest and those of their researchers. If they are not, they can expect that federal oversight, investigative, or prosecutorial bodies will be.

Risk management professionals also should be mindful of the potential for costly civil and criminal litigation growing out of regulatory noncompliance. Numerous well-publicized instances of death or serious injury to human subjects in clinical trials have given rise to costly litigation against institutions, investigators, and individual IRB members. In virtually all instances, civil litigants have raised nondisclosure of prior adverse effects experienced by research subjects or nondisclosure of conflicts of interest as a basis of their causes of action. It is advised that the risk management professionals ensure that IRB procedures and audit mechanisms provide for full disclosure to the IRB and research subjects of all potential risks and complications and all conflicts of interest associated with the research. It is further advised that the risk management professional investigate whether coverage for personal injury and death arising out of administrative actions (such as actions of IRB chairs and members) is included in its insurance portfolio, whether through its professional and general liability coverage or its directors' and officers' (D&O) insurance. Keep in mind that D&O policies traditionally do not include coverage for personal injury and death.

An additional area of potential risk arising out of regulatory non-compliance relates to enforcement activities of the DHHS Office of the Inspector General (OIG) and the U.S. Department of Justice. The risk management professional should be aware that obtaining federal funds in a fraudulent manner, for instance, through billing of the federal government for health care services provided pursuant to a clinical trial for which billing is not permitted; engaging in scientific misconduct in a federally funded research proposal; or improper time and effort and cost reporting in federally funded grants can all serve as the basis for both civil and criminal charges under the federal fraud and abuse laws, including the False Claims Act. In the civil context, the government is entitled to treble damages for successful prosecution. Federal prosecutors have indicated that non-compliance with IRB requirements such as false information or a failure to provide required information to the IRB regarding adverse events, can serve as a basis for prosecution under the fraud and abuse laws.

The Fiscal Year 2005 Work Plan of the DHHS Office of the Inspector General list several research compliance-related areas earmarked for scrutiny, including university administrative and clerical salaries, recharge centers, level of commitment, response of IRBs to adverse event reports, time and effort reporting.

Federal enforcement of regulatory requirements as they apply to research has been and will continue to be aggressive, whether through agency enforcement activities, or application of civil and/or criminal penalties. The cost of non-compliance to the institutions and its employees and agents could be high.

Medical Record Privacy

Under the Common Rule, the IRB must consider whether there are adequate provisions to protect the confidentiality of human subjects. There are additional regulatory requirements for protection of Protected Health Information (PHI), under the privacy provisions of the Health Insurance Portability and Accountability Act (HIPAA) that apply to research. (See 45 C.F.R. Parts 160 and 164.) These privacy protections became effective April 14, 2003, and are enforceable by DHHS through both civil and criminal penalties. HIPAA requirements are discussed in greater detail in Chapter 41; this discussion focuses only on HIPAA and research.

On December 4, 2002, DHHS Office for Civil Rights issued a comprehensive Guidance on the National Standards to Protect the Privacy of Personal Health Information. The Guidance can be found at [www.hhs.gov/ocr/hipaa]; the section on research is found on pages 85–98 of the 123-page document.

Use and Disclosure of Protected Health Information (PHI) for Research Purposes

In general, PHI may be used or disclosed by a covered entity for research if:

1. The covered entity obtains an authorization from the individual to use the individual's PHI.

2. An IRB or Privacy Board waives the need for an individual authorization based on specific criteria set forth in the regulations.

3. The researcher reviews the data "preparatory to research" and does not remove the data from the premises.

4. There is a "data use agreement" between the covered entity and the researcher to obtain a "limited data set" of data that is facially deidentified.

Individually identifiable health information relating to either live or deceased persons that is transmitted or maintained by covered entities in any form or medium is considered PHI and is subject to HIPAA protection. However, under the Common Rule, a human subject is defined as "a living individual" about whom an investigator obtains data through intervention or interaction or obtains identifiable private information. Accordingly, under HIPAA, the IRB or Privacy Board must review and approve the confidentiality provisions of research and must require authorizations or waive the requirement for authorizations for research involving PHI of deceased persons that would not have been reviewed by the IRB under the Common Rule. Risk management professionals should note that the definition of PHI includes the requirement that the information be identifiable. Accordingly, information is not PHI if all specified identifiers are removed as specified in the privacy regulations, or if an expert certifies that the information used alone or in combination with other available information could not identify the individual.

Notwithstanding strong objection from the research community, the final rule issued by DHHS retained the requirements that for information to be de-identified, all of the following information must be removed:

- Names
- Geographic subdivisions smaller than a state except first three digits of ZIP code
- All elements of dates (except year) for those under 89 years
- Telephone numbers
- FAX numbers
- Electronic mail addresses
- Social Security numbers
- Medical record numbers
- Health plan beneficiary numbers
- Account numbers
- Certificate or license numbers
- Vehicle identifiers and serial numbers, including license plate numbers
- Device identifiers and serial numbers
- Web universal resource locators (URLs)
- Internet protocol (IP) addresses
- Biometric identifiers, including finger and voice prints
- Full-face photographic images and any comparable images
- Any other unique identifying number, characteristic, or code, with some exceptions

The rules permit use and disclosure of PHI without an authorization for treatment, payment, and health care operations. However, because research is not considered a health care operation, disclosure without an authorization for research purposes is not permitted, with limited exceptions (for example, research on decedents under certain specified circumstances; reviews preparatory to research; and for research using a limited data set).

A. Authorization for Use and Disclosure of Protected Health Information (PHI) for Research Purposes

To be valid, an authorization for research must include (a) a description of the PHI to be used or disclosed (and this must be the minimum necessary for the research); (b) the person or class of persons who may use or disclose PHI and to whom use or disclosure may be made; (c) the purposes of the use or disclosure; (d) the possibility of redisclosure; (e) an expiration date (end of research study or "none"); (f) signature and date; and (g) a right to revoke. Note also that although research may be conditioned on the subject executing an Authorization to Use and Disclose Protected Health Information for Research Purposes, treatment may not be conditioned on a suject's agreement to participate in research. Refusal to provide treatment if a subject refused to agree to participate in research would be viewed as impermissible coercion.

B. Exceptions from Authorization Requirement

If a researcher requests that authorization be waived for a particular research proposal, the IRB or Privacy Board may waive the authorization only with the following findings:

- The use or disclosure involves no more than minimal risk to the individual's privacy, based on a plan to protect identifiers or a plan to destroy identifiers as soon as possible unless there are research or legal reasons not to do so.
- Assurance that the PHI will not be reused or disclosed to any other person except as required by the research or law.
- The research could not practicably be conducted without the waiver.
- The research could not practicably be conducted without the PHI.

Risk management professionals should note that this analysis is very similar to the analysis currently employed by IRBs when determining whether subject consent for research may be waived. IRB templates can be modified to accommodate the new requirements.

A covered entity may allow access to the PHI of a deceased individual without an authorization or waiver if the researcher represents that the information is sought solely for research on the PHI of decedents. If requested, the researcher provides documentation of the death of the individuals and documentation that PHI is necessary for research purposes.

A covered entity may allow use or disclosure of PHI without an authorization or a waiver for reviews preparatory to research if the researcher represents that (1) the use or disclosure is solely to prepare a research protocol or otherwise preparatory to research; (2) no PHI will be removed from the covered entity; and (3) the PHI is necessary for research purposes.

Compilation of research databases or manipulation of PHI to create a database or to bank tissue also requires an authorization or waiver by an IRB or Privacy Board. This waiver to create the database does not eliminate the requirement for either an authorization to use the data in research or a waiver. An authorization or waiver is required for referral of a patient to a researcher or for a researcher to directly contact a patient. The PHI that the researcher may use or disclose must be defined in the authorization, or, if by waiver, the researcher must specify the minimum information necessary to accomplish the research.

Researchers are not considered business associates under the privacy rules and would not be required to execute business associate agreements with the covered entity to access PHI. The authorization for access to PHI for research must describe the research for which the PHI is to be used. "Future research," although currently a common description used in consent forms, is not an adequate description under HIPAA. Of course, the IRB may waive authorization based on the criteria previously mentioned.

Record-Keeping

If PHI is accessed pursuant to an authorization, the institution is not required to keep a record of that disclosure. If PHI is disclosed pursuant to a waiver, a review preparatory to research or research on decedents, the covered entity must keep a record of disclosures and must provide an accounting when requested. This may be accomplished either through an annotation of the record, which is then provided to the subject, or by providing the subject a list of protocols for which waivers have been granted during the time period involved.

Summary

HIPAA is one more regulatory burden that potentially could delay the review and approval process for research, to the chagrin of researchers and research institutions. However, once it is determined whether the institution will rely on the IRB to make privacy decisions or whether a separate Privacy Board will make such determinations, templates can be developed to facilitate the process and prevent regulatory mistakes.

Risk management professionals should be aware that Fiscal Year 2005 Work Plan of the DHHS Office of the Inspector General indicates an intent to conduct an assessment of the policies and procedures of colleges and universities for protecting the privacy of medical records of people participating in NIH-funded clincal trials and other research, in compliance with the HIPAA privacy standards.

············

PATIENT SELF-DETERMINATION ACT

The federal Patient Self-Determination Act of 1990 (PSDA) [P.L. No.101–508, codified at 42 U.S.C. Sections 1395(c)(c) and 1396(a)(a), Section 4206 of the Omnibus Reconciliation Act of 1990] requires institutional health care providers who receive federal funds, such as hospitals, nursing homes, hospices, and home health agencies, to inform patients of their right to make health care decisions.[9] This includes the right to accept or refuse treatment and the right to formulate advance directives (commonly referred to as living wills and durable powers of attorney).

The law requires hospitals to provide written information to each adult patient at the time of admission concerning the institution's policies for implementing the patient's right to make health care decisions. Advance directives are documents formulated in advance of a period of incapacity in which individuals executing the documents set forth their wishes with respect to treatment options or delineate who should serve as surrogate decision-makers in the event that the individuals become unable to express their own wishes.

The PSDA sets forth a mechanism for educating patients about their constitutional right to self-determination that was recognized by the U.S. Supreme Court in its first "right to die" case, *Cruzan v. Director, Missouri Department of Health,* 497 U.S. 261, 110 S.Ct. 2841, 111 L.Ed. 2nd 224, 58 U.S.L.W. 4916 (1990). In Cruzan, the court held that the due process clause of the Fourteenth Amendment to the U.S. Constitution gives to each person a constitutionally protected liberty interest in refusing unwanted medical treatment, thereby giving constitutional status to the ethical principle of respect for patients' autonomy. In this context, the right of autonomy and the right of self-determination are synonymous.

If a person is incapacitated, and thereby unable to make or express an informed and voluntary choice to accept or refuse treatment, that patient does not lose the right. Rather, the individual's right to make the treatment choices must be exercised by a surrogate. The Durable Power of Attorney for Health Care is the mechanism by which an individual designates who will serve in that surrogate role.[10]

The PSDA focuses on the right of competent patients to determine and direct the future course of their medical treatment. The act seeks to avoid a situation in which the wishes of a patient are not clearly known, or that there is no legally valid surrogate decision-maker available to advise the health care provider what the patient would want under the circumstances. The PSDA does not alter the common law concept of next of kin, nor does it affect substantive state law regarding surrogate decision-making. It sets forth a mechanism whereby patients learn about their rights under state law to make treatment decisions and execute advance directives and are offered the opportunity to take advantage of those rights. Under the PSDA, health care institutions must:

1. Provide written information to all adult patients upon admission or initial receipt of care about their rights to make decisions, including the right to accept or refuse treatment and to execute advance directives, and the written policies of the institution that respect these rights.

2. Comply with state law regarding the rights of patients to make treatment decisions and execute advance directives.

3. Educate the staff and the community about these issues.

4. Document in the patient's medical records whether the individual has executed an advance directive.[11]

5. Not require the execution of an advance directive as a precondition to the provision of care.

Even when an individual has executed an advance directive that sets forth the individual's wishes regarding the acceptance or refusal of treatment, including life-sustaining treatment, it is not always clear to the health care provider or the surrogate what the individual intended under particular clinical circumstances. For example, did the individual who specified that life-sustaining treatment be withdrawn in the event of a terminal, incurable disease or persistent vegetative state intend that mechanical ventilation and artificial hydration and nutrition be withheld, or just the respirator? If the individual did not address a persistent vegetative state, but addressed only a terminal, incurable disease, did that individual intend the treatment choice to be applied to the former, and would state law permit the withdrawal of treatment under these circumstances? State laws differ on the interpretation of when a person is in a terminal, incurable condition so as to invoke the terms of an advance directive. State law may require that an advance directive specify its applicability to a persistent vegetative state for the treatment options to apply. Template Advance directives should be drafted that specifically address treatment options under these different clinical presentations.

In light of court decisions upholding the rights of pregnant women to refuse invasive medical treatment regardless of the gestational age of the fetus, whether or not the treatment is deemed lifesaving or otherwise beneficial (see *Baby Boy Doe v. Mother Doe*, 260 Ill. App.3d 392, 632 N.E.2d 326 [Ill. App. 1994]; In re A.C., 573 A.2d 1235 [D.C. App. 1990]), advance directives that address the treatment wishes of pregnant patients should be considered, particularly for institutions providing tertiary maternal-fetal medicine or perinatology services. The directive should address the provision of life-sustaining treatments for the mother, including artificial hydration, nutrition, and CPR, both before and subsequent to viability of the fetus; and whether or not the patient authorizes a caesarean section if it is deemed to be in the best interest of the unborn child. The directive should provide for authorization or refusal of these treatments, and should specify that failure to provide the treatments may result in the death of, or harm to, the baby.

············
DO NOT RESUSCITATE (DNR)—WITHHOLDING OR WITHDRAWING TREATMENT

It has been said that the paradox of modern medicine is that treatment intended to save life often ends up prolonging the agony of dying.[12] Whether it is due to the clinician's or family's refusal to accept defeat, or the mistaken belief that the withholding or withdrawing of treatment is ethically abhorrent, or the simple discomfort that accompanies a discussion of the inevitability of death, this issue continues to be one of the most difficult and frequent ethical dilemmas confronting health care providers. It is not a new issue. In his treatise *The Art,* Hippocrates defined the purpose of medicine to include the following:

> . . . to do away with the sufferings of the sick, to lessen the violence of their diseases, and to refuse to treat those who are over-mastered by their diseases realizing in such cases that medicine is powerless. . . . Whenever therefore a man suffers an illness which is too strong for the means at the disposal of medicine he surely must not expect that it can be overcome by medicine.[13]

It is clear from the prior discussions of patient autonomy and self-determination that there is a constitutionally protected and ethically sanctioned right to refuse treatment, including life-sustaining treatment. It is important to understand, and to put into practice, a process to determine and implement the treatment decision when the patient cannot make or communicate the choice. Frameworks for decision-making can be found in the 1983 report entitled *The President's Commission for the Study of Ethical Problems in Medicine and Biomedical and Behavioral Research: A Report on the Ethical, Medical, and Legal Issues in Treatment Decisions: Deciding to Forego Life-Sustaining Treatment*[14] and in the Hastings Center's *Guidelines on the Termination of Life-Sustaining Treatment and the Care of the Dying* (1987).[15]

Health care providers should understand that their patients have the right to make health care decisions based on their own values and experiences, and to have their decisions respected. The first step is determining the appropriate decision maker. The competent adult patients, those who can understand the significance of their decisions and can communicate those decisions effectively, have the right to make the decisions. The patients have the right to balance benefits and burdens and decide whether to proceed with treatment, based on their own values and personal preferences. As the commission noted, "The moral claim of autonomy supports acting in accord with the patient's preference."[16] It is ethically appropriate to reject treatment when the burdens of treatment outweigh the benefits of treatment or when treatment is deemed to be futile.

If the patient cannot make or communicate the decision, it is the role of the appropriate surrogate decision-maker to advise the health care provider what the patient would want. This is known as the Substituted Judgment Test. It is not the role of the surrogate to make an independent judgment of what is in the best interest of the patient (the "Best Interest Test"), unless a decision could not otherwise be reached, such as where the patient has never had the capacity to form a judgment (such as a newborn). In general, unless the health care provider has reason to believe that the treatment choice of a legally valid surrogate is inconsistent with that which the patient would make or has set forth in an advance directive, the decision of a surrogate should control.

In the event of a disagreement between clinician and surrogate as to the appropriate course of action, internal mechanisms to resolve the matter, including ethics committee consultation, should be attempted. Resorting to a judicial forum to resolve disagreements between health care providers and decision-makers regarding the appropriate course of treatment for an incapacitated patient is generally unproductive. "Decision-making about life-sustaining care is rarely improved by resort to the courts."[17] It is not the role of the court to substitute its own judgment for the informed substituted judgment of the surrogate, nor will it substitute its own best interest determination for that of the surrogate. Unless the health care provider can establish that the decision of a surrogate to either require or refuse medical treatment, including a do-not-resuscitate order (DNR), constitutes either neglect or abuse, thereby invoking the authority of the state to protect innocent third parties,[18] courts will not override the decisions of legally valid surrogates.

Another example is *In re Baby K,* 16 F.3d 590 (4th Cir. 1994), in which appeals court affirmed the district court ruling was that requiring the hospital to provide full pulmonary resuscitation for an anencephalic infant when requested by the mother, even though the care was deemed futile and outside the scope of the standard of care. The Court of Appeals held that a refusal by emergency room personnel to provide stabilizing resuscitative measures to the infant, if brought to the emergency department in respiratory distress, would constitute a violation of the requirements of the Emergency Medical Treatment and Active Labor Act (EMTALA), 42 USC sec. 1395dd, that all persons seeking emergency medical treatment receive an appropriate medical screening and stabilizing treatment. The lower court ruling that it could not substitute its judgment for the judgment of the mother, who was the legally valid surrogate, was affirmed. The court also stated, with respect to the moral dilemma facing the health care providers who thought the provision of futile care to Baby K was inappropriate:

> . . . to the extent that [Virginia law] exempts treating physicians in participating hospitals from providing care they consider medically or ethically inappropriate, it is preempted . . . it does not allow the physicians treating Baby K to refuse to provide her with respiratory support.[19]

In a recent decision by the District of Columbia Court of Appeals, the court recognized that parents have a fundamental constitutional right to the care, custody, and management of their child that is not absolute, but must yield to the best interest and well-being of the child. In the case of *In Re K.I.,* nos. 98-FS-1683 and 98-FS-1767, 1700–1742 (D.C. App. 1999), the parents disagreed as to the appropriateness of resuscitation for their terminally ill child. The medical evidence established that resuscitation would be futile and would result only in pain and discomfort. The lower court concluded that the mother's refusal to consent to the issuance of the DNR order was unreasonably contrary to the child's well-being. In affirming the lower court ruling that a DNR order should be entered, the Court of Appeals held:

> . . . in cases involving minor respondents who have lacked, and will forever lack, the ability to express a preference regarding their course of medical treatment . . . and where the parents do not speak with the same voice but disagree as to the proper course of action, the best interests of the child standard shall be applied to determine whether to issue a DNR. . . .[20]

In a recent case that reached national prominence, and which involved state and federal government intervention, the husband of a patient determined to be in a persistent vegetative state sought to have life-prolonging procedures terminated, over the objection of her parents.

Michael Schiavo, the husband of Terry Schiavo, petitioned the guardianship court in Florida to authorize termination of artificial hydration and nutrition. The court found by clear and convincing evidence that Terry Schiavo was in a persistent vegetative state and that Terry Schiavo would elect to cease life-prolonging procedures if she were competent to make her own decision. The decisions of the state and federal courts that heard and reviewed this case ultimately supported Terry Schiavo's constitutional liberty interest to accept or refuse treatment, without interference by the legislative and executive branches of government. There were numerous court proceedings related to this matter. (See, in particular, *Jeb Bush v. Michael Schiavo*, No. SC04-925, [Supr Ct of Fla, Sept 23, 2004].)

....

CONCLUSION

It is recommended that risk management professionals become familiar with the ethical issues discussed in this chapter and promote their dissemination to the health care providers who deal with these difficult issues on a regular basis. An ethics consultation mechanism should be made available at any time it is needed to assist health care providers, patients, and their families reach health care decisions that can be implemented with the knowledge that all parties are comfortable with the decision.[21]

Endnotes

1. "Surrogate" refers to the individual who is legally authorized to make health care decisions on behalf of a patient who cannot make or communicate decisions due to incapacity. The surrogate may be the common law next-of-kin or an individual designated by the patient in a Durable Power of Attorney for Health Care to make health care decisions for the patient in the event of temporary or permanent incapacity.

2. Fletcher, J. C. and others. "Clinical Ethics: History, Content, and Resources." In: Fletcher, *Introduction to Clinical Ethics*. Hagerstown, Md. University Publishing Group, 1995, pp. 3–17. The term autonomy derives from the Greek *autos,* meaning self, and *nomos,* meaning rule or law-self-rule, or self-law. The concept of autonomy is associated with privacy, free choice, and personal responsibility for one's choices. Beauchamp, T. L., and L. Walters, *Contemporary Issues in Bioethics*. Belmont, Calif.: Wadsworth Publishing Company, 1994, p. 22.

3. Angell, M. "The Nazi Hypothermia Experiments and Unethical Research Today." *New England Journal of Medicine,* 322, May 17, 1990, 146–64.

4. Jonsen, A. R. "The Ethics of Research with Human Subjects: A Short History." In Jonsen, A. R., R. M. Veatch, and L. Walters. *Source Book in Bioethics*. Georgetown: Georgetown University Press, 1998, pp. 5–9.

5. OPRR is the former federal office with human subject research oversight authority. The office relocated from the National Institutes of Health (NIH) to the Office of Public Health and Science, DHHS, and is now called the Office for Human Research Protection (OHRP). The move was generally accepted as a means of increasing the visibility of federal oversight of human subject protection, and access to the secretary of DHHS.

6. Ellis, G. "Protecting the Rights and Welfare of Human Research Subjects." *Academic Medicine,* 74(9), September 1999, pp. 1008–1009.

7. For particularly sensitive research, such as genetic research when there is a concern that the release of information regarding the results of research could lead to discrimination in the workplace or in the ability of individuals who are found to be carriers of genetic diseases to obtain life or health insurance, there is a mechanism for protection

of data. The secretary of DHHS, or the secretary's designee, may issue a Certificate of Confidentiality "to protect the privacy of research subjects by withholding their identities from all persons not connected with the research. . . . Persons so authorized to protect the privacy of such individuals may not be compelled in any Federal, State, or local civil, criminal, administrative, legislative, or other proceedings to identify such individuals." 42 USC sec. 241(d), Section 301(d) of the Public Health Service Act, Protection of Identity, Research Subjects. For further information, call NIH at (301) 402-7221.

8. For example, is the amount of compensation offered so excessive as to be coercive? Is the subject compensated only at the end of a six-month clinical trial so that the subject cannot withdraw during the trial without loss of all compensation? Or is the compensation prorated for the amount of time the subject participated?

9. Subsequent to enactment of the PSDA, which is enforceable only against institutions that participate in Medicare and Medicaid, the Joint Commission on Accreditation of Health Care Organizations (JCAHO) amended its accreditation standards to require all health care organizations that are accredited by the JCAHO to maintain mechanisms for informing patients about their rights to self-determination and honoring those rights. See JCAHO Comprehensive Accreditation Manual for Hospitals: The Official Handbook, Patient Rights and Organizational Ethics, RI.1.2.4 (1999).

10. This chapter focuses on the rights of patients and their surrogates to make treatment decisions. It is important for the risk management professional to understand that the law presumes consent for medically necessary medical treatment in a medical emergency when consent of the patient cannot be obtained and a surrogate is not available. If the patient's life or future health may be jeopardized if treatment is not instituted immediately, and the treatment has not been refused by the patient, consent will be presumed.

11. While not specified in the law, institutional policies should include a mechanism by which the patient's advance directive is included in the medical record so it is readily available and known to the clinicians before implementation is needed. An advance directive in a safe at the bank or in a drawer at home is not helpful to the health care provider when a decision must be made immediately.

12. Hite, C. A., et al. "Death and Dying." In: Fletcher, et al. *Introduction to Clinical Ethics*, Hagerstown, Md.: University Publishing Group, 1995, pp. 115–138.

13. Hippocrates. The Art. In *Hippocrates* (vol. II). Jones, W.H.S. (trans.). Loeb Classical Library, Cambridge, Mass.: Harvard University Press, 1967. Cited in E. D. Pellegrino, "Withholding and Withdrawing Treatments: Ethics at the Bedside." *Clinical Neurosurgery*, 35, 1989, pp. 164–184.

14. *The President's Commission for the Study of Ethical Problems in Medicine and Biomedical Research: Deciding to Forgo Life-Sustaining Treatment: A Report on the Ethical, Medical, and Legal Issues in Treatment Decisions.* Washington, D.C.: U.S. Government Printing Office, March 1983. Many of the developments during the decade subsequent to the issuance of this report that shape the law and ethics of patient self-determination, as it is understood today, grow out of recommendations of the commission—for example, state enactment of legislation providing for advance directives, and the growth of institutional ethics committees to provide consultation to clinicians and patients and their families on issues that have life-or-death consequences for patients.

15. An excellent summary of the decision-making process described in the ethics literature, including reference to the reports by the Hastings Center and the President's Commission, may be found in Dr. Carol Taylor's 1990 article "Ethics in Health Care and Medical Technologies." *Theoretical Medicine*, 11, 1990, pp. 111–124.

16. The President's Commission, p. 245.

17. *Ibid.,* p. 247.

18. For example, courts have traditionally ordered medically necessary and appropriate treatment of children over parental objections. See *In the Matter of Adam L.,* 111 Wash. L. Rep. 25 (D.C. Sup. Ct., Jan. 6, 1983). However, in instances when treatment is not likely to preserve life, or is itself highly risky, judges generally will not substitute their judgment for the judgment of patients.

19. *Ibid.*

20. *In the Matter of Adam L.,* p. 1,714. The standard for deciding whether and under what circumstances it is legally permissible to forgo life-sustaining treatment for critically ill or handicapped newborns is set forth in the 1984 amendments to the Child Abuse Prevention and Treatment and Adoption Reform Act of 1974. 42 USCA sec. 5102 (3)(A) and (3)(B). Regulations are found at 45 C.F.R. Part 1340. In general, it is not permissible to withhold medically indicated treatment except under certain specified conditions.

   The infant is chronically and irreversibly comatose.

   The provision of such treatment would merely prolong dying.

   Treatment would not be effective in ameliorating or correcting all of the infant's life threatening conditions.

   Treatment would otherwise be futile in terms of the survival of the infant.

   Treatment would be virtually futile in terms of the survival of the infant and the treatment itself would be inhumane.

   To the extent that the law prohibits the withholding of artificial hydration and nutrition from these infants, that portion of the law is inconsistent with the Supreme Court holding in *Cruzan* that affords constitutional status to the right to withhold medical treatment, including artificial hydration and nutrition, which was the medical treatment at issue in that case.

21. Whether an ethics consult note should be entered in the patient record, and what its contents should be, are the subject of ongoing debate in the ethics literature. I generally favor a consult note placed in the chart that outlines the ethical dilemma and sets forth the recommendations regarding whether the various treatment options that are available to the practitioner and the patient or surrogate are ethically or morally permissible under the clinical circumstances, but does not dictate treatment decisions. A record of the consult must be maintained and, in the event of litigation, it is discoverable whether it is in the patient chart or in the records of the consult service. In other words, the content of the note (in terms of objectivity and recognition that the ultimate decision makers are the physician and the physician's patient and surrogate) is more important than its location.

Suggested Readings and Web Sites

American Medical Association, "Current Opinions of the Council on Ethical and Judicial Affairs." [www.ama-assn.org/ama/pub/category/2503.html].

American Medical Association, "Principles of Medical Ethics" (2001). [www.ama-assn.org/ama/pub/category/2512.html].

American Nurses Association, "Code for Nurses with Interpretive Statements," "Position Statement on Forgoing Artificial Nutrition and Hydration," "Position Statement on Nursing and the Patient Self-Determination Act," "Position Statement on Nursing Care and Do-Not-Resuscitate Decisions." [www.NursingWorld.org], or contact the American Nurses Association in Washington, D.C., at (202) 554-4444.

An Investigator 101 CD-ROM human subject protection training program can be obtained from Public Responsibility in Medicine and Research at: [www.PRIMR.org], and distributed by OHRP to institutions with federal assurances.

Conflict of interest standards and recommendations can be found at: [grants1.nih.gov/grants/policy/coi/index.htm].

The "Common Rule" can be found at: [www.hss.gov/ohrp/humansubjects/guidance/45cfr46htm].

Food and Drug Administration, "Guidance for Institutional Review Boards and Clinical Investigators" (1998 Update) [www.fda.gov/oc/ohrt/irbs/default.htm].

Guidelines on the Termination of Life-Sustaining Treatment and the Care of the Dying, The Hastings Center, Indiana University Press, 1987.

HIPAA information available at the American Council on Education (ACE) at: [www.acenet.edu/washington/policyanalysis/HIPAA.pdf].

NIH, Office of Extramural Research, "Conflicts of Interest Information Resources Available on the Web" [grants1.nih.gov/grants/policy/coi/resources.htm].

Office of Human Research Protection Institutional Review Board Guidebook (1993) [ohrp.osophs.dhhs.gov/irb/irb-guidebook.htm].

Office for Protection from Research Risks, Human and Animal Protection [grants.nih.gov/grants/oprr/oprr.htm].

The President's Commission for the Study of Ethical Problems in Medicine and Biomedical and Behavioral Research, Deciding to Forgo Life-Sustaining Treatment: A Report on the Ethical, Medical, and Legal Issues in Treatment Decisions. Washington, D.C.: U.S. Government Printing Office, March 1983.

Readily accessible electronic investigator training programs can be accessed through: [cme.nci.nih.gov] and [ohrp.osophs.dhhs.gov/humansubjects/guidance/local.htm].

Task force recommendations from the Association of American Medical Colleges can be found at: [www.aamc.org].

U.S. Agency for International Development, "How to Interpret the Federal Policy for the Protection of Human Subjects," or "Common Rule" [www.info.usaid.gov].

U.S. Department of Energy, Office of Science, Office of Biological and Environmental Research, Protecting Human Subjects [www.science.doe.gov/production/ober/humsubj].

Recombinant DNA/Gene Therapy research information at: [www4.od.nih.gov/oba/RAC/RAC_FAQs.htm].

Appendix 7.1.

OATH OF HIPPOCRATES

Fourth Century b.c.e.

Attributed to Hippocrates, the oath, which exemplifies the Pythagorean school rather than Greek thought in general, differs from other, more scientific, writings in the Hippocratic corpus. Written later than some of the other treatises in the corpus, the Oath of Hippocrates is one of the earliest and most important statements on medical ethics. Not only has the oath provided the foundation for many succeeding medical oaths, such as the Declaration of Geneva, but it is still administered to the graduating students of many medical schools, either in its original form or in an altered version.

I swear by Apollo Physician and Asclepius and Hygieia and Panaceia and all the gods and goddesses, making them my witnesses, that I will fulfil according to my ability and judgment this oath and this covenant:

To hold him who has taught me this art as equal to my parents and to live my life in partnership with him, and if he is in need of money to give him a share of mine, and to regard his offspring as equal to my brothers in male lineage and to teach them this art—if they desire to learn it—without fee and covenant; to give a share of precepts and oral instruction and all the other learning to my sons and to the sons of him who has instructed me and to pupils who have signed the covenant and have taken an oath according to the medical law, but to no one else.

I will apply dietetic measures for the benefit of the sick according to my ability and judgment; I will keep them from harm and injustice.

I will neither give a deadly drug to anybody if asked for it, nor will I make a suggestion to this effect. Similarly I will not give to a woman an abortive remedy. In purity and holiness I will guard my life and my art.

I will not use the knife, not even on sufferers from stone, but will withdraw in favor of such men as are engaged in this work.

Whatever houses I may visit, I will come for the benefit of the sick, remaining free of all intentional injustice, of all mischief and in particular of sexual relations with both female and male persons, be they free or slaves.

What I may see or hear in the course of the treatment or even outside of the treatment in regard to the life of men, which on no account one must spread abroad, I will keep to myself holding such things shameful to be spoken about.

If I fulfil this oath and do not violate it, may it be granted to me to enjoy life and art, being honored with fame among all men for all time to come; if I transgress it and swear falsely, may the opposite of all this be my lot.

Appendix 7.2.

⋮ THE BELMONT REPORT (APRIL 18, 1979)

············

DEPARTMENT OF HEALTH, EDUCATION, AND WELFARE

Office of the Secretary Protection of Human Subjects

Belmont Report: Ethical Principles and Guidelines for the Protection of Human Subjects of Research, Report of the National Commission for the Protection of Human Subjects of Biomedical and Behavioral Research.

AGENCY: Department of Health, Education, and Welfare.

ACTION: Notice of Report for Public Comment.

SUMMARY: On July 12, 1974, the National Research Act (Pub. L. 93–348) was signed into law, thereby creating the National Commission for the Protection of Human Subjects of Biomedical and Behavioral Research. One of the charges to the Commission was to identify the basic ethical principles that should underlie the conduct of biomedical and behavioral research involving human subjects and to develop guidelines which should be followed to assure that such research is conducted in accordance with those principles. In carrying out the above, the Commission was directed to consider: (i) the boundaries between biomedical and behavioral research and the accepted and routine practice of medicine, (ii) the role of assessment of risk-benefit criteria in the determination of the appropriateness of research involving human subjects, (iii) appropriate guidelines for the selection of human subjects for participation in such research and (iv) the nature and definition of informed consent in various research settings.

The Belmont Report attempts to summarize the basic ethical principles identified by the Commission in the course of its deliberations. It is the outgrowth of an intensive four-day period of discussions that were held in February 1976 at the Smithsonian Institution's Belmont Conference Center supplemented by the monthly deliberations of the Commission that were held over a period of nearly four years. It is a statement of basic ethical principles and guidelines that should assist in resolving the ethical problems that surround the conduct of research with human subjects. By publishing the Report in the Federal Register, and providing reprints upon request, the Secretary intends that it may be made readily available to scientists, members of Institutional Review Boards, and Federal employees. The two-volume Appendix, containing the lengthy reports of experts and specialists who assisted the Commission in fulfilling this part of its charge, is available as DHEW Publication No. (OS) 78–0013 and No. (OS) 78–0014, for sale by the Superintendent of Documents, U.S. Government Printing Office, Washington, D.C. 20402.

Unlike most other reports of the Commission, the Belmont Report does not make specific recommendations for administrative action by the Secretary of Health, Education, and Welfare. Rather, the Commission recommended that the Belmont Report be adopted in its entirety, as a statement of the Department's policy. The Department requests public comment on this recommendation.

National Commission for the Protection of Human Subjects of Biomedical and Behavioral Research.

Members of the Commission

Kenneth John Ryan, M.D., Chairman, Chief of Staff, Boston Hospital for Women.

Joseph V. Brady, Ph.D., Professor of Behavioral Biology, Johns Hopkins University.

Robert E. Cooke, M.D., President, Medical College of Pennsylvania.

Dorothy I. Height, President, National Council of Negro Women, Inc.

Albert R. Jonsen, Ph.D., Associate Professor of Bioethics, University of California at San Francisco.

Patricia King, J.D., Associate Professor of Law, Georgetown University Law Center.

Karen Lebacqz, Ph.D., Associate Professor of Christian Ethics, Pacific School of Religion.

*David W. Louisell, J.D., Professor of Law, University of California at Berkeley.

Donald W. Seldin, M.D., Professor and Chairman, Department of Internal Medicine, University of Texas at Dallas.

Eliot Stellar, Ph.D., Provost of the University and Professor of Physiological Psychology, University of Pennsylvania.

*Robert H. Turtle, LL.B., Attorney, VomBaur, Coburn, Simmons & Turtle, Washington, D.C.

Table of Contents

A. Boundaries Between Practice and Research

B. Basic Ethical Principles

   1. The medical staff on initial appointment and during the reappointment process.
      1. Respect for Persons
      2. Beneficence
      3. Justice

C. Applications

   1. Informed Consent
   2. Assessment of Risk and Benefits
   3. Selection of Subjects

* Deceased.

....

BELMONT REPORT

Ethical Principles and Guidelines for Research Involving Human Subjects

Scientific research has produced substantial social benefits. It has also posed some troubling ethical questions. Public attention was drawn to these questions by reported abuses of human subjects in biomedical experiments, especially during the Second World War. During the Nuremberg War Crime Trials, the Nuremberg code was drafted as a set of standards for judging physicians and scientists who had conducted biomedical experiments on concentration camp prisoners. This code became the prototype of many later codes[1] intended to assure that research involving human subjects would be carried out in an ethical manner.

The codes consist of rules, some general, others specific, that guide the investigators or the reviewers of research in their work. Such rules often are inadequate to cover complex situations; at times they come into conflict, and they are frequently difficult to interpret or apply. Broader ethical principles will provide a basis on which specific rules may be formulated, criticized and interpreted.

Three principles, or general prescriptive judgments, that are relevant to research involving human subjects are identified in this statement. Other principles may also be relevant. These three are comprehensive, however, and are stated at a level of generalization that should assist scientists, subjects, reviewers, and interested citizens to understand the ethical issues inherent in research involving human subjects. These principles cannot always be applied so as to resolve beyond dispute particular ethical problems. The objective is to provide an analytical framework that will guide the resolution of ethical problems arising from research involving human subjects.

This statement consists of a distinction between research and practice, a discussion of the three basic ethical principles, and remarks about the application of these principles.

A. Boundaries Between Practice and Research

It is important to distinguish between biomedical and behavioral research, on the one hand, and the practice of accepted therapy on the other, to know what activities ought to undergo review for the protection of human subjects of research. The distinction between research and practice is blurred partly because both often occur together (as in research designed to evaluate a therapy) and partly because notable departures from standard practice are often called "experimental" when the terms "experimental" and "research" are not carefully defined.

For the most part, the term "practice" refers to interventions that are designed solely to enhance the well-being of an individual patient or client and that have a reasonable expectation of success. The purpose of medical or behavioral practice is to provide diagnosis, preventive treatment, or therapy to particular individuals.[2] By contrast, the term "research" designates an activity designed to test an hypothesis, permit conclusions to be drawn, and thereby to develop or contribute to generalizable knowledge (expressed, for example, in theories, principles, and statements of relationships). Research is usually described in a formal protocol that sets forth an objective and a set of procedures designed to reach that objective.

When a clinician departs in a significant way from standard or accepted practice, the innovation does not, in and of itself, constitute research. The fact that a procedure is "experimental," in the sense of new, untested or different, does not automatically place it in the category of research. Radically new procedures of this description should, however, be made the object of formal research at an early stage in order to determine whether they are safe and effective. Thus, it is the responsibility of medical practice committees, for example, to insist that a major innovation be incorporated into a formal research project.[3] Research and practice may be carried on together when research is designed to evaluate the safety and efficacy of a therapy. This need not cause any confusion regarding whether or not the activity requires review; the general rule is that if there is any element of research in an activity, that activity should undergo review for the protection of human subjects.

B. Basic Ethical Principles

The expression "basic ethical principles" refers to those general judgments that serve as a basic justification for the many particular ethical prescriptions and evaluations of human actions. Three basic principles, among those generally accepted in our cultural tradition, are particularly relevant to the ethics of research involving human subjects: the principles of respect for persons, beneficence and justice.

1. *Respect for Persons*—Respect for persons incorporates at least two ethical convictions: first, that individuals should be treated as autonomous agents, and second, that persons with diminished autonomy are entitled to protection. The principle of respect for persons thus divides into two separate moral requirements: the requirement to acknowledge autonomy and the requirement to protect those with diminished autonomy.

   An autonomous person is an individual capable of deliberation about personal goals and of acting under the direction of such deliberation. To respect autonomy is to give weight to autonomous persons' considered opinions and choices while refraining from obstructing their actions unless they are clearly detrimental to others. To show lack of respect for an autonomous agent is to repudiate that person's considered judgments, to deny an individual the freedom to act on those considered judgments, or to withhold information necessary to make a considered judgment, when there are no compelling reasons to do so.

   However, not every human being is capable of self-determination. The capacity for self-determination matures during an individual's life, and some individuals lose this capacity wholly or in part because of illness, mental disability, or circumstances that severely restrict liberty. Respect for the immature and the incapacitated may require protecting them as they mature or while they are incapacitated.

   Some persons are in need of extensive protection, even to the point of excluding them from activities which may harm them; other persons require little protection beyond making sure they undertake activities freely and with awareness of possible adverse consequences. The extent of protection afforded should depend upon the risk of harm and the likelihood of benefit. The judgement that any individual lacks autonomy should be periodically re-evaluated and will vary in different situations.

   In most cases of research involving human subjects, respect for persons demands that subjects enter into the research voluntarily and with adequate information. In some situations, however, application of the principle is not obvious. The involvement of prisoners as subjects of research provides an instructive example. On the one hand, it would seem that the principle of respect for persons requires that prisoners not be deprived of the opportunity to volunteer for research. On the other hand, under prison conditions they may be subtly coerced or unduly influenced to engage in research activities for which they would not otherwise volunteer. Respect for persons would then dictate that prisoners be protected. Whether to allow prisoners to "volunteer" or to "protect" them presents a dilemma. Respecting persons, in most hard cases, is often a matter of balancing competing claims urged by the principle of respect itself.

2. Beneficence—Persons are treated in an ethical manner not only by respecting their decisions and protecting them from harm, but also by making efforts to secure their well-being. Such treatment falls under the principle of beneficence. The term "beneficence" is often understood to cover acts of kindness or charity that go beyond strict obligation. In this document, beneficence is understood in a stronger sense, as an obligation. Two general rules have been formulated as complementary expressions of beneficent actions in this sense: (1) do not harm and (2) maximize possible benefits and minimize possible harms.

The Hippocratic maxim "do no harm" has long been a fundamental principle of medical ethics. Claude Bernard extended it to the realm of research, saying that one should not injure one person regardless of the benefits that might come to others. However, even avoiding harm requires learning what is harmful; and, in the process of obtaining this information, persons may be exposed to risk of harm. Further, the Hippocratic Oath requires physicians to benefit their patients "according to their best judgment." Learning what will in fact benefit may require exposing persons to risk. The problem posed by these imperatives is to decide when it is justifiable to seek certain benefits despite the risks involved, and when the benefits should be forgone because of the risks.

The obligations of beneficence affect both individual investigators and society at large, because they extend both to particular research projects and to the entire enterprise of research. In the case of particular projects, investigators and members of their institutions are obliged to give forethought to the maximization of benefits and the reduction of risk that might occur from the research investigation. In the case of scientific research in general, members of the larger society are obliged to recognize the longer term benefits and risks that may result from the improvement of knowledge and from the development of novel medical, psychotherapeutic, and social procedures.

The principle of beneficence often occupies a well-defined justifying role in many areas of research involving human subjects. An example is found in research involving children. Effective ways of treating childhood diseases and fostering healthy development are benefits that serve to justify research involving children—even when individual research subjects are not direct beneficiaries. Research also makes it possible to avoid the harm that may result from the application of previously accepted routine practices that on closer investigation turn out to be dangerous. But the role of the principle of beneficence is not always so unambiguous. A difficult ethical problem remains, for example, about research that presents more than minimal risk without immediate prospect of direct benefit to the children involved. Some have argued that such research is inadmissible, while others have pointed out that this limit would rule out much research promising great benefit to children in the future. Here again, as with all hard cases, the different claims covered by the principle of beneficence may come into conflict and force difficult choices.

3. Justice—Who ought to receive the benefits of research and bear its burdens? This is a question of justice, in the sense of "fairness in distribution" or "what is deserved." An injustice occurs when some benefit to which a person is entitled is denied without good reason or when some burden is imposed unduly. Another way of conceiving the principle of justice is that equals ought to be treated equally. However, this statement requires explication. Who is equal and who is unequal? What considerations justify departure from equal distribution? Almost all commentators allow that distinctions based on experience, age, deprivation, competence, merit and position do sometimes constitute criteria justifying differential treatment for certain purposes. It is necessary, then, to explain in what respects people should be treated equally. There are several widely accepted formulations of just ways to distribute burdens and benefits. Each formulation mentions some relevant property on the basis of which burdens and benefits should be distributed. These formulations are (1) to each person an equal share, (2) to each person according to individual need, (3) to each person according to individual effort, (4) to each person according to societal contribution, and (5) to each person according to merit.

Questions of justice have long been associated with social practices such as punishment, taxation and political representation. Until recently these questions have not generally been associated with scientific research. However, they are foreshadowed even in the earliest reflections on the ethics of research involving human subjects. For example, during the 19th and early 20th centuries the burdens of serving as research subjects fell largely upon poor ward patients, while the benefits of improved medical care flowed primarily to private patients. Subsequently, the exploitation of unwilling prisoners as research subjects in Nazi concentration camps was condemned as a particularly flagrant injustice. In this country, in the 1940s, the Tuskegee syphilis study used disadvantaged, rural black men to study the untreated course of a disease that is by no means confined to that population. These subjects were deprived of demonstrably effective treatment in order not to interrupt the project, long after such treatment became generally available.

Against this historical background, it can be seen how conceptions of justice are relevant to research involving human subjects. For example, the selection of research subjects needs to be scrutinized in order to determine whether some classes (e.g., welfare patients, particular racial and ethnic minorities, or persons confined to institutions) are being systematically selected simply because of their easy availability, their compromised position, or their manipulability, rather than for reasons directly related to the problem being studied. Finally, whenever research supported by public funds leads to the development of therapeutic devices and procedures, justice demands both that these not provide advantages only to those who can afford them and that such research should not unduly involve persons from groups unlikely to be among the beneficiaries of subsequent applications of the research.

C. Applications

Applications of the general principles to the conduct of research leads to consideration of the following requirements: informed consent, risk/benefit assessment, and the selection of subjects of research.

1. Informed Consent—Respect for persons requires that subjects, to the degree that they are capable, be given the opportunity to choose what shall or shall not happen to

them. This opportunity is provided when adequate standards for informed consent are satisfied.

While the importance of informed consent is unquestioned, controversy prevails over the nature and possibility of an informed consent. Nonetheless, there is widespread agreement that the consent process can be analyzed as containing three elements: information, comprehension, and voluntariness.

Information. Most codes of research establish specific items for disclosure intended to assure that subjects are given sufficient information. These items generally include: the research procedure, their purposes, risks and anticipated benefits, alternative procedures (where therapy is involved), and a statement offering the subject the opportunity to ask questions and to withdraw at any time from the research. Additional items have been proposed, including how subjects are selected, the person responsible for the research, etc.

However, a simple listing of items does not answer the question of what the standard should be for judging how much and what sort of information should be provided. One standard frequently invoked in medical practice, namely the information commonly provided by practitioners in the field or in the locale, is inadequate since research takes place precisely when a common understanding does not exist. Another standard, currently popular in malpractice law, requires the practitioner to reveal the information that reasonable persons would wish to know in order to make a decision regarding their care. This, too, seems insufficient since the research subject, being in essence a volunteer, may wish to know considerably more about risks gratuitously undertaken than do patients who deliver themselves into the hand of a clinician for needed care. It may be that a standard of "the reasonable volunteer" should be proposed: the extent and nature of information should be such that persons, knowing that the procedure is neither necessary for their care nor perhaps fully understood, can decide whether they wish to participate in the furthering of knowledge. Even when some direct benefit to them is anticipated, the subjects should understand clearly the range of risk and the voluntary nature of participation.

A special problem of consent arises where informing subjects of some pertinent aspect of the research is likely to impair the validity of the research. In many cases, it is sufficient to indicate to subjects that they are being invited to participate in research of which some features will not be revealed until the research is concluded. In all cases of research involving incomplete disclosure, such research is justified only if it is clear that (1) incomplete disclosure is truly necessary to accomplish the goals of the research, (2) there are no undisclosed risks to subjects that are more than minimal, and (3) there is an adequate plan for debriefing subjects, when appropriate, and for dissemination of research results to them. Information about risks should never be withheld for the purpose of eliciting the cooperation of subjects, and truthful answers should always be given to direct questions about the research. Care should be taken to distinguish cases in which disclosure would destroy or invalidate the research from cases in which disclosure would simply inconvenience the investigator.

Comprehension. The manner and context in which information is conveyed is as important as the information itself. For example, presenting information in a disorganized and rapid fashion, allowing too little time for consideration or curtailing opportunities for questioning, all may adversely affect a subject's ability to make an informed choice.

Because the subject's ability to understand is a function of intelligence, rationality, maturity and language, it is necessary to adapt the presentation of the information to the subject's capacities. Investigators are responsible for ascertaining that the subject has comprehended the information. While there is always an obligation to ascertain that the information about risk to subjects is complete and adequately comprehended, when the risks are more serious, that obligation increases. On occasion, it may be suitable to give some oral or written tests of comprehension.

Special provision may need to be made when comprehension is severely limited—for example, by conditions of immaturity or mental disability. Each class of subjects that one might consider as incompetent (e.g., infants and young children, mentally disabled patients, the terminally ill and the comatose) should be considered on its own terms. Even for these persons, however, respect requires giving them the opportunity to choose to the extent they are able, whether or not to participate in research. The objections of these subjects to involvement should be honored, unless the research entails providing them a therapy unavailable elsewhere. Respect for persons also requires seeking the permission of other parties in order to protect the subjects from harm. Such persons are thus respected both by acknowledging their own wishes and by the use of third parties to protect them from harm.

The third parties chosen should be those who are most likely to understand the incompetent subject's situation and to act in that person's best interest. The person authorized to act on behalf of the subject should be given an opportunity to observe the research as it proceeds in order to be able to withdraw the subject from the research, if such action appears in the subject's best interest.

Voluntariness. An agreement to participate in research constitutes a valid consent only if voluntarily given. This element of informed consent requires conditions free of coercion and undue influence. Coercion occurs when an overt threat of harm is intentionally presented by one person to another in order to obtain compliance. Undue influence, by contrast, occurs through an offer of an excessive, unwarranted, inappropriate or improper reward or other overture in order to obtain compliance. Also, inducements that would ordinarily be acceptable may become undue influences if the subject is especially vulnerable.

Unjustifiable pressures usually occur when persons in positions of authority or commanding influence—especially where possible sanctions are involved—urge a course of action for a subject. A continuum of such influencing factors exists, however, and it is impossible to state precisely where justifiable persuasion ends and undue influence begins. But undue influence would include actions such as manipulating a person's choice through the controlling influence of a close relative and threatening to withdraw health services to which an individual would otherwise be entitled.

2. Assessment of Risks and Benefits—The assessment of risks and benefits requires a careful arrayal of relevant data, including, in some cases, alternative ways of obtaining the benefits sought in the research. Thus, the assessment presents both an opportunity and a responsibility to gather systematic and comprehensive information about proposed research. For the investigator, it is a means to examine whether the proposed research is properly designed. For a review committee, it is a method for determining whether the risks that will be presented to subjects are justified. For prospective subjects, the assessment will assist the determination whether or not to participate.

The Nature and Scope of Risks and Benefits. The requirement that research be justified on the basis of a favorable risk/benefit assessment bears a close relation to the principle of beneficence, just as the moral requirement that informed consent be obtained is derived primarily from the principle of respect for persons. The term "risk" refers to a possibility that harm may occur. However, when expressions such as "small risk" or "high risk" are used, they usually refer (often ambiguously) both to the chance (probability) of experiencing a harm and the severity (magnitude) of the envisioned harm.

The term "benefit" is used in the research context to refer to something of positive value related to health or welfare. Unlike "risk," "benefit" is not a term that expresses probabilities. Risk is properly contrasted to probability of benefits, and benefits are properly contrasted with harms rather than risks of harm. Accordingly, so-called risk/benefit assessments are concerned with the probabilities and magnitudes of possible harms and anticipated benefits. Many kinds of possible harms and benefits need to be taken into account. There are, for example, risks of psychological harm, physical harm, legal harm, social harm and economic harm and the corresponding benefits. While the most likely types of harms to research subjects are those of psychological or physical pain or injury, other possible kinds should not be overlooked.

Risks and benefits of research may affect the individual subjects, the families of the individual subjects, and society at large (or special groups of subjects in society).

Previous codes and Federal regulations have required that risks to subjects be outweighed by the sum of both the anticipated benefit to the subject, if any, and the anticipated benefit to society in the form of knowledge to be gained from the research. In balancing these different elements, the risks and benefits affecting the immediate research subject will normally carry special weight. On the other hand, interests other than those of the subject may on some occasions be sufficient by themselves to justify the risks involved in the research, so long as the subjects' rights have been protected. Beneficence thus requires that we protect against risk of harm to subjects and also that we be concerned about the loss of the substantial benefits that might be gained from research.

The Systematic Assessment of Risks and Benefits. It is commonly said that benefits and risks must be "balanced" and shown to be "in a favorable ratio." The metaphorical character of these terms draws attention to the difficulty of making precise judgments. Only on rare occasions will quantitative techniques be available for the scrutiny of research protocols. However, the idea of systematic, nonarbitrary analysis of risks and benefits should be emulated insofar as possible. This ideal requires those making decisions about the justifiability of research to be thorough in the accumulation and assessment of information about all aspects of the research, and to consider alternatives systematically. This procedure renders the assessment of research more rigorous and precise, while making communication between review board members and investigators less subject to misinterpretation, misinformation and conflicting judgments. Thus, there should first be a determination of the validity of the presuppositions of the research; then the nature, probability and magnitude of risk should be distinguished with as much clarity as possible. The method of ascertaining risks should be explicit, especially where there is no alternative to the use of such vague categories as small or slight risk. It should also be determined whether an investigator's estimates of the probability of harm or benefits are reasonable, as judged by known facts or other available studies.

Finally, assessment of the justifiability of research should reflect at least the following considerations: (i) Brutal or inhumane treatment of human subjects is never morally justified. (ii) Risks should be reduced to those necessary to achieve the research objective. It should be determined whether it is in fact necessary to use human subjects at all. Risk can perhaps never be entirely eliminated, but it can often be reduced by careful attention to alternative procedures. (iii) When research involves significant risk of serious impairment, review committees should be extraordinarily insistent on the justification of the risk (looking usually to the likelihood of benefit to the subject—or, in some rare cases, to the manifest voluntariness of the participation). (iv) When vulnerable populations are involved in research, the appropriateness of involving them should itself be demonstrated. A number of variables go into such judgments, including the nature and degree of risk, the condition of the particular population involved, and the nature and level of the anticipated benefits. (v) Relevant risks and benefits must be thoroughly arrayed in documents and procedures used in the informed consent process.

3. Selection of Subjects. Just as the principle of respect for persons finds expression in the requirement for consent, and the principle of beneficence in risk/benefit assessment, the principle of justice gives rise to moral requirements that there be fair procedures and outcomes in the selection of research subjects.

    Justice is relevant to the selection of subjects of research at two levels: the social and the individual. Individual justice in the selection of subjects would require that researchers exhibit fairness: thus, they should not offer potentially beneficial research only to some patients who are in their favor or select only "undesirable" persons for risky research. Social justice requires that distinction be drawn between classes of subjects that ought, and ought not, to participate in any particular kind of research, based on the ability of members of that class to bear burdens and on the appropriateness of placing further burdens on already burdened persons. Thus, it can be considered a matter of social justice that there is an order of preference in the selection of classes of subjects (e.g., adults before children) and that some classes of potential subjects (e.g., the institutionalized mentally infirm or prisoners) may be involved as research subjects if at all, only on certain conditions.

    Injustice may appear in the selection of subjects, even if individual subjects are selected fairly by investigators and treated fairly in the course of research. Thus injustice arises from social, racial, sexual and cultural biases institutionalized in society. Thus, even if individual researchers are treating their research subjects fairly, and even if IRBs are taking care to assure that subjects are selected fairly within a particular institution, unjust social patterns may nevertheless appear in the overall distribution of the burdens and benefits of research. Although individual institutions or investigators may not be able to resolve a problem that is pervasive in their social setting, they can consider distributive justice in selecting research subjects.

    Some populations, especially institutionalized ones, are already burdened in many ways by their infirmities and environments. When research is proposed that involves risks and does not include a therapeutic component, other less burdened classes of persons should be called upon first to accept these risks of research, except where the research is directly related to the specific conditions of the class involved. Also, even though public funds for research may often flow in the same directions as public funds for health care, it seems unfair that populations dependent on public health care constitute a pool of preferred research subjects if more advantaged populations are likely to be the recipients of the benefits.

One special instance of injustice results from the involvement of vulnerable subjects. Certain groups, such as racial minorities, the economically disadvantaged, the very sick, and the institutionalized may continually be sought as research subjects, owing to their ready availability in settings where research is conducted. Given their dependent status and their frequently compromised capacity for free consent, they should be protected against the danger of being involved in research solely for administrative convenience, or because they are easy to manipulate as a result of their illness or socioeconomic condition.

[FR Doc. 90-12065 Filed 4-17-79; 8:45 am]

Endnotes

1. Since 1945, various codes for the proper and responsible conduct of human experimentation in medical research have been adopted by different organizations. The best known of these codes are the Nuremberg Code of 1947, the Helsinki Declaration of 1964 (revised in 1975), and the 1971 Guidelines (codified into Federal Regulations in 1974) issued by the U.S. Department of Health, Education, and Welfare Codes for the conduct of social and behavioral research have also been adopted, the best known being that of the American Psychological Association, published in 1973.

2. Although practice usually involves interventions designed solely to enhance the well-being of a particular individual, interventions are sometimes applied to one individual for the enhancement of the well-being of another (e.g., blood donation, skin grafts, organ transplants) or an intervention may have the dual purpose of enhancing the well-being of a particular individual, and, at the same time, providing some benefit to others (e.g., vaccination, which protects both the person who is vaccinated and society generally). The fact that some forms of practice have elements other than immediate benefit to the individual receiving an intervention, however, should not confuse the general distinction between research and practice. Even when a procedure applied in practice may benefit some other person, it remains an intervention designed to enhance the well-being of a particular individual or groups of individuals; thus, it is practice and need not be reviewed as research.

3. Because the problems related to social experimentation may differ substantially from those of biomedical and behavioral research, the Commission specifically declines to make any policy determination regarding such research at this time. Rather, the Commission believes that the problem ought to be addressed by one of its successor bodies.

⋮ NUREMBERG CODE 1946

The Nuremberg Military Tribunal's decision in the case of the *United States v. Karl Brandt et al.* includes what is now called the Nuremberg Code, a ten-point statement delimiting permissible medical experimentation on human subjects. According to this statement, humane experimentation is justified only if its results benefit society and it is carried out in accord with basic principles that "satisfy moral, ethical, and legal concepts." To some extent, the Nuremberg Code has been superseded by the Declaration of Helsinki as a guide for human experimentation.

1. The voluntary consent of the human subject is absolutely essential.

   This means that the person involved should have legal capacity to give consent; should be so situated as to be able to exercise free power of choice, without the intervention of any element of force, fraud, deceit, duress, over-reaching, or other ulterior form of constraint or coercion; and should have sufficient knowledge and comprehension of the elements of the subject matter involved as to enable him to make an understanding and enlightened decision. This latter element requires that before the acceptance of an affirmative decision by the experimental subject there should be made known to him the nature, duration, and purpose of the experiment; the method and means by which it is to be conducted; all inconveniences and hazards reasonably to be expected; and the effects upon his health or person which may possibly come from his participation in the experiment.

   The duty and responsibility for ascertaining the quality of the consent rests upon each individual who initiates, directs or engages in the experiment. It is a personal duty and responsibility which may not be delegated to another with impunity.

2. The experiment should be such as to yield fruitful results for the good of society, unprocurable by other methods or means of study, and not random and unnecessary in nature.

3. The experiment should be so designed and based on the results of animal experimentation and a knowledge of the natural history of the disease or other problem under study that the anticipated results will justify the performance of the experiment.

4. The experiment should be so conducted as to avoid all unnecessary physical and mental suffering and injury.

5. No experiment should be conducted where there is an a priori reason to believe that death or disabling injury will occur; except, perhaps, in those experiments where the experimental physicians also serve as subjects.

6. The degree of risk to be taken should never exceed that determined by the humanitarian importance of the problem to be solved by the experiment.

7. Proper preparations should be made and adequate facilities provided to protect the experimental subject against even remote possibilities of injury, disability, or death.

8. The experiment should be conducted only by scientifically qualified persons. The highest degree of skill and care should be required through all stages of the experiment of those who conduct or engage in the experiment.

9. During the course of the experiment the human subject should be at liberty to bring the experiment to an end if he has reached the physical or mental state where continuation of the experiment seems to him to be impossible.

10. During the course of the experiment the scientist in charge must be prepared to terminate the experiment at any stage, if he has probable cause to believe, in the exercise of the good faith, superior skill and careful judgment required of him that a continuation of the experiment is likely to result in injury, disability, or death to the experimental subject.

["Permissible Medical Experiments." Trials of War Criminals before the Nuremberg Military Tribunals under Control Council Law No. 10: Nuremberg October 1946–April 1949. Washington: U.S. Government Printing Office (n.d.), vol. 2, pp. 181–182.]

Appendix 7.4.

ON THE PROTECTION OF HUMAN SUBJECTS: U.S. DEPARTMENT OF HEALTH, EDUCATION, AND WELFARE'S INSTITUTIONAL GUIDE

In 1971, the Department of Health, Education, and Welfare (DHEW), now known as the Department of Health and Human Services (DHHS), issued institutional guidance designed to safeguard the rights and welfare of human subjects of federally funded medical research. This document expanded and formalized guidelines that the National Institutes of Health published in 1966 and revised in 1969. The policies in the DHEW document were also reviewed, and a revised version was published in the Code of Federal Regulations (45 CFR 46) in May 1974. These regulations, the 1974 version of the Guide, were likewise reviewed and revised—this time on the basis of recommendations from the National Commission for the Protection of Human Subjects of Biomedical and Behavioral Research (1974–1978)—and officially promulgated in 1981. The DHEW guidance document remains the bedrock of federal regulations governing the protection of human subjects in research.

············
POLICY

Safeguarding the rights and welfare of human subjects involved in activities supported by grants or contracts from the Department of Health, Education, and Welfare is the responsibility of the institution which receives or is accountable to the DHEW for the funds awarded for the support of the activity. In order to provide for the adequate discharge of this institutional responsibility, it is the policy of the Department that no grant or contract for an activity involving human subjects shall be made unless the application for such support has been reviewed and approved by an appropriate institutional committee.

This review shall determine that the rights and welfare of the subjects involved are adequately protected, that the risks to an individual are outweighed by the potential benefits to him or by the importance of the knowledge to be gained, and that informed consent is to be obtained by methods that are adequate and appropriate.[1]

In addition the committee must establish a basis for continuing review of the activity in keeping with these determinations.

The institution must submit to the DHEW, for its review, approval, and official acceptance, an assurance of its compliance with this policy. The institution must also provide with each proposal involving human subjects a certification that it has been or will be reviewed in accordance with the institution's assurance.

No grant or contract involving human subjects at risk will be made to an individual unless he is affiliated with or sponsored by an institution which can and does assume responsibility for the protection of the subjects involved. Since the welfare of subjects is a matter of concern to the Department of Health, Education, and Welfare as well as to the institution, no grant or contract involving human subjects shall be made unless the proposal for such support has been reviewed and approved by an appropriate professional committee within the responsible component of the Department. As a result of this review, the committee may recommend to the operating agency, and the operating agency may require, the imposition of specific grant or contract terms providing for the protection of human subjects, including requirements for informed consent.

APPLICABILITY

A. **General**   This policy applies to all grants and contracts which support activities in which subjects may be at risk.

B. **Subject**   This term describes any individual who may be at risk as a consequence of participation as a subject in research, development, demonstration, or other activities supported by DHEW funds.

This may include patients; outpatients; donors of organs, tissues, and services; informants; and normal volunteers, including students who are placed at risk during training in medical, psychological, sociological, educational, and other types of activities supported by DHEW.

Of particular concern are those subjects in groups with limited civil freedom. These include prisoners, residents or clients of institutions for the mentally ill and mentally retarded, and persons subject to military discipline.

The unborn and the dead should be considered subjects to the extent that they have rights which can be exercised by their next of kin or legally authorized representatives.

C. **At Risk**   An individual is considered to be "at risk" if he may be exposed to the possibility of harm—physical, psychological, sociological, or other—as a consequence of any activity which goes beyond the application of those established and accepted methods necessary to meet his needs. The determination of when an individual is at risk is a matter of the application of common sense and sound professional judgement to the circumstances of the activity in question. Responsibility for this determination resides at all levels of institutional and departmental review. Definitive determination will be made by the operating agency.

D. **Types of Risks and Applicability of the Policy**

1. Certain risks are inherent in life itself, at the time and in the places where life runs its course. This policy is not concerned with the ordinary risks of public or private living, or those risks associated with admission to a school or hospital. It is not concerned with the risks inherent in professional practice as long as these do

not exceed the bounds of established and accepted procedures, including innovative practices applied in the interest of the individual patient, student or client.

Risk and the applicability of this policy are most obvious in medical and behavioral science research projects involving procedures that may induce a potentially harmful altered physical state or condition. Surgical and biopsy procedures; the removal of organs or tissues for study, reference, transplantation, or banking; the administration of drugs or radiation; the use of indwelling catheters or electrodes; the requirement of strenuous physical exertion; subjection to deceit, public embarrassment, and humiliation are all examples of procedures which require thorough scrutiny by both the Department of Health, Education, and Welfare and institutional committees. In general those projects which involve risk of physical or psychological injury require prior written consent.

2. There is a wide range of medical, social, and behavioral projects and activities in which no immediate physical risk to the subject is involved; e.g., those utilizing personality inventories, interviews, questionnaires, or the use of observation, photographs, taped records, or stored data. However, some of these procedures may involve varying degrees of discomfort, harassment, invasion of privacy, or may constitute a threat to the subject's dignity through the imposition of demeaning or dehumanizing conditions.

3. There are also medical and biomedical projects concerned solely with organs, tissues, body fluids, and other materials obtained in the course of the routine performance of medical services such as diagnosis, treatment and care, or at autopsy. The use of these materials obviously involves no element of physical risk to the subject. However, their use for many research, training, and service purposes may present psychological, sociological, or legal risks to the subject or his authorized representatives. In these instances, application of the policy requires review to determine that the circumstances under which the materials were procured were appropriate and that adequate and appropriate consent was, or can be, obtained for the use of these materials for project purposes.

4. Similarly, some studies depend upon stored data or information which was often obtained for quite different purposes. Here, the reviews should also determine whether the use of these materials is within the scope of the original consent, or whether consent can be obtained.

E. **Established and Accepted Methods**　Some methods become established through rigorous standardization procedures prescribed, as in the case of drugs or biologicals, by law or, as in the case of many educational tests, through the aegis of professional societies or nonprofit agencies. Acceptance is a matter of professional response, and determination as to when a method passes from the experimental stage and becomes "established and accepted" is a matter of judgement.

In determining what constitutes an established and accepted method, consideration should be given to both national and local standards of practice. A management procedure may become temporarily established in the routine of a local institution but still fail to win acceptance at the national level. A psychological inventory may be accepted nationally, but still contain questions which are disturbing or offensive to a local population. Surgical procedures which are established and accepted in one part of the country may be considered experimental in another, not due to inherent deficiencies, but because of the lack of proper facilities and trained personnel.

Diagnostic procedures which are routine in the United States may pose serious hazards to an undernourished, heavily infected, overseas population.

If doubt exists as to whether the procedures to be employed are established and accepted, the activity should be subject to review and approval by the institutional committee.

F. **Necessity to Meet Needs**   Even if considered established and accepted, the method may place the subject at risk if it is being employed for purposes other than to meet the needs of the subject. Determination by an attending professional that a particular treatment, test, regimen, or curriculum is appropriate for a particular subject to meet his needs limits the attendant risks to those inherent in the delivery of services, or in training.

On the other hand, arbitrary, random, or other assignment of subjects to differing treatment or study groups in the interests of a DHEW supported activity, rather than in the strict interests of the subject, introduces the possibility of exposing him to additional risk. Even comparisons of two or more established and accepted methods may potentially involve exposure of at least some of the subjects to additional risks. Any alteration of the choice, scope, or timing of an otherwise etablished and accepted method, primarily in the interests of a DHEW activity, also raises the issue of additional risk.

If doubt exists as to whether the procedures are intended solely to meet the needs of the subject, the activity should be subject to review and approval by the institutional committee.

•••••••••••

INSTITUTIONAL REVIEW

A. **Initial Review of Projects**

1. Review must be carried out by an appropriate institutional committee. The committee may be an existing one, such as a board of trustees, medical staff committee, utilization committee, or research committee, or it may be specially constituted for the purpose of this review. Institutions may utilize subcommittees to represent major administrative or subordinate components in those instances where establishment of a single committee is impracticable or inadvisable. The institution may utilize staff, consultants, or both.

The committee must be composed of sufficient members with varying backgrounds to assure complete and adequate review of projects and activities commonly conducted by the institution. The committee's membership, maturity, experience, and expertise should be such as to justify respect for its advice and counsel. No member of an institutional committee shall be involved in either the initial or continuing review of an activity in which he has a professional responsibility, except to provide information requested by the committee. In addition to possessing the professional competence to review specific activities, the committee should be able to determine acceptability of the proposal in terms of institutional commitments and regulations, applicable law, standards of professional conduct and practice, and community attitudes [note to 21 CFR 130 omitted]. The committee may therefore need to include persons whose primary concerns lie in these areas rather than in the conduct of research, development, and service programs of the types supported by the DHEW.

If an institution is so small that it cannot appoint a suitable committee from its own staff, it should appoint members from outside the institution.

Committee members shall be identified by name, occupation or position, and by other pertinent indications of experience and competence in areas pertinent to the areas of review such as earned degrees, board certifications, licensures, memberships, etc.

Temporary replacement of a committee member by an alternate of comparable experience and competence is permitted in the event a member is momentarily unable to fulfill committee responsibility. The DHEW should be notified of any permanent replacement or additions.

2. The institution should adopt a statement of principles that will assist it in the discharge of its responsibilities for protecting the rights and welfare of subjects. This may be an appropriate existing code or declaration or one formulated by the institution itself [note omitted]. It is to be understood that no such principles supersede DHEW policy or applicable law.

3. Review begins with the identification of those projects or activities which involve subjects who may be at risk. In institutions with large grant and contract programs, administrative staff may be delegated the responsibility of separating those projects which do not involve human subjects in any degree; i.e., animal and nonhuman materials studies. However, determinations as to whether any project or activity involves human subjects at risk is a professional responsibility to be discharged through review by the committee, or by subcommittees.

   If review determines that the procedures to be applied are to be limited to those considered by the committee to be established, accepted, and necessary to the needs of the subject, review need go no further; and the application should be certified as approved by the committee. Such projects involve human subjects, but these subjects are not considered to be at risk.

   If review determines that the procedures to be applied will place the subject at risk, review should be expanded to include the issues of the protection of the subject's rights and welfare, of the relative weight of risks and benefits, and of the provision of adequate and appropriate consent procedures.

   Where required by workload considerations or by geographic separation of operating units, subcommittees or mail review may be utilized to provide preliminary review of applications.

   Final review of projects involving subjects at risk should be carried out by a quorum of the committee. . . . Such review should determine, through review of reports by subcommittees, or through its own examination of applications or of protocols, or through interviews with those individuals who will have professional responsibility for the proposal project or activity, or through other acceptable procedures that the requirements of the institutional assurance and of DHEW policy have been met, specifically that:

   a. The rights and welfare of the subjects are adequately protected.

      Institutional committees should carefully examine applications, protocols, or descriptions of work to arrive at an independent determination of possible risks. The committee must be alert to the possibility that investigators, program directors, or contractors may, quite unintentionally, introduce unnecessary or unacceptable hazards, or fail to provide adequate safeguards. This possibility is particularly true if the project crosses disciplinary lines, involves new and untried procedures, or involves established and accepted procedures which are new to the personnel applying them. Committees must also assure themselves that proper precautions will be taken to deal with emergencies that may develop even in the course of seemingly routine activities.

When appropriate, provision should be made for safeguarding information that could be traced to, or identified with, subjects. The committee may require the project or activity director to take steps to insure the confidentiality and security of data, particularly if it may not always remain under his direct control.

Safeguards include, initially, the careful design of questionnaires, inventories, interview schedules, and other data gathering instruments and procedures to limit the personal information to be acquired to that which is absolutely essential to the project or activity. Additional safeguards include the encoding or enciphering of names, addresses, serial numbers, and of data transferred to tapes, discs, and printouts. Secure, locked spaces and cabinets may be necessary for handling and storing documents and files. Codes and ciphers should always be kept in secure places, distinctly separate from encoded and enciphered data. The shipment, delivery, and transfer of all data, printouts, and files between offices and institutions may require careful controls. Computer to computer transmission of data may be restricted or forbidden.

Provision should also be made for the destruction of all edited, obsolete or depleted data on punched cards, tapes, discs, and other records. The committee may also determine a future date for destruction of all stored primary data pertaining to a project or activity.

Particularly relevant to the decision of the committees are those rights of the subject that are defined by law. The committee should familiarize itself through consultation with legal counsel with these statutes and common law precedents which may bear on its decisions. The provisions of this policy may not be construed in any manner or sense that would abrogate, supersede, or moderate more restrictive applicable law or precedential legal decisions.

Laws may define what constitutes consent and who may give consent, prescribe or proscribe the performance of certain medical and surgical procedures, protect confidential communications, define negligence, define invasion of privacy, require disclosure of records pursuant to legal process, and limit charitable and governmental immunity.

b. The risks to an individual and outweighed by the potential benefits to him or by the importance of the knowledge to be gained.

The committee should carefully weigh the known or foreseeable risks to be encountered by subjects, the probable benefits that may accrue to them, and the probable benefits to humanity that may result from the subject's participation in the project or activity. If it seems probable that participation will confer substantial benefits on the subjects, the committee may be justified in permitting them to accept commensurate or lesser risks. If the potential benefits are insubstantial, or are outweighed by risks, the committee may be justified in permitting the subjects to accept these risks in the interests of humanity. The committee should consider the possibility that subjects, or those authorized to represent subjects, may be motivated to accept risks for unsuitable or inadequate reasons. In such instances the consent procedures adopted should incorporate adequate safeguards.

Compensation to volunteers should never be such as to constitute an undue inducement.

No subject can be expected to understand the issues of risks and benefits as fully as the committee. Its agreement that consent can reasonably be sought for subject participation in a project or activity is of paramount practical importance.

The informed consent of the subject, while often a legal necessity is a goal toward which we must strive, but hardly ever achieve except in the simplest cases.

   Henry K. Beecher, M.D.

c. The informed consent of subjects will be obtained by methods that are adequate and appropriate [note to 21 CFR 130 omitted].

Informed consent is the agreement obtained from a subject, or from his authorized representative, to the subject's participation in an activity.

The basic elements of informed consent are:

1. A fair explanation of the procedures to be followed, including an identification of those which are experimental;
2. A description of the attendant discomforts and risks;
3. A description of the benefits to be expected;
4. A disclosure of appropriate alternative procedures that would be advantageous for the subject;
5. An offer to answer any inquiries concerning the procedures;
6. An instruction that the subject is free to withdraw his consent and to discontinue participation in the project or activity at any time.

   In addition, the agreement, written or oral, entered into by the subject, should include no exculpatory language through which the subject is made to waive, or to appear to waive, any of his legal rights, or to release the institution or its agents from liability for negligence (the use of exculpatory clauses is contrary to public policy [*Tunkl v. Regents of University of California*]).

   Informed consent must be documented. . . .

   Consent should be obtained, whenever practicable, from the subjects themselves. When the subject group will include individuals who are not legally or physically capable of giving informed consent, because of age, mental incapacity, or inability to communicate, the review committee should consider the validity of consent by next of kin, legal guardians, or by other qualified third parties representative of the subjects' interests. In such instances, careful consideration should be given by the committee not only to whether these third parties can be presumed to have the necessary depth of interest and concern with the subjects' rights and welfare, but also to whether these third parties will be legally authorized to expose the subjects to the risks involved.

The review committee will determine if the consent required, whether to be secured before the fact, in writing or orally, or after the fact following debriefing, or whether implicit in voluntary participation in an adequately advertised activity, is appropriate in the light of the risks to the subject, and the circumstances of the project.

The review committee will also determine if the information to be given to the subject, or to qualified third parties, in writing or orally, is a fair explanation of the project or activity, of its possible benefits, and of its attendant hazards.

Where an activity involves therapy, diagnosis, or management, and a professional/patient relationship exists, it is necessary "to recognize that each patient's mental and emotional condition is important . . . and that in discussing the element of risk, a certain amount of discretion must be employed consistent with full disclosure of fact necessary to any informed consent" (*Salgo v. Leland Stanford Jr. University Board of Trustees* [154C.A.2nd 560; 317 P.2d 1701]).

Where an activity does not involve therapy, diagnosis, or management, and a professional/subject rather than a professional/patient relationship exists, "the subject is entitled to a full and frank disclosure of all the facts, probabilities, and opinions which a reasonable man might be expected to consider before giving his consent" (*Halushka v. University of Saskatchewan* [1965] 53 D.L.R. [2d]).

When debriefing procedures are considered as a necessary part of the plan, the committee should ascertain that these will be complete and prompt.

B. **Continuing Review**   This is an essential part of the review process. While procedures for continuing review of ongoing projects and activities should be based in principle on the initial review criteria, they should also be adapted to the size and administrative structure of the institution. Institutions which are small and compact and in which the committee members are in day-to-day contact with professional staff may be able to function effectively with some informality. Institutions which have placed responsibility for review in boards of trustees, utilization committees, and similar groups that meet on frequent schedules may find it possible to have projects reviewed during these meetings.

In larger institutions with more complex administrative structures and specially appointed committees, these committees may adopt a variety of continuing review mechanisms. They may involve systematic review of projects at fixed intervals, or at intervals set by the committee commensurate with the project's risk. Thus, a project involving an untried procedure may initially require reconsideration as each subject completes his involvement. A highly routine project may need no more than annual review. Routine diagnostic service procedures, such as biopsy and autopsy, which contribute to research and demonstration activities generally require no more than annual review. Spot checks may be used to supplement scheduled reviews.

Actual review may involve interviews with the responsible staff, or review of written reports and supporting documents and forms. In any event, such review must be completed at least annually to permit certifications of review on noncompeting continuation applications.

C. **Communication of the Committee's Action, Advice, and Counsel** If the committee's overall recommendation is favorable, it may simultaneously prescribe restrictions or conditions under which the activity may be conducted, define substantial changes in the research plans which should be brought to its attention, and determine the nature and frequency of interim review procedures to ensure continued acceptable conduct of the research.

Favorable recommendations by an institutional committee are, of course, always subject to further appropriate review and rejection by institution officials.

Unfavorable recommendations, restrictions, or conditions cannot be removed except by the committee or by the action of another appropriate review group described in the assurance filed with the Department of Health, Education, and Welfare.

Staff with supervisory responsibility for investigators and program directors whose projects or activities have been disapproved or restricted, and institutional administrative and financial officers should be informed of the committee's recommendations. Responsible professional staff should be informed of the reasons for any adverse actions taken by the institutional committee.

The committee should be prepared at all times to provide advice and counsel to staff developing new projects or activities or contemplating revision of ongoing projects or disapproved proposals.

D. **Maintenance of an Active and Effective Committee** Institutions should establish policy determining overall committee composition, including provisions for rotation of memberships and appointment of chairmen. Channels of responsibility should be established for implementation of committee recommendations as they may affect the actions of responsible professional staff, grants and contracts officers, business officers, and other responsible staff. Provisions should be made for remedial action in the event of disregard of committee recommendations.

Endnote

1. Reprinted from The Institutional Guide to DHEW Policy on Protection of Human Subjects. DHEW Publication No. NIH 72-102, December, 1, 1971 (Washington, D.C.: U.S. Government Printing Office, 1971), pp. 2–11.

8

Interpersonal Communication Skills: The Ultimate Loss Control Technique

Geri Amori

Effective communication as a basic requirement for safe health care is a concept that has always been acknowledged, but only in recent years fully appreciated. Risk managers have long cited communication breakdown as a factor in malpractice litigation. Studies by Beckman,[1] Colon,[2] Eastaugh,[3] Levinson,[4] Vincent,[5] Wood,[6] and others support the fact that patients and families often decide to sue based more upon communication issues than on unexpected outcomes.

Although effective communication is essential to good relationships with patients and families, it is also a key to safe patient care. The Joint Commission on Accreditation of Healthcare Organizations (JCAHO) has cited communication as the root cause for approximately 65 percent of the 2,966 sentinel events reported between 1995 and 2004.[7] Breakdown in communication among caregivers is attributed to those situations in which there are transfers, hand-offs, or multiple disciplines involved in the care of a patient. In addition, the difficulty in communicating during highly chaotic, intense situations speaks to the need for training in teamwork.

Furthermore, although the JCAHO Patient Safety Goals have consistently included goals to improve communication among providers, in 2006 the Joint Commission has added a thirteenth goal encouraging active communication with patients to improve the safety of care.[8] The goal states: "Encourage the active involvement of patients and their families in the patient's care as a patient safety strategy." It also states: "Define and communicate the means for patients to report concerns about safety and encourage them to do so." Although in 2006 this subsection applies only to Assisted Living, Disease-Specific Care, Home Care, and Laboratory, it is a generally applicable goal that may likely apply to all settings.

Communication among caregivers, and with patients and families, is clearly key for safe care. Safe care delivered in respectful relationships, as demonstrated through highly developed interpersonal skills, is the greatest opportunity for reduction of losses and decreased litigation. Although abundant literature supports the effect of communication in relation to care interactions or to families and patients, far less is found about the effect of poor communication with those outside the direct care relationship, such as the effect of communication in community relations, or with respect to the media. Regardless of the presence of specific supportive literature, the general literature shows that effective communication is crucial to the reduction of risk in all aspects of the enterprise, including operations, personnel issues, and strategic positioning in the community.

Despite the emphasis on effective communication in health care, the specifics of how and what to communicate, and the unique aspects of communication that influence patient satisfaction, malpractice reduction, and loss prevention are rarely discussed and even less understood. Complicating the efforts of organizations to improve communication is the lack of tools that can easily and reliably measure communication skills.[9,10] Nevertheless, communication skills are the building blocks for all true loss control. Interpersonal communication skills influence the way patients perceive our organizations and the care they receive. Their perceptions of our concern for their well-being and their value as humans and as customers, influences the ultimate decision whether to sue in the face of a negative unanticipated outcome. Effective communication among staff influences trust in the organization, willingness to cooperate as a team, and organizational loyalty.[11] In the strict loss control sense, employees who feel cared about by the organization and their coworkers because of respectful, inclusive, and open communication are less likely to abuse the workers' compensation system or to have stress-related illness that influences use of the employer's health plan. Furthermore, costly staff turnover is minimized. Providers—a vulnerable and yet essential component of our health care systems—require true respect in our communications to feel compelled to cooperate with the growing complexity of health care administration.

The discrepancy between effective and ineffective communication is a major frustration for the risk manager. The risk management professional is often in the position of coaching or facilitating communication among individuals or groups of individuals. The ability to recognize, facilitate, coach, and teach effective communication can make the difference between circumstances that result in large financial losses and those in which reasonable compensation is made.

Given this role, it is important for the risk management professional to have teaching tools to support and evaluate effective communication. How do we know when we have communicated effectively? Does it primarily mean having interpersonal verbal and nonverbal techniques, writing skills, or computer skills? Is it simply being "nice"? It is, in fact, all these things. A key factor, however, is the use of the term "skill" or "technique." Communication techniques can be taught as a skill. Just as in a sport, technique must be paired with practice and desire. Nonetheless, specific approaches and techniques have been proven to create more effective communication encounters.

GENERAL PRINCIPLES OF EFFECTIVE COMMUNICATION

In its simplest form, effective communication is the process of transmitting information from one person to another in a way that can be understood. For that to happen, several key things must occur:

● The sender (transmitter of information) must create the message in words or symbols that the recipient can understand.

- The message must move or be transmitted from one person to another via some medium (air, paper, computer, or other medium).
- The recipient must interpret the message and process it.
- The recipient must create a response.
- The response must move from one person to another.
- To be effective, the original sender must know that the message has been received and that it is understood as it was intended.

Most communication training focuses on the first step of the process: How to put the message into meaningful words or symbols. Nevertheless, this is the area in which most people feel least confident. Although the ability to properly create a message is essential, it is during the final step, the receiving of feedback, where most communication falls apart.

For example, suppose that the physician tells a patient with viral-induced asthma to begin taking the prescribed medication at the first sign of a cold; however, the patient associates asthma with a cough, not specifically a cold. The patient might reasonably believe that he has heard to begin the medicine at the first sign of a cough. The physician may ask if the patient has any questions. The patient, believing that he understood, reports no questions and leaves the appointment. One might argue that the physician has asked for feedback ("Do you have any questions?") and the patient has provided that feedback ("No."). In fact, no feedback has been given.

The sender has no greater awareness of whether the patient understood than if the question had not been asked. This matter is further complicated if the physician, unaware of the patient's medical literacy, has phrased the directions using terminology that the patient does not fully understand. Perhaps the physician was distracted and not looking at the patient, so the patient felt as though the physician were in a hurry. Perhaps the patient looked confused, but the physician, thinking about something else, didn't notice the nonverbal cue. If the physician had elicited useful feedback and had "listened" with eyes and ears, there would have been the opportunity to rephrase the instructions so that the patient could understand the directions. Effective communication, which would have enhanced the potential for compliance and cooperative care, would have occurred.

The feedback portion of communication is what we hard-wire when we institute "read backs" and other procedures to affirm that a message is received. Nevertheless, it is unwise to rely only on feedback to create effective communication. Each step of the communication process contributes to the clarity of the message and the ease (or difficulty) with which it is understood. These elements apply to any effective communication, whether verbal or written, with patients, families, colleagues, or the community.

Key Principles for Creating a Message

The following key principles apply to creating any message:

- Use simple language, avoiding medical jargon. (For example, the average person believes that a "throbbing" headache means a "painful" headache, not one that intensifies with the heartbeat—although the term "throbbing" is familiar to almost everyone in our culture.)
- Ensure that the recipient has the emotional and medical capacity to comprehend. Patients who are frightened or distraught, just out of anesthesia, or in the midst of psychosocial transitions may lack their usual capacity to comprehend information. Individuals with physical or mental disabilities, or cultural or religious perspectives

that differ from the communicator, might be unable to hear the message at the time the communicator delivers it.

- The communicator should not use words that trigger defensive reactions in the recipient. As soon as the recipient hears a message that can imply that the sender is not accepting of the recipient's belief systems or is critical of the person, the ability of the sender to transmit the message effectively is terminated.

- When providing comfort, use words that convey empathy, not sympathy. Empathy is letting the patient or the patient's family know that the communicator understands how the patient or family might feel the way they do, even if the communicator has never had the experience. For examples, a statement such as: "I understand how it might feel to have a bad outcome to your surgery" is far more meaningful than "I know just how you feel." The only way to know exactly how the person feels would be if the communicator had had exactly the same experience as the patient or a very similar psychosocial background. On the other hand, a statement such as "I feel sorry for you" implies to the recipient that the communicator is in a position of granting sympathy. The unspoken message is, "I'm glad it's not me," whereas, "I'm so sorry this has happened to you" expresses the communicator's sadness.

Key Principles for Transmitting a Message

In messages delivered verbally, nonverbal qualities affect the interpretation of the message more than words do. Nonverbal behaviors that reduce the ability of the recipient to receive information include:

- Rate of communication (distressed people cannot comprehend quickly)
- Tonal pitch of communication (talking in a lower pitch also slows down the rate of speech, which can affect comprehension)
- Standing when the patient is sitting (can communicate dominance over the recipient)
- Looking over rather than through glasses (patients can read this as "looking down her nose at me")
- Sitting on the patient's bed (can be interpreted as invading the patient's space)
- Talking while simultaneously walking out the door (can be interpreted as uncaring)

Key Principles for Understanding the Interpretation Process

All individuals interpret messages through biases and beliefs created by their cultural, religious, and personal experiences; there is no absolute way to predict how any recipient will interpret a message.

The individual's state of physical and emotional health also plays a role. Even the surroundings can affect individuals' ability to hear—and thereby how well they actually understand.

Individuals' responses to the original message are based upon their understanding of the message and their beliefs about the sender. Many patients are in awe of health care professionals, or fear losing access to care if they appear "difficult." Other patients fear appearing unintelligent or illiterate to providers and do not wish to lose their pride or "take too much time." Still other patients fear that if they do not stand up for themselves, they will not get their health care or personal needs met. Fear of being passive drives them to behave aggressively with providers. In each of these situations, patients' internal drivers affect not only how they receive the original message, but also how they respond.

Nonverbal attributes of the sender that are beyond the sender's control also might affect how the recipient receives the message, including the following:

Authority   How the recipient feels about and responds to authority figures will influence the value or threat of the message.

Gender   How a message is received can be greatly influenced by the recipient's biases about the ability of the gender of the sender to be knowledgeable about the information being transmitted.

Age   The ages of both the sender and the recipient influence the reliability attributed to the message. Is the sender of a perceived "age" to be able to have this level of knowledge? Does the recipient feel respected and accepted by the sender?

Appearance   Not only the sender's physical appearance, but also the appearance of the environment in which the message is transmitted can influence the perceived reliability and credibility of the message.

Gestures and Actions   The sender's nonverbal habits influence the recipient because of the contextual interpretation. Even involuntary mannerisms such as an eye tic or a post-Bell's neuropathy might unwittingly influence message interpretation by the recipient. Although communicators cannot alter these attributes, they should remain aware of their potential to be distracting. The wise communicator is willing to address personal attributes if they appear to be affecting the communication process.

Key Principles of the Communication Feedback Process

The message sender is responsible for eliciting feedback. No message is delivered until there is assurance that it has been understood. The method for eliciting feedback is more than asking simple questions with a yes or no answer. "Do you have questions?" is insufficient because it gives the message sender no information about what parts of the message were inadequately understood. "What didn't you understand?" is also insufficient because it implies that the recipient understood a sufficient amount of the message to be able to verbalize what parts of the message were unclear.

More effective means of eliciting feedback include using statements and questions such as the following:

- "Help me ensure that I've been clear with you."
- "Tell me what you understood."
- "From your response, it sounds as if you feel I've been critical of you personally."
- "Let me try to rephrase this in a way that is more helpful."
- "I've given you lots of information. Why don't you give me back what you felt were the key points? That way I can make clear any that may be fuzzy."

CREATING RELATIONSHIP THROUGH EFFECTIVE COMMUNICATION IN A PATIENT- AND FAMILY-CENTERED SYSTEM

The term "patient-centered care" is increasingly used in different settings to denote a focus on the patient and family as the compass for care delivery. In patient-centered care, the needs of the patient and family, not the needs of the provider or the health care delivery system, dominate what care is provided, how it is provided, and the look and feel of the physical environment in patient care areas, in addition to the educational materials, patient information, and other communication tools used by patients and their families.

Health care organizations approach the process of becoming patient- and family-centered in several different ways. Many institute formal mechanisms to engage families and patients. One such mechanism is the use of a patient-family council, which serves as a sounding board for hospital staff on proposed changes, new initiatives, and improvements. Families are also being brought into the health care process through participation in quality improvement teams and safety committees, as mentors to patients in certain high-risk treatment processes, and through other formal mechanisms.

Effective communication lies at the heart of high-quality patient- and family-centered care. Every visit can work toward building relationships. During a patient-centered visit, the clinician uses effective communication techniques to understand the effect of the disease or condition on the life of the patient from the patient's perspective and with a realistic view. Rather than "prescribe" activities and treatments, the physician and patient together explore the options and patient preferences for care. The commitment to a treatment plan is generated from the patient's perspective. The provider helps the patient understand the choices, engages the patient in conversation about how to avoid errors, and coaches in preventing the condition from worsening or returning.[12,13]

Patient Rights

Nowhere is the need for effective communication so substantiated as in the discussion of patient rights. First developed by the American Hospital Association in 1973, *A Patient's Bill of Rights* was an effort to apply the precepts of consumer activism to health care. States then began promulgating legislation establishing similar patients' bills of rights. The early versions were applicable primarily in the inpatient setting, most often designed to protect patients from unscrupulous health care organizations allowing the needs of the system to override the needs of the patient. Such documents informed patients that it was their right to know who was providing care to them, to have their care explained to them, and to have a choice in their treatment. They were also apprised of their right to privacy, respect, care without discrimination, and to have their complaints resolved.

The Advisory Commission on Consumer Protection and Quality in the Health Care Industry was established by Executive Order 13017, dated September 5, 1996, to advise the President on changes occurring in the health care system and, where appropriate, to make recommendations on how best to promote and assure consumer protection and health care quality. President Clinton appointed the Advisory Commission on March 26, 1997. The commission issued a document intended to improve care and protect consumers. The document had three goals:[14,15]

- "To strengthen consumer confidence by assuring that the health care system is fair and responsive to consumers' needs, provides consumers with credible and effective mechanisms to address their concerns, and encourages consumers to take an active role in improving and assuring their health

- "To reaffirm the importance of a strong relationship between patients and their health care professionals

- "To reaffirm the critical role consumers play in safeguarding their health by establishing rights and responsibilities for all participants in improving their health"

Patient Responsibility

A more recent evolution in the patients' rights movement has been the expansion to include patients' responsibilities. The Advisory Commission on Consumer Protection and Quality in the Health Care Industry report: "Quality First: Better Health Care for All Americans" was published in March 1998. A summary of recommendations from that report can be found at (www.hcqualitycommission.gov/prepub/recommen.htm). As part of its work, President Clinton asked the Commission to draft a consumer bill of rights. This consumer bill of rights not only sets out patients' rights, but also includes the following list of thirteen responsibilities:[16]

- "Take responsibility for maximizing healthy habits, such as exercising, not smoking, and eating a healthy diet.

- "Become involved in specific health care decisions.

- "Work collaboratively with health care providers in developing and carrying out agreed-upon treatment plans.

- "Disclose relevant information and clearly communicate wants and needs.

- "Use the health plan's internal complaint and appeal processes to address concerns that may arise.

- "Avoid knowingly spreading disease.

- "Recognize the reality of risk and limits of the science of medical care and the human fallibility of the health care professional.

- "Be aware of a health care provider's obligations to be reasonably efficient and equitable in providing care to other patients and the community.

- "Become knowledgeable about his or her health plan coverage and health plan options (when available) including all covered benefits, limitations and exclusions, rules regarding use of network providers, coverage and referral rules, appropriate processes to secure additional information, and the process to appeal coverage decisions.

- "Show respect for other patients and health workers.

- "Make a good-faith effort to meet financial obligations.

- "Abide by administrative and operational procedures of health plans, health care providers, and government health benefit programs.

- "Report wrongdoing and fraud to appropriate resources or legal authorities."

Similarly, the American Hospital Association in its most recent edition of *A Patient's Bill of Rights*, now entitled *The Patient Care Partnership: Understanding Expectations, Rights and Responsibilities,* has expanded the focus to include responsibilities and reasonable expectations on the part of patients.[17]

Communicating with Patients with Cultural or Physical Challenges

In a patient- and family-centered system, the provider will encounter patients with physical or cultural needs that challenge the organization's ability to communicate effectively. Clinicians and staff must be trained to recognize obstacles in communication before the patient either does not comply with treatment or demands the support. The organization also must provide readily accessible qualified interpreters for several languages and sign language experts who are trained in medical terminology. In addition, the organization should have identified individuals who are educated in and knowledgeable about the beliefs and perceptions of the cultural and religious constituents of the community. These individuals should be available for consultation prior to any significant interaction with patients or families.

Awareness of the cultural and physical influences on communication is essential for the organization to address patient needs for effective communication. Lack of systems to ensure early and adequate evaluation of patient communication needs, and systems to address these needs, is often missed as a risk exposure.

Cultural Challenges to Communication   The cultural challenges to communication have received much publicity and attention in the past fifteen years. By 2050, Hispanics are predicted to constitute 24 percent of the U.S. population, and Asians will constitute approximately 8 percent. Caucasian whites are anticipated to total approximately 50 percent of the population.[18] Effective risk management means being aware of the cultural composition of the organization's service area and remaining apprised of changing demographics.

Among the factors for an organization to consider in evaluating its cultural competency is the educational program on communication for all staff. Important issues that address the unique cultural differences among the prevalent cultural and religious communities in the area should be discussed and illuminated in an academic and nonjudgmental manner. The goal is to reduce the potential for miscommunication by recognizing and addressing the influence of cultural factors on the interpretation of spoken and written communications. For example, it is important to recognize key variables in cultural interpretation of messages and situations, such as beliefs about the following:

- Health and illness
- Gender roles and how those might be affected by treatment and by examination by providers of the opposite gender
- The role and value of children in the family
- Personal responsibility for illness and treatment, including beliefs about autonomy and authority figures
- The meaning and process of death
- The role of family in helping maintain one's health
- The role of spirituality in both illness and healing

It is also important to recognize the following culture-influenced differences in communication:

- Nonverbal communication and the meaning of gesture
- Proxemics and appropriate distances for communication
- Language that might affect interpretation of dialogue
- Clinicians should consult with identified resources in the facility before engaging in difficult conversations where cultural interpretation could affect the therapeutic relationship. When uncertain of cultural implications and when no cultural educational resource is available, clinicians should always ask a same-gender physician to examine patients of the same sex (female physician to examine female patients). Also, they should always speak respectfully to the husband of a patient.

- It is important that providers ask the patient or patient's family about beliefs concerning the patient's illness, health and how it is achieved, and any religious, cultural, or familial traditions, rites, or sacraments that might be helpful or comforting to them. It is particularly important that providers ask patients whether they would like the provider to communicate about health and health decisions with them alone, with their spouse, or with some other family member.

More than ever, it is essential to use open-ended questions to elicit feedback about what is transpiring in the health care process.

Physical Challenges to Communication   Individuals with different physical challenges also create unique communication issues. Whereas patients with hearing or speaking disabilities are readily recognized as having special communication needs, the spectrum of those with communication challenges is far broader than that addressed by the Americans with Disabilities Act. Older individuals might not recognize that they are missing important communication if they are as yet unaware of (or unwilling to deal with) incremental hearing loss. The natural loss of hearing or eyesight is a slow process that will affect individuals at differing times in life. The provider or health care giver might not be aware that the individual is not hearing accurately, or patients with early cataracts might not recognize subtle changes in their ability to see or to differentiate medications.

Ultimately, it is in the best interest of the health care organization to ensure that any potential impediments to communication be addressed in advance. The Americans with Disabilities Act requires that the organization provide appropriate, respectful tools and assistance for individuals with physical disabilities. This includes hearing assistance or interpreters for those with hearing or speaking disabilities. In addition, the needs of those with sight-related disabilities must be addressed with appropriate signage, educational information, and other written materials. In addition, the Civil Rights Act prohibits discrimination against individuals because of their race, religion, age, or sexual orientation. Both laws seek to address, among other things, the ethical dilemma of supporting the right of the individual to direct the course of care.

Provider Cultural and Physical Communication Challenges   The cultural and physical attributes of providers can create risk exposure—for example, a provider with an accent indigenous to a region other than where the provider is practicing. Not only is the potential for miscommunication increased, but there is also the potential for a clash of provider and patient beliefs or prejudices.[19–21] Furthermore, providers with undiagnosed hearing loss, early-stage mental disabilities, and other impairments create the risk of practice judgment limitations in addition to the risk of communication disruption. Although many organizations have plans for dealing with such impairments when they become obvious, the organization that is communication-sensitive will find ways to address these issues early, without creating prejudice toward the providers, and will control the potential risk exposure.

COMMUNICATING WITH PATIENTS AND FAMILIES

Establishing a communication link with patients and their families is the linchpin of liability reduction techniques. Efforts to create and maintain this link start with the office visit.

The Initial Office Visit

The tone set in the first scheduling phone call, followed by the first visit, establishes the patient's belief about the efficiency and patient-centeredness of the practice. Often support staff is the patient's first contact. The telephone scheduler, the receptionist, and the medical assistant will influence the direction of the patient-provider relationship before the physician ever meets the patient. Staff communication skills are vital to ensure optimal opportunity for establishing a positive working relationship. Failure in those first encounters will set the stage for future misperceptions and potential anger.

Because staff members provide the patient's first impression of the office, they should be taught:

- To use surnames until patients give permission to be addressed by their first names
- To wait for a response to the question, "May I put you on hold?"
- To communicate that the first appointment is for assessment and evaluation, not ongoing treatment

The communication goal of the initial visit is to establish the basis for future encounters. With a firm basis for effective communication established at the first office visit, the patient might be more able to admit deviation from the prescribed regimen, if necessary, when meeting with the physician on subsequent visits, and the provider is relieved of having to guess about the reasons that the treatment failed to work. Furthermore, when a procedure is being considered, rapport has already been established for informed treatment plan development and consent. It is therefore essential that the provider establish reasonable patient expectations. This visit provides the opportunity to talk about acceptable and unacceptable behaviors, including after-hours requests, children in the waiting room, expectations about bill payment, and handling disagreements and complaints.

The initial visit is also important in establishing the level of trust that sets the stage for future potential consent and disclosure discussions. Although many providers find these discussions distasteful, they form the basis for potential discussions about unanticipated events, difficult diagnoses, or objectionable behavior and the possible need to terminate the relationship.

During the first scheduling phone call, a staff member might make a statement such as, "You'll love Dr. Jones! All his patients do. Of course he can treat your problem." This can create an expectation that the patient will like the provider and that the provider is not only the appropriate person to treat the specific problem, but also will provide a cure.

At the first office visit, the provider should elicit and discuss patient expectations. If the patient has unrealistic ideas about access or treatment, the provider can dispel these. At the first visit, the provider should also observe new patients for indications of their understanding of medical systems and problems; for their educational background; and for any cultural, religious, gender, or other influences to which the provider might wish to be sensitive in future interactions.

Subsequent Visits

Different challenges exist for establishing communication, depending on whether the patient needs primary care or specialty care.

With primary care, the provider might see the patient only during an annual physical exam, so the relationship being built could form the basis for years of interactions. The dialogue is often prescriptive, and the opportunity to establish an ongoing personal connection is limited.

Conditions requiring treatment in specialty care are usually specific and often urgent. The relationship may be limited to one or two visits.

To build partnership in both primary and specialty care, the provider should:

- Note personal information about patients, such as hobbies or interests, and allude to those during the course of visits
- Develop the treatment plan in partnership with patients, even for conditions considered mild or relatively innocuous
- Ask patients what they are willing to do to participate in the self-care process
- Tell patients they should be willing to speak up if they recognize that they are not going to follow provider recommendations so that together, they and the provider can develop a feasible care plan
- Tell patients that if they find that they have been unable to comply with recommendations made at an earlier visit, they should feel free to discuss this with the provider without fear of retribution

Informed Consent

Although a complete discussion of informed consent is beyond the scope of this chapter, the principles of truly informed consent are based on the principles of effective communication. Only when the patient is informed and educated about the available options for treatment, including the option of no treatment, can there be an honest dialogue about the risks and benefits of treatment.

The foundation for consent originates in both the science of ethics and in the principles of patient rights. Ethically, the basis of consent is the doctrine of autonomy, which supports the right of the individual to make choices about the direction of care without coercion or deception.[22] Consent may be defined as "the willing acceptance of a medical intervention by a patient after adequate disclosure by the physician of the nature of the intervention, its risk, and benefits, as well as of alternatives with their risks and benefits."[23] It also constitutes the ongoing process of discussion about the meaning of health to the patient, self-care approaches, and treatments, including noninvasive tests and medications.[24,25]

At times, patients might make decisions counter to those that providers believe are reasonable. They also might be influenced by cultural factors or beliefs about health and wellness that conflict with those of the provider. They might even refuse information.[26] Families also might influence a patient's autonomy by subtle—or sometimes not so subtle—coercion to take action perceived as best from their perspective, even if it fails to meet the patient's values and health care goals. Complicating this array of barriers is the essential question of capacity: Is the individual even able to make a decision of this type at this time?

In a litigious society, informed consent is often considered simply the form the patient signs, rather than the discussion and process between the patient and physician. However, case law has defined what providers must tell patients: the risks and benefits of the procedure, alternatives and their risks, and the details of how, when and who can obtain the informed consent. Unfortunately, there is no one specific consent conversation that will fit all situations or patients. The inadequacy of legislation, regulation, health care guidelines and policies, and professional ethical standards to address consent, is an indication of the importance of communication as an essential component of truly informed consent.

The skills required for a provider to enter into a consent dialogue are similar to those required for effective communication and relationship building. The provider must be able to assess the patient's level of understanding, the patient's values, and which aspects of the potential risks and benefits might be most important to that person's situation. The provider must also use language that is truly "informing" to the patient and the patient's family.[27] Consequently, training staff in how to participate in a consent dialogue is as essential as the elements to be included in the consent itself.

Consent is not meant just for those procedures and medications for which the potential for injury is high. Health care has generally used the terms "invasive" or "medically complex" to identify procedures that require consent. From a legal perspective, that is a sufficient guideline. However, from the perspective of building effective relationships with patients and families, the consent process should be used throughout every health care relationship.

By making the discussion of alternatives, risks, and benefits related to every care decision a regular part of visits, providers have the opportunity to educate patients. Using this approach, the discussion about a more invasive procedure is not a new process or language. Patients learn to see the consent process as a routine part of what happens during care and not as an event that either happens or doesn't happen. By creating a practice in which consent discussions are integral components, the provider reduces the likelihood of unanticipated events or rare complications creating a rift in the relationship.

Although the requirements and conditions are delineated in Volume II, Chapter 4 on informed consent in this series, there are considerations that apply whether consent is being discussed as part of a formal process for invasive procedures, or is a component of the informal treatment plan development process that occurs at every office visit. The communication considerations for procuring valid consent include:

- An assessment of the individual's ability and readiness to enter the dialogue (Is the patient on medications, delirious, or experiencing an emotional or psychiatric trauma? Is the patient in denial of the diagnosis or urgency of need for treatment?)

- The ability of the provider to present the information in a comprehensible manner. (Can the provider explain the condition requiring treatment in lay terms with sufficient information that the patient can understand the need for treatment and ramifications of non-treatment? Can the provider explain the proposed treatment in a way that someone with no education can understand the essential points of the risks, benefits, and alternatives? Can the provider engage in a simple discussion about the options available, including allopathic and alternative approaches? Can the provider discuss in simple, nonjudgmental terms the implications of herbal and other self-directed treatments, including possible interactions between methods that could result in delay of healing at best, or life-threatening interactions at worst?)

Disclosure of Unanticipated Events

Since the JCAHO in 2001 under the Ethics, Rights ad Responsibilities (RI) Standards (RI 1.2.2) required that patients be advised of all unanticipated outcomes, the issue of disclosure has taken on increasing importance. In the past, efforts to communicate uncomfortable information to patients have been seriously lacking. Historically, providers have believed that they were protecting patients by not disclosing disturbing news, such as a cancer diagnosis.[28] Physicians have been reluctant to share medical errors or deviations. In fact, neither providers nor organizations have demonstrated the skills, techniques, or support for effective disclosure. A study published in 2001 implies that this lack of training is experienced even during medical residency.[29] Whether new or experienced, providers are still often ill-prepared for this most difficult interpersonal encounter.

The initiators of the conversation have uncomfortable information to divulge, so they are in a vulnerable psychological, emotional, and potentially legal position. Providers often experience fear of litigation, of reprisal from the organization, and of being ostracized by peers. Thus they may have a tendency to shift blame to others, reveal incomplete information, or "fill in the blanks" with facts that support their beliefs. Because of these human tendencies, organizational infrastructures that support the willingness of providers and staff to be open and honest with patients must be designed, supported, and implemented.

Why should the organization be open and honest with patients? At the most basic level, patients have the right to understand everything that is applicable to their own health and well-being, to be empowered to participate in care decisions. Furthermore, the physician's role is not passive. It goes beyond delivering care to promoting the patient's interests and working with the patient to achieve the patient's health care goals.[30] If a patient cannot receive the information because of health status, it is the right of the proxy to be able to make decisions in concert with the patient's wishes. None of this can happen without complete and truthful disclosure.

The risk management professional must recognize that not all providers or employees will be able to, or should, participate in disclosure conversations. Although any person can improve skills in almost any area, not all individuals have the same facility for human connection. It is unfair to expect all providers to behave the same way or to develop the same ability to participate in disclosure conversations. Nonetheless, it is essential for the organization to ensure that providers are trained in effective disclosure techniques. Furthermore, when the provider or the risk management professional recognizes that a provider is not equipped, whether psychologically or interpersonally, to lead a disclosure discussion, the organization has an obligation to support the provider by supplying an effective communicator as part of the disclosure team.

One approach is that the delivery of bad news is not a one-step process. It is an event that will likely happen several times over the course of the relationship with the patient. At the least, the organization should consider disclosure a two-step process. The first step is the discussion in which the unexpected outcome is revealed or disclosure has occurred. The second meeting explains the basis for the event and begins the discussion of appropriate compensation if applicable to the situation.

Furthermore, organizations must learn to treat each circumstance of disclosure with sensitivity and concern. If staff and providers take the time to build honest communication with patients and their families, the foundation for disclosure discussions has been built.

Conveying the News   The skills for disclosing unanticipated events such as a devastating diagnosis, an unanticipated treatment outcome, the failure to achieve a hoped-for outcome, or a medical error, are generally similar to those for discussing any uncomfortable news, and they constitute many of those skills previously discussed in this chapter. The first skill is to send the message in a manner in which the individual can hear it. Also, the active solicitation of feedback is essential. Without verifying patient understanding, it is impossible to assess the needs of patients and their families for additional information and for emotional support.

To impart unexpected news that is negative, sad, or discouraging in a manner that is respectful of the recipients and sensitive to their needs and reactions, it is important to hold the disclosure meeting in a neutral place whenever possible. Water and tissues should be pre-set in the room to avoid having to break the conversation to procure them.

Appropriate staff, the attending physician, and, whenever possible, the person(s) with whom the patient or family has the closest relationship should be involved in the meeting. It is essential that the family not be outnumbered by hospital staff. However, at least one member of the team should be an effective communicator.

In difficult conversations, the range of readiness is narrower than for other types of communication. Hospitalized patients are likely worried or frightened and might be under the influence of medication that impairs their ability to think and respond clearly. Also, the family may be in an emotional or physical state that limits their ability to process information. They might have been long hours at the bedside and are frightened, worried, and tired.

If further medical decisions are required or the poor outcome is already known to the patient and family, disclosure may have to be made before the parties are fully ready and willing to hear the news. In this case, it is essential that the recipients be asked how much information they would like at the first, then subsequent, disclosure discussions. The deliverer of the message must recognize that the imparting of bad news is often a multi-step process that might involve different hospital staff, and should communicate that to the recipient. The full process of disclosure often involves:

- The initial broaching of the issue and revelation of the problem
- The next meeting for clarification of findings and resolution of the situation
- Another meeting to talk about negotiation of emotional and possibly financial interests

    The disclosure conversation should include:

- The facts, described in short sentences and in simple, lay terms
- The outcomes of the event and diagnosis described in short, simple sentences
- The next steps for treatment or closure
- What the facility is doing to investigate
- Concern and regret for the situation
- An apology when appropriate

Handling Crying   Most often, anger, sadness, and fear will elicit tears during the disclosure conversation. The patient and family should be permitted to cry for as long as necessary. Verbal permission can be given directly by such statements as, "I would cry, too." "It's OK to cry. It's absolutely understandable in your situation."

Out of respect, the person delivering the message should not touch the patient or family physically unless there has been a long-term or emotionally close relationship such that the person is certain that touch is acceptable or there is permission.

Handling Anger   Anger is often difficult to handle in disclosure discussions because the individual doing the disclosing might not have been involved in the event.

Nonetheless, the deliverer of bad news is often the target of an angry tirade. Effective methods for dealing with angry people include:

- Acknowledging the anger
- Accepting the anger, but not accepting responsibility for it. (This involves responding respectfully, but not accepting abusive discussion.)
- Allowing sufficient time for the angry person to fully express anger and frustration
- Accepting that the person may be angry with the person delivering the message and associate that person with the news.

   If the patient and family cannot continue the discussion, it is essential to schedule another meeting to continue the conversation to discuss next steps and follow-up.

Handling Denial   Depending upon the nature of the information being given, many people shut down receptivity to information that is emotionally threatening. This is not a purposeful behavior, but a reaction to hearing information with implications so great that the individual cannot cope with it at the time. People will often find evidence to support their perceptions that the information is not accurate. This can happen when there is a devastating diagnosis or a death. The method for dealing with denial is much like dealing with anger, and requires a more active stance on the part of the news deliverer. The person relaying the news should:

- Acknowledge the reasonableness of the denial
- Allow the person to present a rationale for the denial
- Slowly and simply repeat the facts of the situation
- Repeat the information several times until the recipient hears it
- Refrain from giving in to the denial as an easy "out" from the difficult nature of the situation or an opportunity for the discloser to abdicate responsibility for ensuring that the recipient understands the full ramification of the situation

Closing the Conversation   Many people let disclosure conversations extend beyond the time when it is useful to the recipient. By the same token, individuals who are uncomfortable with expressed emotion, or very upset by the information they are called upon to disclose, might end the conversation prematurely. The meeting should end when:

- All appropriate information has been communicated
- All reactive emotions have been expressed
- The recipient is ready to begin planning next steps

   At this point, the discloser should reiterate:

- The facts in simple, summary terms
- Any important questions the patient or family has asked
- The answers to important questions

Planning for Follow-up   The discloser should ask the patient or family:

- If there is anyone for them to be with
- If there is another person with whom the discloser should talk about the situation

- If they have a place to stay
- If there is someone who can drive them where they need to go
- If they would like to speak with their spiritual leader or helping persons from the hospital
- If they need something to eat

The discloser should also tell them when and from whom they will hear next.

Apologies

Legal implications of admitting involvement in an unanticipated outcome have been ascribed with inhibiting providers and organizations from expressing legitimate human sorrow.[31] States are beginning to respond by promoting legislation that does not include apology as an admission of culpability. In 1986, Massachusetts was the first state that precluded an apology of sympathy from being admitted as evidence of liability in a civil action. Colorado in 2003 has passed legislation (Colorado Revised Statute §13–25–2003) that allows a fully admitting apology ("I'm sorry I hurt you") without the fear that it can be used in court.[32] California, Florida, Texas, Tennessee, Washington, Missouri, Louisiana, Florida, Maryland, Tennessee, Texas, Montana, New Jersey, Georgia, Oklahoma, Ohio, Wyoming, Illinois, and Oregon have laws that protect expressions of sympathy and many other states are quickly following suit.[33]

Michigan?

People are afraid to apologize when there is fear of retribution or no hope of forgiveness. However, apology has been linked with more rapid repair of trust so long as the apology was appropriate to the involvement, and when the apology was made for an actual error.[34] The implications for apology in health care are great. Admitting participation in an error when an error was made, or gently stating that no error was made (if certain no error has been made), is most likely to generate forgiveness and restoration of trust.

In addition, apology does not replace accountability. Research shows that organizations that hold people accountable without offering genuine forgiveness are punitive, and ultimately reduces the accountability they claim to demand, and yet forgiveness without accountability results in complacency.[35] Apology that does not include accountability is likely to be taken as insincere. The balance that is likely to invoke forgiveness is a sincere apology coupled with an acceptance of the responsibility to follow through with actions designed to ensure personal and organizational accountability.

From a communication perspective, this raises an interesting dilemma. How should an apology be worded? Should you as a provider apologize for mistakes that might be the responsibility of others? Is it ever appropriate for a person other than the responsible party to acknowledge an error and take responsibility?

The purpose of apology is to rebuild trust, not to avoid litigation. Words should be chosen carefully and delivered simply and sincerely. It doesn't matter whether the apologizer says, "I'm sorry," "I apologize," or "I wish it weren't so." It is important to use the word "I"—"I apologize"; "I'm sorry"; "I feel terrible that . . ."

The apologizer should speak slowly and use a lower tone of voice. Use empathic nonverbal skills (sit at the same level or lower than the message recipient, uncross arms and legs, show that you are listening). Give the person time to respond, do not react defensively to whatever is said. Acknowledge the recipient's right to feel a full range of emotions. Acknowledge the recipient's perspective and, if blamed, feel free to disagree with respect and calm. Allow silence at the end of the apology.

Apology is a powerful communication and human tool. Whenever possible, the apologizer should practice the apology before the discussion. The ability to forgive and to regain trust rests with the person to whom the apology is owed. A sincere apology enhances the possibility that the person will be able to regain trust, and that both parties will be able to move on and heal.

Patient Complaints

There are times when patients are unhappy with their care, although there has been no error, nor any other action which reasonably places the organization or provider at risk for legal action. Often these are the most frustrating types of situations to manage because the ramifications seem minimal in comparison to many issues with which risk management professionals must deal daily. However, the danger in the unsubstantiated complaint is the potential for the patient's future negative perceptions and feelings. Hence, managing patient complaints at every step of the relationship in a positive and effective manner is essential to the partnering relationship and key to effective risk management.

Every complaint, regardless of the lack of direct ramifications, contains valid feedback and should be addressed by the organization. The feedback might be seemingly insignificant. It might be information about staff response to workload, the receptionist desk set-up, or the telephone routing system. Nonetheless, this is information about how systems and individuals are influencing the external perception of the organization. Ultimately, this is a reflection of the degree to which the organization is seen as patient-oriented.

Although the system and hierarchy for managing patient complaints must be captured in organizational policies and procedures, the skills for discussing complaints with patients should be acquired by anyone who works with patients. This includes administration, clinicians, and staff. There is no substitute for effective communication and genuine interest in the concerns of patients and their families.

The key to resolving a complaint is for patients or family members to feel that their concerns are considered valid by the organization and that the organization will take steps to remedy the underlying causes of the problem. Fortunately, most patients are reasonable. Vincent's seminal study clearly established that patients and families desire to be treated with respect and dignity; to have their fears acknowledged and not held against them; to have their complaints taken seriously; and to feel as if they have contributed to improving the situation.[36] By allowing patients and families to express themselves without defensive reactions, the organization acknowledges patient-family dignity. By sharing organizational challenges to provide consistent customer service with patients and families, the organization communicates that it trusts and values their judgments and perceptions. Finally, by apologizing and asking how patients and families believe the organization can improve, the organization is taking the needs of patients and families into consideration.

In managing complaints, the communication goal is to gather information to determine areas for further investigation without making promises for specific action of compensation, and without raising the defense mechanisms of the complainant. Staff members meeting with complainants should:

- Review the patient's record
- Talk with anyone who may be aware of the patient's concerns
- Determine ahead of time the medical and educational sophistication of the complainant and the nature of the complaint itself
- Whenever possible, select a neutral location
- Select a time when the conversation can occur without interruption If only ten minutes are available and the patient has a strong need to talk immediately, an acceptable way to

approach the situation might be to say, "I'm sorry. I really have only ten minutes right now. Those ten minutes are yours, and then, perhaps, we can make an appointment for another meeting." For the ten minutes available, the patient deserves undivided attention.

- Avoid debating the merits of the complaint
- Recognize the signs of being led into debate and deflect the process

Under the Interpretive Guidelines for Medicare Conditions of Participation at: §482.13(a)(2), the hospital must establish a process for prompt resolution of patient grievances and must inform each patient whom to contact to file a grievance. A patient grievance is described as a written or verbal complaint (when the verbal complaint about patient care is not resolved at the time of the complaint by staff present) by a patient, or the patient's representative, regarding the patient's care, abuse or neglect, issues related to the hospital's compliance with the CMS Hospital Conditions of Participation (CoP), or a Medicare beneficiary billing complaint related to rights and limitations provided by 42 CFR §489.

Any process is limited in its efficacy by the skill of the individuals who are responsible. Without solid conflict resolution, negotiation, and interpersonal communication skills, the most complex system is doomed to result in patients and families who remain angry and marginalized. It is essential that the system not be seen as a substitute for skillful communication and that the system is designed to find the truth in every complaint and to find respectful ways to manage patient expectations.[37]

Patients Who Are Difficult to Manage

There are patients who are difficult to work with. Patients sometimes see providers as "one size fits all." They believe that they should be able to go to any provider and receive similar expressions of warm, caring interaction. However, providers are different, and sometimes the pairing of personalities makes it impossible for specific people to work together. Furthermore, many providers come from socioeconomic and educational backgrounds very different from the people they serve. Cultural differences based upon family of origin and early moral teachings might result in personality clashes.

Often, the behavioral standards and decision-making standards of the two parties are in such conflict that communication becomes almost impossible. Before a provider makes a decision not to work with any given individual, the risk management professional should ensure that the provider has the requisite communication skills. Poorly handled interactions or termination of the relationship with patients can foster animosity that frequently leads to claims and potential claims. The most frequently encountered types of behaviors and attitudes that result in difficult communications follow.

Entitled or Demanding Behavior   Patients who behave in a way that is interpreted as "entitled" or "demanding" frequently feel powerless. They might believe that unless they make demands, they will not be heard, nor will their needs be given consideration. Unfortunately, many staff and providers prefer not to accommodate individuals who exhibit demanding behavior. The demanding position elicits the most reaction when matched with other individuals who are afraid of what will happen if the demands are not met. Most individuals get annoyed and wish to be rid of the demanding patients. However, there are ways to work with people who feel a need to place demands on the system or staff.

When conversing with demanding patients and families, the goal is to communicate respect and acceptance of the patient's and family's perspective while setting limits on behavior.

A demand is usually a metaphor for what the person wants. A patient who says, "I demand that I be seen today" is most likely saying they are afraid they will wait for weeks to learn about a condition that is worrying them. An appropriate response could be: "I understand your desire to be seen today. We have limited times available. Tell me your thoughts for wanting to be seen today so we can see about making the best effort to get your needs met."

- Acknowledge their desire to be seen.
- Try to ascertain the reasons beneath the expressed reasons.
- Set reasonable parameters for what can and cannot be accommodated.

The same principle may apply to patients who demand certain tests or medications. Patients pick up bits of information that they believe might be appropriate for them. Anxious patients might not believe that the provider will not consider all tests and medications, and therefore they will demand them. Ask the patient what it is about the medicine or test that they believe will be better than other choices for their condition. Engage the patient in your thought processes about the tests and medications and how they may or may not be appropriate.

Create an agreement with the patient about conditions under which you will consider the medication or tests they are requesting, and keep your agreement.

Demeaning or Rude Behavior   Demeaning or rude behavior may range from children misbehaving in the waiting room to patients who use obscenities when they believe their demands are thwarted. Although actions for managing rude behavior can include anything from simple dialogue to the procurement of a restraining order, basic communication techniques for addressing the behavior remain the same.

The rude or demeaning individual is similar to the demanding individual. The behavior feels aggressive and sometimes hostile to the listener, yet the underlying emotion of the sender is often one of fear or threat. Much like the complaining or demanding individual, there is rarely any benefit to provoking the rude individual into a defensive posture. When the agitated person is provoked, the provider or staff loses control over the situation. There is the risk that a patient or family could become agitated to the point of physical response. Consequently, it is in the best interest of the organization that staff maintain equilibrium while attempting to address the unacceptable behavior.

This is not to say that a patient who behaves persistently in demeaning or rude ways should not be terminated from the physician's practice or dealt with in the hospital setting. Persistent or physically endangering behavior must be addressed expeditiously and firmly. The preferred approach to managing and defusing the behavior, however, offers patients the opportunity to recognize and change their conduct. This response enables more extreme actions to be a part of a process that preserves patient dignity.

The communication goal is to manage behavior and create a respectful environment for other staff and patients while conveying respect for the patient and family and not eliciting an escalation of the behavior. Understanding the following techniques and principles will assist in managing the disruptive or rude patient and family:

- Approach the individual with a simple description of the unacceptable behavior.
- State the reason that the behavior is not acceptable. For example, "I am sorry. It is important that the children lower the volume of their voices in this office. Our patients are cancer patients, like you, and many of them are feeling very ill. The

children's loud voices make it very uncomfortable for everyone. What can we do about this?" or, "I'm sorry. The language you are now using with staff is unacceptable. Therefore, I will have to ask you to consider your language before we can continue this conversation."

- Separate the judgment of the behavior from judgment of the individual.

- The individual receiving the message must recognize that the behavior is the problem—not the person or the person's dignity.

- Where the behavior persists, state consequences clearly and calmly, even to the point of calling security or police.

- The person managing the conversation must never lose control, nor resort to labeling the patient or family.

- If the behavior should escalate physically, ensure that there are witnesses, that there is a way out of the room, that there are no sharp objects easily accessible, and that there is a plan for contacting security.

Uncooperative Behavior   The term "uncooperative patient" may be ascribed to a wide variety of behaviors, from the patient who cancels visits regularly or does not keep referral appointments, to the patient who fails to comply with the treatment regimen. Often these patients have good intentions, but fail to see the importance of the expected behavior. Other patients simply might believe that ignoring health issues will make them go away. In either case, these are usually not malicious intentions, but actions that require dialogue and management.

Patients often misunderstand that missed appointments might affect the provider's ability to give high-quality care. They also might not realize that medications must be taken consistently for efficacy. Communication with these patients frequently takes on an educational function. The provider should clarify the patient's expectations in the absence of the patient's cooperation with the plan.

Communication with the uncooperative patient must be clear, concise, and specific. "I am very worried about trying to provide care for you when I cannot trust that you will show up for visits or take your medicine. It puts both you and me at risk. You are at risk for getting worse, and I am at risk for not being able to provide you adequate care. What are we going to do about it?" Sometimes these patients will be unable to change their behavior because their disorganization or denial is deep-rooted. This must be managed so that the patient feels that the behavior is at issue and not the person. Discussions about lack of cooperation should be documented completely and non-judgmentally in the record. Often the lack of behavior change subsequent to the discussion becomes the basis for later termination of the patient-provider relationship. Consequently, it is essential that the process be documented should there be a later allegation of patient abandonment or failure to diagnose or treat a patient's condition.

Behavior that Does Not Fit the Provider's Beliefs about Allopathic Medicine   One physician was concerned about liability and called risk management because his patient wanted to go to Mexico for an alternative treatment to chemotherapy. Not only was he worried about the portal for chemotherapy becoming occluded or contaminated, but also he thought the patient was "nuts" to pursue this approach to therapy. He called the risk manager ostensibly for advice, knowing full well that what he wanted to hear was that he should forbid the action.

When this event occurred, complementary and alternative medicine (CAM) approaches to medicine were not as popular as they are now. As of 1999, it was estimated that up to 43 percent of Americans had used complementary and alternative approaches to health care.[38] That number is projected to grow. No longer can the provider claim ignorance of alternative approaches and categorically dismiss them as ineffective. It is essential that providers explore and be aware of their beliefs about complementary approaches to health care. Providers who are unwilling to understand the perspectives of many of today's patients should recognize and be clear that they are not the right providers for patients who prefer to augment their care with herbal treatments, acupuncture, chiropractic, or other forms of complementary or alternative treatments. Providers must be open with patients about their inability to work with complementary or alternative modalities; however, they must be able to express that inability in a way that does not judge the patient.

This is a difficult communication encounter. Therefore, any conversation between a provider and a patient with conflicting perspectives about the correct approach to a health care problem has the possibility of conflict. Nevertheless, providers should share with patients the rationale behind their differing beliefs. At the same time, they must communicate, directly and indirectly, the patient's right to select the treatment approach that is in alignment with the patient's own beliefs.

Communicating about Differing Beliefs about Medicine and Moral Behavior   The communication goal is to retain integrity as a provider, and adhere to one's personal ethical and moral value system, while permitting the patient and family to express differing values in an environment of respect and trust, and ensuring that they receive the type of care that fits their philosophical framework.

The patient's perspective should be acknowledged by the following:

- Express a sincere wish to be able to share that perspective.
- Express a perspective that differs from that of the patient.
- Offer to help the patient find someone whose philosophies and perspective more closely align with those of the patient.
- The sentiment must be genuine and must be focused on the needs of the patient.

Behavior that may be Ethically Disturbing to the Provider   Beliefs about alternative approaches to medicine and what is medically permissible may differ among both providers and patients. The most obvious examples are beliefs about abortion and organ donation. These procedures or treatments are legal, but may have moral implications depending upon the cultural and religious beliefs of the patient and the provider.

On a more mundane basis, some patients might desire surgeries that a physician perceives as unnecessary or dangerous and in which the physician might not want to participate. Some patients might feel it is their right to demand treatments, much like purchasing a car or house. Providers must not feel morally obligated to provide services that they believe would betray the Hippocratic Oath. In cases of moral disagreement, providers must be willing to own their own beliefs, acknowledge that patients have the right to their personal beliefs, and be willing to refer patients to someone who shares the same beliefs. These dialogues involve the same skills as those for working with patients whose views might differ on the use of complementary and alternative treatments.

The organization's policy for addressing the moral and ethical dilemmas of staff should include empathic communication as part of the process. The risk management professional, along with members of the institutional ethics committee, are in the best positions to provide this guidance.

Terminating the Patient Relationship

The termination of the patient relationship should never be a surprise to the patient. [Refer to Volume II, Chapter 8 for more information on termination of the patient relationship.] This can occur only if the communication has been open, honest, and direct at every step of the relationship. If expectations are set at the beginning of the relationship that unacceptable behaviors will be addressed and documented during the relationship, the dialogue or letter that announces the need to terminate the relationship will be seen as a logical conclusion.

White Paper

30 days

Frequently, a discussion about the need to terminate the relationship is documented by a certified letter. The discussion should follow the same tenor and form as discussions about unacceptable behaviors. The major difference between a dialogue about termination of the relationship and dialogues about unacceptable behavior is the outcome of the discussion and the follow-up. In the termination dialogue, the provider needs to ensure that the patient is able to hear the reasons for the termination and the provider's parameters for interim behaviors. Often the interim plan includes emergency care, the names of potential providers, and an expressed willingness to forward copies of records to the new provider at no charge to the patient. In many cases, the patient may be terminated from a single provider, in other cases from an entire practice or group of practices. Finally, the dialogue, the rationale for the termination, and all previous stated patient behavior conversations should be documented in the medical record non-judgmentally and factually.

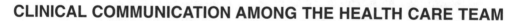

CLINICAL COMMUNICATION AMONG THE HEALTH CARE TEAM

The issues of communicating with staff and physicians on a more general level are discussed later in this chapter. In this section, the communication model is applied to the tools known to improve communication in handoffs, transfers, urgent situations, and on teams.

Human factors engineering—the study of the interface of humans with machines—teaches that under less than ideal conditions, humans are more likely to make mistakes. Conditions that are considered "human factors" include environmental and equipment design features, such as cell phones with screen backlighting that makes the print too hard to read. Also, personal conditions such as fatigue, sleep deprivation, biorhythm disturbance, medication effects, illness, distraction, stress, and environmental conditions such as heat or cold, noise, and chaos affect the way a human can perform tasks. Some conditions are temporary, such as environmental conditions; other conditions are permanent, such as features on equipment or the design of the building, unit, or section.[39]

Hardwiring the Communication Model

Recognizing the link between the communication cycle and human factors, the method for improving communication in hand-offs, transfers, and chaotic situations such as surgery or trauma care is to address those human factors. This can be accomplished by hard-wiring communication techniques into the system. Popular tools for improving communication in patient care include such systems as the Situation/Background/Assessment/Recommendation (SBAR) Situational Briefing Model. In addition, by understanding the relationship of human factors to the communication model, the risk management professional can design tools internally to address communication issues in clinical care.

Hardwiring the Message   The key to creating an understandable message is twofold: developing a common vocabulary and scripting. For communication to be hardwired, the entire group must understand what key words mean in that environment. When applying the communications model to improving a clinical situation, assess what terms are frequently used and determine if there is a common understanding about the meaning and implications of those terms. If not, the meaning should be developed and posted. Common vocabulary is an essential component of precise communication. The Institute for Safe Medical Practices list of unacceptable abbreviations, high alert medications, and a list of drug names which are easily confused is available at (www.ismp.org/Tools/default.asp). It offers a good start to the development of a common vocabulary.

Coupled with precise communication is the need for scripting. Scripting is particularly important in situations where variation can cause confusion or where a consistent message is necessary. Scripting has been used successfully in registration functions, where presenting a consistent message to the public is considered essential. Scripting has less often been used in the clinical setting.

The Situational Briefing Model developed by Michael Leonard, MD, and Suzanne Graham at Kaiser Permanente is an excellent example of clinical scripting and standardization of communication.[40] In the model, the mechanism for contacting the physician, the checklist to ensure proper preparation, and a scripted communication that covers the situation, the background, the assessment, and the recommendation are all defined. The communication format is scripted so that each important information factor is prompted by a cue in the script. Despite clarity of the model, there are still requisite conditions for success. The information must be transmitted clearly, and physicians must accept the format as the method used by the organization to communicate important information. Messages received in this format must be recognized as representing important communication not to be dismissed. Physicians also must be willing to listen and respond to the information in a way that demonstrates that the information was heard and understood.

Hardwiring the Method of Transmission   Transmitting information is more difficult to hardwire because of the many conflicting factors that can affect transmission. However, employee empowerment to take action when communication is unclear is an initial step. Often those on the front line of care recognize unclear or distorted communication before those communicating are aware of the problem. Staff should be empowered to terminate care if the care seems unsafe, or if there is a lack of understanding about the actions to be taken. Furthermore, messages should be conveyed using consistent mechanisms and methods of handling messages. Illegible handwriting, unclear speaking skills, malfunctioning telephone equipment, and other such transmission impediments should not be tolerated. With hardwired methods of transmission, the possibility of a message being ignored because it comes via a different route of communication is reduced.

occupational therapists — something to improve handwriting?

Hardwiring the Reception and Interpretation of the Message   Interpretation of a message is tied to the encoding and transmission of the message. In situations in which the vocabulary is defined and messages are scripted or delivered using the organizationally accepted mechanisms, the opportunity for misinterpretation is greatly reduced. Nonetheless, members of the health care team might be expecting a different message, or they might ignore the message through distraction or a belief that the message has been received. These constraints cannot be eliminated; consequently, it is essential that the feedback loop is hardwired into each communication situation.

Hardwiring Feedback   Risk management professionals are familiar with hardwired feedback. The read-back of verbal orders—that is, the recipient's iteration to the original communicator of what was received and understood by the recipient—is one form of hardwired feedback. Most communication falls apart in this portion of the communication cycle. In interpersonal communication, this happens because the receiver's interpretations are different from the sender's. The lack of feedback to the sender misleads him or her to believe that the message was understood.

The same is true for clinical interaction. Unless the originator of the order, direction, or clinical information knows what has been received by the person for whom the message was intended, the message was not delivered. This is the area where handoffs and transfers are most vulnerable. Systems of transfer and handoff assume that the recipient has read, heard, or understood the information.

A common misunderstanding in communication is that the message, once delivered, is complete. However, until the original sender is assured that the message was received and understood in the manner in which it was intended, the communication cycle is incomplete. Incomplete communication has critical implications in clinical care. Too often, the method of communicating consists of writing a "note in the chart" or leaving a written message. This method does not complete the communication process, and the potential for error is great. Risk management professionals should consider the hardwiring of feedback into any hand-off or transfer process improvement. This might require a change in accountability for the assurance of the message delivery.

Communication in the Care Team

The ability to work as an effective team is unquestionably important in the current health care environment. Nonetheless, much is still being learned about teams in health care. At the most basic level, a team is a group of people with a common goal and high levels of self-direction, interreliance, and accountability. Although the terms are used interchangeably, teamwork is different from being a team; it is the ability to work together cooperatively.[41]

There is a vast amount of literature on groups, group dynamics, and teams. Some basic principles apply to all groups and are essential in a discussion about teamwork or teams. Individuals in groups behave in ways that are similar to their normal interpersonal patterns and in other ways that are markedly different. The sociology of a group environment fosters freedom in some to act out their anger through lack of cooperation or demanding behavior; in others, the public nature of groups fosters a more reticent reaction. In addition, power and leadership in groups evolves differently. Although an individual might have the power of authority, another individual who is well-liked or respected might have power because of the group's desire to follow a leader. Group dynamics influences committees, working groups, administrative teams, or clinical care teams. Team skill-building should focus on these dynamics and on self-understanding for team members. In addition, an effective team-training course should hardwire some of the communication transactions to ensure precise interaction.

The introduction of flight recorders and cockpit voice recorders into modern jet aircraft generated insights about the communication failures that often led to accidents. The inability to respond appropriately to the situation due to lack of awareness and the interpersonal dynamics that inhibited effective communication led to the development of Crew Resource Management (CRM).[42] In recent years, CRM has been applied successfully in health care. The success of CRM in high-risk situations has led to its application in emergency departments, operating rooms, and other high-risk clinical areas. A feature of CRM is situational awareness training—that is, the hardwiring of communication patterns and scripting of communication for high-risk situations so that attention is drawn to the critical message. Empowerment and scripting are provided for communicating across the authority gradient. CRM training includes cognitive skills such as situational awareness, planning and decision-making skills, interpersonal skills such as communication and teamwork dynamics, and handling the emotional climate and stress. Although CRM is only one model, it is one that has worked in aviation and is widely applied in high-risk clinical areas.

OTHER INTERNAL COMMUNICATION

It is easy to forget that customers include not only external but also internal relationships. Staff and providers sometimes assume that because they are working in the same environment, they interpret events and situations in similar ways. However, this assumption can lead to miscommunication, mistrust, and a breakdown of patient information handoffs.

Communication with Staff

Historically, organizations have accomplished communication with employees using a top-down approach. Memos sent by leadership often are considered "communication" with all staff. The fallacy in this approach rests in the belief that 1) the memo recipient appreciates the importance of the information; 2) leadership fully understands who needs which pieces of information; and 3) the information is transmitted in a manner that will be understood and remembered. In health care organizations, the goal is to create an environment of patient safety—part of which is trust. Trust starts at the top of the organization and permeates through staff, ultimately affecting care. The basis of trust is transparency, defined as "allowing others to see the truth without trying to hide or shade the meaning, or altering the facts to put things in a better light."[43] The mechanism for creating that transparency is effective, frequent, and honest communication.

For employees to feel valued as integral members of the health care team, information about all aspects of the organization should be communicated to every person in the organization. Information that could affect employee activity or community issues should be communicated in a manner that can be easily understood by staff of differing cultural, generational, ethnic, and educational backgrounds. Written materials should be printed in at least 12-point type and should be provided at the fifth-grade level for nonprofessional staff and at no higher than an eighth-grade level for professional staff.[44] At the same time, written materials must not appear patronizing nor diminishing. The goal is for staff to be able to explain information to others, in addition to understanding it themselves. Staff at all levels should be able to discuss the basic activities and positions of the organization in simple language. By ensuring that staff are well informed about the organization's activities and status, the organization creates an environment in which employees believe they are valued and knowledgeable.

The most difficult component of communication with staff is the recognition of one's own biases and filters, which influence the ability to be effective. If communicators believe that employees are self-motivated to perform well for intrinsic reasons, those people will communicate in a different style than if they believe that employees need structure, strong supervision, and concrete direction to perform well. Neither of these beliefs is inherently inaccurate. However, each results in a different style of management that yields a different reaction from employees.

Communicators must also recognize and appreciate differences in attitudes toward work. Often, conflicts that arise among nursing staff, support staff, and even physician staff can be traced to a misunderstanding of the goals and motivations for workplace behaviors. If risk management professionals are to communicate effectively among all levels of the organization, they must recognize the different filters through which messages are being received and should formulate spoken and written messages to address a variety of needs and receiving filters.

The communication goal is to share information and gain cooperation in a manner that respects the intellectual and affiliation needs of staff while conveying complex business information and expectations for behavior.

Guidelines include the following:

- Keep messages simple and clear. Use uncomplicated, basic lay language that all levels of staff can comprehend.

- Express expectations. Do not assume that individuals will know what the expected behaviors are, no matter how clear they seem.

- Communicate everything that is influencing the organization's environment, regardless of whether it appears to affect the staff.

- Ensure that all methods of communication are understood. For example,

- Ensure that the staff understands that e-mail is being used as a form of ongoing communication and that it is important to attend to such e-mails. In regard to memos, ensure that staff understands that a memo from the risk manager's office is not routine and should be read carefully. Whenever possible, build in the need for a response to the message. For example:

  - Ask staff to respond to e-mails. What do they think about the information delivered? How do they think the information will alter their work or their work situation? Do they have suggestions for smooth implementation of new policies, and so on?

  - Ask the staff to pose questions about the information contained in memos.

- In verbal presentations, ensure that staff members understand they have a responsibility to ask questions, just as the communicator has a responsibility to communicate clearly and elicit feedback. Ask them to provide a re-cap of information presented verbally in a meeting.

Communicate Expectations Prior to Corrective Action   Staff should not be surprised by corrective action in response to their infractions of policy or acceptable behavior. Staff members of differing cultural, generational, or socio-economic backgrounds might have differing ideas about acceptable workplace behaviors, which should be addressed proactively. Corrective action should be communicated in a manner that respects the employee's beliefs and perspective while describing the unacceptable behavior. Corrective messages should be couched within a statement of the value that the employee brings to the organization. Use "I" rather than "you" statements when discussing employee behavior. For example:

- "I was disappointed that you were late again after our conversation because I thought we had developed a plan."

- "I am concerned about what patient families are telling me about their conversations with you because you have always been such a helpful staff person."

- "I am worried about your health. You appear tired and distracted. How can I help?"

- "Is there anything I can do to help ensure your timeliness?"

- "Is there anything going on in your life that is affecting your work that it would help for me to know about?"

- "Is there a way we can support you to help ensure that your performance stays at its usual level?"

Emphasize to all the staff the importance of each individual's role in the patient care continuum, and the role of each individual in making the patient care team function as a whole. Frontline staffs frequently believe that they have little influence over the patient experience and feel devalued by the organization. In all departments of the organization, leaders have the ability to make staff feel valued and important through their willingness and ability to communicate appreciation. The willingness of leadership to engage employees at all levels in the organization and to communicate simply about the issues creates an environment in which trust can be developed.

Communication with Physicians

Physicians create a special type of communication challenge within the health care organization. In communicating with physicians, risk management professionals must recognize the potential for physicians' fear and frustration to result in behaviors that resemble anger and denial. Studies show that physicians today are experiencing a high degree of burnout.[45] Also, physician suicide rates are significantly greater than those of the average population.[46] Physician behavior perceived as obstreperous or self-involved simply might be the symptom of concern about their ability to maintain professional and personal credibility and control.

Whereas risk management professionals pursue education about the most current legal and regulatory implications for health care, physicians feel pressured to remain current in the technology and treatment approaches in their specialties. Many physicians believe that professional competence is equal to technical competence, and might believe that technical competence will protect them from the professional and personal humiliation and devastation of a lawsuit. Consequently, communication with physicians about regulatory, legal, or even interpersonal aspects of health care is often met with resistance. To facilitate effective communication, risk management professionals must be aware of the issues that physicians are facing and address the underlying fear or concerns with respect and without blame.

The communication goal is to gain physicians' cooperation and trust, and to convey respect while providing support in risk exposure situations, providing legal and regulatory guidance, and coaching in effective communication with patients, families, and staff.

Risk management professionals should never assume that physicians have the same background knowledge or frame of reference as the risk manager. The job of the risk management professional is to educate, while recognizing the fact that change is difficult and might feel burdensome to physicians.

The risk manager should never assume that physicians will support changes in policies or practices because they "should." Just as risk management professionals have experienced an ever-proliferating array of regulatory change, so have physicians. They might believe that "all those administrators" are there to take care of "this stuff." It feels overwhelming. Physicians should be given room to vent frustration and then given help with adjusting to necessary changes and new regulations.

- Recognize that physicians often feel like the least important member of the team—and yet the member of the team held legally responsible for the outcome of care. In that position, the physician might justifiably feel the need to lash out.
  - Acknowledge the physician's frustrating position.
  - Acknowledge the complexity of the system and how overwhelming it must feel at times.
  - Without eliciting defensive reactions, try to elicit information about the ways physicians believe the system could be improved.
  - Convey your message in a respectful, simple manner.
  - Deliver your message slowly, in a warm vocal tone, and with positive body language (no hands on hips, no tight lips, and so on.).
  - Ask for feedback. Allow any tirade to happen, and wait patiently. Acknowledge the frustration. Use encouraging phrases, such as, "It must feel like every time you turn around, there's a new regulation or policy."
- If all else fails, acknowledge the difficulty and let the conversation go until a later time.
- Make a follow-up plan to revisit and discuss the matter again.
- Ask the provider to consider ways to work together to address the issue.

....
COMMUNICATION WITH OTHER KEY CUSTOMERS

Although the guidelines for permissible disclosures to patient representatives are thoroughly discussed in Volume III, Chapter 18 on HIPAA in this series, the interpersonal techniques for communicating with patient representatives (ministers, insurers, attorneys, and so on) are a separate issue. As in any communication with family, community, or the press, the goal is to convey only permissible information while protecting the rights of the patient. Decisions about what is permissible to disclose might be a fine line, especially when the patient has limited mental or physical ability to communicate. Nevertheless, it is essential that the patient, or the patient's proxy, have the ability to control the nature and amount of information given.

Religious

With regard to ministers, the JCAHO states that patients have a right to have their spiritual needs met.[47] For this reason, patients are queried about their religious preference at admission. The revised HIPAA regulations do not prohibit communication with religious leaders in the community, unless the patient has specifically requested that no information be given. In many communities, the local clergy have daily access to admission lists to scan for admission of members of their congregation to provide religious counseling. Nevertheless, this permissible action under HIPAA prompts two considerations. First, who in the community falls under the definition of "religious leader?" How is the organization defining and controlling to whom patient admission information is given? Second, do the clergy adhere to maintaining confidentiality? The health care organization has an ongoing responsibility to ensure that clergy understand and remember the purpose of allowing information to be shared: The patient is to receive clerical visitation during hospitalization, not for patient information to be shared with the congregation. This concept is true even if the intent of the sharing is to generate prayers or other types of support for the patient. The secondary sharing of patient information must be predicated on the specific request of the patient or the patient's proxy and is not at the discretion of the religious leader.

Attorneys

Attorneys present an even more complex challenge. Patients employ attorneys to represent them in different situations. It behooves the risk manager to determine the purpose of the attorney's request for information. If the risk manager determines that the attorney is preparing a claim against the hospital, it is in the best interest of the institution for the risk manager to remain calm and respectful in all communication. Attorneys may behave in an adversarial manner in hopes of intimidating the organization into providing information that the risk manager might not otherwise feel compelled to reveal.

Concern about release of records is worth mentioning because attorneys often give patients blanket release forms to complete to obtain as much information as possible. Depending upon the nature of the legal issue, much of the information in the record is not pertinent to the situation. Some of the information might be sufficiently sensitive that the patient would not want the attorney to have it. In the spirit of partnership with the patient and communicating concern about the patient's privacy, health care staff and risk managers should ensure that patients understand the breadth and ramifications of releases they have signed. This provides patients with an additional opportunity to confirm or refine the amount of information that they want released.

Community and Visitors

Communication happens not only in individual conversations but also through the actions of the organization and staff. Visitors and the community thus have a perception about the organization's willingness and ability to communicate, which determines the level of trust in the organization. It is important that discussions with the community share the positive things done to enhance patient safety, and the organization's concern about the relationship with the community. Marketing materials must be simple and truthful without elaborate claims. Management of patient complaints must be caring and consistent. Interactions with the community must include positive participation in community activities and reports to the community in the local media about ways that staff works to enhance care for patients. However, it is important that the organization and employees be able and willing to live up to the images they portray. If not, the communication not only fails, but also is seen as duplicitous and damages the reputation of the organization.

The Media

The media are looking for information that the community will find interesting and intriguing, not necessarily for information that protects the rights of patients. Regardless, they are part of the community and are often the most visible way that the organization communicates externally. The media can be the risk management professional's ally or foe. Effective communication and positive relationships with the media can foster a partnership that is effective and meets the needs of both parties. Above all else, the organization should have a plan for responding to the media and a proactive position on the image it wishes to portray. The communication goal is to work with the media to ensure that information that is published or released about the organization and its staff is fair and accurate.

- The best approach is to learn to work with the media.
- The health care organization should identify the newspaper and broadcast journalists most willing to work with it in accurately communicating health news.
- The organization should invite those individuals into the facility and educate them about health care and the organization.
- When a crisis develops, the organization might consider offering those reporters an exclusive in the hope that they are likely to get the story right and that other media will follow their lead.

SUMMARY

Effective communication is based upon a cycle of encoding, transmission, decoding, and feedback. Each message must be put into a format that can be sent to another individual. Effective messages are stated simply, without jargon or pretense, and recognize the different ways that words can be interpreted. Transmission of the message should be done with recipient needs in mind. Spoken messages should be clear, stated slowly, using simple language, with the recognition of recipient needs and potential responses to the message. Written messages should use short sentences and simple educational approaches, and must be visually designed with sharp contrast and printed in at least 12 point font. The sender must recognize that decoding will occur through the filters of the recipient. The recipient brings a host of filters: cultural (ethnic, religious, gender, generational), physical (hearing, visual, and sensory), and experiential (childhood experiences, previous experiences with health care or work) through which the message is interpreted. No message received is ever completely the intended message sent, because the transmitter and the recipient are not the same person. Consequently, it is essential that the sender of the message elicit information from the recipient that allows the sender to know whether the message was understood.

When dealing with angry, difficult, or upset people, the primary goal must be to elicit information about how the message or the situation is affecting the recipient without generating a defensive reaction. This is best done by assuming a respectful, calm position and by acknowledging the legitimacy of the recipient's beliefs and feelings. This must be done even if the feelings do not seem legitimate to the risk management professional. Acknowledging that interpretation in a manner in which a person is allowed to retain self-respect in the face of difficult situations is essential to effective communication.

To convey respect in communication, the message sender attends to physical and vocal actions in addition to words. Communication is always a combination of both the words and the message medium.

Finally, it is imperative to document important communication. Effective documentation should follow the pattern of effective communication. It should summarize the message stated, and with respectful terminology free of judgment. Finally, all significant questions or clarifications should be stated in the record. Often these clarifications are areas of vulnerability and might emerge later as continued misperceptions.

There is no such thing as bad communication or good communication. Effective communication elicits mutual respect among the parties and greater understanding of the issues and concerns. Less effective communication promotes misunderstanding and anger and often leads to lawsuits and claims. Effective communication is a highly effective loss control technique. The ability to both use and coach effective communication is a tool that risk management professionals should strive to possess.

Endnotes

1. Beckman, H. B., K. M. Markakis, A. L. Suchman, and R. M. Frankel, "The Doctor-Patient Relationship and Malpractice. Lessons from Plaintiff Depositions." *Archives of Internal Medicine,* 1994, 154 (12): 1365–70.

2. Colon, V. F. "10 Ways to Reduce Medical Malpractice Exposure." *Physician Executive,* 2002, 28(2): 16–8.

3. Eastaugh, S. R. "Reducing Litigation Costs through Better Patient Communication." *Physician Executive,* 2004, May–June (3): 36–8.

4. Levinson, W. "In Context: Physician-Patient Communication and Managed Care." *Journal of Medical Practice Management,* 1999, 14(5): 226–30.

5. Vincent, C., M. Young, and A. Phillips. "Why do People Sue Doctors? A Study of Patients and Relatives Taking Legal Action." *Lancet,* 1994, 343(8913): 1609–13.

6. Wood, H. "Managing Malpractice Liability: Tips to Limit Your Risk." *Journal of the Indiana Dental Association,* 2001, 80(3): 12–4.

7. Joint Commission on Accreditation of Healthcare Organizations. "Sentinel Event Statistics: Root Causes of Sentinel Events." [jcaho.org/accredited+organizations] 2005.

8. Joint Commission on Accreditation of Healthcare Organizations. "Facts About 2006 Patient Safety Goals." [jcaho.org/accredited+organizations/patient+safety/06_npsg/06_facts.htm] 2005.

9. Dannefer, E. F., Henson, L. C., Bierer, S. B., Grady-Weliky, T. A., Meldrum, S. Nofziger, A. C., Barclay, C., and Epstein, R. M. "Peer Assessment of Professional Competence." *Medical Education,* 2005, 39(7A): 713–22.

10. Gordon, G. H. "Defining the Skills Underlying Communication Competence." *Seminars in Medical Practice,* 2002, 5(3): 21–8.

11. Reina, D. S., and Reina, M. L. *Trust and Betrayal in the Workplace.* San Francisco, CA: Berrett-Koehler Publishers, Inc., 1999.

12. Agency for Healthcare Research and Quality, *Expanding Patient-Centered Care to Empower Patients and Assist Providers.* Research in Action, Issue 5, AHRQ Publication No. 02–0024. May 2002. [www.ahrq.gov/qual/ptcareria.htm]

13. Gray, G. R. Teaching Patient-centered Care. *Family Medicine,* 2002, 34(9): 644–5.

14. The Quality Interagency Coordination Task Force (QuIC). *Patient Rights and Responsibilities.* [www.consumer.gov/qualityhealth/rights.htm], last revised 3/2005.

15. The Advisory Commission on Consumer Protection and Quality in the Health Care Industry. Charter of the Advisory Commission found at: [www.hcqualitycommission.gov/charter.html], Objectives of the Consumers Bill of Rights can be found at: [www.hcqualitycommission.gov/cborr/preamb.html]

16. The Advisory Commission on Consumer Protection and Quality in the Health Care Industry Consumer Rights and Responsibilities Executive Summary, VIII Consumer Responsibilities (can be accessed at [www.hcqualitycommission.gov/cborr/exsumm.html] Late date accessed 12/22–24/05.

17. American Hospital Association,. The Patient Care Partnership: Understanding Expectations, Rights, and Responsibilities. Chicago, IL: American Hospital Association, 2003.

18. Population Reference Bureau. [www.prb.org]. June 2005.

19. Crisp, A. H., and Edwards, W. J. "Communication in Medical Practice across Ethnic Boundaries." *Postgraduate Medical Journal,* 1989, 65: 150–155.

20. David, R. A., and Rhee, M. "The Impact of Language as a Barrier to Effective Health Care in an Underserved Urban Hispanic Community." *Mount Sinai Journal of Medicine,* 1998, 65(5–6): 393–7.

21. Murray-Garcia, J. L., Garcia J. A., Schembri, M. E., and Guerra, L. M. "The Service Patterns of a Racially, Ethnically, and Linguistically Diverse Housestaff." *Academic Medicine,* 2001, 76(12): 1232–40.

22. Ahronheim, J. C., J. D. Moreno, C. Zuckerman. *Ethics in Clinical Practice.* Gaithersburg, MD: Aspen Publishers, Inc., 2000. p. 35.

23. Jonson, A. R., M. Siegler, and W. J. Winslade. *Clinical Ethics.* New York: McGraw Hill, 1998, p. 55.

24. Braddock, C., and others. "Informed Decision Making in Outpatient Practice: Time to get Back to Basics." *JAMA: the Journal of the American Medical Association,* 1999, 282(24): 2313–20.

25. Elwyn, G. Edwards, A. and Kinnersley, P. "Shared Decision-Making in Primary Care: The Neglected Second Half of the Consultation." *British Journal of General Practice,* 1999, 49(443): 477–82.

26. *Ibid.*, p. 80.

27. Agard, A. *Informed Consent: Theory Versus Practice.* Nature Clinical Practice, Cardiovascular Medicine. 2005, 2(6): 270.

28. Grassi, L., et al. "Physicians' Attitudes to and Problems with Truth-Telling to Cancer Patients." *Supportive Care in Cancer,* 2000, 8(1): 40–5.

29. Dosanjh, S., J. Barnes, and M. Bhandari, "Barriers to Breaking Bad News Among Medical and Surgical Residents." *Medical Education,* 2001, 35(3): 197–205.

30. Hobgood, C., Hevia, A., and Lemon, M. R. Disclosing Medical Error: A Professional Standard. Seminars in Medical Practice, 2004, 7: 12–23.

31. Zimmerman, R. "Doctors' New Tool to Fight Lawsuits: Saying 'I'm Sorry;' " "Malpractice Insurers Find Owning Up to Errors Soothes Patient Anger 'The Risks are Extraordinary'." *Journal of the Oklahoma State Medical Association,* 2004, 97(6): 245–7.

32. Cohen, J. R. "Toward Candor after Medical Error: The First Apology Law." *Harvard Health Policy Review,* 2004, 5(1): 21–4. Other states with Apology Statutes include: Oregon (2003) Or. Rev. Stat. § 677.082, Massachusetts (1986) Mass Gen Laws ch.233, § 23D, Texas (1999) Tex Civ Prac and Rem Code §18.061, California (2000) Cal Evid Code § 1160, Florida (2001) Fla Stat §90.4026, Washington (2002) Rev Code Wash §5.66.010, Tennessee (2003) Tenn Evid Rule §409.1, Ohio (2004) ORC Ann §2317.43, Wyoming Wyo. Stat. §1–1–130, Oklahoma 63 OKL. St. § 1–1708.1H, (Colo. Rev. Stat. § 13–25–135)., Oregon (2003) Or. Rev. Stat. § 677.082.

33. Keeva, S. "Law and Sympathy." *ABA Journal,* 2004, August: 74–5.

34. Kim, P. H., D. L. Ferrin, C. D. Cooper, and K. T. Dirks. "Removing the Shadow of Suspicion: The Effects of Apology Versus Denial for Repairing Competence- Versus Integrity-Based Trust Violations." *Journal of Applied Psychology,* 2004, 89(1): 104–18.

35. Fritz, R. E., and S. P. Fitzgerald. *Forgiveness and Accountability*. USA: BrownHerron Publishing, 2003.

36. Vincent, C., M. Young, and A. Phillips. "Why do People Sue Doctors? A Study of Patients and Relatives Taking Legal Action." *Lancet,* 1994, 343(8913): 1609–13.

37. Baker, S. K. *Managing Patient Expectations: The Art of Finding and Keeping Loyal Patients*. San Francisco, CA: Jossey-Bass Publishers, 1998.

38. White House Commission on Complementary and Alternative Medicine Policy. "Final Report." [www.whccamp.hhs.gov/finalreport.html] March 2002.

39. Civil Aviation Authority—Safety Regulation Group "Fundamental Human Factors Concepts." [www.caa.co.uk].

40. SBAR Technique for Communication: A Situational Briefing Model. [www.ihi.org/IHI/Topics/PatientSafety/SafetyGeneral/Tools/SBARTechniquesfor CommunicationASituationalBriefingModel.htm].

41. Hays, J. M. *Building High Performance Teams: A Practitioner's Guide*. Australia: Argos Press, 2004. p. 1.

42. Royal Aeronautical Society. Crew Resource Management. [www.raes-hfg. com/reports/crm-now.htm].

43. Oliver, R. W. *What is Transparency?* New York: McGraw Hill, 2004. p. 3.

44. National Institutes of Health. "Clear and to the Point: Guidelines for Using Plain Language at NIH." [www1.od.nih.gov/execsec/guidelines.htm]. August 2000.

45. Bruce, S. M. H. M. Congalen, J. V. Congalen. "Burnout in Physicians: A Case for Peer Support." *Internal Medicine Journal,* 2005, 35(5): 272–8.

46. Schernhammer, E. "Taking their Own Lives—The High Rate of Physician Suicide." *New England Journal of Medicine,* 2005, 352(24): 2473–6.

47. Joint Commission on the Accreditation of Healthcare Organizations. 2002 Hospital Accreditation Standards. USA: JCAHO, 2002.

Suggested Readings

Baker, S. *Managing Patient Expectations: The Art of Finding and Keeping Loyal Patients*. San Francisco, CA.: Jossey-Bass Publishers, 1998.

Banja, J. *Medical Errors and Medical Narcissism*. Sudbury, MA: Jones and Bartlett Publishers, 2005.

Brewin, T., and Sparshott, M. *Relating to the Relatives: breaking bad news communication and support*. Abingdon, Oxon, UK: Radcliffe Medical Press, Ltd., 1996.

Buckman, R. *How to Break Bad News: A Guide for Health Care Professionals*. Baltimore, MD: The Johns Hopkins University Press, 1992.

"Health Literacy: Report of the Council on Scientific Affairs. Ad Hoc Committee on Health Literacy for the Council on Scientific Affairs, American Medical Association." *JAMA: The Journal of the American Medical Association,* 1999, 281(6): 552–7.

Heymann, J. *Equal Partners: A Physician's Call for a New Spirit of Medicine.* Pennsylvania: University of Pennsylvania Press, 1995.

Lloyd, M., and Bor, R. *Communication Skills for Medicine*. New York: Churchill Livingstone, 1996.

Luckmann, J. *Transcultural Communication in Health Care*. Canada: Delmar Thomson Learning, 2000.

Osborne, H. *Health Literacy from A to Z: Practical Ways to Communicate Your Health Message*. Sudbury, MA: Jones and Bartlett, 2005.

Patterson, K., J. Grenny, R. McMillan, and A. Switzler. *Crucial Conversations: Tools for Talking When Stakes are High*. New York: McGraw-Hill, 2002.

Reina, D., and Reina, M. L. *Trust and Betrayal in the Workplace: Building Effective Relationships in Your Organization*. San Francisco, CA: Berrett-Koehler Press, 1999.

Spector, R. E., *Cultural Diversity in Health and Illness*. New Jersey: Prentice Hall, 2004.

9

Physician and Allied Health Professional Credentialing

Mark A. Kadzielski

Credentialing is an area in which risk management professionals can significantly minimize the liabilities inherent in the health care industry. To do so, the risk management professional documents credentialing policies and procedures, periodically reviews a facility's policies on credentialing, and keeps abreast of current developments in health care. Risk management professionals also should be prepared to function proactively by continually discovering new methods to prevent or minimize the potential liabilities associated with the provision of health care.

Historically, increased regulation has proven to be costly and also has tended to bring increased scrutiny by entities or individuals entrusted with the function. Even though credentialing increases costs and scrutiny (as do malpractice awards), the institution and maintenance of written credentialing policies and procedures by a health care facility are among the most effective preemptive risk management tools available. Although facilities have little, if any, control over the practice of medicine, they can exercise substantial control over the qualifications and competence of physicians and allied health professionals (AHPs). Credentialing is a necessary and vital tool with which facilities can make strides in utilization patterns and quality outcomes. The concomitant costs and inconveniences are clearly outweighed by the benefits.

This chapter discusses aspects of credentialing for both physicians and allied health professionals (AHPs), including sources of potential liability, state and federal credentialing provisions, and accreditation standards. It also describes AHP qualifications and scope of authority, and laws and regulations regarding AHP scope of practice.

....

CREDENTIALING OF PHYSICIANS

Credentialing is the process by which health care organizations review applicant physicians' licensure, certification, references, and other professional information pertaining to their qualifications and ability to provide health care services. It entails a decision by a health care delivery system that determines whether an applicant is qualified to provide health care services for that organization.

Credentialing involves granting medical staff membership to physicians or granting them clinical privileges, two diverse concepts that require the analysis of different criteria. Accordingly, health care delivery systems should clearly differentiate between them. Membership provides practitioners with a voice in the governance of the health care delivery system, whereas clinical privileges provide physicians with the opportunity to practice their clinical skills without being embroiled in the delivery system's affairs.

From a risk management perspective, granting privileges is more critical than granting membership alone, because significant potential liability accompanies the ability to perform surgical or nonsurgical procedures. But, as set forth in this chapter, such liability may be minimized by competent risk management. Likewise, medical staff membership without clinical privileges can be an effective risk management tool for health care organizations.

The Joint Commission on Accreditation of Healthcare Organizations (JCAHO) defines credentialing as "(t)he process of obtaining, verifying, and assessing the qualifications of a health care practitioner to provide patient care services in or for a health care organization."[1] JCAHO further defines the process as a "series of activities designed to collect relevant data that will serve as the basis for decisions regarding appointments and reappointments to the medical staff, as well as delineation of clinical privileges for individual members of the medical staff."[2] The National Committee for Quality Assurance (NCQA), a private, not-for-profit organization that assesses and reports on the quality of managed care plans broadly defines *credentialing* as "the process (by which managed care organizations) select and evaluate the practitioners who practice within its delivery system."[3]

Credentialing is a multi-step process that must be tailored to fit the specific needs of each health care organization, whether a hospital, a managed care organization (MCO), an integrated delivery system (IDS), an independent practice association (IPA), or some other type of delivery system. Tailoring can be accomplished by documenting credentialing processes in bylaws, rules and regulations, and policies and procedures, as applicable. However, facilities should not attempt to cut costs by applying another organization's bylaws, rules and regulations, or policies and procedures to their own operations. This practice can result in the application of inappropriate and inconsistent policies that can negatively affect accreditation status and the quality of care provided in the facility.

Credentialing standards ensure the uniform treatment of all staff members being considered for appointment and reappointment and provide the individual staff member with a fair, known, and systematic information collection process. Further, strict adherence to a documented credentialing system can protect a facility in credentialing disputes. Health care institutions should not fall prey to the mistaken belief that only large organizations with plentiful resources can afford to scrutinize applicants' credentials carefully and discipline errant physicians in a uniform and systematic manner. No organization, large or small, should underestimate the importance of the credentialing function.

Federal Law on Credentialing

An integral part of risk management is a working familiarity with federal and state laws concerning credentialing and accreditation standards specific to the health care delivery system in which they will be applied. Below, various credentialing laws and accreditation standards are set forth.

The Medicare Conditions of Participation for Hospitals provide that "(t)he medical staff must examine credentials of candidates for medical staff membership. . . ."[4] They also require the collection of credentialing information for purposes of reappointment to the medical staff.[5] The Medicare Conditions of Participation for Long Term Care Facilities provide that "(p)rofessional program staff must be licensed, certified, or registered, as applicable, to provide professional services by the State in which he or she practices."[6] The Conditions of Participation for Home Health Agencies provide that "(p)ersonnel practices . . . are supported by appropriate, written personnel policies. Personnel records include qualifications and licensure that are kept current."[7] The Medicare Conditions of Participation for Comprehensive Outpatient Rehabilitation Facilities provide that "(p)ersonnel that provide service must be licensed, certified, or registered in accordance with applicable State and local laws."[8] Medicare also prescribes similar Conditions of Participation for Critical Access Hospitals,[9] and for Clinics, Rehabilitation Agencies, and Public Health Agencies as Providers of Outpatient Physical Therapy and Speech-Language Pathology Services.[10]

State Law on Credentialing

To varying degrees, most states supplement federal statutory credentialing provisions with their own legislative pronouncements on credentialing. Through the enactment of regulations, many states require a health care facility to credential its physicians before granting clinical privileges. For example, in California, "all members of the medical staff (are) required to demonstrate their ability to perform surgical and/or other procedures competently and to the satisfaction of an appropriate committee . . . at the time of application for appointment to the staff and at least every two years thereafter."[11] Further, the doctrine of corporate liability for negligent credentialing, a state law tort theory, necessitates implementing and maintaining written credentialing policies and procedures.

Accreditation Standards

Accreditation standards require that physicians be credentialed before being granted privileges to practice medicine at a facility. Apart from state law and the Medicare Conditions of Participation for Hospitals, a governing body's responsibility for credentialing physicians who practice in its hospital is established by accrediting bodies such as the JCAHO. The JCAHO standards require that the mechanisms for appointment or reappointment to the medical staff and the initial granting and renewal or revision of clinical privileges be fully documented in the medical staff bylaws, rules and regulations, and policies.[12]

Outside the hospital context, similar standards exist for MCOs and ambulatory surgery centers (ASCs) through accrediting bodies such as the NCQA and the Accreditation Association for Ambulatory Health Care (AAAHC), in addition to several others. For example, the NCQA requires that "(t)he managed care organization document the mechanism for the credentialing and re-credentialing of MDs, DOs, DDSs, DPMs, DCs, and other licensed independent practitioners with whom it contracts or employs who treat members outside the inpatient setting and who fall within its scope of authority and action."[13]

Internet Credentialing

With the advent of the Internet, new opportunities are available for facilities in their ongoing efforts to credential practitioners. Online databases, such as the Office of Inspector General's (OIG) List of Excluded Individuals/Entities (LEIE) and Web sites maintained by state licensing authorities, provide additional information regarding practitioners to the public, including consumers and individuals not otherwise entitled to similar information maintained by the National Practitioner Data Bank (NPDB) or the Healthcare Integrity and Protection Data Bank. The existence of these databases may also establish a new standard of care regarding the frequency of checking whether practitioners have been disciplined. The OIG may impose a Civil Monetary Penalty of up to $10,000 for each item or services furnished by an individual excluded from participation in a federal health care program (for example, Medicare, Medicaid, and so on) *on any individual or entity which contracts with the excluded individual.* For liability to be imposed, the provider submitting the claims for health care items or services furnished by an excluded individual must either "know or *should* know" that the person was excluded.[14] Thus, the OIG "urges health care providers and entities to check the OIG List of Excluded Individuals/ Entities on the OIG Web site (www.hhs.gov/oig) prior to hiring or contracting with individuals or entities."[15] Providers should also "periodically check the OIG Web site for determining the participation/exclusion status of current employees and contractors." Although the OIG does not expressly state how often providers should check the Web site, one may infer the appropriate frequency from the fact that the OIG updates the LEIE *monthly.*

....

DOCUMENTATION OF CREDENTIALING CRITERIA

Key to the uniform application of credentialing criteria is *documentation of the criteria in a facility's governance documents,* such as the bylaws, rules and regulations, and policies, procedures, and protocols. Each of these documents serves a different function. Generally, the *bylaws* provide an organization's basic framework. In the hospital context, medical staff bylaws delineate the staff's responsibilities, the basic framework for committees and members, the process by which staff members are disciplined, and the delegation of functions. The *rules and regulations* provide additional details on operational aspects of performing the responsibilities assigned by the bylaws. At a minimum, documentation of, and adherence to, written credentialing criteria delineated in governance documents invalidates the argument that a facility randomly and discriminatorily applies its credentialing criteria. A health care organization's *policies, procedures, and protocols* contain the detailed rules and regulations that govern day-to-day operations. These documents can contain as much detailed information as is deemed necessary. In fact, it is advisable in many circumstances that they contain the most detailed information available in order to guide the medical staff and ensure consistency in the day-to-day decision making of the organization's physicians.

Written credentialing criteria should be directly related to patient care and based on objective factors such as education, experience, and current competence rather than on arbitrary distinctions based on title. If distinctions are to be made between the types of services that can be provided by two groups of practitioners (for example, radiologists and emergency department physicians, orthopedists and podiatrists, or psychiatrists and psychologists), they should derive from *objective criteria* and the *standard of care in the community* to avoid the appearance of discrimination based solely on profession. Properly developed and documented credentialing criteria that are applied appropriately should withstand the strictest scrutiny.

In addition, written credentialing criteria should be facility-specific and based upon such factors as a facility's license capacity and availability of equipment, personnel, and services. Physicians should not be granted privileges to perform procedures that exceed the facility's financial and personnel resources. Drafters and reviewers of credentialing criteria should be cognizant of the health facility's assets and limitations when reviewing the credentialing criteria.

Documentation of credentialing criteria should not be done haphazardly, at the last minute, or after the fact. Credentialing criteria must be reviewed by committees or bodies that are responsible for establishing those criteria, such as a credentialing committee, an executive committee, and the hospital governing body. To minimize legal liabilities, it is vital for leadership such as the executive committee and the governing body to provide oversight and input, and final approval.

············

POTENTIAL LIABILITIES RELATED TO CREDENTIALING

Risk management professionals play an important role in minimizing potential liabilities. Specifically, they must be vigilant in advocating the establishment and maintenance of written policies and procedures. Health care facilities that credential physicians might be liable to those very same physicians for discrimination; restraint of trade; economic credentialing; violation of the facility's bylaws, rules and regulations, and policies and procedures; and many other actions or inactions. Risk management professionals must be wary of not only the acts or omissions for which a facility might be liable to physicians who exercise privileges there, but also of the potential liabilities a facility may have to patients, their families, estates, or legal representatives.

Early implementation of written policies and procedures or protocols can be accomplished only when risk management professionals keep abreast of the rapidly evolving health care sector and can identify potential liabilities before they occur. Failure to perceive potential liability issues early will result in a lack of written policies and procedures and the absence of a uniform and sound approach to risk issues, thus increasing the risk of litigation.

Almost all risk management professionals and health care providers are familiar with the liability associated with less than optimal outcomes and the importance of maintaining guidelines intended to minimize such liability. Sometimes overlooked, however, is the need to advocate the implementation of policies to minimize the legal risk associated with negligent credentialing, economic credentialing, breach of privacy, violation of the Americans with Disabilities Act (ADA), and a physician's breach of a "duty to warn."

Negligent Credentialing

Traditionally, there was no institutional liability for the negligence of individual providers. However, beginning in 1965 with *Darling v. Charleston Community Memorial Hospital,* various state courts began recognizing a new doctrine called "hospital corporate liability."[16] In *Darling,* the Supreme Court of Illinois held that the hospital had an independent duty to ensure that high-quality care was rendered at its facility, and held the hospital accountable for negligently screening the competency of its medical staff. Numerous states have adopted some form of the hospital corporate liability theory, thereby providing some legal relief for the tort of negligent credentialing, including Arizona, California, Colorado, Georgia, Michigan, Nebraska, Nevada, New Jersey, New York, North Carolina, North Dakota, Pennsylvania, Rhode Island, Texas, Washington, West Virginia, and Wisconsin.[17]

Health care facilities and providers should not be surprised to see the doctrine of corporate liability extended to MCOs, IPAs, and IDSs in the near future.[18] Like hospitals, courts will likely conclude that such entities have a duty to credential and re-credential affiliated physicians and monitor the quality of care provided by affiliated physicians. And if health care delivery systems credential physicians, such systems have a duty to credential them thoroughly and properly. If an MCO, IPA, or IDS breaches its duty to provide high-quality care to a patient by failing to screen out incompetent physicians or take appropriate measures against physicians who are providing substandard medical care, the entity might be negligent based on a theory of corporate liability.

The nexus between the health care delivery system and the medical care provided may be based on a health care system's advertising claims. Advertising campaigns used by health care entities to attract new consumers generally contain representations regarding the qualifications of affiliated physicians and the high quality of care that patients can expect from a particular plan's physicians. Representations regarding the quality of care to be provided by physicians affiliated with MCOs, IPAs, and IDSs are much more direct than the implied representations attributed by courts to hospitals upon which corporate liability was based in the 1960s. Thus, based on the same theoretical underpinnings, liability may be easily extended to MCOs, IPAs, and IDSs.[19]

Moreover, we may see corporate liability further extended to management services organizations (MSOs) and other independent contractors that credential physicians on behalf of a hospital, MCO, IPA, or IDS. Risk management professionals in MSOs must be aware of such potential liability and should advocate the institution and maintenance of uniform written credentialing procedures if the facility has contracted for, or is entrusted with, credentialing functions.

Economic Credentialing

Currently, economic credentialing is a bone of contention between some physicians and health care institutions. The term *economic credentialing* has been used to denote a credentialing, selection, or termination action based, at least in part, on economic considerations. The current absence of a definitive determination by state legislatures, courts, and professional associations on the parameters of using economic criteria in credentialing decisions, and the legal and medical communities' failure to provide an acceptable definition of the term, may render the use of economic criteria a double-edged sword with costly consequences.

In simple terms, *economic credentialing* is the use, in the credentialing of a physician, of data that indicate that physician's effect on the financial success of a facility. This term also refers to the use of data that reflect the proportion of indigent patients admitted or treated by a particular physician at a facility. The economic factors generally relate to a physician's utilization of health care resources and a provider's profits for the facility resulting from the physician's payer mix, market share, charges, and collections.

Apart from the position (or lack thereof) of professional associations, the legislatures, and the courts on economic credentialing, the economic pressures on health care systems make it probable that economic factors will continue to be used in credentialing decisions. To minimize potential liability, risk management professionals who are employed by facilities that use economic credentialing should advocate and assist in the development of a written protocol addressing the use of economic credentialing.

Hospital-based risk management professionals must be familiar with Medicare's position on the use of economic credentialing by hospitals. The Medicare Conditions of Participation for Hospitals provide that "(t)he governing body must . . . (e)nsure that under no circumstances is the accordance of staff membership or professional privileges in the hospital dependent solely upon certification, fellowship, or membership in a specialty body or society."[20] Accordingly, if economic criteria are to be used in hospital credentialing decisions, they should not be the *sole* basis for terminating or granting medical staff privileges. If this does occur, the risk management professional should be alert to the possibility of not merely civil liability, but also potential administrative penalties that the Health Care Financing Administration can impose, such as exclusion from the Medicare program.

Using economic criteria in a uniform, reasonable manner to educate practitioners and to identify the links between economic factors and quality of care may minimize potential liability. For example, disclosure of reasons for refusal to grant privileges or for termination of privileges may diminish the legal liability associated with economic credentialing. Risk management professionals also may advocate educating physicians about the efficient use of health care resources. One such approach is to use physician profiling of cost, quality, and utilization data. Sharing profiled information with physicians allows them to change their approach to a more cost-effective one while preserving the quality of care. Furthermore, challenges to economic credentialing may hinge on inclusion of these procedures in written governance documents such as the bylaws, especially in states such as Florida, where bylaws are deemed to be a contract between facility and physician.

Breach of Patient Privacy

A breach of a patient's privacy rights may occur in several ways, ranging from intrusion on a patient's privacy in the patient's room to the unauthorized disclosure of patient-identifiable medical information. Although it might be relatively easy to prevent intrusion into a patient's room, other breaches of privacy, such as improper disclosure of either patient information or individual providers' quality outcome information, can be much more difficult to control. As a result, it is essential that a facility implement and maintain written policies and procedures pertaining to disclosure. Accordingly, the risk management professional should be familiar with state law regarding privacy rights.

In addition, Medicare's recently added "Patients' Rights" Condition of Participation for Hospitals *expressly* states that the "patient has the right to personal privacy" and "the right to confidentiality of his or her clinical records."[21] Although Medicare has yet to explain how it will interpret this Condition of Participation, it is certain that patient privacy has become a top concern among government investigators, due in part to the advent of the Internet and the increased accessibility of information via such developments as the electronic medical record.

Disclosure of Patient-Identifiable Information

In this era of managed care, compliance with state law regarding disclosure of patient-identifiable information is becoming increasingly difficult because of the proliferation of contracts between individuals and entities pertaining to medical or administrative support functions. Further, the proliferation of complicated delivery systems that affiliate with different types of providers has made it more difficult to determine to whom medical records may be released. And in most states, state law has failed to keep pace with the rapid changes in the health care sector, thus increasing the risks associated with the provision of health care.

Although the disclosure of patient-identifiable information might be an unavoidable reality in the race for managed care contracts, facilities should not risk the liability associated with the wrongful disclosure of patient-identifiable information in contravention of applicable state law. Any disclosure of patient-identifiable information should be reviewed, in detail, by legal counsel before executing agreements containing promises regarding disclosure of such information. Risk management professionals should notify and assist in educating the medical records department—and all other appropriate departments—about the liability associated with wrongful disclosure and identify the release of medical information as an area of risk. Further, facilities should maintain written guidelines on disclosure of such information.

Disclosure of Individual Providers' Quality Outcome Information

Driven by the need to compete in a changing health care market, many different entities, such as managed care plans, payers, and employers, may seek quality outcome information from a health care delivery system. The quantifiable nature of such information renders it an effective marketing tool that can be easily disseminated to the public, which can then compare individual providers and make informed choices about the quality of the providers associated with a managed care plan. Quality outcome information also allows employers to easily ascertain which managed care plan will be the best one for its employees.

However, legal and regulatory constraints are often imposed on health care delivery systems that can result in the nondisclosure of information or the limitation of the types of information that can be disclosed. The entities to whom quality outcome information can be disclosed should be independently determined by each health care facility with the assistance of its legal counsel, which will play a crucial role in maneuvering the facility through the quagmire of legal and regulatory provisions. By creating written protocols and guidelines for disclosure, the risk management professional can assist the organization in handling such highly sensitive and confidential information.

First, such protocols should be based on applicable state law—if it exists. Second, facilities should determine whether quality outcome information is protected from discovery. Statutory privileges accorded to peer review information may protect quality outcome information if such information is discussed and analyzed in the peer review process for peer review purposes. Whether a facility is willing to disclose such information should be dependent, in part, on whether the information is protected by state law. Third, if a facility's written policy permits the release of such information, the facility should obtain written authorization from physicians that allows its release. Preferably, such release should be obtained upon the physician's membership in the organization rather than at the time that such information is requested.

Depending on the scope of payers' requests, facilities might want to consider disclosing quality outcome information—provided that patient and physician anonymity are maintained. Disclosure of provider-specific quality outcome information, however, is plagued with peril. The provider whose quality outcome information is released might have some legal rights. The wrongful disclosure of provider-specific quality outcome information could embroil a facility in costly litigation. Accordingly, quality outcome information should be released only in accordance with a written policy based on applicable state law and reviewed by the appropriate facility departments and individuals.

Violation of the Americans with Disabilities Act or the Rehabilitation Act

As of 1999, the impact of the Americans with Disabilities Act (ADA) and Section 504 of the Rehabilitation Act on the credentialing of health care practitioners remains unclear. The ADA prohibits discrimination based on the physical or mental status of an individual.[22] Section 504 of the Rehabilitation Act similarly prevents discrimination based on the physical or mental status of an individual in any program or activity receiving federal financial assistance, and thus Section 504 presumably applies to any health care facility "participating" in either Medicare or Medicaid.[23]

Courts have begun to address the applicability of the ADA to credentialing decisions at private hospitals or other nonpublic health care facilities. In *Menkowitz v. Pottstown Mem'l Med. Ctr.*, the Third Circuit held that both the ADA and Section 504 of the Rehabilitation Act prohibits disability discrimination against a medical doctor with staff privileges at a hospital. In *Menkowitz*, a physician claimed that he had been discharged in violation of the ADA and Section 504 of the Rehabilitation Act when his clinical privileges were summarily suspended after he disclosed to the medical staff that he had been diagnosed with attention-deficit disorder. More recently, on June 13, 2005, the Federal District Court in South Dakota granted summary judgment to a hospital being sued for violations of the ADA and the Rehabilitation Act by a cardiac surgeon with severe manic-depressive disorder. The court held that a member of the medical staff was an independent contractor who was not entitled to claim the benefits of either federal law, and directly disagreed with the *Menkowitz* ruling.[24] Obviously, this issue is far from clearly resolved.

Facilities are granted broad discretion to collect and verify different types of information in the credentialing process. According to the JCAHO, each facility must independently determine the applicability of the ADA to its medical staff.[25] Thus, a facility has the discretion to determine whether it will require information pertaining to the physical or mental condition of the medical staff applicant.

The NCQA similarly gives MCOs the following guidance on questioning applicants regarding their physical and mental health status: "A practitioner completes an application for membership. . . . The application includes a current and signed attestation and addresses: reasons for any inability to perform the essential functions of the position, with or without accommodation; (and the) lack of present illegal drug use. . . ."[26] The NCQA further provides that "(t)he exact statement or inquiry may vary depending on applicable legal requirements such as the Americans With Disabilities Act."[27]

Clearly, the JCAHO explanation of intent behind the standard—"the act does not appear to prohibit inquiry as to the ability of the applicant . . . to perform the specific privileges requested"[28]—is ambiguous. The NCQA similarly provides little guidance on the issue of the applicability of the ADA. Whether the ADA is applicable to health care facilities, and exactly when a facility can inquire about applicants' mental and physical health status, will remain unclear until the ADA's applicability to the credentialing process is further clarified by legislative or judicial intervention.

For guidance, facilities may review the Equal Employment Opportunity Commission (EEOC) enforcement guidelines on ADA applicability. Although these guidelines do not provide guidance on ADA applicability to health care facilities, they might help determine what types of health status questions can be posed to applicants and when.

Based on accreditation standards and the EEOC enforcement guidelines, it appears reasonable to request information from practitioners regarding their physical and mental ability to perform the clinical privileges requested in connection with their application to the facility. However, ideally the information should be considered *only after* the applicant has otherwise been approved for medical staff membership or clinical privileges, to avoid the inference that an adverse decision was based solely on the disclosed disability. If the practitioner discloses a disability covered under the ADA (or Section 504 of the Rehabilitation Act), the facility should assess whether reasonable accommodation would allow the practitioner to exercise clinical privileges or perform medical staff duties consistent with the standards imposed upon non-disabled practitioners. The facility should also carefully consider the manner in which questions regarding physical and mental ability are phrased. As a result, all policy documents and applications addressing health status inquiries should be reviewed by legal counsel. Risk management professionals may, however, minimize liability by warning appropriate departments and individuals of such perils and advocating a review of existing bylaws, rules and regulations, and applications.

Breach of Duty to Warn

At first blush, the doctrine of a physician's duty to warn appears rather simple: physicians must discuss their patients' medical condition and course of treatment with them or their legal representatives. Often, however, facilities fail to implement written protocols pertaining to a physician's duty to warn. At times, physicians also neglect to carry out that duty.

In 1995, the health care industry eagerly awaited adjudication of *Reisner v. Regents of the University of California.*[29] In *Reisner,* a physician and a hospital were sued by the sexual partner of a teenager who had died of AIDS—contracted after receiving a transfusion. Although the hospital and the physician knew of the patient's exposure to HIV within days of its occurrence, the physician apparently failed to warn her. Three years later, the patient, unaware that she had contracted the virus, engaged in sexual relations with the plaintiff and exposed him to the virus. A California court held the hospital liable for the physician's failure to warn his patient that she had contracted HIV. (*Reisner* should not be confused with *Tarasoff v. Regents of the University of California,* in which a psychiatrist was sued because he failed to warn a third party of potential harm from his patient.[30])

Such liability might have been avoided by implementation of, and adherence to, a carefully drafted protocol pertaining to effective communication between physician and patient or the patient's legal representative. Although the *Reisner* decision is not applicable outside California, risk management professionals should: (1) be familiar with a physician's duty to warn patients; (2) advocate and assist their facilities in developing and implementing written policies and procedures aimed at minimizing such risks through notification and counseling of patients, including exposed or infected patients, in accordance with state law; and (3) advocate educating physicians regarding their duty to warn and the liability associated with the failure to do so.

············

INFORMATION SHARING AND THE CONTRACTUAL ALLOCATION OF RISK

The proliferation of IDSs and the continuing consolidation of health care facilities raise issues of information sharing between affiliated health care facilities. The development of credentialing policies and procedures for physicians and AHPs, and the actual credentialing of health care providers, is costly and time-consuming. Health care facilities can decrease the time spent on such activities and the associated costs and can eliminate duplication by engaging in information sharing. Nevertheless, although information sharing is efficient and cost-effective if executed correctly, facilities must consider some accreditation limitations and legal concerns when determining the extent of information sharing and the protection and use of the shared information.

Initially, analyzing, and implementing an information-sharing system will require a commitment of significant time and resources. If such a system is to be implemented, it should be documented in a written agreement. Also, bylaws, rules and regulations, and appointment and reappointment applications of all participating facilities should be reviewed and amended to reflect the information-sharing system and to ensure a certain degree of consistency between facilities. Confidentiality agreements also should be executed and enforced between facilities and their peer review members, and issues pertaining to the release of patient-identifiable medical information, fraud and abuse, and National Practitioner Data Bank and Healthcare Integrity and Protection Data Bank issues should be analyzed. Proper implementation of an information system can be efficiently accomplished with the assistance of risk management personnel who can identify and analyze facility-specific risk issues that may arise before, during, and after implementation of an information-sharing system.

Contractual Provisions for the Confidentiality of Information

Sharing confidential peer review information poses questions regarding the discoverability of this sensitive information. Some states, including California, protect peer review documents of licensed health facilities such as hospitals and federally certified ASCs. Based on a state's definition of a health care facility and the concomitant protections that may be available, myriad health care entities, ranging from hospitals to MCOs and ASCs, can share information.

Notwithstanding the statutory protections afforded peer review documents, facilities should be wary of sharing confidential peer review information because any subsequent disclosure of peer review committee records could result in a loss of this protection. Clearly, providing an entity with confidential information makes it harder to control its dissemination. The risk of such disclosure and the possible loss of statutory protection, if it is available, can be reduced if health care facilities enter into written agreements limiting the sharing of such information for the purpose of peer review. Moreover, contract provisions should prohibit the further release of such information, identify the parties entitled to review it, identify the method in which it should be maintained, and delineate a facility's liability for failing to comply.

Facilities engaged in information sharing can mitigate the risk of voluntary disclosure of peer review information by executing confidentiality agreements between not only the health care facilities, but also each health care facility and each of its peer review committee members. To avoid dissemination of additional information, facilities also should consider removing identifying information on practitioners (other than the practitioner under consideration) and patients' names from shared peer review documents.

Obtaining Appropriate Releases

Practitioners who are damaged professionally by an unauthorized release of confidential peer review information may have some legal rights. To avoid any such risk, facilities should require providers to sign a release specifically authorizing the sharing of credentialing information between facilities. Execution of such a release is particularly important because it serves as documentation of authorization, notifies the physician of the conditions for release of information, and provides a facility with a certain degree of immunity from liability. In addition, the facility's bylaws should contain a provision which infers consent to release such information from an application for clinical privileges or medical staff membership.

Release of Patient-Identifiable Medical Information

Another concern with information sharing is the release of patient-identifiable medical information, which is governed by state law. Unless state law provides that a health care facility may release patient-identifiable information without the patient's written consent, a facility should remove patient-identifiable information from medical records and peer review documents before releasing them to another health care facility.

Fraud and Abuse Concerns

Risk management professionals also must be aware that fraud and abuse concerns might arise because the responsibilities undertaken by one facility for the benefit of another could be viewed as a benefit. To comply with applicable state and federal laws, any information-sharing arrangement should be undertaken in an arm's-length transaction and pursuant to a written agreement. (An *arm's-length transaction* pertains to a relationship between two or more contracting parties unblemished by any other connections or relations that might bias the judgment of the contracting parties.) Such an agreement should specify the responsibilities of the parties, the term of the agreement, and the fair market-value cost(s) associated with performing such services.

National Practitioner Data Bank (NPDB) and the Healthcare Integrity and Protection Data Bank (HIPDB)

Finally, federal law prohibits the release of National Practitioner Data Bank (NPDB) reports except to hospitals.[31]

The NPDB contains adverse *licensure* action reports on physician and dentists (including revocations, suspensions, reprimands, censures, probations, and surrenders for quality purposes); adverse *clinical privilege* actions against physicians and dentists; adverse *professional society membership* actions against physicians and dentists; and *medical malpractice payments* made on all health care practitioners. Groups that have access to this data system include: (1) hospitals; (2) other health care entities that conduct peer review and provide or arrange for care; (3) state boards of medical or dental examiners; (3) other health care practitioner state boards; and (4) practitioners conducting a self-inquiry. Unauthorized release of information contained in the NPDB can result in an $11,000 fine for each individual and entity involved in the release. However, a hospital can be appointed as an agent of another health care facility and then obtain such information on its behalf without violating federal law. Any such principal-agent relationship should be formally documented to avoid any disputes between facilities and claims by physicians about the unauthorized release of information. Under such circumstances, an agent must submit a separate request for information for each entity on whose behalf it is acting.

Federal law also prohibits the release of information contained in the Healthcare Integrity and Protection Data Bank (HIPDB), opened in 1999, to anyone except Federal and State government agencies, health plans, and self queries from health care suppliers, providers, and practitioners.[32] However, hospitals *do not* have direct access to the HIPDB. The HIPDB contains information regarding certain final adverse actions against health care providers, suppliers, or practitioners. Final adverse actions include: (1) civil judgments against a health care provider, supplier, or practitioner in federal or state court related to the delivery of a health care item or service; (2) federal or state criminal convictions against a health care provider, supplier, or practitioner related to the delivery of a health care item or service; (3) actions by federal or state agencies responsible for the licensing and certification of health care providers, suppliers, or practitioners; (4) exclusion of a health care provider, supplier, or practitioner from participation in federal or state health care programs; and (5) any other adjudicated actions or decisions that the Secretary establishes by regulations. Settlements in which no findings or admissions of liability have been made are excluded from reporting. However, any final adverse action emanating from such settlements and consent judgments otherwise reportable under the statute will be reported in the data bank. All final adverse actions are required to be reported *regardless of whether such actions are being appealed by the subject of the report.*

To ensure that the NPDB and HIPDB contain all relevant information, federal law imposes specific reporting requirements on entities which collect information on practitioners.[33] Failure to report such information can lead either to the imposition of severe monetary sanctions or to the withdrawal of immunity under federal law for peer review activities.[34] *It is therefore crucial that any facility required to report information to either the NPDB or HIPDB maintain policies and procedures that ensure that reporting is timely.*

CREDENTIALING OF ALLIED HEALTH PROFESSIONALS

In today's rapidly evolving health care market, facilities might be motivated to extend the role of AHPs such as nurse midwives, physician assistants (PAs), nurse anesthetists, and nurse practitioners. The rapid push of AHPs to the forefront of medicine has been motivated by not only the advent of managed care, social reform, economic pressures, and financial concerns, but also by AHPs eager to assume the tasks and responsibilities for which they have been trained. However, such forces must be tempered by progression based on qualifications, training, experience, and current competence.

Licensure, certification, and registration are three forms of credentialing mechanisms that assist facilities in defining AHP qualifications and competence. Risk management professionals must be familiar with these mechanisms and the role they play in credentialing AHPs.

Registration is mutually exclusive of licensure, whereas certification is interdependent with licensure. Unlike licensure and certification, registration is devoid of any nexus to the provision of high-quality services or an attempt to standardize the profession to allow for the production of benchmarks linking education, training, and experience to high-quality services. In contrast, certification is a method of not only distinguishing members within a profession but also of providing facilities, employers, patients, and the public with a valid mechanism by which to identify the level of training a particular AHP has received.

Decisions to delegate responsibilities to AHPs that are not within the scope of their licensure or are outside the facility's protocol can have serious civil, criminal, and financial ramifications. For example, if a service or treatment that can be performed only by a physician is delegated to an AHP, a violation of the state's medical practice act might have occurred. Depending on the facility's marketing and advertising strategies and oral representations—made to patients—such conduct also might result in claims of misrepresentation.

Sources of Potential Liability

Risk management professionals must be familiar with the circumstances under which liability may be imputed to health care facilities, supervising physicians, and AHPs resulting from the provision of services by AHPs. For example, a facility might expose itself to liability if it fails to ensure adequate physician supervision, or if it permits an AHP to perform procedures outside the scope of the AHP's license or outside the facility's approved protocols. Supervising physicians likewise face exposure should they fail to adequately supervise. AHPs face exposure if they fail to exercise appropriate clinical judgment, and facilities can be exposed to liability if they do not rigorously enforce the standards established in their protocols.

Another source of potential liability is a facility's failure to educate AHPs about risk management issues. According to a study conducted by the American Academy of Physician Assistants Risk Management Task Force in 1992, 40 percent of survey respondents indicated that they did not receive orientation in risk management issues.[35] Accordingly, investing resources in orienting AHPs, including PAs, about risk management issues specific to the setting in which they practice may reduce liability.

Dependent versus Independent AHPs

There are two categories of AHP—dependent and independent. *Dependent AHPs,* or practitioners, cannot provide patient care services without direction or suspension by a physician. For example, PAs are dependent AHPs. In the hospital context, dependent AHPs may not be members of the medical staff and are not required to have prerogatives. On the other hand, *independent AHPs* may provide patient care services without direction or supervision by a physician. Nurse midwives are an example of independent AHPs. In the hospital context, although independent AHPs must have delineated clinical privileges, certain classes of them may be members of the medical staff. For example, clinical psychologists are often medical staff members.

The credentialing of independent AHPs differs markedly from the credentialing of dependent AHPs. Most facilities recognize that federal law, state law, and accrediting bodies do not require that dependent AHPs be credentialed. Thus, facilities generally do not expend scarce resources on credentialing this class of practitioner. However, they should maintain a written dependent AHP credentialing policy because these individuals provide patient care services. In addition, the OIG can impose severe civil monetary penalties for submitting claims for services provided by AHPs whom the facility "knows or should have known" have been excluded from participation in Medicare. (See previous section on "Internet Credentialing.") The JCAHO, among others, requires periodic verification of competence using clinically valid, objective criteria.

Laws Regarding Scope of Practice

Scope-of-practice issues are almost exclusively within a state's domain, codified in state law and regulations; federal law does not address scope of practice. Guidelines promulgated by licensing boards and associations are additional sources of information that can be used in determining a class of AHPs' scope of practice. However, distinctions must be clearly drawn between legal authority that is enforceable by the state and that might result in criminal or civil sanctions if violated, and guidelines that are merely recommended by professional associations. AHPs' scope of practice within a facility should be based on the interrelation of various factors such as state law, regulations, accreditation standards, and association guidelines.

Accreditation Standards Regarding Scope of Practice

Whether an AHP functions in an acute care hospital, a psychiatric hospital, an ASC, or some other health care facility will dictate which accreditation standards are applicable to the exercise of that AHP's practice privileges. Generally, scope-of-practice issues either will not be addressed in accreditation standards or will be deferred to state law and regulations governing the practice. For example, the JCAHO *Comprehensive Accreditation Manual for Hospitals* provides that "(i)ndividuals are granted the privilege to admit patients to inpatient services in accordance with state law. . . ."[36]

Although accrediting bodies generally do not limit the independent AHPs' scope of practice, the accreditation guidelines may expressly reference the type of patient care that may be appropriately provided by independent AHPs. The JCAHO manual provides that ". . . licensed independent practitioners who are permitted to provide patient care services independently may perform all or part of the medical history and physical examination, if granted such privileges."[37]

In contrast, dependent practitioners generally are not addressed by accrediting bodies such as the JCAHO, NCQA, AAAHC, and others. Thus, each facility must determine the scope of dependent practitioners' practice in its protocols based on state laws, regulations, and the licensing board's guidelines, if any; AHPs' functions within the clinical setting; the degree of supervision required; and the facility's needs.

Identification of Clinical Services to Be Provided

All individuals who are permitted by law and by a hospital to provide patient care services independently must have delineated clinical privileges, whether or not they are medical staff members.[38] Thus, whenever a request is received from an AHP for medical staff membership or practice privileges, the health care facility should have a documented procedure that it follows as early as forwarding the application.

If a class of AHP that currently is not employed at a hospital applies for practice privileges, a hospital should investigate whether there is a need for the services of this class of AHP, document its findings, and make recommendations based on objective findings. Similarly, other types of health care organizations should investigate and document their need for AHPs.

The following issues are paramount in determining whether to allow a particular class of AHP to practice at a facility:

- The education, training, and skills that such a class of AHP must possess to perform patient care services
- The legal scope of practice for the applicable class of AHP
- A determination of the necessity of supervision of the AHP and the extent of such supervision
- The number and types of facilities in the area that provide the services offered by such AHPs
- The extent of demand for such services at this facility
- The criteria that will be used to credential this class of AHP

Additionally, all facilities, including hospitals, should identify the qualifications that a supervising physician must possess to oversee the AHP, if applicable. Some states even require specific licensure for supervisors. Apart from identifying whether a sufficient number of physicians are available and willing to supervise dependent AHPs, input from physicians regarding the credentialing of AHPs should be limited to information pertaining to matters that affect the quality of care and the operation of the facility to avoid any semblance of protectionism of existing economic interests, conspiracy, claims of antitrust, and defamation.

QUALIFICATIONS AND SCOPE OF ALLIED HEALTH PROFESSIONAL AUTHORITY

Nurse midwives, PAs, clinical psychologists, physical therapists, nurse anesthetists, and nurse practitioners are representative of different classes of AHPs. Educational requirements vary for each class of AHP, as do the clinical practice and degree of autonomy each class of AHP can exercise based on state law and the setting in which the AHP practices. Although each enumerated class of AHP (and several other classes of AHPs that have not been mentioned) is worthy of evaluation, the scope of this chapter does not permit a complete listing. Only nurse midwives, PAs, and nurse anesthetists are discussed herein.

Nurse Midwives

The practice of midwifery is composed of two distinct components. Some states recognize both lay midwives and nurse midwives. *Lay midwives* are those individuals who perform midwifery services but do not possess a nursing degree. Whether they can practice midwifery and the types of services they can provide depend on state law. *Nurse midwives,* on the other hand, are registered nurses who have completed a state-mandated course of formal education after basic nursing education. They possess the advanced formal training, knowledge, and ability to provide gynecological care, prenatal care, and low-risk obstetrical care such as delivery and postpartum care.

To minimize risks, facilities should maintain written policies addressing the credentialing of nurse midwives, with particular emphasis on scope of practice issues. Liability also can be minimized by implementing written protocols, based on state law, regarding the prescription and administration of medication by midwives. Further, to reduce risks, midwives should be required to document thoroughly all patient care and comply with a facility's consultation and referral policies.

Scope of Practice

Nurse midwifery practice is legal in all 50 states and the District of Columbia. However, the scope of nurse midwifery practice is dependent on state law and the clinical setting in which midwives practice. For example, in California, nurse midwives may provide care and advice in several different settings during the antepartal, intrapartal, postpartal, inter-conceptional, and family planning stages. More specifically, they can conduct deliveries on their own responsibility and care for newborns, including preventive measures and the detection of abnormal conditions in the mother and child.[39]

Prescriptive Authority

Nurse midwives have prescription-writing authority in 41 states.[40] Risk management professionals should be familiar with the statutory limitations that apply to nurse mid-wives' prescriptive authority. For example, nurse midwives cannot prescribe controlled substances in California, Idaho, Nevada, New Mexico, Tennessee, and Virginia. Other states maintain different restrictions on nurse midwives' prescriptive authority. Failure to be familiar with the limitations of midwifery can result in the imposition of significant liability on a facility.

Physician Assistants

Physician assistants (PAs) are health professionals licensed to practice medicine with physician supervision. Except for Mississippi (the only state that does not recognize PAs), each state requires PAs to be licensed, certified, or registered before they can engage in the practice of medicine. Approximately 21 states require PAs to pass a national certifying examination administered by the National Commission on Certification of Physician Assistants before commencing practice. Passing the examination entitles the PA to use the title of physician assistant-certified.

Based on state law, PAs may be able to perform clinical services such as patient evaluation, patient monitoring, and diagnosis; to provide therapeutic treatment such as administering injections; to provide immunizations and suture; to provide wound care; to manage certain conditions produced by infection or trauma; and to counsel patients on complying with therapeutic regimens and injection of medications. The physician-PA relationship, however, is a dependent one that requires supervision by a physician. A PA is an agent of the supervising physician. Accordingly, physicians may be liable for the negligent acts of PAs because they select or supervise PAs and exercise control over them.

Sources of Liability Specific to Pas

Facilities may be liable for less than optimal care rendered by PAs and for negligently credentialing PAs. Such potential liability illustrates the importance of professional liability insurance for PAs and for physicians. Facilities may be held responsible for paying a judgment against a physician or the PA if either of the individuals is uninsured or underinsured. Accordingly, the scope of coverage and policy limitations also must be reviewed and understood before granting practice privileges to PAs.

Some states also require that a physician obtain licensure as a PA supervisor before supervising PAs. As part of the credentialing process, before allowing a physician and the physician's assistant to provide direct patient care, a facility should establish mechanisms to ensure that a supervising physician maintains appropriate current licensure as a PA supervisor.

Prescriptive Authority

Currently, approximately 38 states grant prescriptive-writing authority to PAs. Prescriptive authority can encompass prescribing, dispensing, or merely transmitting prescriptive orders. Familiarity with the degree of prescriptive authority that PAs are legally permitted to exercise is essential. For example, in the District of Columbia, PAs are limited to prescribing non-controlled substances. In California, hospital regulations provide that PAs are limited to transmitting, orally or in writing, a prescription from the supervising physician, and that such transmission, if written in the patient's medical record, must be reviewed, dated, and countersigned by the supervising physician within seven days of transmission.[41] To minimize liability, it is necessary to be familiar with the degree of prescriptive authority that PAs may exercise.

Accordingly, facilities should implement and maintain written protocols regarding PAs' prescriptive authority, transmittal authority (oral or written), and dispensing authority, if any. Pharmacy personnel and PAs should also be provided with such written protocols.

Nurse Anesthetists

Nurse anesthesia is an advanced clinical nursing specialty. Nurses can become certified registered nurse anesthetists (CRNAs) after attending an accredited nurse anesthesia education program and passing a national certification exam. CRNAs practice in settings ranging from hospitals, ASCs, and pain clinics to physicians' offices. CRNAs can manage patients' operative anesthesia needs as well as pre- and post-operative needs. Depending on state law and the clinical setting, they may be legally authorized to perform physical assessments, prepare patients for anesthetic management, administer anesthesia, maintain anesthesia intraoperatively, oversee recovery from anesthesia, and manage the patients' postoperative course. Proper utilization of CRNAs subject to strict controls through proper credentialing can result in high-quality and cost-effective care, thus benefiting facilities, employers, physicians, and patients alike.

The issue of CRNA supervision continues to be hotly debated in the health care sector. Statutory requirements regarding the degree of supervision and supervisors' qualifications vary among states. Many states, such as California, recognize the independent practice of CRNAs. In California, absent any restrictions that may be imposed by a facility, CRNAs may lawfully perform all anesthesia service without physician supervision after the physician has ordered the administration of anesthesia. However, the area of supervising physicians' qualifications is less clear. Some states require CRNAs to be supervised by a physician, although such supervision does not necessarily need to be provided by an anesthesiologist. Accordingly, risk management professionals should be familiar with whether limited-license practitioners, such as dentists and podiatrists, can supervise CRNAs, and the degree of independence that CRNAs are legally authorized to exercise.

Although the battle lines have been drawn for years and many can predict which side each camp will take, it is likely that the issue of CRNA supervision will remain hotly debated. Based on financial pressures that are continually being exerted on health care systems nationwide, however, it also is likely that CRNAs who provide high-quality care will gain a stronger foothold in today's health care market.

Verification of Credentials

It also is important to re-verify AHPs' credentials vigilantly, including PAs, after the initial grant of practice rights. According to the American Academy of Physician Assistants Risk Management Task Force study mentioned earlier, 96 percent of the respondents indicated that hospitals required initial verification of PAs' credentials, but only 81 percent re-verified them.[42]

There should be *no* discrepancy between verification rates during credentialing and re-credentialing. Re-verification of pertinent information such as current licensure; current competency; maintenance of malpractice insurance; initiation of legal actions or judgments against AHPs, including PAs; verification of current participation-exclusion status regarding federal health care programs; and other such malpractice information is an important risk management tool. A facility's failure to diligently maintain current credentialing information on all those who practice in its midst can affect its accreditation rating, quality outcomes, and reputation in the community.

....

MINIMIZING POTENTIAL LIABILITY IN THE COURSE OF CREDENTIALING

Several steps can be taken to reduce the risk of liability associated with credentialing. First and foremost, developing a risk management plan that addresses qualifications, credentials, and practice guidelines should eliminate a substantial degree of inconsistency and minimize liability. A risk management plan should be based on a state's licensure laws, state and federal regulations, and the facility's needs. In addition to risk management plans for different liability issues and different classes of practitioners, facilities must institute and maintain written protocols. Written protocols provide systematic guidance to administrators, surveyors, physicians, and other entities and individuals who are entrusted with credentialing functions.

After implementing credentialing protocols, compliance with such protocols should be sought. For example, credentialing decisions should be clearly delineated in an applicant's file. The denial and granting of practice privileges should be based on objective factors that are documented in an applicant's file. Justification of credentialing decisions, as opposed to conclusory statements such as "practice privileges granted" or "practice privileges denied," will support a facility's claim that a practitioner's privileges were denied based on objective factors used to evaluate members of such class of AHP.

As a rule, facilities should not communicate credentialing decisions orally. Statements made by facility employees may be admissible in a hearing challenging the facility's credentialing decision. All employees involved in the credentialing process should be aware that any and all information regarding credentialing should be communicated only in writing by individuals with the authority to do so.

Too often, in today's extremely competitive health care market, decision makers fail to take necessary actions in accordance with their facility's written protocols or make exceptions for practitioners who are well respected in the community or who have been on the hospital staff for many years. However, such a practice is hazardous, to not only patients but also the facility's licensure, Medicare and Medicaid certification, accreditation status, and financial condition. Uneven application of rules and policies is likely to result in legal liability.

Implementing effective communication strategies is also an important risk management tool. Effective communication strategies should be implemented to provide prompt reporting and resolution of problems. Facilities should be careful not to implement policies, procedures, and protocols with which the staff cannot or will not comply. Implementation of written standards that are not strictly followed might expose facilities to liability for failure to comply with their own standards.

············
CONCLUSION

Credentialing poses several potential sources of liability for the health care organization. Discrimination, restraint of trade, inadequate supervision of allied health professionals, negligent credentialing, failure to check whether the practitioner has been excluded from participation in federal health care programs, and wrongful disclosure of peer review and quality outcome information are among the most serious.

Risk management plays a significant role in minimizing those sources of potential liability. By documenting and ensuring adherence to the health care organization's credentialing policies and procedures, and periodically reviewing them, the risk management professional can minimize potential liabilities associated with this process. Also, the ongoing and rapid changes in health care are bringing changes in potential sources of liability. By staying familiar with current developments in health care, the risk management professional will be better able to foresee new areas of potential liability and address them early.

Endnotes

1. Joint Commission on Accreditation of Healthcare Organizations. *JCAHO Comprehensive Accreditation Manual for Hospitals* ("JCAHO Comprehensive Accreditation Manual for Hospitals") Oakbrook Terrace, IL: JCAHO, 2005.
2. *Ibid.*
3. National Committee for Quality Assurance. Standards for the Accreditation of Managed Care Organizations ("NCQA Standards for Accreditation") Washington, DC: 2004.
4. 42 CFR § 482.22(a)(2).
5. 42 CFR § 482.22.
6. 42 CFR § 483.430(b)(5).
7. 42 CFR § 484.16.
8. 42 CFR § 485.54(b).
9. 42 CFR § 485.604.
10. 42 CFR § 485.705.
11. 22 CCR § 70701 (a)(7).
12. JCAHO Comprehensive Accreditation Manual for Hospitals.
13. NCQA Standards for Accreditation.
14. 42 CFR § 1003.102(a)(2).
15. 64 Fed. Reg. 52791, 52793 (September 30, 1999) (OIG Special Advisory Bulletin).

16. 211 N.E.2d 253 (Ill. 1965).

17. See, Kadzielski, "Provider Deselection and Decapitation in a Changing Healthcare Environment," 41 St. Louis L. J. 891 (Summer, 1997), and cases cited at footnote 12. In California, the theory of corporate liability for negligent credentialing was established in *Elam v. College Park Hospital,* 132 Cal.App.3d 332 (1982).

18. In *McClellan v. Health Maintenance Organization,* 604 A.2d 1053, *allocatur denied,* 616 A.2d 985 (Pa. 1992), the court held that an HMO may be held liable under the theory of ostensible corporate liability for failing to "select and retain only competent individuals."

19. In *Petrovich v. Share Health Plan,* 188 Ill.2d 17 (1999), the Illinois Supreme Court considered portions of the health plan's member handbook that referred to the "comprehensive high quality services" purportedly provided by plan physicians to hold that an HMO could be held vicariously liable under an apparent authority theory for the malpractice of its independent contractor physicians. See also, *Villazon v. Prudential Health Care Plan,* 843 So.2d 842, 854 (Fla. 2003), where the Florida Supreme Court held that the totality of the evidence led to the conclusion that the HMO had the "right to control" the means by which plan physicians rendered medical care to enrollees.

20. 42 CFR § 482.12(a)(7).

21. 42 CFR § 482.13, as reported in 64 Fed. Reg. 36070 (July 2, 1999).

22. 42 U.S.C. §§ 12101–12213.

23. 29 U.S.C. § 794.

24. *Menkowitz v. Pottstown Mem'l Med. Ctr.,* 154 F.3d 113, 123–24 (3d Cir. 1998) and *Wojewski v. Rapid City Regional Hospital,* 2005 WL 1397000 (D.S.D. 2005).

25. JCAHO Comprehensive Accreditation Manual for Hospitals, (MS. 5.4).

26. NCQA Standards for Accreditation (CR 4).

27. NCQA Standards for Accreditation (CR 4 & footnote).

28. JCAHO Comprehensive Accreditation Manual for Hospitals. (MS. 5.4–5.4.3 and accompanying "Intent").

29. 37 Cal.Rptr.2d 518 (1995).

30. *Tarasoff v. Regents of the University of California,* 551 P.2d 334 (1976).

31. 45 CFR § 60.13. See, generally, Kadzielski, "A New Quality Challenge: Coordinating Credentialing and Corporate Compliance," 14 *Annals of Health Law* 409 (Summer, 2005).

32. 45 CFR § 61.14.

33. 45 CFR § 60.4–9; 45 CFR § 61.4–11.

34. 45 CFR §§ 60.7, 60.9; 45 CFR §§ 61.9, 61.11.

35. American Academy of Physician Assistants Risk Management Task Force. *Hospital Practice Survey.* Alexandria, VA: AAPA, Apr. 1992.

36. JCAHO Comprehensive Accreditation Manual for Hospitals (MS. 6.1).

37. JCAHO Comprehensive Accreditation Manual for Hospitals (MS. 6.2.2).

38. JCAHO Comprehensive Accreditation Manual for Hospitals (MS. 5.14).

39. 16 CCR § 1463.

40. American College of Nurse Midwives. *A Handbook of State Legislation.* Washington, DC: ACNM, 1995.

41. 16 CCR § 1399.541(h).

42. AAPA. Hospital Practice Survey.

10

Documentation and the Medical Record

Sandra K. Johnson
Leilani Kicklighter
Pamela J. Para

The medical record is important as a tool of effective communication. It facilitates continuous performance improvement, supports reimbursement of services provided, and provides clinical data for research and education. The purpose of a medical record is to document the course of a patient's care and treatment. Documentation is the essence of the medical record, and risk management professionals have a vested interest in preserving the record and in enhancing the quality of documentation.

Medical records can take many forms, such as paper, electronic, microfiche, and fax, depending on the setting and culture of the organization. The health care industry's move to electronic medical records is generating new risks. For example, computer physician order entry (CPOE) has created challenges related to documentation and efficiency during conversions from paper-based systems to CPOE systems. The health care risk management professional's organizational risk assessment should identify the methods by which patient care is documented throughout the health care system.

It is important for the health care risk management professional to remember that although the medical record is the central repository for the documentation of all health care delivery segments, it is not the only important business document. The business aspects of health care require the same recordkeeping and documentation as other businesses. Retention and easy retrieval of any business document is important.

Medical records also take various forms in different types of health care settings (i.e., acute care, long-term care, and ambulatory care). Depending on the environment, regulatory and accreditation requirements may specify the contents of the medical records as well as retention and other requirements. To see what constitutes a medical record, refer to Table 10.1.

TABLE 10.1   What Constitutes a Medical Record?

Standard Medical Record Components	*Other Components (Depending on the Circumstances)*
Admission/Identification/Face Sheet	Electrocardiogram (ECG, EKG)
Vital Signs/Graphic Sheet	Imaging and X-Ray Reports
Physicians' Orders	Lab Reports
Medical/Surgical/Health History and Physical	Emergency Department Record
Problem List	Operative Report
Medication Record	Consult Reports
Progress Notes	Autopsy Report
Discharge Notes/Summary	Transfer Records
Authorization Forms (consents for admission, treatment, surgery, and release of medical records)	Anesthesia Record
	Recovery Room Record
	Labor and Delivery Record
	Fetal Monitoring Strips
	Non-stress Test Reports

While there are several types of documents with which health care risk management professionals should be aware, the purpose of this chapter is to emphasize and reinforce the role of risk management in the need for proper systems and processes for documentation and maintenance of the medical record. The medical record is a well-established communication link benefiting both patients and health care providers in any health care setting. For a sampling of documents of interest to the risk management professional, see Table 10.2.

DOCUMENTATION

Documentation may be defined as the recording of pertinent facts and observations about an individual's health history, including past and present illnesses, tests, treatments, and outcomes. Documentation is the basis for reimbursement, establishes a medical history, and creates a legal record in the event of a claim. Other purposes of documentation include, but are not limited to:

- Chronologically documenting the care rendered
- Planning and evaluating the patient's treatment
- Facilitating communication among all caregivers
- Providing continuity of care for the patient
- Providing evidence of care and treatment in legal actions and reimbursement purposes
- Meeting the standard of care
- Meeting accreditation and licensure requirements

The challenge of using documentation as a tool of communication across different types of health care settings is to connect all entities in an efficient way.

TABLE 10.2   Types of Documents of Interest to Health Care Risk Managers

Medical records	Financial records
Employee health records	Billing records
Corporate and organizational policies and procedures	Minutes of Board and committee meetings
Licenses, certificates, and permits	Personnel files (including documentation of competencies and job descriptions)
Incident and occurrence reports	OSHA records
Electronic correspondence and backup tapes	Insurance policies
Contracts and agreements	Fetal monitoring strips
ECG/EKG reports	Radiology films (i.e., x-ray, CT, MRI)
Patient logs (i.e., surgery, labor and delivery, emergency department)	Accreditation and other inspection reports
Patient transfer forms	Consultation reports
Lab reports	Autopsy reports
Credentialing files	Claims files and legal records
Advance directives	Consent forms
Medical staff bylaws	Equipment maintenance records
Patient education materials	Staff training manuals and records
Record of patient's valuables	Discharge reports/forms (with patient's/resident's signature of understanding of any discharge instructions provided; AMA forms)
Checklists (i.e., falls, restraints, activity, dietary, preoperative, sponge and needle counts)	Non-stress test results
Care plan	Medication administration record

Accreditation, Licensure, and Regulatory Requirements

Health care is a highly regulated business that requires documentation to support compliance. Recent federal regulations affecting documentation, maintenance, and release of health information include the Health Insurance Portability and Accountability Act of 1996 (HIPAA). HIPAA affects confidentiality and authorized access to personal health information (PHI). For more details about HIPAA, see Chapter 18 in Volume III.

The rules that govern documentation and medical record management come from several sources:

- Federal—Centers for Medicare and Medicaid Services (CMS) documentation requires:

  a) Records document evidence of a physical examination, including a health history, performed no more than seven days before admission or within forty-eight hours after admission

  b) Admitting diagnosis

  c) Results of consultative evaluations of the patient and appropriate findings by clinical and other staff involved in the patient's care

  d) Documentation of complications, hospital-acquired infections, and adverse reactions to drugs and anesthesia

  e) Properly executed informed consent forms for procedures and treatments specified by the medical staff, or by federal or state law if applicable, to acquire patient consent

f) All practitioners' orders; nursing notes; medication records; radiology, treatment, and laboratory reports; and vital signs and other information necessary to monitor the patient's condition

g) Discharge summary with outcome of hospitalization, disposition of care, and provisions for follow-up care

h) Final diagnosis with completion of medical records within thirty days following discharge

- State statutes and state licensure requirements: These vary from state to state and address such things as content, timeliness, retention procedures, maintenance, destruction, and signing of medical records.

- Professional practice standards: Organizations such as the American Nurses Association (ANA), American Health Information Management Association (AHIMA), Health Information Management Systems Society (HIMSS), Health Insurance Association of America, and the American Medical Association (AMA), identify specific standards for documentation. The American Nurses Association has introduced a new tool to streamline the nursing documentation process. Available in a brochure titled *Principles for Documentation,* this new guide includes policy statements, principles and recommendations to assist nurses with documentation and to comply with institutional and regulatory requirements.

- Specific health care facility protocols: Although not laws, they can be used as evidence in civil litigation to establish the facility's acceptable standard of practice.

- Insurance companies, managed care organizations, and other third-party organizations: These parties may refuse to pay claims if the care rendered is not properly or thoroughly documented.

- Joint Commission on Accreditation of Healthcare Organizations (JCAHO): Information Management (IM) standards focus on hospital-wide information planning and management processes to meet the hospital's internal and external information needs. The JCAHO standards are designed to be equally compatible with paper-based, electronic, or hybrid systems. JCAHO standards specify the following elements of documentation:[1]

a) The hospital has a complete and accurate medical record for every individual assessed, cared for, treated or served.

b) The medical record thoroughly documents operative or other high risk procedures and the use of moderate or deep sedation or anesthesia.

c) For patients receiving continuing ambulatory care services, the medical record contains a summary list of all significant diagnoses, procedures, drug allergies, and medications.

d) Designated qualified personnel accept and transcribe verbal orders from authorized individuals.

e) The hospital can provide access to all relevant information from a patient's record when needed for use in patient care, treatment, and services.

According to hospital survey results posted for 1,453 organizations by the end of 2004, some of the most frequent "Not Compliant" standards were:

a) IM.3.10: 27 percent of hospitals (abbreviations, symbols, acronyms are standardized);

b) IM.6.10: 12 percent of hospitals (medical record delinquency rate); and

c) IM.6.50: 10 percent of hospitals (verbal orders including "read-back").[2]

Documentation may also be used to demonstrate compliance with the JCAHO National Patient Safety Goals for handoffs through a Continuity of Care Record.

- Individual State Nurse Practice Acts
- Textbooks and articles

Charting and Documentation Models

Organizational policy should specify the charting style and documentation model to meet the specific needs of the particular environment. However, some standard charting components apply throughout the health care industry.

Essential Charting Components

JCAHO Standard IM.6.20 specifies that each medical record contains, as applicable, the following clinical and case information:

- Emergency care, treatment, and services provided to the patient before the patient's arrival, if any
- Documentation and findings of assessments
- Conclusions or impressions drawn from medical history and physical examination
- The diagnosis, diagnostic impression, or conditions
- The reason(s) for admission or care, treatment, and services
- The goals of the treatment and treatment plan
- Diagnostic and therapeutic orders
- All diagnostic and therapeutic procedures, tests, and results
- Progress notes made by authorized individuals
- All reassessments and plan of care revisions, when indicated
- Relevant observations
- The response to care, treatment, and services provided
- Consultation reports
- Allergies to foods and medicines
- Every medication ordered or prescribed
- Every dose of medication administered, including the strength, dose, or rate of administration, administration devices used, access site or route, known drug allergies, and any adverse drug reaction
- Every medication dispensed or prescribed on discharge
- All relevant diagnoses or conditions established during the course of care, treatment, and services
- Each medical record contains, as applicable, the following demographic information:
  - The patient's name, sex, address, date of birth, and authorized representative, if any
  - Legal status of patients receiving behavioral health care services

- Each medical record contains, as applicable, the following information:
  - Evidence of known advance directives
  - Evidence of informed consent patient care
  - Records of communication with patient regarding care, treatment, and services, for example, telephone calls or e-mail, if applicable
  - Patient-generated information (for example, information entered into the record over the Web or in previsit computer systems), if applicable
- For patients receiving continuing ambulatory care services, the medical record contains a summary list including the following information:
  - Known significant medical diagnoses and conditions
  - Known significant operative and invasive procedures
  - Known adverse and allergic drug reactions
  - Known long-term medications, including current prescriptions, over-the-counter drugs, and herbal preparations[3]

Documentation requirements will differ depending on the setting—in a hospital, nursing home, home health care agency, or other community facility. For example, perioperative, critical, and emergency care areas have specialized criteria and forms for documenting nursing care. Additionally, requirements may change depending on the patient population (that is, requirements in obstetric settings differ from those in geriatric settings).

Documentation Models

There are several documentation models that can be used, depending on the culture and needs of the organization:

- Charting by exception: encourages documentation of only abnormal findings, significant changes, and unusual occurrences. Although originally intended to reduce the length and repetitiveness of the narrative note, it creates the perception that care proceeded from one bad event to another.[4] Documentation sources have cited *Lama v. Borras* (1994), a case in which the court stated that there was evidence to suggest that charting by exception did not regularly record information important to an infection diagnosis, such as the changing characteristics of the surgical wound and the patient's complaints of postoperative pain. One of the attending nurses conceded that under the charting by exception policy, she would not report a patient's pain if she did not administer medicine or if she gave the patient only aspirin-type medication. The court also concluded that the intermittent charting of possible signs of infection failed to record the sort of continuous danger signals that would most likely spur early intervention by a doctor.[5]
- Narrative charting: a chronological account of the patient's status, the interventions performed, and the patient's responses.[6] Handwritten or computer-generated narrative notes summarize information obtained by general observation, the health history interview, and a physical examination. The current trend in hospitals and home care agencies is to avoid writing long narrative note entries.[7] Because nursing documentation is judged more for quality than quantity, the narrative note should be concise, pertinent, and evaluatory. If it is too lengthy, it will interfere with efficient data retrieval.

- AIR (Assessment-Intervention-Response): a narrative charting format that synthesizes major nursing events while avoiding repetition of information found elsewhere in the medical record.[8]

- Flow sheets: also called abbreviated progress notes, flow sheets have vertical or horizontal columns for recording dates, times, and interventions. Data can be inserted quickly and concisely, preferably at the time care is given or when a change in the patient's condition is observed. An advantage of this model is that all members of the health care team can compare data and assess the patient's progress over time. However, using flow sheets does not exempt an organization from narrative charting to describe observations, patient teaching, patient responses, detailed interventions, and unusual circumstances.

- Checklists: tasks that need to be accomplished by the staff member or the patient.

- Computerized charting system: consists of a complex, interconnected set of software applications that process and transport data that are input by the health care team; categorizes the patient's data and stores the health care history, including inpatient and outpatient records from various facilities; helps guide the health care team in providing care and identifying patient education needs.[9] An effective computerized documentation system must have the capacity to record and send data to the appropriate departments; adapt easily to the health care facility's needs; display highly selective information on command; and provide easy storage access and retrieval for all trained personnel, while maintaining the highest standards of patient confidentiality.[10]

- Focus charting: based on patient-centered problems; tends to rely only on individual occurrences or significant changes. This often eliminates positive notes that are useful in documenting care that is outcome-based; works best in acute care settings and on units where the same care and procedures are repeated frequently.[11]

- POMR (Problem-Oriented Medical Record System): describes specific patient problems on multidisciplinary progress notes. The POMR is most effective in acute care and long-term care settings.[12]

- PIE (Problem, Interventions, Evaluations of Interventions): organizes information according to patients' problems; integrates a plan of care into the nurses' progress notes.[13]

- FACT (Flow sheets individualized to specific services; Assessment features standardized with baseline parameters; Concise, integrated progress notes and flow sheets documenting the patient's condition and responses; Timely entries recorded when care is given): documents only exceptions to the norm or significant information about the patient incorporates charting by exception principles; developed to help caregivers avoid the documentation of irrelevant data, repetitive notes, inconsistencies among departments, and to reduce the amount of time spent charting.[14]

- Core: focuses on the nursing process; most useful in acute care and long-term care facilities.[15]

- Critical pathway: an interdisciplinary care plan that describes assessment criteria, interventions, treatments, and outcomes for specific health-related conditions (usually based on a DRG) across a designated timeline; usually organized according to categories, such as activity, diet, treatments, medications, patient teaching, and discharge planning.[16]

- S.O.A.P.: A popular method of charting, this method of documentation originated in the 1960s from a problem-oriented medical record format. S.O.A.P. is now used in acute care, long-term care, home care, and ambulatory clinic settings. The problem-oriented medical record defines and follows each clinical problem individually and organizes them for solutions. The S.O.A.P. model is used for the progress notes section of this type of medical record, and may be used as S.O.A.P. or S.O.A.P.I.E.R.

S = Subjective

Principal complaint or history

Symptomatic

In the patient's own words whenever possible

O = Objective

Measurable, observable, what the provider observes and inspects

May include a physical exam, diagnostic test results, and so on

A = Assessment

Diagnostic

Determination of the problem

Interpretation or impression of the current condition

What the provider thinks is going on based on the data

P = Plan

Plan of action for each problem

I and E = Interventions and Evaluation

Specific interventions implemented

Patient's response to interventions

R = Revision

Any changes from the original care plan (interventions, outcomes, or target dates).

See Table 10.3 for the advantages and disadvantages of using the S.O.A.P. model of documentation.

Many health care facilities have adapted the source-oriented or problem-oriented method to better meet their documentation needs. In the home health care setting, for example, nurses have created many documentation forms, including the initial assessment form, problem list, day-visit sheet, and discharge summary, to better reflect the services and essential aspects of care they provide. Whichever documentation model is selected, policies and procedures should determine the approved method for the individual health care organization or system. The use of checklists and flow sheets also needs to be described in policies and procedures. Policies and procedures set minimum requirements that can be used as a guideline for quality improvement criteria. The chosen documentation model must meet documentation needs while complying with organizational policy, state and federal laws, and other regulations or accreditation requirements. Compliance and consistency is paramount, and staff education is the key.

Sample Documentation Techniques

Risk management strategies include several documentation techniques that can facilitate accurate communication through and support the core purposes of the medical record.

TABLE 10.3   **Advantages and Disadvantages of the S.O.A.P. Model of Documentation**

Advantages	*Disadvantages*
All of a patient's problems are considered in total context	Requires training and commitment of entire professional staff
The record clearly indicates the goals and methods of the patient's treatment	If not implemented in its pure form, modifications of the S.O.A.P. format can diminish the original goal of structured and logical entries
Facilitates interdisciplinary communication	
Easier to track corrective actions for purposes of quality improvement monitoring	Potential redundancy among flow sheets, care plans, and S.O.A.P.(I.E.) note
Structure: each entry contains information in a predetermined format, which lends consistency to the documentation of patient care	S.O.A.P.(I.E.) charting may not meet the needs of organizations who are searching for a less time-consuming method of documentation
Reflects the nursing process by encompassing assessment, nursing diagnosis, planning, interventions, and evaluation of nursing care	May meet resistance from other health care professionals
Can be used effectively with standard care plans	Routine care may remain undocumented
Can be incorporated within integrated medical record documentation, to foster collaboration and enhance communication among health care professionals	Need to make sure to close the problems if the format is truly problem oriented
Organizes problems into specific categories	
Promotes continuity of care	
Minimizes non-essential data	
Factual	
Facilitates follow-up care	
Compliance with recognized standards and an accepted format	

Correcting Errors in the Medical Record

The acceptable method for correcting an error is to draw one line through the entry, initial or sign it, date it, and place the correct information above the drawn-through entry. If space is not available or if the corrected information is too lengthy to place adjacent to the incorrect entry, the corrected note should be placed in the appropriate place on the record (progress notes, nursing notes, and so on) and it should be contemporaneous with that date's notes. It should be dated and signed and the reason for the correction noted. Incorrect entries should not be obliterated, erased, nor should correction fluid be used, as these methods of correction might appear to be an attempt to conceal the entry. It is strongly recommended that additions to the record after an adverse outcome, patient complaint, or request for records be avoided.

Hearsay

The risk management professional should advise staff that "hearsay," or statements made by persons other than the author of the entry, should not be documented as if they were fact. Instead, the method by which the author of the entry heard the statement and the fact that it was heard from another source should be documented with the actual statement documented in quotation marks.

Telephone Calls and Telephone Advice in Physician Office Practices

It is recommended that medical advice not be given over the phone unless the identity of the receiving party is known. However, this is a common occurrence for the physician who receives calls from patients. All health care organizations should have clearly documented policies governing who may give what type of advice over the phone other than the physician. In those instances when medical advice is provided, documentation is imperative. Emphasis should be placed on those organizations or areas that are more prone to receive patient calls, such as outpatient clinics, physician offices, home health agencies, and emergency departments.

Patients often call their physicians' offices during the day or after hours. A duplicate phone message pad (even at the bedside at home) is one way to keep a back-up log of who called, the date and time, and the reason. In the clinic or office, the original copy should go to the physician to return the call and the conversation should be added to the note for filing in the patient's medical record. Such documentation will reflect the initial reason for the call, the further description of the problem as described to the physician, and the physician's response or recommendation. Documentation of this information might prove to be invaluable if the quality of care is called into question. At a minimum, the date, time, and content of the discussion should be documented. All telephone messages must be filed in the medical record in chronological order.

Physician Notification

Whenever a call or page is made to a physician, the date and time should be carefully documented. The conversation with the physician should include the date and time if different from the call, and should include the content of the conversation. This conversation should include the exact signs and symptoms, lab results, and other details conveyed to the physician and the response, including additional information requested and given to the physician. Responses from the physician need to be similarly documented. If the situation is serious and the physician has not responded in a timely manner, the nurse must follow the "chain of command" procedures and contact the nursing supervisor or other appropriate person, in accordance with facility procedures. In addition, notice should also be provided to the chief of the physician's specialty. Regardless of the setting or the reason, when the patient care staff has a need to make contact with a physician, especially in the acute-care high-risk units, time is of the essence. Each health care setting should have policies governing expected response time and steps to take if response is not received within policy parameters.

Many physicians use an answering service to take calls. The service, in turn, pages the physician. The answering service should keep a log of the time the call was received for the physician and the time the physician returned the call to the service. Staff who reach an answering service when calling a physician should document the name of the person taking the call and the phone number of the answering service for potential future reference.

Countersignatures

Countersignatures imply that the health care provider has done more than just read and sign an entry or order. The countersignature connotes that the health care provider agrees with the patient care described or transcribed. Whenever a health care provider signs an entry in a medical record, the provider is responsible for whatever is contained in the entry.

History and physical (H&P), operative note, admission note, and discharge summaries are often dictated and transcribed. When completing charts, the physician signs these transcribed documents, authenticating the contents. As often as possible, the risk management professional should emphasize to the medical staff the significance of reading, verifying, and correcting transcribed notes before authenticating them with their signatures.

Those who use electronic medical records should be assigned electronic signatures, which should never be given to anyone to use; for instance, the radiologist should not give the electronic signature to the radiology transcriptionist to bypass verifying and authenticating the transcription. In some states this could be construed as fraud, which is an offense reportable to the state licensing board.

CMS requires documentation of verbal orders or entries requiring countersignatures be signed as soon as possible. One physician cannot sign for another, unless both share joint responsibility. Facility policies and medical staff bylaws should define whether documentation by house staff and allied health professionals requires countersignatures. In some instances this is governed by specific state law.

Medical students and nursing students' documentation should be countersigned by a supervisor. Check state statutes for specifics.

Abbreviations

The use of abbreviations saves time; however, they may be misinterpreted if they are ambiguous. Health care providers should be instructed to use universally accepted, standard medical abbreviations and those specifically approved by the individual health care facility. Abbreviations can vary by setting. For those facilities employing traveling nurses, there should be a process for all providers to have the same understanding where abbreviations are concerned. The JCAHO Sentinel Event Alert Number 23 and National Patient Safety Goals have addressed the use of abbreviations to prevent medication errors.

Authentication

JCAHO provides that entries in medical records may be made only by individuals given that right, as defined in facility policies and procedures and medical staff bylaws. All entries should be dated and signed by the author. In addition to the full name, the professional title should be reflected, such as MD (medical doctor), PA (physician's assistant), APRN (advanced practice registered nurse), RN (registered nurse), and so on. It is suggested that policies, procedures, and bylaws be reviewed to ensure that there is no conflict among these authorizing documents. JCAHO will survey a facility's performance against its own guidelines, and discrepancies can result in conditional or preliminary denial of accreditation.

Documentation of Termination of Care

When dealing with non-compliant patients and families (those who fail to follow instructions on diet, medications, use of safety devices, or who tamper with medical equipment), the risk management professional should advise staff to thoroughly document these issues objectively, including all education and reinforcement provided. If it becomes necessary to "administratively or permanently discharge" or refuse further care, the usual practice is to advise the patient and family of the intent to do so orally, followed immediately by written notice, sent by certified mail, with return receipt. This written notice should give a timeframe (usually thirty days) for continued care (sometimes limited to emergency care during the timeframe). Included should be either prescriptions for the timeframe (thirty days) or a reference that if a refill prescription is needed during the thirty days it will be provided. It should also include referrals for continued care, such as several names and phone numbers of physicians in the same specialty and the names and phone numbers of the local or regional medical and osteopathy (DO) societies. A copy of correspondence with the patient should be maintained in office files and in the medical record. It is recommended that the risk management professional check with legal counsel to verify that such a termination process complies with specific state statutes and case law.

Documentation Challenges

It is the responsibility of each health care professional to comply with the facility's policies and procedures for documentation. Documentation must be objective and free of speculation.

Verbiage

Plaintiffs' attorneys look for gaps and inappropriate language to discredit or cast doubt on the credibility of medical records. Verbiage such as "unintentionally," "inadvertently," and "unexpectedly" is not appropriate, because it reflects a judgment that something untoward happened. Words such as "appeared," "apparently," and "seems to be" are not specific, and can be used by plaintiffs' attorneys to cast doubt. Additionally, many words can have different meanings, and misuse might leave the author open to criticism. If it is necessary to use these words, then supplemental information is needed to provide clarity.

It is also important not to, inadvertently or intentionally, imply that a fellow provider was negligent. Here are some ways to avoid raising a "red flag" for being drawn into a lawsuit with another provider:

- Do not place blame for an unsatisfactory outcome.
- Empathize, don't apologize.
- Do not comment before having all the facts.
- Don't write in the medical record that someone was negligent.
- Do not prematurely document a corrective action plan.
- Discuss differences of opinion in a private environment away from patients.[17]

Legibility

The biggest documentation challenge is legibility. Documentation should be able to be read without needing interpretation. In a legal proceeding, a jury will need to make a determination based on their interpretation. Poor handwriting leads to misunderstandings among health professionals and patients. Studies report that illegible notes also lead to poor communication among specialties.

In 1994, the American Medical Association reported that medication error secondary to misinterpreted physicians' prescriptions was the second-most prevalent and expensive claim in 90,000 malpractice claims over a period of seven years. In 1994, the average indemnity payment for the 393 most recent medication-error claims was $120,722, with a range of $5,000 to $2.2 million per claim.[18]

Legibility has likewise affected litigation. In a widely publicized 1999 case in Odessa, Texas, a jury awarded $450,000 to the widow and children of a patient who died after a pharmacist dispensed the wrong drug after misreading the physician's handwriting.[19] Half of the judgment was assigned to the pharmacy, leaving the physician responsible for paying the other half. The defense attorney believes that the jury was trying to send a message to the medical community that in the computerized age there is no reason for doctors to create the potential for error by writing out their prescriptions instead of typing or printing them out. On August 12, 2004, a 41-year-old in Redwood City, California, received a lethal chemotherapy overdose, ten times the proper dosage, allegedly attributed to the doctor's illegible handwritten prescription. The family has asked the County Counsel's Office for $1 million and a written apology.[20]

There may be regulatory and accreditation implications to illegible handwriting. The Conditions of Participation for Hospitals: Medical Record Services (Section 482.24(c)[1]) state "all entries must be legible and complete, and must be authenticated and dated promptly by the person (identified by name and discipline) who is responsible for ordering, providing, or evaluating the service furnished." Criteria for quality medical records at the state level are commonly addressed in state licensing acts. Additional sources of handwriting legibility compliance can be found in JCAHO Medical Staff Standards, Management of Information Standards, and Performance Improvement Standards. It is incumbent upon the risk management professional to be familiar with associated regulatory and accreditation requirements, and to facilitate compliance throughout the health care organization.

In consideration of the real and potential threats to patient safety posed by illegible medical records, experts predict that JCAHO surveyors will check medical records more thoroughly for compliance with pertinent JCAHO standards and requirements. During a JCAHO survey, a hospital in Kentucky received a citation for illegible handwriting primarily because "neither the surveyor nor anyone in the room could determine (whether) the order for a medication was for 50 mg or 5.0 mg," according to the hospital's director of performance improvement.

Poor handwriting has been attributed to time pressure. Another reason is that handwriting instruction in Europe and in the United States has used models and teaching methods that do not hold up under any degree of speed.[21]

Three solutions have been identified for the problem of illegibility. The medical staff of Cedars-Sinai Medical Center decided to offer a special class in handwriting for members of the medical staff, which they speculated would be "raising the bar for other medical institutions."[22] Salem Hospital recently held a handwriting class for area medical professionals by instructors who teach penmanship to doctors and nurses around the world, because "improving handwriting among medical professionals can greatly reduce the risk of medical errors."[23] Second, studies reveal that transcription services are not only faster than writing but also improve physician productivity, satisfaction, and legibility of medical records.[24] Finally, computers already play a major role in solving handwriting problems. To minimize the potential for adverse drug reactions and miscommunicated orders, many hospitals are using computers for decision support and to order medications. Computers also note potential drug interactions, allergies, and side effects, suggesting dosage adjustments based on patient data such as age, weight, and height. These systems can also provide detailed therapy recommendations from a database of commonly prescribed drugs.[25]

Whereas one of the numerous goals for converting to an electronic medical record is to resolve legibility issues, the acute-care setting is probably further along in the conversion process. Long-term care facilities, home health agencies, outpatient clinics, physician offices, and other health care settings might not be as far along in that process, because it is costly, both in terms of financial and human resources.

Reimbursement

Today's health care system includes multiple, complex structures with multiple, complex requirements for reimbursement. Caregivers and health care organizations are not only accountable to internal quality management teams, case managers, and required reimbursement structures, but also to federal and state agencies, HMOs, preferred provider organizations (PPOs), and independent practice associations (IPAs), among others. Documentation is scrutinized by Medicare, Medicaid, and insurance company reviewers, among others, for the quality of care, patient outcomes, and the need for continued treatment. Reviewers from these groups examine the medical record for discrepancies. They look for differences in the treatment ordered and the treatment provided. If a discrepancy cannot be explained satisfactorily or reconciled reasonably, payment may be denied.

Payments by Medicare and Medicaid are sources of operating revenue for the health care organization. Although both Medicare and Medicaid were established in 1966 under the Social Security Act, the two organizations differ in their reimbursement policies, regulations, and documentation guidelines. Under Medicare, documentation is required to support the need for skilled medical and nursing care and its delivery. For example, a record for a Medicare Part A skilled facility resident must support not only the direct skilled services provided, but also the assessment and oversight that skilled services require. In the home care setting, Medicare has tied reimbursement to OASIS regulations that require that nurses complete an assessment and that agencies transmit the assessment and other data within strict timeframes. Under Medicaid, documentation is required to ensure payment, but required content varies according to setting. Lack of documentation as to the medical necessity of a test procedure or service could prove troublesome to defend should a claim arise in which this issue is in question.

Besides a lack of documentation, especially in the long-term care environment, there needs to be congruence among the various documents within the medical record, without which the credibility of the care might be compromised, not to mention cause for suspicion of fraud and abuse.

Documentation discrepancies identified by reviewers can also be "red flags" if the medical record becomes evidence in litigation. Inconsistencies in documentation leave both the caregiver and health care organization open to accusations of incompetence and fiscal irresponsibility. Ultimately, a medical record containing inconsistencies can be difficult or impossible to defend in court. Risk and health information management professionals must establish a partnership to communicate such findings and act upon them in an expedient manner.

Documenting a Medical Error

Documentation of patient care and events in the medical record is mandated by state and federal laws, accrediting organizations, professional organizations, and clinical standards of practice. Medical records may be used for legal proceedings including, but not limited to, state board disciplinary proceedings and during negligence actions filed against the facility or specific health care providers when a patient injury or death occurs. The assumption is the testimony documentation that will be following such an event will be based on factual documentation in the medical record.[26]

Although it is not appropriate to make the incident report itself a part of the medical record, the facts about the incident and how it was resolved should be documented. Neither the completion of an incident report nor reference to risk management should be referenced in the medical record because it is considered confidential and privileged under many state laws, and might unnecessarily raise a red flag. Here are some tips for health care professionals who need to document a medical error:

- Refer to organizational policy about what is classified as a medical error.
- Document the actual time of the event.
- Do not refer to the event as a "medical error."
- Objectively document what happened in the accepted charting model for the organization.
- Document who was notified.
- Document the response received to notifications and any other interventions.
- Document the patient's, resident's, and family's understanding of the event and how questions were answered.
- Document the outcome and treatment plan as indicated.
- Document the disclosure discussion (see Chapter 8 for more information on disclosure).

Physician and Allied Health Chart Completion Issues

Not only do delinquent or incomplete medical records compromise reimbursement, they are also an obstacle to providing quality care. The standard is that records are to be completed within thirty days after discharge. If the period of completion is longer, those numbers count against the facility when surveyed by JCAHO, and the physician is not in compliance with the Medical Staff Bylaws and risks being suspended from admitting privileges. In addition, should the record be requested by an outside party, that is, a third-party payer or an attorney, issues could arise from sending an incomplete record, especially if additions or changes are made to the record when the chart is finally completed.

Dictated notes reflect the date and often the time of dictation and of transcription. It is preferable to time the dictation as close as possible to the date of the action, that is, surgical procedure, consultation, history, and physical. Dictations dated after the date of a request from a third party can be looked upon with suspicion.

Physicians and others who dictate reports or notes should be reminded that their signature is evidence that they have read and agreed that the transcription is correct, thereby authenticating the note or report. Notes and reports sometimes have references to the wrong side or wrong site, to an antibiotic or other medication that sounds alike but is incorrect because the physician did not spell the drug. Further, there might be blanks in the transcription because the transcriber could not understand the word. Sometimes a physician whose first language is not English can dictate with an accent that results in errors in transcriptions. In such cases, physicians should take extra care to review carefully their transcribed reports and summaries. When physicians sign a report or summary with blanks or other errors as above, they are authenticating that the contents are correct, only to have this raised as an issue in a deposition or other legal proceeding.

Because turnaround time of the transcribed reports and summaries can be a deterrent to timely chart completion, risk management should work closely with health information management to monitor controls. Strategies for encouraging chart completion include, but are not limited to, the suspension of privileges and imposition of fines.

Risk management professionals need to work with organizational and medical staff leaders to prepare a fair procedure for enforcing compliance with timely and appropriate chart completion.

Medical Record Alterations

If the medical record is altered, unintentionally or purposefully, it can be misleading to others, and documentation as to the actual care provided may be disputed. In *Pyle v. Morrison,* 716 S.W. 2d 930 (1986), a malpractice suit was brought against doctors for their treatment of a child's fractured arm. The jury decided in favor of the plaintiffs—$400,000 for the child and $15,000 for the father. The deciding factor was the testimony of a nurse who said that she thought a portion of the medical record had been altered after the child's surgery. Tampering with the medical record is both unethical and illegal. Falsification, including alteration of medical records, can also be grounds for a criminal indictment or a civil claim for damages. Even with the best of intentions, changing inaccurate information, filling in omissions, altering dates and times, rewriting text, destroying records, adding to someone else's notes, and correcting or amending notes in violation of the facility's policy can be construed as "tampering with medical records." This can expose the health care organization and health care provider to many different types of claims, raise many other issues, and, quite possibly, could result in the loss of affirmative defenses in a negligence claim. Additionally, tampering may be reportable to external agencies and professional licensing boards. All known cases of tampering should be reported to the corporate compliance officer.

In the state of Florida, the Agency for Health Care Administration has provided: "The Board of Nursing shall impose disciplinary penalties upon a determination that a licensee . . . (d) Has falsely represented the patient's chart, patient flow sheets, narcotic records, or nursing progress records, or otherwise misrepresented the facts on records relating directly to the patient."[27] Although this illustrates a specific state's handling of this issue, risk management professionals should be thoroughly familiar with their respective states' disciplinary rules, promulgated by professional regulatory and licensing boards.

The risk management professional should be notified and should assist in the investigation whenever it is suspected or determined that a record has been altered. Reports should be filed with the external licensing board as appropriate. In addition, the risk management professional can assist in the preservation of records and deter alterations. Having a policy and procedure on the early sequestering of medical records after a significant incident will decrease the probability that the records will be released and altered.

If a patient experiences a poor or unexpected outcome, the urge to alter the record to make the care appear more appropriate might be overwhelming. With this in mind, the risk management professional should rely on established policy and procedures (developed in conjunction with legal counsel and the medical records department) to preserve the current in-use record. Refer to Table 10.4 for Documentation Do's and Don'ts.

One effective way to decrease alterations is to copy the current record that discusses the poor outcome for the medical record file and put the original in the "legal file" under the care and control of the medical records director. The copy on the shelf is available for patient care reference. Should the original need to be reviewed or

TABLE 10.4   Documentation Do's and Don'ts

Documentation Do's	*Documentation Don'ts*
Complete record as soon as possible	Use vague/ambiguous subjective terms
Use a ballpoint pen, not pencil or felt tip	Make statements against a colleague's interests
Be neat and write legibly	Change a record, post date an entry, or record false information
Sign/date/time/and sign each entry with professional designation	Use "white-out" or erase an entry
Document facts, observations, patient's condition, complications	Skip lines or leave blank spaces between entries
Show thought process—know what you plan to do and why	Use abbreviations that offend or are misunderstood
Be accurate—use clear and concise language that can be explained later	Criticize another practitioner's judgment or recommendations
Chart both positive and negative findings	Refer to incident reports or to risk management, quality assurance, and peer review activities or meetings
Correct errors by lining through them once, initialing, and writing the correct word or statement	Release the original copy of the medical record
Give all information on drugs—name, dosage and strength, route, time	Alter, destroy, or otherwise tamper with a medical record
Chart anything unusual or unexpected	Make subjective statements, other than those quoted from a patient or resident
Follow an established/accepted method of charting	
Use only accepted standard abbreviations	
Make sure the patient's name is on the top of each new page	
Use clear and concise language—avoid ambiguous terms and phrases	
Make sure that verbal orders are documented and co-signed according to hospital policy	
Record pertinent laboratory results	
Record patient response to medication and treatment	
Avoid improper corrections, erasures, or obliterations	
Avoid accusatory language	
Avoid time gaps and omissions	
Follow protocol for late entries	
Document patient and family education	

completed, a representative of the medical records department should sit with the individual to prevent alterations. It is the medical records department personnel who must testify or sign affidavits to the effect that the original record has been in their care, control, and custody. Should the original record be sent to risk management or legal counsel for safe-keeping, the medical records department personnel would not be able to make such statements. If this policy is consistently followed for potentially serious incidents and events, the likelihood of alterations should be prevented because no one would have unfettered access to the original record. Usually, when a serious incident has occurred, the risk management professional asks for a copy to begin an early investigation, which would be another copy available for comparison should alterations after the fact be suspected.

Omissions

Entries holding the distinction of being the most frequently omitted might be some of the most important to the overall record. For example, some of the most frequently omitted entries in the long-term care setting include:

- Resident and family education
- Conversations with family
- Cues and redirection of the resident[28]

....

RECORD RETENTION

How long a record should be kept depends on factors such as:

- Statutes of limitations
- Individual state statutes
- Standards and regulations—those that have medical record retention requirements include, but are not limited to:[29]

    a) Joint Commission on Accreditation of Healthcare Organizations (JCAHO)

    b) Centers for Medicare and Medicaid Services (CMS): for hospitals, home health agencies, state and long-term care facilities, comprehensive outpatient rehabilitation, organ procurement, rural primary care

    c) Occupational Safety and Health Administration (OSHA)

    d) The Public Health Services Act: Immunization Program and National Childhood Vaccine Injury Act

    e) The National Commission on Correctional Health Care for Health Services in Jails and Prisons

    f) Federal reimbursement requirement guidelines

    g) Institutional record retention policies

Clear and complete recordkeeping guidelines must be developed and implemented for every health care organization. Although most records are maintained in one location, recordkeeping guidelines should also address all departments that maintain separate files. In addition, recordkeeping guidelines must address the review of all medical records shortly after the patient or resident is discharged, to ensure that the record is complete. Records that are involved in pending or threatened legal action should be segregated.

Destruction of patient health information is carried out in accordance with federal and state law and pursuant to a proper written retention schedule and destruction policy approved by the health information manager, chief executive officer, medical staff, and legal counsel. Records involved in any open investigation, audit, or litigation should not be destroyed.[30]

·············
RELEASE OF RECORDS

Records should be released only as authorized by state and federal laws and by the organization's policies and procedures. Policies and procedures for the release of medical records should address:

- Who may request and secure a copy of a patient's medical record (in the acute-care setting, it is most often the patient or authorized representative who requests the record; in the long-term care setting, it is more often the resident's Power of Attorney, guardian, or surrogate)

- Who is authorized to release records and to whom (such as patients, another staff member, attorneys, insurance company representatives)

- How access to medical records is monitored and documented (who checks out and returns records and when)

- Appropriate mechanisms to protect sensitive patient and employee health information (such as information related to HIV results, lifestyle, substance abuse, psychological profiles, or behavioral health records)

Failure to follow proper release procedures can result in significant liability. To minimize opportunities for liability, records should not be removed from the central location. Alternatively, only a copy of the record should be released so that the original records are always maintained within the records retention area.

The American Health Information Management Association (AHIMA) has recently defined the legal health record for disclosure purposes. The legal health record is generated at or for a health care organization as its business record, and it is the record that will be disclosed upon request. It does not affect discoverability of other information held by the organization. It is imperative that health care organizations define their legal health records, because the content is governed by laws and regulations that vary by practice setting and state. For further information on the updated AHIMA guidelines, visit [library. ahima.org/xpedio/groups/public/documents/ahima/pub_bok1_027921.html] (last visited September 2005).

·············
OWNERSHIP OF MEDICAL RECORDS

The medical record is an unusual type of property, as both the patient and the health care facility or provider have an ownership interest. The health care facility or provider owns the actual record, but the patient owns the information contained therein. The record must remain in the facility or doctor's office; therefore, the facility or office has the responsibility to exercise control in the release of the document itself or the information contained therein. Patients and others who have a vested interest have a right to access the information contained in the record; but there are limitations on this right, which vary by state.

In today's environment, medical record ownership issues arise relative to mergers, acquisitions, divestitures, and HMO provider contracts. This is illustrated by a case from the Florida Fourth District Court of Appeals in *Humana Medical Plan v. Fischman*, decided in December 1999. Humana terminated an agreement with a physician provider. This decision was based on a contract provision, which stipulated that the medical records relating to Humana members, during the term of their enrollment, would be the property of Humana. Despite many requests, the physician provided only those records for which he had received prior written consent from his patients. The physician argued that, according to Florida Statute (F.S.) 455.667, governing the disclosure of patient medical records, Humana did not qualify as the "owner" of the records. Humana conceded that F.S. 455.667 did not authorize it to obtain these records and admitted it did not obtain written authorization from the insured in advance. The Florida Appeals Court upheld the lower court's decision in favor of the physician. Cases such as this demonstrate the importance of reviewing contract language, in advance, regarding the issue of ownership of the medical record.

For records that are stored in the medical records department, it is prudent to have a policy and procedure on the release or availability of records to requesting and appropriate parties. Depending on the status of an identified event (incident, notice of intent to sue, claim being made, lawsuit, and so on), the record could be sequestered with the original not being made available unless under direct supervision. This policy will prevent the inadvertent alterations or misplacement of the record (see Exhibit 10.1).

MEDICAL RECORD AUDITS

Compliance with documentation standards and expectations can be verified through regular medical record audits. Typical questions to be answered with a medical record audit are included in Exhibit 10.2. Medical records may be audited by examining the following organizational processes:

- Is the reason for the patient encounter documented?
- Is there a process to verify that services that are provided are documented?
- Does the record clearly explain why support services, procedures, and supplies were provided?
- Is the assessment of the patient's condition apparent in the record?
- Does the record contain information on the patient's progress and on the results of treatment?
- Does the record include a plan for care?
- Does the information in the record describing the patient's condition provide reasonable medical rationale for the services?
- Does the information in the record support the care given in case another health care professional must assume care or perform medical review?
- Is the documentation in compliance with established policies and procedures, and local, state, and federal requirements?

DOCUMENTATION AND RISK MANAGEMENT

The medical record has historically been a tool of risk management. Appropriate documentation promotes quality of care, preserves the financial integrity of the organization, and maintains competitiveness in the marketplace. Documentation is multidisciplinary and a way for all members of the patient care team to work together for the patient's benefit.

EXHIBIT 10.1   **Sample Request for Records Form**

North Broward Hospital District
Risk Management Department
REQUEST FOR RECORDS

☐ IPMC Region   ☐ NBMC Region   ☐ CSMC Region   ☐ BGMC Region   ☐ Western Region

TO: ☐ Pathology
             ☐ Central Business Office
             ☐ Radiology
             ☐ QA/UR
             ☐ Medical Records
             ☐ Other _____

FROM: Risk Management: _____ _____ _____
                                    Name   Telephone #   Location

RE: Patient:_____ Medical Record #_____

        Admitted: _____ Discharged: _____ DOB: _____

In anticipation that the above patient may file a claim against his/her health care providers:

☐ Secure all specimens, slides and blocks (itemize below)
☐ Secure all films, scans and x-rays (itemize below)
☐ Prepare   ☐ One   ☐ Two itemized copy(ies) of bill
            ☐ One   ☐ Two copy(ies) of Detailed Billing notes; forward all to Risk Management
☐ Forward a copy of the QA/UR review on this patient to the person identified above.
☐ Forward _____ copy(ies) of the medical records to: ☐ District   ☐ Regional Risk Management

              ☐ Number the pages of the original medical record prior to copying

DATE DONE	NUMBER	TYPE

Secured originals are not to be released out of your department or viewed without authorization by Risk Management.

Please complete and return to Risk Management within 5 days of receipt

EXHIBIT 10.2   Questions for Medical Record Review

- If the patient alleged some deficiently in patient care, could the record negate the patient's story?
- Is there a logical process presented in the record for coming to a decision about the course of treatment?
- Would any reasonable physician be likely to come to the same conclusion?
- Were the appropriate tests ordered in a timely manner?
- Do test results verify the course of treatment?
- Was appropriate consultation obtained?
- Do the consultants' reports agree with the course of treatment?
- If not, were the differences clearly explained and justified in the record?
- Did the physician comment on the interventions and results of treatments provided by other professionals (e.g., nurses and therapists) that may have affected the condition of the patient or the treatment regimen?
- Do the progress notes indicate that the patient knew about the benefits and reasonably expected risks and alternatives before giving consent to high-risk or invasive procedures?
- Are the entries accurately times, dated, signed, and above all, legible?
- Do they reflect professionalism (for example, no evidence of infighting with other members of the care team)?
- Is there any evidence of alteration of the record? (Even if this was done innocently, juries frown on even the appearance of fraud or cover-up.)
  a) Looked at in its entirety, does the medical record present a complete picture of the care provided with no ambiguity, no unexplainable gaps in time for treatments or medications, no illegible entries, and so on?

Reprinted with the permission of the American Society for Healthcare Risk Management.

Liability Exposures

A discussion of legal considerations pertaining to documentation must reflect the changing demands of the health care environment. More elderly people are receiving medical care, and medical conditions are more acute. There are constantly new procedures, drugs, and equipment introduced to provide medical care. There is more emphasis on consumers' rights, and the media's heightened interest attracts even further attention and scrutiny of the provision and quality of health care services.

One only needs to attend a professional liability trial or read a malpractice case transcript to realize how much a jury relies on documentation. What the providers document or fail to document will certainly influence the outcome of any case.

Plaintiffs' attorneys have erroneously promoted that an action that is not documented is not performed. Health care providers know that this old adage is incorrect, as much patient care is rendered that is never documented. However, documentation is especially significant in cases of informed consent, medication, treatment entries, and also "routine" observations. For a listing of what plaintiffs' attorneys look for in the medical record, refer to Table 10.5.

When there is no recorded continuity of the patient's status and deterioration occurs, absence of documentation will be used to support a claim of negligence. Other ways that medical records can be used adversely in the event of a claim include but are not limited to:

- A series of events leading up to a patient's injury in the hospital
- Failure of the staff to use information available in the patient's record
- Failure to impart important information from one department to another
- Failure to write legible medical orders

One way for health care providers to evaluate their charting is to view it as an attorney might ask, if it were presented as evidence to a jury, would it be thorough and convincing?

TABLE 10.5   What Plaintiffs' Attorneys Look For in the Medical Record

Vague, ambiguous, or contradictory statements open to interpretation

Incomplete or sparse records that fail to demonstrate consistent, attentive care

Failure to address discrepancies in observations made by other clinicians

Failure to follow up on recommendations made by other clinicians

Failure to address signs or complaints of distress

Criticisms of the care rendered or perceived mistakes made by other practitioners

References to incident reports, risk management activities, quality assurance meetings, or peer review procedures

Omissions, including but not limited to missing laboratory test results, radiology results, EKG strips, etc.

Erasures, use of liquid correction fluid, or any other attempt to alter the record

Inaccuracies or inconsistencies that can be used to infer substandard care

Words and phrases with multiple meanings or possible interpretations

Any loose ends that can be used to imply negligence or substandard care

Lack of supervision

Alterations

Lack of informed consent documentation

Lack of patient education documentation

Illegible entries/signatures

Time delays and unexpected time gaps

Liability issues specifically concerning medical records include but are not limited to:

- Record authentication
- Record retention
- Record destruction
- Access to medical records
- Release of confidential information
- Release of information in litigation
- Electronic record security

Documentation issues that help jurors make decisions about cases include:

- What is reasonably expected of the health care professional's peers?
- What is in accordance with the standard of care?
- How does it reflect upon the quality of care provided?

A medical record can be used in the affirmative defense of a claim if it:

- Documents all relevant medical information
- Substantiates the rationale for care provided or not provided
- Highlights the interaction between professionals
- Creates a timeline for care rendered
- Documents the psychosocial needs and concerns of the patient and relevant others

- Preserves the medical history of patient care
- Is more reliable than personal recollection
- Demonstrates good communication
- Demonstrates quality medical care

Protecting Privileged Information

Documents that can remain protected from discovery in legal proceedings are defined by each individual state. Risk management professionals should explore state statutes for particular information about which documents are considered privileged information. Types of records that can be privileged include, but are not limited to:

- Incident reports
- Risk and quality management committee minutes
- Incident investigations
- Corrective action plans
- Root cause analyses

The specifics of whether or not a particular document remains privileged also should be explored. For example, if the document is typically protected from discovery, or if it is shared with a third party, the privilege may be waived. Risk management professionals and medical records personnel should coordinate efforts to ensure that the proper protections are effective and in compliance with federal and state statutes.

Forensic Documentation Examination

For many years forensic documentation techniques have been used to analyze handwriting, signatures, and chronology of entries. The techniques have not changed, but the scope of the analysis has broadened. The following is a brief list of such forensic methods, which can be used in support or defense of a claim. For more information, a knowledgeable defense attorney should be contacted.

Electrostatic Detection Apparatus   This equipment can detect latent impressions on the underlying pages of a document that have been amended. The advantage is that it provides a hard copy; the disadvantage is that the equipment is not portable.

Ink Analysis   This technique can be used if there is a possibility that the medical record was altered. It is the only method to establish identifiers of the ink type used for entry. The advantage is that it may provide conclusive evidence of fabrication if the ink contains certain markers; the disadvantage is that because tiny ink samples are lifted from the original document, damage does occur. Many types of ink have not been tagged and there is no standardization.

Infrared Exams   This type of tool is used to identify ink types but cannot be used to show that inks are the same. The advantage is that it does not destroy the document. The disadvantages are that the equipment is not transportable, so original documents must go to a laboratory, and the exam cannot distinguish among all ink types.

Identification of Date Markers Date markers can identify most paper copy machines, printers, and typewriter ribbons. An advantage is that it is objective and reliable; however, it is very time-consuming.

Handwriting Analysis If an expert handwriting analysis is undertaken, risk management professionals must ensure the integrity of the chain of custody of evidence. Often, this requires hand-carrying the original medical record or documents to the analyst and remaining with them until they are returned to the original custodian. The custodian may be called upon to testify to the maintenance of this chain of custody of evidence.

Documentation and Litigation

The medical record is a critical legal document. In a malpractice lawsuit, the patient's medical record demonstrates the quality of care provided. It describes (or fails to describe) acts, events, conditions, diagnoses, and opinions at or near the time of the alleged malpractice event. The following cases illustrate the medical record's importance in the courtroom:

- In *Cruz v. West Volusia Hospital Authority d/b/a West Volusia Memorial Hospital,* Volusia County, Florida Circuit Court No. 95–10313 (1997), the nurse failed to inform the obstetrician of fetal distress or document it. As a result, the baby suffered hypoxic ischemic encephalopathy. The parties reached an out-of-court settlement for $2,425,000.

- In *Cloughly v. St. Paul Fire and Marine Insurance Company, Washington County,* Arkansas Circuit Court, Case No. C1V95–996 (1997), neither the hospital nor the nurse documented how a portable ventilator was set up, and there was no record that oxygen saturation readings had been taken. A $2,125,000 settlement was reached before trial.

- In *Toinkham, Administrator of Estate of Muncey, v. Mt. Carmel Health d/b/a Mt. Carmel East Hospital,* Franklin County, Ohio, Court of Common Pleas, Case No. 94CVA-09–6736 (1997), the plaintiff's attorney alleged that the nurses did not properly assess, monitor, and care for the patient before and after the injection of morphine because these actions were not documented in the medical record. The patient was later found in total cardiac arrest and could not be revived. A $433,415 verdict was returned at trial.

Table 10.6 will identify for the risk management professional, chart components that may be of interest when evaluating liability.

In Anticipation of Legal Action

The following tips may be useful if legal action is anticipated:

- Follow the organization's claim reporting procedures.
- Secure all pertinent records.
- Release a copy of the record only after receiving a written request and signed authorization, in accordance with organizational policy.
- Before releasing the medical record, seek to obtain the specific components of the medical record that are needed by the requestor and only release those portions that are requested.
- Never change a record in any way once a copy has been released.

TABLE 10.6   Essential Charting Components of Interest to the Health Care Risk Management Professional

Nursing observations and assessments	General demeanor/affect
Appearance	Activity and restrictions
Height and weight	Vital signs
General physical condition	Mental state
History of past hospitalizations	Medication administration record (MAR)
History of past surgery, anesthesia, and any complications	Discharge plan
Allergies	Dietary restrictions
Reason for admission/presenting complaint	Physical or cultural disabilities
Preferred language	Skin condition
Instruction provided to patient/resident and family (including opportunities for them to ask questions, return demonstrations, any specific instructional materials provided)	Discharge instructions: diet, activity, medications, skin care and hygiene, specific treatments indicated, referrals, follow-up appointments
Problem list	Consents
Physicians' orders	Ancillary provider notes/consultation reports
Relevant health risk factors	The patient's progress, including response to treatment, change in treatment, change in diagnosis, and patient non-compliance
Intake and output	

··········

EMERGING RISK EXPOSURES

Although the basic principles of documentation remain the same, new forms of documentation require an examination of related risk exposures.

Electronic Recordkeeping

Department of Health and Human Services Secretary Mike Leavitt told the House Appropriations Committee that he "sees a day when every American can have access to an electronic health record."[31] This commitment is also reflected in President Bush's fiscal year 2006 budget proposal that includes $125 million for health information technology.

Electronic medical records are discussed in more detail in Chapter 14. It is sufficient to mention that electronic medical records have been developed to help reduce costs and improve care. This type of database will eliminate the need for physicians to repeat certain tests, and it will allow them to find out which medication a patient is taking.[32] Nevertheless, hospitals are challenged with making the transition. Cedars-Sinai Medical Center in Los Angeles, California, shelved its $34 million computer system after three months, following "full-blown staff rebellion in the fall of 2002." Some of the barriers identified with implementation included:

- Poor technology ("clunky and slow");
- Only a few of the 2,000 doctors with privileges at the hospital were involved in developing the system;
- Training was insufficient; and
- Culture change.[33]

With the advent of electronic medical records, policies and procedures need to be reviewed to accommodate new considerations, such as corrections in the medical record. Hospitals must be able to strike a balance between the benefits of the technology and the method and pace of implementation, always with an eye on safety.

Computerized Physician Order Entry (CPOE)

Today, about 6 percent of hospitals nationwide have computerized systems for doctors' orders.[34] Hospitals that are complying with the Leapfrog Group's recommendation that hospitals issue voluntary reports on progress in implementing computerized order entry systems and other measures to improve safety have reported that they have eliminated virtually all transcription errors by going to electronic physician ordering.[35]

However, more than 90 percent of prescriptions are still written by hand, and researchers have found that computer systems are prone to make twenty-two types of medication errors (for example, selecting the wrong patient file because names and drugs are close together or because patients' names do not appear on screens; different doctors using the same terminal, so if one fails to log off, a prescription could go to the wrong patient).[36]

As reported in 2005, a study that analyzed the effect of computerized order entry systems on medical errors at the Veterans Administration Medical Center in Salt Lake City found that the VA's CPOE system was able to eliminate mistakes from illegible handwriting and could offer simple advice, such as avoiding drug interactions, but it was not "designed to provide more sophisticated advice on drugs, dosages and patient-monitoring strategies that might have averted harm." Another study at the University of Pennsylvania hospital corroborated these findings. The studies highlighted "strikingly high numbers of adverse drug events" and "many potential glitches" in a CPOE system.[37]

Risk management professionals are cautioned to carefully evaluate the risks and flaws of any CPOE system and encouraged to contribute to contingency solutions.

Medical Record Database Privacy Issues

In May, 2005, California health officials notified 21,600 Medi-Cal beneficiaries that a laptop containing their personal information had been stolen. In response, state Sen. Jackie Speier (D) said she will introduce a bill that would require California agencies and contractors to encrypt all personal information stored on laptops.[38]

....
RISK MANAGEMENT PROFESSIONAL'S ROLE

The risk management professional should be vigilant in assessing the quality of medical record documentation, looking for opportunities to enhance the value and quality of the medical record.

The following are some suggestions to the risk management professional for addressing documentation issues:

- Review incident patterns and trends for documentation issues and problems throughout the organization.

- Evaluate on a regular basis the effectiveness of the organization's documentation style and format.

- Review annually all forms, policies, procedures, protocols, and standards relating to documentation in the medical record.

- Review the minutes of the medical records committee and closed records review proceedings to assess the response to previously identified concerns.
- Contact defense counsel for advice on documentation issues that have been identified in claims, and obtain a copy of pertinent documentation case law.
- Review the protocol for handling inappropriate documentation.
- Familiarize yourself with current federal and state statutes, Medicare Conditions of Participation, and other standards regarding documentation.
- Develop a collaborative relationship with the medical records department personnel responsible for coding medical records and for responding to subpoenas and requests for records.
- Incorporate risk management and documentation issues as part of the general orientation for all new employees.
- Conduct random audits of medical records to identify documentation issues.
- Develop a collaborative relationship with transcription services and include them in the auditing process.

With the increased pressure to be cost efficient, the necessity for real-time access to information, the advent of telemedicine, the development of the electronic medical record, all coupled with an increasing array of delivery sites, the risk management professional is required to maintain an understanding of evolving documentation risks and challenges.

CONCLUSION

As one of many health care business documents, the medical record can be the organization's strongest ally in providing quality care. It can also be its worst enemy if improperly prepared or maintained. Ensuring the appropriateness, thoroughness, and timeliness of medical record documentation is a significant loss prevention activity that should be undertaken by the risk management professional. The medical record leaves the one lasting documentation of patient care. It is the primary document in which health care information about a patient is recorded.

Proper documentation enhances good health outcomes. Patients and residents receive quality nursing and medical care based on a documented assessment of their needs. Medical records can be more than the sum of their parts.

Endnotes

1. *Hospital Accreditation Standards,* Joint Commission on Accreditation of Healthcare Organizations, 2005.
2. *Joint Commission Update,* American Hospital Association, 2005.
3. *Hospital Accreditation Standards* I.M.6.10, I.M.6.20, I.M.6.30, I.M.6.40, I.M.6.50, and I.M.6.60, Joint Commission on Accreditation of Healthcare Organizations, 2005.
4. Beicher, T., et al. *Defensive Documentation for Long-Term Care: Strategies for Creating a More Lawsuit-Proof Resident Record,* HcPro, Inc., 2003, p. 10.
5. Beverage, D., et al. *Charting Made Incredibly Easy,* Third Edition, Lippincott Williams & Wilkins, 2006, p. 137.
6. Holmes, H. N., et al. *Documentation,* Second Edition, Springhouse Corporation, 1999, p. 67.

7. *Ibid.,* p. 107.

8. *Ibid.,* p. 70.

9. Beverage, *op. cit.,* p. 97.

10. Holmes, *op. cit.,* p. 11.

11. Beverage, *op. cit.,* p. 70.

12. *Ibid.,* p. 63.

13. Holmes, *op. cit.,* p. 74.

14. Beverage, *op. cit.,* p. 81.

15. *Ibid.,* p. 85.

16. *Ibid.,* p. 50.

17. Worsley, B., "Pointing Fingers is Risky Business," *Medical Liability Monitor,* Nov. 2004, Vol. 29, No. 11, p. 8.

18. MSJAMA Online, "Poor Physician Penmanship," vol. 278, pp. 1116–1117, Oct. 1, 1997.

19. *Vasquez et al. V. Kolluru,* A-103 TX 042 (2000).

20. Friedland, N. "Chemo overdose result of illegible prescription," *The San Francisco Examiner,* April 26, 2005.

21. "Back to the Blackboard: Physicians Must Improve Handwriting Skills." HCPro, 2002. www.msleader.com. Last visited June 2005.

22. "'Handwriting Challenged' Doctors to Take Penmanship Class at Cedars-Sinai Medical Center," *Science Daily Magazine,* April 27, 2000.

23. Monaghan, M. "Physicians get help with poor pen skills," StatesmanJournal.com, March 16, 2005.

24. "Back to the Blackboard: Physicians Must Improve Handwriting Skills," HCPro, 2002, www.msleader.com. Last visited June 2005.

25. MSJAMA Online, "Poor Physician Penmanship," vol. 278, pp. 1116–1117, Oct. 1, 1997.

26. Brent, N. "How Should I Document a Med Error?" *Nursing Spectrum*—Career Fitness Online, March 3, 2005.

27. Florida Administrative Code 59S-8.005.

28. Beicher, T., et al. "Common Medical Record Omissions and Pitfalls of the Pen," *Defensive Documentation for Long-Term Care: Strategies for Creating a More Lawsuit-Proof Resident Record,* Chapter 8, HcPro, Inc., 2003.

29. "Practice Brief: Retention of Health Information." *The Journal of AHIMA,* American Health Information Management Association, Chicago, IL, 1998.

30. *Ibid.*

31. "HHS Secretary Touts EHRs, Telemedicine," iHealthbeat, California Healthcare Foundation [www.ihealthbeat.org/index.cfm?Action=dspItem&itemID=109414]. March 4, 2005. Last visited June 2005.

32. "Blue Cross, Cerner Plan Tennessee EMR Database," iHealthbeat, California Healthcare Foundation, May 26, 2005 [www.ihealthbeat.org/index.cfm?Action=dspItem&itemID=111721] Last visited June 2005.

33. Connolly, C. "Cedars-Sinai Doctors Cling to Pen and Paper," Washingtonpost.com, March 21, 2005.

34. *Ibid.*

35. "HHS Secretary Touts EHRs, Telemedicine," iHealthbeat, California Healthcare Foundation, March 4, 2005 [www.ihealthbeat.org/index.cfm?Action=dspItem&itemID=109414] Last visited June 2005.

36. Ritter, J. "Docs' Scrawl Can Endanger Patients," *Chicago Sun-Times,* May 8, 2005.

37. "Wall Street Journal Examines Impact of Computerized Physician Order Entry Systems on Medical Error Rate," kaisernetwork.org Daily Reports, June 1, 2005 [www.kaisernetwork.org/daily_reports/rep_index.cfm?DR_ID=30456]. Last visited June 2005.

38. "Stolen Laptop Contains Information on Medi-Cal Beneficiaries." iHealthbeat, California Healthcare Foundation, May 31, 2005 [www.ihealthbeat.org/index.cfm?Action=dspItem&itemID=111790] Last visited June 2005.

Suggested Reading List and Web Sites (last visited June 2005)

American Health Information Management Association, Documentation for Ambulatory Care.

American Health Information Management Association, Documentation and Reimbursement for Behavioral Healthcare Services.

American Health Information Management Association [www.ahima.org].

American Hospital Association [www.aha.org].

American Medical Association [www.ama-assn.org].

American Nurses Association [www.nursingworld.org].

Beicher, T., *Defensive Documentation for Long-Term Care: Strategies for Creating a More Lawsuit-Proof Resident Record,* HcPro, Inc., Marblehead, MA, 2003.

Beverage, D., Editor, *Charting Made Incredibly Easy,* 3rd edition, Lippincott Williams & Wilkins, 2006.

Centers for Medicare and Medicaid Services [www.cms.hhs.gov/default.asp].

Clark, J. S., RHIA, Technical Editor, AHIMA, Documentation for Acute Care.

Ella, J., RHIT, CPHQ, AHIMA, Documentation and Reimbursement for Behavioral Healthcare Services

Getty, B. and others. "Rx for Handwriting Success: A Handwriting Seminar for Medical Professionals." [http://www.handwritingsuccess.com].

Health Insurance Association of America [www.hiaa.org].

Holmes, H. N., Managing Editor. *Documentation,* 2nd edition. Springhouse Corporation, Springhouse, Pennsylvania, 1999.

Institute for Safe Medication Practice [www.ismp.org].

Joint Commission on Accreditation of Healthcare Organizations [www.jcaho.org].

NSO Risk Advisor [www.nso.com].

Office of Inspector General [www.oig.gov].

Priny Rose Abraham, RHIT, CPHQ, AHIMA, Documentation and Reimbursement for Home Care and Hospice Programs.

11

Basic Claims Administration

Ellen L. Barton

"There is always a great deal at stake in a health care professional liability claim: large sums of money of course, but also professional reputations and even individual careers. With the crisis in medical malpractice and health care liability growing more severe daily, the stakes have never been higher and the need for professionalism in claim management has never been greater."[1]

Given this environment, it is incumbent on the "new" risk management professionals to understand basic claims administration, because they are likely to be involved, at least to some degree, in the process. The purpose of this chapter is to introduce the principles of claims administration and highlight best practices for risk managers new to the process. More detailed information is contained in Volume III, Chapter 10—Claims and Litigation Management.

THE CLAIMS ENVIRONMENT

One only has to read the local newspaper on a regular basis to understand that our society has adopted what some would call "a lottery mentality." Some buy lottery tickets in hopes of winning big money and others sue whomever they can for whatever "wrong" they have incurred in hopes of winning big money. Unfortunately, the latter behavior dramatically affects the health care industry. Although the health care industry is working hard to ensure the delivery of safe care (see Volume II, Chapter 1—Patient Safety), we must continue to deal with claims of patient injury due to the alleged negligence of a health care provider or delivery system.

Commercial Insurance

When a facility is commercially insured for medical professional and general liability, the insurance company generally provides complete claims management services. Such services may include: claims investigation, assignment of a claims adjuster, medical records production, claims management (including the strategy for handling a claim), setting reserves, assignment of legal counsel, settlement discussions, and litigation management (if after suit has been filed, a decision is made to defend the claim). Even if the company retains an outside claims service, it is still the company's responsibility to provide these services. Although it is likely that the risk management professional will be involved in various aspects of the process, the insurance company manages the process.

Self-Insurance

When a facility is self-insured for health care professional and general liability, it is the facility's responsibility to provide the services necessary to manage such claims. The facility may decide to retain a third-party administrator (TPA) to perform some or all of a set of identified services. For instance, the facility may decide to hire a TPA to investigate and manage the claim, including settlement discussions until a lawsuit is filed. Then the facility may assign the case to legal counsel with the TPA having no further responsibility. TPAs generally employ trained individuals who are qualified to investigate claims, review medical records, engage in settlement discussions, and maintain appropriate documentation. Another facility may decide to outsource the entire claims process to a law firm or TPA, and yet another facility may decide to manage the entire claims process internally with appropriately trained personnel. Whatever approach is adopted by a particular facility, it is important for the facility to employ effective claims management practices.

THE CLAIM PROCESS

The first step in the claims process is a *coverage determination.* Just as the owner of a new automobile buys an auto insurance policy to provide coverage for accidents involving injuries to third parties, a health care organization buys medical professional and general liability insurance to provide coverage for medical incidents involving injuries to patients. However, after an auto accident, a determination must be made that the auto accident was indeed covered under the policy. Likewise, when a patient is injured at a health care facility and a claim is reported, it is first necessary to determine that there is coverage. If the facility is commercially insured, the insurance company will make the determination. If the facility is self-insured (through a trust fund, a captive insurance company, or through designated operating funds), an appropriately designated individual will determine coverage in accordance with the facility's policies and procedures. Coverage determinations are important for several reasons: first, to ensure the integrity of the policy language (commercial insurance or captive insurance company), the trust document (self-insurance), or other specified parameters when operating funds are used; and second, to comply with the terms of the facility's or insurance company's excess carriers or reinsurers (see Chapter 15—Introduction to Risk Financing). It cannot be emphasized enough that understanding coverage and reporting requirements is critical to a successful claims management program. The following questions must be answered to determine whether a loss is covered:

Is the Person Involved Covered?   Is the physician employed and thus covered under the facility's medical professional liability policy, or is the nurse working for an agency whose contract requires the agency to provide coverage?

Is the Time of the Loss within the Policy Period?   This is particularly critical with "claims-made" professional liability policies, especially where the policy requires that the date when the loss occurred and the date when the claim was made fall within a particular time period for coverage to apply. (For further discussion on coverage forms, see Chapter 16 on Insurance: Basics Principles and Coverages.)

Is the Cause of the Loss Covered?   For instance, was the injury caused by medical negligence (a "covered loss") or assault and battery, an intentional tort excluded from coverage?

Are the Types and Amounts of Damages Covered?   This specifically refers to compensatory and punitive damages. Many insurance policies exclude punitive damages. Others are silent on the issue, thus allowing state law to allow or deny punitive damages coverage. Compensatory damages are those that compensate claimants for injuries and might include such items as lost wages, medical bills, expected future medical costs, pain and suffering, and so on. The policy, however, will not pay more than the stated limit under any circumstance.

Is the Location Covered?   Most medical professional liability policies will provide coverage anywhere in the world as long as the activities of the "covered" individuals are within the scope of their employment. However, there might be situations where an employed resident physician "moonlights" at a non-affiliated, competing hospital in a neighboring community and the policy does not extend coverage to such situations.

Do any Exclusions Apply?   For example, most if not all professional liability insurance policies exclude assault and battery as mentioned previously, and sexual abuse (or perhaps even allegations of sexual abuse), and other defined causes of loss.

Is there Other Insurance that would Apply to the Loss?[2]   This question is important to answer because many health care professionals purchase their own medical professional liability insurance regardless of their employment situation. Nurses often subscribe through a state or national association program for medical professional liability coverage and might have limits of coverage available separate and apart from the facility's policy. Because of potential coverage conflicts, it is "best practice" for a risk management professional to review specific medical professional liability policy and coverage language as respects the section on *other insurance*. In most instances, this section will dictate how other policies or coverages will be treated for the claim in question. Risk management professionals should develop a complementary policy and procedure addressing how such *personal* (other) coverage will be treated. Within the facility, the primary question to answer is "will the personal coverage be considered *primary* or *excess* to the facility's coverage or will both carriers share in the loss proportionally?" The thought of having additional limits available to pay the claim might be appealing to the risk management professional, but senior management needs to make this clarification known, to avoid causing a serious employee relations issue. The facility's policy on personal coverage should be clearly articulated to avoid any misunderstanding or potential conflicts in the management of the claim.

If a facility is commercially insured and the insurer makes a preliminary determination that there is likely no coverage, the carrier will often undertake to investigate and defend the claim, but issue a "Reservation of Rights" letter in an attempt to preserve the company's right to deny coverage at a later date.

. . . .

THE RISK MANAGEMENT PROFESSIONAL'S RESPONSIBILITIES

The risk management professional's responsibilities in managing claims will depend on a variety of factors: If the facility is commercially insured or self-insured, if the facility chooses to outsource the claims management function, or if the facility has assigned responsibility for the claims process to the legal department. Regardless of the specific responsibilities, the risk management professional should have a thorough understanding of the entire process to assure that claims are appropriately resolved. Thus, the risk management professional needs to ensure that the following functions are appropriately performed:

1. Claims Reporting

- Primary insurer, if commercially insured
- Internal mechanism, if self-insured
- Excess carrier or reinsurer, if applicable

2. Claim Investigation

- Medical record review
- Interviews (coordinate with legal counsel to interview patient, health care provider, witness, and so on)
- Expert review of case
- Initial assessment
- Reserve setting

3. Claims Management Strategy

- Liability determination
- Settle or defend decision
- Claims committee review. (Such review can serve as a quality control mechanism to be certain that the liability determination is accurate and that the decision to settle or defend is prudent.)

4. Settlement

- Documentation (supporting the payment amount)
- Documentation that the approval process was followed

5. Litigation

- Pre-trial and trial strategy
- Coordination on public relations concerns
- Witness preparation
- Decisions and information exchanged during trial
- Post-trial strategy

Claims Adjuster's Responsibilities

Just as risk management professionals' responsibilities vary, so too do claims adjusters' responsibilities, depending on the service agreement between the adjusters and either the insurance company or the health care facility. In most cases, however, if claims adjusters have been assigned to handle claims, their responsibilities will include steps 1 through 5 as outlined above.

Claims Identification and Investigation

The organization's risk management plan will include mechanisms to identify and report potential and actual claims and a method as to how those claims will be investigated and managed. Identification mechanisms include formal systems such as the incident reporting system or informal mechanisms such as information received from surveys, questionnaires, and so on. The initial investigation is an important aspect of claims handling. Regardless of the risk financing mechanism chosen, the risk management professional plays an important role in the investigative process.

Reporting of Claims The reporting of claims is the single-most important step in the process of assuring coverage for any payments that may be required. This reporting happens on multiple levels. First, there is the report of a potential claim from within the facility to the risk management professional. Next, if the facility is commercially insured, there is the report from the facility to its insurance carrier. This reporting requirement and its timing are critical to ensure compliance with the terms and conditions of the insurance policy. Similarly, there also might be instances when reporting to excess carriers or reinsurers (for captive insurance companies) is necessary. Risk management professionals first must understand the facility's risk financing program and then design a process that facilitates the facility's ability to adhere to various reporting requirements. Insurance policies specify the circumstances that require reporting. Unfortunately, the policy wording in the insurance policy that specifies the circumstances for which reporting is required is not always clear and easy to understand. Therefore, the risk management professional, in conjunction with the insurance agent or broker, should clarify the reporting requirements to avoid situations that could result in lack of coverage for failure to report or late reporting. Finally, there is the reporting of a claim that is in the form of a written demand for compensation from a claimant or the claimant's attorney. To avoid these surprises, the facility needs an *early warning claim reporting system* that provides the risk management professional with immediate information regarding facts and circumstances that have caused, or are likely to cause, injury to a patient and may likely lead to payment of money. A facility's incident reporting system may also serve as the claims reporting system. The best results occur when the risk management professional has the trust and confidence of the health care facility and its medical staff and employees regardless of the reporting system. It is generally the phone call or e-mail from within the facility that will signal the need for a formal investigation. Regardless of how the information is relayed, the key is to establish a communication link with the medical and nursing staff and all ancillary personnel. Once the risk management professional has been alerted to an incident or situation that needs further attention, there is a need for a greater formality in communication.

Initial Investigation   If the risk management professional is going to conduct the initial investigation, it is important for any such investigation to be done at legal counsel's direction in order to provide the greatest protection possible for the information gathered. Generally, TPAs working either for insurance companies or for health care facilities will instruct claims adjusters to operate under the direction of legal counsel to gain protection afforded by the attorney-client privilege. Initial investigations play a critical role in determining liability and the anticipated amount of damages. Such investigations should be done as soon as practicable after notice of an occurrence or claim. That is when the most information will be available regarding the facts and circumstances surrounding the injury or potential for injury. This reinforces the importance of *timely* internal notice—notice simultaneous with the occurrence itself, which will provide the best opportunity for a thorough investigation. Witnesses, patients, the medical records, and other necessary documentation are more likely to be available near the time of the occurrence rather than days, months, or even years later.

Interviews and Evidence   "Investigation means assembling, with maximum accuracy and minimum effort, the information and evidence on which the insurer (commercial company or self-insurance trust fund) can determine the position it should take in respect to its legal obligation—or to put it in practical terms, whether to settle, compromise, or deny the claim."[3]

Probably the most common technique to gather information and evidence is interviewing. Interviewing is a skill that can be learned. It is incumbent upon the risk management professional to learn it well, given what is at stake for those involved in the claim. All witnesses—meaning all those who are in a position to provide information that is both relevant and material to the claim—should be interviewed. Thus, the first task is to identify all possible witnesses and obtain contact information. Contact information should include the following: name, address, age, sex, name and address of "emergency" contact (that is, someone who will always know the witness's whereabouts), nationality, phone number, Social Security number, occupation, and current employment. It is also "best practice" to inform witnesses who are also insureds as to the status of the coverage determination and their rights and responsibilities as insureds. Finally, all insureds should be cautioned not to discuss the facts and circumstances of the case with anyone without prior authorization from the risk management professional or legal counsel. Because a claim's life is generally at least several years, it is also "best practice" to regularly update the involved parties as to the status of the case. Doing so also allows the risk management professional or claims adjuster to update contact information that might be needed later.

If an interview is undertaken at the direction of legal counsel, it is important to preserve the information in the most authentic manner possible. The use of an outline or guidelines on questions to ask may prove helpful. The use of *signed* or *recorded* statements, although routinely used in adjusting auto claims, is rare in the context of health care professional liability claims. In interviewing witnesses, the goal is to understand what happened from the witness's perspective. When documenting an interview, it is important for the risk management professional or adjuster to document the witness's view as objectively as possible and without drawing conclusions. This is particularly important because negligence in a health care setting involves the applicability of various standards of care that are usually determined by expert testimony. When interviewing witnesses, the risk management professional or adjuster can take witnesses through the preliminary information by asking a series of questions. Then, the interviewer should allow the witness to tell what happened in the witness's own words. As the witness relates the information, the interviewer can clarify various aspects by asking various *why* questions. For example, if the claim involves a medication overdose and the nurse who administered the overdose is being interviewed, it is important to understand why the nurse failed to adhere to the appropriate protocol. The gentle use of *why* questions is the best method for getting the full explanation. Often initial interviews in health care professional liability claims are not documented simply because many defense attorneys do not want to create a record at this time. Thus, documentation should be undertaken carefully.

Evidence generally refers to medical records, pathology slides, x-rays, and other similar radiographic images. It would also include photographs, diaries or journals, employment records, income tax returns, and physical objects (such as the piece of equipment that is suspected to have malfunctioned). Gathering evidence is particularly important for several reasons: It will help determine liability, it may also help evaluate damages, and it will provide the basis for an *expert* opinion. All evidence in a medical professional liability claim should be sequestered by the risk management professional, and accessed only by authorized personnel. Although interviews of the claimant will produce information regarding the injury (and hence, damages), it will also be necessary to have medical reports written by care providers that define in more objective terms the extent and permanency of injuries and what, if any, additional treatment might be necessary.

Should a lawsuit be filed involving a claim that was previously filed, reported, and investigated, it is incumbent upon those supervising the claims management process to give all appropriate materials from the initial investigation to defense counsel, so that duplication of effort is avoided and conflicting information does not impede the evaluation of the claim.

Claims File Management

Regardless of whether a health care organization is commercially insured or self-insured, it is important for the organization to maintain a claims file. If the organization is commercially insured, there should be agreements about what documents will be kept in which file. For example, if a case is in litigation, the decision might be that all depositions will be maintained by defense counsel, and copies of deposition summaries will be maintained by the risk management professional and the insurance company. There should be a system for naming and numbering the files for easy access for several reasons, including claim audits, auditor's reports, and so on.

Contents   It will be helpful to maintain a sense of order in the file. Regardless of how the claims file is organized, there are distinct general categories of materials that should be maintained as follows:

- Correspondence
- Investigation documentation
- Medical records

- Expert reports
  - Medical research
  - Damages
- Legal papers
- Expenses
- Reserve history

The manner in which the materials are filed should be consistent for all claims files to facilitate retrieval and review. In addition, it might be helpful to prepare a cover sheet for each claim that contains up-to-date information regarding what the claim is about, the status of the claim or litigation, and expense and indemnity history, including payouts, remaining reserves, and reserve dollar change with dates.

Documentation   All documentation maintained in a claim file should be legible and clearly identified. If a risk management professional is uncertain about exactly what materials should be maintained in the claim file, a review with defense counsel should provide the necessary guidance.

Claims Reserving   A loss reserve is simply an estimate of how much it will cost to pay the claim. In addition, reserves need to be calculated for "loss adjustment expenses" (LAE)—the amount of money it will cost to "adjust the claim"—conduct the investigation, review medical records, hire a TPA, pay legal fees, and so on. There is no real science to reserving, and although many insurance companies and TPAs have developed "worksheets" in an attempt to make the process "objective," there is no definitive method to reserving losses. Most often, health care facilities use the individual case method. That is, the claims adjuster, insurance company, or risk management professional sets a dollar amount based on the facts and circumstances of the particular claim. In such cases, the following should be considered:

- Demographics: What is the claimant's age, gender, occupation, level of education, number of dependents?
- Nature and extent of injury: Is it permanent? Was there significant pain and suffering?
- Damages: What are the total medical bills? What type of care or treatment might be needed in the future? Were there any lost wages?
- Is the claimant represented by legal counsel? Does the attorney have a good reputation?
- Liability factors: Was the standard of care breached? If so, do the actions go beyond negligence? Would the facts support a claim for punitive damages? Did the claimant contribute to the injury?
- Are there any comparable verdicts? Are there any legal limits to recovery, such as a cap on pain and suffering?[4]

Obviously it is important to place some monetary value on a claim, to reserve such funds for when payment is due. However, there is another equally important reason to reserve claims: to allow actuaries for both commercial and self-insureds to predict losses into the future and thereby set premiums or funding contributions for alternative risk financing arrangements.

There is a practice called *"stairstepping,"* in which loss reserves are periodically increased by set amounts in the absence of any circumstance that would support such an increase. This practice should be discouraged, because it might improperly inflate not only individual case reserves but also aggregate reserves and *"incurred but not reported"* (IBNR) reserves—those amounts set aside for claims that have occurred but have not been reported yet.

Claims Management Strategy

Although a health care facility may be commercially insured, it is equally important for the risk management professional to be involved in claim management strategy in those situations as when the facility is self-insured because, quite simply, no matter who pays the claim, the *loss history* belongs to the facility. Thus, while a commercial insurance company might argue that a good business decision might involve paying a nominal amount of money to settle the claim, a risk management professional might argue that the good reputation of the facility is worth defending the claim.

Settlement

There is general agreement that when a determination of liability has been made (that is, a duty to adhere to a standard of care existed, the duty was breached, and damages resulted directly from the breach of the duty) it is far better for all parties to reach a settlement agreement. This generally includes paying money, providing additional treatment, and having the claimant sign a release of future liability. It is in everyone's best interest to settle legitimate claims as soon as possible. This generally follows a thorough investigation and appropriate communication with the involved health care professionals, the facility's senior management, and any insurance carrier involved. It is equally important to defend claims that are found to be baseless. This approach supports the integrity of the facility and of the health care professionals who practice within it. Unfortunately, even though there might be a determination of liability, the parties might not agree on the amount of damages, and thus might become unable to reach settlement.

Alternative Dispute Resolution

When settlement between or among the parties is not reached through informal discussions, there are a variety of mechanisms available to facilitate resolution of the claim before filing suit and using the legal system. Among the alternative dispute resolution mechanisms are the following:

- Mediation
- Arbitration
- Private judging
- Neutral fact finding
- Ombudsman
- Minitrial
- Summary jury trial
- Moderated settlement

These mechanisms may be binding or non-binding and some may, in fact, be prescribed by state law as part of tort reform legislation. Remember that using any of these alternative dispute resolution mechanisms is more likely to provide a satisfactory conclusion than would litigation.

The Legal System

The use of the legal system as a claims management strategy should be reserved for those cases in which suit has been filed and the health care facility has made a determination that it has no legal liability for the injuries claimed. Defending such cases sends an important message to the plaintiff's bar and supports the integrity of the claims management process.

. . . .

REGULATORY REPORTING OF CLAIMS

Health care professionals are under enormous scrutiny in the practice of medicine and the delivery of health care. In addition to a facility's peer review and quality improvement committees, there are other entities that are entitled to information regarding the quality of a health care professional's practice.

National Practitioner Data Bank

Organizations and insurance companies who pay money on behalf of a health care provider (physicians, dentists, or other licensed practitioners, such as nurses, or nurse midwives) for injuries sustained by a patient during the course of medical treatment are required to report such information to the National Practitioner Data Bank. (see Volume I, Chapter 9—Physician and Allied Health Professional Credentialing and Volume III, Chapter 16—Statutes, Standards, and Regulations)

Governmental Agencies

The National Practitioner Data Bank also requires the payments described previously to be reported to the appropriate state licensing agency within thirty days of the date the payment was made. Patients might also file claims against physicians at the State Medical or Nursing Board. Such claims are taken very seriously and are generally investigated by members of the Medical or Nursing Board similar to a "peer review" process.

. . . .

CONCLUSION

Once a claim is resolved, it is important to review the various aspects of the case with the involved individuals and others (such as members of a claims committee or patient safety committee) to identify whatever risk management issues might be the basis of future educational sessions, new or revised policies and procedures, or significant systemic change. Thus, risk management professionals' roles in claims administration becomes a necessary component of their responsibilities to promote practices that support patient safety. Health care providers are trained to learn from their mistakes and the risk management professional can play a vital role in assessing the systems that support the practice of medicine and ensure that an atmosphere of continuous quality management with a focus on safe patient care prevails.

Endnotes

1. Cambridge Professional Liability Brochure. [www.cambridgeintegrated.com/claims_svcs/files/CISG_ProfLiab.pdf], Rosemont, IL: Cambridge Integrated Services Group, 2004, p. 17.

2. Hoopes, D. *The Claims Environment,* 2nd Edition. Malvern, Pennsylvania: American Institute for Chartered Property Casualty Underwriters/Insurance Institute of America, 2000, p. 2.8.

3. Johns, C. T. *An Introduction to Liability Claims Adjusting,* 2nd Edition. Cincinnati, OH: The National Underwriting Company, 1972, p. 111.

4. Hoopes, D., *op. cit.* p. 2.18.

Suggested Reading

Hoopes, D. *The Claims Environment,* 2nd Edition. Malvern, PA: American Institute for Chartered Property Casualty Underwriters/Insurance Institute of America, 2000.

Johns, C. T. *An Introduction to Liability Claims Adjusting,* 2nd Edition. Cincinnati, OH: The National Underwriting Company, 1972.

12

A Contract Review Primer for Risk Management Professionals

Peggy L. B. Nakamura

In the ever-changing world of health care organizations, knowledgeable risk management professionals involved in the contract review process are a valuable resource to senior management. The risk management professional protects the assets of the organization through involvement in the contracting process, regardless of when that process begins. Contract review is a proactive risk control activity that uses a systematic approach to minimize the potential for problems. Risk management professionals are best suited for this task based on their training, experience, and knowledge of internal operations. This enables them to focus on areas of liability, insurance, hold-harmless and indemnification, and other risk elements common to many health care contracts such as qualifications of service providers or reporting claims and lawsuits. This systematic approach does not eliminate the need to involve competent counsel in major contracts; rather, the involvement of the risk management professional augments thoughtful consideration of all contractual relationships placing the organization at risk.

To accomplish an efficient review of a contract, the risk management professional must understand the type of contract being considered, the contractual responsibilities (performance) of the various parties, and the importance of identifying the negative consequences if a poorly drafted contract is executed.

This chapter provides the health care risk management professional with basic tools to develop a systematic approach to the contract review process that includes the major areas of liability assumption and transfer through indemnification and hold-harmless provisions, insurance requirements, and standard contract terminology.

....

CONTRACT STRUCTURE

A contract, according to *Black's Law Dictionary,* is defined in part as "an agreement between two or more parties creating obligations that are enforceable or otherwise recognizable at law."[1] A contract can also be construed as an agreement, letter contract, letter of intent, memorandum of understanding, lease, purchase agreement or order, or oral contract.

A contract contains legally binding obligations between two or more parties, and provides one or more of the parties with a legal remedy if another party fails to perform as specified in the document. For a contract to exist, all the legal essentials must be included. The essentials are:

- The parties to the contract are legally (competent) to enter into a valid contract, as individuals or as business entities.
- The contract represents a "meeting of the minds" between the parties.
- There is consideration; a bargained-for exchange of legal value exists between the parties.
- The purpose or object of the contract is legal.
- The contract is documented in writing if required for legal enforcement in that state.

A well-written contract serves to confirm the understanding between the parties and avoids future disagreements about terms, conditions, and definitions critical to the relationship. Contract terms should always be clear should and contain adequate detail to avoid subsequent misunderstandings.

Parties to the Contract

The legal names of all parties to the contract should be listed in the opening paragraph. Once the parties are identified by legal name, a shortened name (for example, "facility," "entity," "contractor," and so on) can be identified and used. The use of this shortened name also should be identified clearly in the opening paragraph and should be used consistently throughout the document. Changing identifying terms (for example, "contractor" to "vendor") within the body of the contract should be avoided. Also, it is advisable to determine the proper contracting party on behalf of the organization (such as subsidiary, affiliate, corporate, or parent) before drafting the contract so that the legal names accurately reflect the entities involved in the contract relationship.

The risk management professional should have ready access to current listings of all subsidiaries, affiliates, joint ventures, and other legal partnerships, that identify the correct legal names and incorporation dates for all potential contracting parties. Articles of incorporation are particularly helpful documents to have available. As DBAs ("doing business as") become more plentiful within health care, it is necessary to know of their existence and basic legal structure. To minimize the potential for new liability created upon incorporation of a DBA, the risk management professional should be notified upon the incorporation of this legally distinct entity.

Performance Expectations

Written performance expectations for both parties, including definitions and timeframes for completion, are key to a successful business relationship and should be memorialized in the contract. The description should be easily understood by both parties, should cover standards for performance, and should contain specific remedies for non-performance. It is important to quantify and qualify, to the extent possible, standards that the receiver of the services will use to determine whether the anticipated service quality has been met. In certain situations, failure to meet the "quality standard" should result in automatic termination of the contract without financial penalty to the receiver of such services.

The performance area is an appropriate section for requiring the contractor to meet Joint Commission on Accreditation of Healthcare Organizations (JCAHO) standards if considered a contract service (for example, security, nutritional services, biomedical engineering, reference laboratory, or temporary staffing agency) affecting patient care delivery in the hospital.

For example, JCAHO standards specify that when patient care services are provided by another source, a patient should receive the same level of performance from that source as from the organization. Leaders must also participate in the selection of sources for needed services not provided by the department or organization.[2] Additional standards apply to quality control processes required in clinical laboratory services, radiology, dietetic services, nuclear medicine, and radiation oncology.

Any health care organization anticipating a JCAHO accreditation survey should consider contract services as a potential—and probable—area of scrutiny. The risk management professional can provide invaluable assistance in this area through:

- The development of requirements for all contracted services and the implementation of a system for contract maintenance.

- A current, well-written contract for each contracted service that includes a requirement for the contractor to meet JCAHO standards, applicable state or federal standards, and licensure requirements or laws, and provision that the contract may be terminated for failure to meet those standards.

- A written job description and a completed competence assessment, evaluation, or appraisal tool for personnel provided through contractual arrangements.

- Clinical privileges for physicians or other eligible individuals to admit and treat patients that are defined by the medical staff when delivering services by contract.

- The contractor's qualifications and competency as they relate to the type of services delivered, and ongoing education or training necessary to maintain the requisite skills (for example, licensure, basic life support, or continuing education), provided and documented.

- The contractor's performance of background screening, including criminal background checks, verification of current licensure, and applicable certifications for all employees performing contract services.

The risk management professional might also consider the addition of appropriate quality control or performance improvement activities, after consultation with knowledgeable professionals in that particular field. These may include specific measurable performance standards and a requirement for the contractor to meet employee health requirements for the organization.

CRITICAL CONTRACT PROVISIONS

Most contracts encountered in health care organizations contain section headings (or provisions) that organize the document and make it easier to review. It is important for the risk management professional to have a basic understanding of "contract vocabulary" before beginning a meaningful review.

Term and Termination

The *effective date* of the contract is the date on which the contract becomes operative, meaning that it has legal force and that the parties are required to perform the contract provisions. The termination date is the date the contract has been fully performed or completed. The period of time between the effective date and the termination date equals the contract term. The beginning, end, and date of signing the contract (execution date) should be readily apparent in the document.

Within this section, the risk management professional should carefully consider automatic extensions or renewals to the contract term. For instance, the following typical provision should warrant further scrutiny:

> This contract shall have an initial term of three years commencing on the date first written above, and shall automatically renew for successive three-year terms.

The risk management professional, when confronted with this provision, should ask the following questions:

1. Is there a provision permitting the termination of the contract before the end of the term?
2. Is there a termination "without cause" clause so that the contractual relationship can be cancelled in the event the business climate has changed?
3. If a termination "for cause" provision exists, does it clearly specify what constitutes "for cause?"

The termination provision should allow as much flexibility as possible, enabling the organization to terminate the contract for reasons of changing need or poor performance.

However, there might be contractual relationships that necessitate financial penalties if a party cancels the contract before expiration of the term. A common example is one in which a party incurs significant costs at the beginning of the term with the anticipation of a long-term commitment, warranting the outlay of "up-front" services such as major equipment installations or relocation costs for individuals recruited to assume a critical role.

Insurance and Indemnification

From a risk management professional's perspective, insurance and indemnification requirements may be among the most critical provisions to review.

Insurance Requirements   Requiring the party(ies) to a contract to procure and maintain insurance is one way to ensure that the indemnifying party (indemnitor) can satisfy the financial obligations arising from the indemnification or hold-harmless provisions. In large part, the type of contract dictates the specific types of insurance that should be required by the contracting parties. For instance, any contract covering professional services should require the service provider to have minimum amounts of professional and general liability insurance. Property, business automobile, fidelity, workers' compensation, and major medical health coverage also are reasonable insurance requirements for many service and maintenance contracts. It is important to consider the possible losses or claims that might arise from the contract performance, and then specify the various insurance coverages necessary to cover them.

The key elements to review whenever insurance requirements are contemplated include: limits of coverage, cancellation provisions, evidence of coverage, financial security of the insuring company,[3] whether parties are named as additional insureds or certificate holders, and whether self-insurance will be accepted in lieu of a commercial insurance policy.

A sample insurance requirement might be that the contractor agrees to secure and maintain in effect, at its own expense, the following insurance:

1. *Commercial General Liability Insurance* for damage to property and injury to, or death of, third parties at limits of at least $1 million for each occurrence of bodily injury and property damage, combined single limits (CSL), subject to aggregate limits of not less than $2 million with an additional insured endorsement naming (ENTITY) as an additional insured on Contractor's policy as respects the contract at hand. Contractor's policy is to provide primary coverage as respects the additional insured (ENTITY), and no contributions will be sought from the additional insured's policies. However, if such insurance is written on a claims-made form, following the termination of this Agreement, coverage shall survive for a period of no less than five years. Coverage evidence shall include a retroactive reporting date preceding or coinciding with the effective date of this Agreement. Contractor shall notify the additional insured of any change in limits, coverage, insurer, or any other change which could diminish the protection afforded as an additional insured on the contractor's policy.

2. *Professional Liability Insurance* with annual limits of not less than $1 million per occurrence and $3 million aggregate. If such insurance is written on a claims-made form, following termination of this Agreement, coverage shall survive for the maximum reporting period available from insurance sources at each anniversary date of such insurance. Coverage shall also provide for a retroactive reporting date preceding or coinciding with the effective date of this Agreement.

3. *Workers' Compensation Insurance* (a) covering all personnel employed to perform services pursuant to this Agreement in accordance with any applicable Workers' Compensation Law and (b) Employers Liability Insurance with a limit of $1 million for each occurrence. Contractor agrees to indemnify and hold harmless (ENTITY) for any and all claims arising out of any injury, disability, or death of any of Contractor's employees, and will request its insurer to issue an endorsement waiving rights of subrogation against the entity.

4. *Business Automobile Liability Insurance* or an equivalent program of self-insurance (owned, non-owned, and hired automobiles included) with a combined single limit (CSL) with no less than $1 million per occurrence.

5. *Fidelity Bond* coverages to cover all acts of dishonesty perpetrated by Contractor's employees or agents, while acting alone or in collusion with others. Fidelity coverage is to be provided on a Commercial Crime Coverage Form A—Blanket coverage basis or its equivalent with limits of at least $500,000. Contractor agrees that to the best of its knowledge all employees working to fulfill this contract are eligible for coverage under said bond.

6. *Commercial Property Insurance* covering its own property on an all risk basis. Contractor waives its right of subrogation against (ENTITY).

Contractor further agrees to secure and maintain in effect for its interest only, contractual liability insurance covering its assumption of liability under this Agreement at a limit of not less than $1 million for each occurrence of bodily injury and property damage CSL.

The foregoing insurance shall be maintained with carriers licensed to do business in the State of _____, and the terms of coverage shall be evidenced by certificates furnished to (ENTITY) along with a copy of the additional insured endorsement.

Both parties agree to comply with all applicable local, state, and federal laws including OSHA.

Insurer Solvency

Within the insurance requirement section, a few phrases may be added to ensure, to the greatest extent possible, that the insurer used by the contracting party will remain financially solvent and able to pay any claims on behalf of its insureds. Language for insurance requirements might be:

> Acceptability of Insurers Prior to commencement of services, CONTRACTOR shall furnish ENTITY with evidence of insurance coverage as required in this CONTRACT and agree that all insurance has been placed with insurers with an A. M. Best rating of no less than A-VII and are also licensed and/or authorized to do business in the state in which services will be rendered.

Amending the Contract

Contracting parties can amend contracts, but the new requirements or contract language should *always* be in writing and signed by both parties. The original contract provisions that now are deleted or changed should be noted in the amendment in addition to a statement in the original contract that all amendments must be in writing and signed by both parties.

From a practical standpoint, many contractual relationships do not always proceed as specified in the contract, and yet the parties are satisfied with the arrangement. For instance, the services provided might change in focus or scope during the contract term and without benefit of a written amendment to the original contract and as signed by both parties. If the receiving party continues to compensate the other party according to the contract terms, a strong argument could be made that the receiving party had given implied consent to the changes in performance and would have difficulty later pleading breach of contract. Contract litigation is expensive and rarely rewarding. Therefore, any changes in the contractual relationship during the term should be mutually acknowledged in writing to avoid subsequent disputes or misunderstandings.

Inspection of Books and Records

Federal law [42 U.S.C. section 1395x(b)(1)(I)] requires that contracts covering services provided to health care entities with a value greater than $10,000 or more during any twelve-month period allow the government access to all pertinent books and records. Sample contract language might be:

> Until the expiration of four (4) years after the furnishing of any services pursuant to this Agreement with a value or cost of $10,000 or more over a twelve (12) month period, CONTRACTOR shall make available, upon written request, to the Secretary of the United States Department of Health and Human Services or the United States

Controller General, or any of their duly authorized representatives, this Agreement, and such books, documents, and records of CONTRACTOR as are necessary to certify the nature and extent of the reasonable costs of services to (ENTITY).

Choice of Law

It is common, and preferable, to have a provision specifying which state law will govern the construction and interpretation of the contract. An example of such a provision is:

This Agreement shall be governed by, subject to, construed, and enforced in accordance with the laws of the state of _____.

Exhibits, Schedules, and Appendices

Often, significant terms of an agreement will be set forth in exhibits, schedules, or appendices to be attached at the end of the agreement. Proper reference must be made to these documents in the body of the agreement. All such attachments should be complete in detail and affixed to the agreement at the time of its execution.

Assignment

Consideration should be given, on a case-by-case basis, as to whether the contract performance can be assigned to another party. If the agreement covers professional, or unique, services, it is often preferable to disallow assignment by the party whose services are sought. Or, organizations within a system might want to preserve their right to assign contractual obligations to a parent or subsidiary entity.

Compliance with Laws and Regulations

This type of contract provision typically specifies the effect that changes in statutes, laws, or regulations might have on the performance of the parties to the contract, and the requirement that the contracting parties comply with applicable laws and regulations. An example, as affecting the Emergency Medical Treatment and Active Labor Act (EMTALA) or state laws regarding the transfer of patients from an emergency department, might be:

The parties to this Agreement shall comply with all applicable federal, state, and local statutes, regulations, and ordinances. To the extent that any provision of this Agreement conflicts with EMTALA or state licensing laws for the provision of Emergency Medical Services and Care or such laws as are amended, the provisions of EMTALA or the state licensing laws, as applicable, shall take precedence over and/or automatically supersede any inconsistent provisions of this Agreement.

Alternative Dispute Resolution

In many business relationships, the parties to the contract may benefit from resolving legal disputes outside the courtroom. Alternative dispute resolution (ADR) is an alternative to conventional litigation. It includes negotiation, mediation, and arbitration. (Chapter 10, Claims and Litigation Management, in Volume III of this series, discusses ADR in more detail.) In many instances, the parties to a contract may insert a clause within the contract requiring mediation of any disputed terms and conditions. Legal counsel should be consulted prior to developing, accepting, or modifying ADR provisions.

············

CONTRACTUAL RISK TRANSFER

One of the most important concepts for a risk management professional to master concerns the transfer (or assumption) of financial risk through contractual provisions. In essence, the contract becomes the governing law with respect to the risks assumed by the parties to the contract. Therefore, understanding the contractual methods of transferring risk is the crucial first step in the process of risk management's review.

Contractual risk transfer may occur in the following provisions of a contract:

- Indemnification or hold-harmless
- Liability limitations
- Subrogation clauses
- Insurance requirements

Each of these provisions serves to restrict, transfer, or require financial risk assumption in a manner specific to the particular relationship embodied in the contract. Careful attention to detail is required as each provision is considered.

Indemnification or hold-harmless provisions contractually require one party (the promisor or indemnitor) to save or hold harmless the other party (the promisee or indemnitee) against the legal consequences of the conduct of another. Generally, any assumption of risk should be limited to actions or activities within the control of the indemnifying party.

Indemnification Provisions

Indemnification provisions may range from the basic and easy to understand to the legally complex, many with confusing terms and responsibilities. However, most provisions can be dissected as to the indemnitor's scope of responsibility and the reasonableness of the risk assumption in the particular contract.

A few considerations for the risk management professional in reviewing the contract include:

- Can the assumption of risk fit into the insurance or self-insurance coverages available?
- What risks can the health care organization afford to assume if coverage is unavailable?
- Will the insurance policy or self-insurance document allow coverage for liability assumed by contract?
- Will the risk assumed through indemnification requirements affect coverage limits for the organization?

In most situations, it is appropriate for each party to the contract to retain responsibility and liability for those contract activities and operations under its control. This includes acts of omission or commission by employees or agents. An ideal contract provision specifies that each party is responsible for its own actions and that the indemnifying party will reimburse the second party for costs incurred as a result of the indemnifying party's negligence.

One example of basic mutual indemnification language follows:

> Each party, Health Care Entity and Contractor, agrees that with respect to any claim or lawsuit arising out of the activities described in this contract, each party shall only be responsible for that portion of any liability resulting from the actions or omissions of its own directors, officers, employees, and agents.
>
> Each party, Health Care Entity and Contractor, and its respective directors, officers, employees, and agents, shall defend, indemnify, and hold harmless the other party from and against any and all liability, loss, expense, reasonable attorneys' fees, or claims for injury or damages arising out of the performance of this contract, but only in proportion to, and to the extent that, such liability, loss expense, attorneys' fees, or claims for injury or damages are caused by or result from the acts or omissions of the indemnifying party.

The risk management professional is well advised to work with legal counsel to develop basic indemnification language, as appropriate, that might serve as a template for contract review. Many contractors or companies are amenable to alternate contract language, if it is provided in a timely and professional manner.

In general terms, there are three types of indemnification and hold-harmless provisions:

1. *Limited*—One party agrees to indemnify the other party if it is sued or incurs expense because of something the indemnifying party did or should have done.

2. *Intermediate*—One party agrees to pay losses and defense costs of the other party if both parties to the contract are liable for the damages.

3. *Broad*—One party agrees to indemnify the other party despite the other party being solely responsible for the loss.

Indemnification and hold-harmless provisions assign to one or both parties the legal consequences arising from the contract performance. Generally, however, it is in the best interests of the parties to the contract that each party is responsible for its own actions, errors, and omissions and that the indemnifying party (indemnitor) reimburses the other party (indemnitee) for losses or damages incurred on behalf of the indemnitor.

Liability Limitations

A liability limitation provision (most often found in architecture, construction, supplier, or manufacturing contracts) transfers risk by limiting the liability of one party in favor of another party. This provision limits the party's liability to a predetermined level or amount of damages, thereby transferring the liability exposure beyond that level to the other party.

Assuming that the health care provider is the recipient of this provision in a contract, it is prudent to consider the reasonableness of the liability limitation and the risk being assumed by the entity. Particular attention should be given to liability limitation provisions regarding errors and omissions, professional acts, breach of contract, personal injury, and property damage. One example of this is when a physician is underinsured (coverage limits are less than the damages awarded against the physician) and the hospital or other health care provider must assume a greater share of the costs due to joint and several liability statutes.

Subrogation Rights

In a subrogation action, an insurer attempts to recover the amount paid to an insured pursuant to an insurance policy from a third party. A waiver-of-subrogation provision in a contract relinquishes the insurer's right to recover from the third party. One common subrogation situation occurs when a contractor's employee is injured on the health care organization's premises while performing services under the contract. When the contractor's workers' compensation carrier receives the claim, it will often pursue a premises liability or negligence cause of action against the organization. A waiver of subrogation would "relinquish" the workers' compensation carrier's right to pursue subrogation against the organization.

As is obvious in this example, the insurer's "rights" are affected. Therefore, parties to the contract should notify their insurer anytime that a waiver of subrogation is included in the contract and obtain authority or approval from the insurer before proceeding.

Implications and Issues for Tax-Exempt Organizations

Internal Revenue Service Revenue Procedure 93–19 has particular significance in contract review involving a tax-exempt-bonds-financed facility and a non-governmental service provider. IRS guidelines set forth its view on the compensation of a *service provider* providing services under a *service contract* to a 501(c)(3) organization. Service contracts may involve all, a portion, or any function of a facility, such as a contract for the provision of management services for an entire hospital or specific department, janitorial services at a facility, or physician services to patients of a hospital.

According to the procedure, the service provider must receive *reasonable* compensation for services rendered, which may not be based on a share of net profits. In addition, at least 50 percent of the compensation must be based on a periodic fixed fee. In the term and termination areas, the term of the contract, including renewal options, must not exceed five years. After three years into the term, the facility owner must be able to cancel the contract for any reason without penalty. And last, the facility owner and the service provider cannot be members of the same controlled group or related parties as defined in the regulations.

As the risk management professional assumes greater responsibility in the area of contract review and file maintenance, it is essential to recognize if the facility is covered by this IRS procedure, and to establish close communication with knowledgeable counsel. It is conceivable that a seemingly innocuous service contract might result in the IRS imposing sanctions on the errant facility.

············

MANAGED CARE CONTRACTS

Many health care organizations now have administrative staff assigned to draft, negotiate, and review managed care contracts. However, this area requires a coordinated approach to best consider the multitude of requirements and provisions that affect the financial viability and operational units of the organization.

What role do risk management professionals play in the managed care-contracting environment? First and foremost, they must be conversant about the expansive risks that an organization assumes when it enters into a managed care contract relationships. Of particular concern are the requirements related to:

- Utilization management and quality assurance (QA) protocols
- Provision for medical screening examination (MSE) in an emergency department (ED) as required under EMTALA.
- Credentialing and privileging of physicians and mid-level practitioners by the managed care organization (MCO)
- Reporting of professional liability claims and lawsuits
- Reporting of actions related to licensure of privileges of facility, staff, and physicians
- Release of historical claims data
- Insurance and indemnification requirements
- Access to peer review and QA committee proceedings
- Financial responsibility in the event of health plan insolvency
- Ability of health plan to remove providers from provider panel
- Appeal processes
- Stop-loss provider excess or risk-limiting protection arrangements

Many health care organizations, particularly those that encompass acute care facilities, fail to consider managed care liability as a significant exposure. However, as health care providers form integrated delivery systems or networks (IDSs or IDNs) or establish business partnerships, ventures, or networks for contracting purposes, the potential for managed care liability expands significantly. For instance, a health care organization that develops an exclusive provider organization (EPO) for its own employees has in essence created its own MCO. The health plan coverage document, pre-authorization requirements, establishment of "exclusive providers" from which the employees must choose, and other administrative processes related to traditional health plans now are a part of the organization's administrative responsibility.

Another example of significant managed care liability exposure is when the health care organization assumes *by contract* delegated functions from a health plan, such as utilization management or provider credentialing. The organization's staff assuming this delegated role must meet the accrediting agency's requirements (for example, the National Committee for Quality Assurance [NCQA]), in addition to any managed care provider manual or policies or procedures detailing the delegated function. Does the contract limit the liability assumed by the organization to that delegated function only? How will this professional service be covered under existing insurance or self-insurance programs? Is the staff that performs this service properly trained, credentialed, and qualified?

Unfortunately, many managed care business liability exposures are not properly identified in the organization's risk-financing program. Once again, the risk management professional can be a valuable resource, identifying new and expanding areas of risk exposure for the organization and integrating risk management concepts, strategies, and techniques into the managed care contracting arena. (Refer to Chapter 2 on Managed Care in Volume III of this series.)

·············
HIPAA: BUSINESS ASSOCIATE REQUIREMENTS

The Health Insurance Portability and Accountability Act (HIPAA) Pub. L. No. 104–191 contains provisions requiring *covered entities* to enter into agreements with their *business associates* whenever *protected health information* (PHI) is disclosed by the covered entity to the business associate. (See Chapter 18, Volume III—HIPAA for an expanded discussion.)

Key Definitions

A *covered entity* is defined in the Final Privacy Standards of HIPAA[4] as a health plan, health care provider, or health care clearinghouse that processes or facilitates the processing of non-standard data elements into standard data elements, or vice versa. A *business associate*[5] can be a person who performs or assists in the performance of a function or activity on behalf of the covered entity involved in the use or disclosure of individually identifiable health information, or a person who provides one of the following services to or for a covered entity if the service involves the disclosure of individually identifiable health information: legal, actuarial, accounting, consulting, data aggregation, management, administrative, accreditation, or financial.

There are several important exceptions to the business associate status requiring a business associate agreement with the covered entity. Members of the covered entity's workforce (employees, volunteers, and trainees), entities that perform services as part of an organized health care arrangement (OHCA), entities that are merely conduits for information (such as the U.S. Post Office), and financial institutions that process consumer payments for health care are all excepted from the business associate definition.

Business Associate Requirements

Each business associate agreement:

- Must establish the permitted and required uses and disclosures of Protected Health Information (PHI)
- May not authorize the business associate to use or further disclose the information in a manner that would violate HIPAA if done by the covered entity[6]

    The business associate must:

- Not use or further disclose the information other than as permitted or required by the contract or as required by law
- Use appropriate safeguards to prevent use or disclosure of the information other than as provided for by the contract
- Report any use or disclosure of the information not provided for by the contract of which it becomes aware
- Ensure that agents and subcontractors agree to the same provisions
- Make protected health information available to the individual who is the subject of the health information
- Make protected health information available for, and incorporate any, amendments as required
- Provide an accounting of disclosures upon an individual's request
- Make its internal practices, books, and records relating to the use and disclosure of protected health information available to the Secretary of the U.S. Department of Health and Human Services

    The business associate agreement must also:

- Authorize termination by the covered entity if the covered entity determines that the business associate has violated a material term

- If feasible, return or destroy all PHI received from the covered entity. If not feasible, the agreement must extend protection of the contract to the information and limit further uses and disclosures to those purposes that make return or destruction impractical.

Risk Management Considerations

The risk management professional is well-advised to actively participate in HIPAA compliance activities related to business associate agreements. Key issues to address include:

1. Is there a current inventory of all covered entity contracts in which PHI is used or disclosed?
2. Is there a written contract in place between each business associate and covered entity?
3. Are there particular provisions in the existing contracts that should be modified or amended to address the use and disclosure of PHI?
4. Is there standard contract language that can be used that includes all of the business associate agreement requirements?
5. Should indemnification and insurance requirements be added to the business associate agreements to reflect this new liability exposure?

Business Associate Contracting Challenges

In addition to the risk management considerations mentioned above, contracting challenges include:

- Identifying all individuals or business relationships falling under the business associate definition
- Developing and implementing a business associate agreement filing system that incorporates file maintenance, monitoring, and sound retention policies
- Modifying the contracting processes to include the negotiation of business associate agreements
- Evaluating the covered entity and business associate relationship so as to properly allocate risk and incorporate contract provisions accordingly

SPECIFIC RISK ISSUES IN HEALTH CARE CONTRACTING RELATIONSHIPS

Additional areas of a health care organization's contractual relationships require the risk management professional's particular attention. These include clinical affiliations, arrangements with temporary or independent contractors, supplemental staffing agencies, consulting services, equipment purchases, construction contracts, and building leases.

Clinical Affiliations

Health care organizations offer students educational affiliations in many departments with a wide variety of clinical experiences. For instance, nursing, occupational therapy, physical therapy, advanced professional training for licensed providers, and other dependent or independent practitioner "on-site" programs occur in many locations every day. There are a few key issues to consider:

- The sponsoring educational institution should specify responsibility for health plan coverage, workers' compensation, and professional liability coverage. Although students may be required to obtain their own professional liability coverage, the limits of coverage and liability responsibility for professional acts should be clearly defined.

- The health care organization cannot transfer responsibility or accountability for the care of its patients to an educational institution despite the presence of students in a clinical area. Therefore, although a student might be assigned patient care duties, the organization's staff must supervise and monitor all care delivered to the patient and not use students as "replacement staff."

This should be reflected in the contract, as in the following wording: "The health care organization retains full administrative and clinical responsibility for the care of its patients. Students and faculty, as participants in this education program, will not replace organization staff and will follow organization policies and procedures in the rendering of patient care."

Additional considerations are:

- The health care organization should be allowed to remove any student from the patient care area for infractions of policy or procedure. Protecting patients from potential injury is of paramount importance.

- The ratio of instructor to student and supervisory responsibility should be clearly noted. For instance, does the facility provide a dedicated individual to fulfill this obligation? Will the school provide faculty on-site to supervise the students?

- Both students and faculty should abide by the facility's policies and procedures including dress code, employee health requirements, confidentiality, and behavior.

- Responsibility for lost or damaged property should be listed in the agreement, with the school reimbursing the facility for lost or damaged equipment or property as a result of student or faculty actions.

- The contract should specify whether the school or facility will be responsible for completing the background criminal screening required by state or federal law.

Temporary or Independent Contractors

Under certain circumstances and applicable federal or state law, an organization may become liable for injuries sustained by a temporary or independent contractor while performing the contract services, particularly in the area of hazardous materials or medical waste handling. Responsibility for the safe handling and disposal of hazardous materials or other medical waste rests with the organization or individual producing such materials, unless noted in the contract. The contract should clearly delineate responsibilities for the handling and disposal of hazardous materials and, if possible, require the employer of the temporary or independent contractor to train its employees accordingly. The organization must decide whether health plan coverage and workers' compensation insurance are to be required for temporary and contract workers, given the scope of services provided.

The contract should also specify that the organization is not liable for any employee benefits, workers' compensation, payroll taxes, and so on for the independent contractor.

However, it might be wise to require the "solo" contractor to have health plan coverage if an accident occurs during contract performance, or to require a company of multiple employees to maintain workers' compensation insurance limits as required by state law.

Temporary Staffing Agencies

Critical to this type of contract is the responsibility of the staffing agency to ensure the competency and qualifications of the staff that it sends to the organization. For instance, a temporary staffing employee previously convicted of a felony assault might create a significant problem for the organization if the agency has failed to "uncover" that employee's history. The unsuspecting health care organization might now expose its patients to a convicted felon and, potentially, an unsafe situation. If the temporary staffing agency has minimal or inadequate coverage for the negligent acts of its employees, or if the contract fails to specify which party has responsibility for claims arising from the services provided by the agency, the organization may become the "deep pocket" or inadvertent responsible party in any subsequent civil action involving the patients.

The staffing agency should perform the initial licensure and competency evaluation of all employees that it sends to facilities under the terms of the contract. However, the receiving facility has a duty to supervise, monitor, and intervene in the temporary staff's patient care activities once they arrive for duty.

Consulting Services

Many contracts for specific consulting services fail to properly quantify the performance expectations as originally intended by the health care organization. Consultants should provide evidence of professional liability, or errors and omission coverage, for their consulting services. Of greater importance, however, is the need for the organization to clarify or articulate its expectations of the consultant's performance. Undoubtedly, many organizations have incurred great expense for consulting services, yet when the consultant's report arrives and the recommendations simply gather dust on a manager's shelf, any benefit to the organization is lost. At the root of this problem lies the inadequate preparation on the part of the health care organization to arrive at a clear understanding of needed services before the contract was drafted or negotiations completed. In addition, the organization should have a clear understanding of how the consultant's recommendations will be used when received. Expectations and performance standards must be clearly articulated and documented before signing any consulting service contract to avoid this frustration and unnecessary expense.

Equipment Purchases

Risk management professionals should become familiar with the process followed in ordering, receiving, and installing new equipment within the organization. In addition, they should understand the organization's equipment exposure by considering the answers to the following questions:

- What warranties does the vendor supply?
- Who, how, and where will the service and maintenance be provided on this equipment?
- If a new upgrade is developed, who pays?

- Who is responsible for patient injury from equipment failure?
- Can the organization pay, at least in part, *after* the equipment is installed and operating as intended?
- Who pays if the equipment malfunctions and no facility services can be provided?
- What would negate a warranty?
- Will the vendor provide emergency service? At what cost?
- What type of notice is required before a service repairman will respond? What is the timeframe?
- Will the vendor train facility staff in the proper use of equipment?
- Can the contract be terminated (the equipment returned) if it fails to produce as advertised? Are there any penalties involved?
- What is the responsibility of biomedical engineering vendors in the area of preventive maintenance and documentation?

Construction Contracts

Because of financial ramifications and local and state building code requirements, among other considerations, the majority of construction contracts will be negotiated and implemented apart from the risk management professional. For purposes of this discussion, the risk management professional is encouraged to request the services of the property insurer, insurance broker, facility operations manager, and local counsel to evaluate the adequacy of the commercial insurance requirements to obtain bonds and secure necessary permits, dispute resolution requirements, and indemnification and hold-harmless provisions. Many property insurers will provide valuable review of construction plans upon request.

Building Leases

A simplistic approach to reviewing a building lease is to ask the following questions and consider whether the "responsible" party in the lease is appropriate:

- Which party is responsible for damage to the building, contents, surrounding property, and so on?
- Who is responsible for pre-existing conditions, such as toxic waste?
- Does each party grant a waiver of subrogation rights?
- Who is responsible for sprinkler damage, fire, earth movement, or flooding?
- If the organization is leasing space to physicians, does the lease meet all necessary requirements?

Once again, building leases most often will involve legal counsel in drafting and negotiating terms. If presented with a lease, the risk management professional is best served by contacting legal counsel for assistance.

Home Care Agencies

A common practice is for the home care agency to subcontract for certain services, particularly when the service volume does not reasonably afford the hiring of such staff (for example, occupational or physical therapy). Therefore, the use of an independent contractor in home care is common, and the provider must be qualified by licensure, education, and training to provide such services. The provider should produce evidence of current professional liability coverage by a certificate representing the amount of coverage and the insured's name. An additional area to consider is the IRS's scrutiny of independent contractor arrangements as it relates to the "control" of the provider's services.

It is important that the home care agency not be misled concerning the qualifications or liability coverage for the contractor, subcontractors, and employees. For instance, an occupational or physical therapist must be knowledgeable and must agree to meet the accreditation requirements of the home care agency. After all, the contractor is representing itself to the agency as being in a provider business and should be held to the provider's standard. Also, it is best to specify the amount of coverage required and to maintain a certificate of coverage with the contract file. In certain instances, the organization may request that the provider's professional liability insurer include the organization as an additional insured with respect to the provider's activities under the contract. This is particularly helpful if the provider is performing direct patient care.

Additional areas of concern in home care are the agency's requirements for client education in relation to medical equipment usage, a medical director's review of practices and policies within the agency, and the safety of employees in the client's home and community. Additional requirements for home care agency contracting may be found in the Community Health Accreditation Program (CHAP) or JCAHO standards, which list contract requirements for the many areas mentioned here, such as applicable standards, licensure required, and evaluation of the independent contractor's services.

....

CONTRACT FILE MANAGEMENT

The key to success in contract review is to establish an efficient system for managing the renewal process and for categorizing the type of contract being reviewed or filed. One suggestion is to develop contract files under the following names: management services, home health, maintenance and repair, temporary staffing, consulting services, professional services, leases, purchase agreements, construction, clinical affiliation agreements, physician-related, managed care, and pending mergers or acquisitions. Within each file, all contracts should be listed by contracting party name, time period, and anniversary date. All requested documentation regarding insurance coverages (such as certificates and additional insured endorsements) should be maintained with each contract in an easily retrievable manner.

A tickler (or diary) system should help the risk management professional to review pending contracts for required certificates of insurance (or coverage) or additional-insured endorsements *prior* to the contract effective date, and should have a process for reviewing contracts well in advance of any anniversary renewal or termination date with applicable notice requirements. Tickler systems can be complex or simple, and can range from sophisticated computer software contract management programs to an entry date on a paper desk calendar. At a minimum, they should list the anniversary date and notice requirement prior to renegotiation or termination. It should allow for adequate time to involve the necessary parties in reviewing the terms and suggesting improvements in performance expectations.

At the time of renewal or renegotiation, the risk management professional should impart to the negotiating parties any newly enacted or contemplated legislation, statutes, or regulations affecting the contract. For instance, Safe Medical Device Act (SMDA) reporting obligations affect many health care organizations, providers, and vendors, yet they rarely are included in the contract specifications.

It is advisable to include a statement in the contract that each party agrees to comply with all applicable federal and state laws, and local ordinances or regulations. However, certain federal or state mandates (for example, SMDA, Patient Self-Determination Act [PSDA],

---

EXHIBIT 12.1   Policy: Contract Review and File Maintenance

POLICY SUMMARY/INTENT:

The process of contract review and contract maintenance is an organized, coordinated process involving affected department managers, responsible directors, and system-wide executives. Contracts are a necessary and important component of health care business relationships and require diligent and thorough review prior to execution and filing.

DEFINITIONS:

1. **Contract:** An agreement between two or more persons (entities, organizations, corporations) that creates an obligation to do or not to do a particular thing. A contract may also be titled: agreement, lease, memorandum of understanding, letter agreement, and purchase order.
2. **Corporate Compliance Program, Contract, and Approval Guidelines:** Entity's policies and procedures regarding compliance with laws governing financial relationships and referrals between affiliates and physicians or other sources of patient referrals or other business.

AFFECTED DEPARTMENT/SERVICES:

1. All system-wide facilities.

POLICY: COMPLIANCE—KEY ELEMENTS

A. Policy:
  1. It is the policy of this facility to comply with the Corporate Compliance Program Contract and Approval Guidelines in their entirety.
  2. It is the policy of this facility to commit to writing all lease, purchase, affiliation, professional service, consulting, independent contractor, and vendor agreements with third parties and to have responsible administrative personnel review critical terms and conditions before signing by a corporate officer.
  3. It is the policy of this facility to maintain all fully executed original contracts in a secure, identified location.

PROCEDURE: COMPLIANCE—KEY ELEMENTS

A. Procedure:
  1. The department manager, or designated contract manager, shall review the proposed contract as supplied by the third party or discuss the critical provisions related to the particular type of contractual relationship under consideration. All questionable or problematic areas shall be highlighted. Any remaining questions shall be referred to legal counsel.
  2. After the above issues have been resolved, the contract will be referred to the appropriate *corporate officer* for signature.
  3. As soon as the necessary signatures have been obtained from all contracting parties, a copy shall be retained in the affected department manager's files and the original sent to the *designated office* for the facility. Contracts shall be retained for the life of the contract plus six years.
  4. The *designated office* will maintain, in a secure filing cabinet, a sequenced list of all contracts, leases, and agreements. The list shall contain: the name of the contracting party, effective date, expiration date, and category of contract.
  5. Responsible department managers shall maintain a tickler file in order to review and renegotiate contracts at least 90 days prior to expiration. During the respective contract periods, key issues and concerns should be referred to the responsible department manager for consideration during renegotiations.

EXHIBIT 12.2   Contract Review and File Maintenance

Type of Contract	Original to:	Duplicate to:
Business Associate		
Construction		
Consulting		
Corporate Compliance		
Equipment Maintenance		
Equipment Purchase		
Independent Contractor		
Leases		
Managed Care		
Professional Services		
Service Agreements		
Student Affiliation		
Supplemental Staffing		
Transfer Agreements		

Occupational Safety and Health Administration [OSHA]) have such a major impact that it is best to delineate each party's actions, to comply with the law and alleviate any misunderstandings as to the appropriate party's responsibility for compliance.

Developing a policy or procedure for the organization related to who may sign contracts on its behalf, maintenance of the contract document, appropriate parties who must review the contract before signing, and the contracts that warrant risk management and legal review is particularly beneficial. Involved managers should participate in the process to some degree because they are key organizational contacts for the contracting party. Further, the person responsible for insurance programs or self-insurance coverages must be included in the process of contract review, preferably before signing the document, to ensure that appropriate insurance or coverage language is used. Refer to Exhibits 12.1–3 and Table 12.1 for sample forms, a contract review and file maintenance policy, and an evaluation tool for service provided by contract.

CONCLUSION

Contracts should not intimidate risk management professionals. By carefully reviewing contracts, considering the language and reasonableness of the provisions, and developing a system for filing and analyzing key contract provisions, the risk management professional will contribute significantly to the avoidance or mitigation of liability for the health care organization. The contract review described in this chapter is limited in scope and in no way purports to replace legal counsel's involvement in contract drafting or negotiating. However, the risk management professional is trained to identify risk exposures for the organization, which should include exposures contained in contracts. The greater the risk management professional's expertise and skill in contract review, the greater the savings to the organization due to decreased use of legal services and decreased liability exposure for the organization.

EXHIBIT 12.3   **Annual Evaluation of Service Provided By Contract**

(Patient Care or Other Outsourced Service)

CONTRACT: _____

INVOLVED DEPARTMENT(S): _____

DATE OF EVALUATION: _____ REVIEWER: _____

REQUIRED ELEMENT/ISSUE	YES	NO	N/A	COMMENTS
Insurance: The service has maintained and provided current information about coverage for the contract service and all providers under the service (Professional, General and Workers' Comp.)				
The service has provided and maintained current information on each provider including:				
Curriculum Vitae/Resume				
License/Certification/Registration				
Evidence of annual updates on OSHA requirement, infection control, etc.				
Other certificates required by position(s) are currently maintained. Please specify: _____ _____ _____				
The contract service has maintained current, comprehensive and appropriate policies and procedures that cover the full scope of services provided.				
Information submitted by the contract service shows that the competency of all contract service providers has been evaluated and the basis upon which the evaluation was conducted.				
Human Resources has verified that the performance evaluation exists.				
The system meets Entity standards.				
Provider-specific monitoring and evaluation results were included in the performance evaluation process.				
Managers of units where contract services are provided contributed information that was used in the performance evaluation process.				
*Contract service providers have received required education regarding blood borne pathogens.				
**Contract service providers have received other annual education updates as appropriate to the services provided.				
***Contract service has provided information, as required by hospital's performance improvement program, in regard to quality control and quality improvement activities.				

(Continued)

EXHIBIT 12.3   Annual Evaluation of Service Provided By Contract *(Continued)*

*If appropriate, contract service providers may participate in Entity-provided annual updates or education provided by contract service will be reviewed by Infection Control Practitioner to assure that Entity standards are met.

**If appropriate, information to be reviewed by individual responsible for Entity education program to assure the Entity standards are met and providers are given necessary education to perform their functions.

***If appropriate, information to be provided by individual who is responsible for oversight of performance improvement activities.

OVERALL EVALUATION OF CONTRACT SERVICE:

_____

_____

_____

_____

_____ Contract to be renewed without changes.   Forward to: _____

_____ Contract to be renewed with changes (see above).

_____ Contract not to be renewed.

Reviewer's Signature: _____   Date: _____

TABLE 12.1   Components of Contract Review

Issue	*Yes*	*No*	*Comments*
IDENTIFICATION OF THE PARTIES			
1. Are all of the parties to the contract identified and are the *legal* names used?	_____	_____	_____
EFFECTIVE/EXECUTION DATE			
1. Can you identify the date the contract terms go into effect and the date it is signed?	_____	_____	_____
TERM			
1. Is the length of the contract specified?	_____	_____	_____
2. Does it renew automatically with mutual party agreement?	_____	_____	_____
TERMINATION			
1. Is the termination without cause?	_____	_____	_____
2. Is it possible to cancel/terminate the contract for failure to perform?	_____	_____	_____
INSURANCE/LIABILITY ISSUES			
1. Are the insurance requirements written to permit self-insurance programs?	_____	_____	_____
2. Are the *types* of insurance applicable to the business relationship?	_____	_____	_____
a. Comprehensive General Liability	_____	_____	_____

(Continued)

TABLE 12.1   Components of Contract Review *(Continued)*

Issue	Yes	No	Comments
b. Professional Liability/E & O	_____	_____	_____
			_____
c. Workers' Compensation	_____	_____	_____
			_____
d. Property	_____	_____	_____
			_____
e. Business Auto	_____	_____	_____
			_____
f. Bonds	_____	_____	_____
			_____
3. Does the contract require that the contracting party (contractor) provide insurance?	_____	_____	_____
4. Are the types of insurance specified, and if so, are the specified types appropriate to the contract services to be provided?	_____	_____	_____
5. Are the required limits of insurance coverage specified, and if so, are the limits appropriate to the potential liability exposure?	_____	_____	_____
6. Does the contract require that the contracting party provide evidence of insurance or a certificate of insurance for each insurance required?	_____	_____	_____
7. Does the contract require that the entity be notified of material change or cancellation of the contracting party's coverage?	_____	_____	_____
8. Does the contract give the entity the right to cancel the contract in the event of insufficient or lack of appropriate insurance coverage as required?	_____	_____	_____
9. Does the contract specify that the insurance requirement will outlive the term of the contract?	_____	_____	_____
10. Is there an appropriate indemnification/ hold-harmless clause based on which party has "control" or ownership of the liability exposure?	_____	_____	_____

(Continued)

TABLE 12.1   **Components of Contract Review** *(Continued)*

Issue	*Yes*	*No*	*Comments*
INDEMNIFICATION/HOLD-HARMLESS			
1. Is the indemnification *mutual*?	_____	_____	
2. Are the parties assuming liability for *only* their own negligent acts?	_____	_____	
PERFORMANCE OF THE PARTIES			
1. Is there a full description of each party's obligations and responsibilities?	_____	_____	
2. Are the financial arrangements understandable and reasonable?	_____	_____	
AMENDMENTS/EXHIBITS			
1. Are all reference documents ("amendments" or "exhibits") attached?	_____	_____	
GOVERNING LAW			
1. Is the state in which the contract terms are implemented or executed the governing law?	_____	_____	
CONTRACT SIGNATORIES			
1. Are the names, signatures, and titles of the parties represented on the signature page?	_____	_____	

Endnotes

1. Black, H. C. *Black's Law Dictionary.* Abridged, Eighth Edition, St. Paul, MN.: West Publishing Co., 2005.

2. Joint Commission on Accreditation of Healthcare Organizations. *2005 Comprehensive Accreditation Manual for Hospitals.* Oakbrook Terrace, IL.: JCAHO, 2005.

3. A. M. Best Company, an independent analyst of the insurance industry, uses financial criteria to rate insurance companies. Factors including profitability leverages, liquidity, assets, and spread of risk are used to determine the rating.

   Every state has a guaranty or insolvency fund to protect insureds and claimants if an insurer becomes insolvent or otherwise unable to fulfill its financial obligations. The funds generally cover only the failure of insurers licensed to do business in that state and offer limits lower than the defunct policy provided. However, such insurer insolvency protection is the best available at this time.

4. 45 C. F. R. 160.103.

5. 45 C. F. R. 160.103.

6. 45 C. F. R. 164.504(e).

Suggested Readings

Benda, C. G., and F. A. Rozovsky. *Managed Care and the Law, Liability and Risk Management: A Practical Guide.* Boston: Little, Brown and Company, 1996.

Clifford, R. C., and B. Sleeth. *Insurance Law Handbook.* Carlsbad, Calif.: Parker and Son, 2005.

ECRI (Emergency Care Research Institute). "Contract Review and Liability Issues: An Overview," *Healthcare Risk Control,* Penn. 2005.

Hall, J. L., and T. A. Williams. "Important Provisions and Features of Any Contract Involving Health Care Providers." *Health Law Handbook,* 1998, pp. 309–341.

Hillman, D. C. "A Primer on PHO Capitation Contracts." *Journal of Health and Hospital Law, American Academy of Healthcare Attorneys.* 29(5), April. December 1996, p. 288.

Ino, A. W. *Managed Care and Capitation Contracting for Home Health Agencies.* Gaithersburg, MD.: Aspen Publishing, 1996.

Keckeissen, F. G., and K. S. Grube. "Independent Contractor or Employee? The Rules and Ramifications of Worker Classification in the Health Care Industry." *Health Law Handbook,* 1998, pp. 413–441.

Miller, T. R., and J. E. Belt. "Conducting a Managed Care Contract Review." *Healthcare Financial Management,* 52(1), Jan. 1998, pp. 40–41.

Pozzar, G. D. *Legal Aspects of Health Care Administration* (9th ed.). Gaithersburg, MD.: Aspen Publishing, 2004.

Wielinski, P. J., W. J. Woodward, and J. P. Gibson. *Contractual Risk Transfer: Strategies for Contract Indemnity and Insurance Provisions.* Dallas: International Risk Management Institute, Inc., 2005.

13

Information Technologies and Risk Management

Ronni P. Solomon
Madelyn S. Quattrone

Health care risk management professionals are witnessing a revolution in health information technology (IT) that is expected to fundamentally transform the delivery of health care and the work processes of health care risk management professionals.

As the patient safety movement gained momentum, the Institute of Medicine's (IOM) 2001 report titled *Crossing the Quality Chasm* recognized that information technology must play a central role in the redesign of the health care system to support substantial improvements in quality and patient safety. "Many medical errors, ubiquitous throughout the health care system, could be prevented if only clinical data were accessible and readable, and prescriptions were entered into automated order entry systems with built-in logic to check for errors and oversights," the report stated.[1] Although it was not the first organization to call for greater automation of clinical data, IOM recommended national health information infrastructure to establish what it called the "rules for the road" for distributing health care data.

Three years later, in the spring of 2004, President George W. Bush, calling for an electronic health record (EHR) for most Americans within a decade, established a new office within the U.S. Department of Health and Human Services (HHS) called Office of the National Coordinator for Health Information Technology (ONC) to coordinate and promote health information technology. Headed by David J. Brailer, M. D., Ph.D., national coordinator for health information technology, the office identified four goals and twelve strategies to guide the adoption of information technology (IT) in the nation's private and public health care sectors. The goals are 1) the adoption of electronic health records; 2) the development of a secure national health information network to permit the exchange of health information among clinicians; 3) the use of personal health records; and 4) the improvement of public health through quality measurement, research, and

CDC

dissemination of evidence. Indeed, HHS envisions the years ahead as "the decade of health information technology."[2]

In May 2005, the U.S. Government Accountability Office (GAO) reported on HHS's efforts to develop a national health IT strategy and to identify lessons learned from the Department of Defense (DOD), Department of Veterans Affairs (VA), and other nations' experiences in implementing health care IT. States are also beginning the process of building health IT networks to share health information statewide, raising concern that different health IT systems in different states and in different hospitals may not be able to "talk to each other." In June 2005, a bipartisan legislative initiative, Senate Bill 1262, known as the "Health Technology to Enhance Quality Act of 2005," was sponsored by Rep. Sen. Bill Frist and Dem. Sen. Hillary Rodham Clinton to spur the development of national health IT standards for the electronic exchange of health information. The bill would also provide financial grants to measure the quality of care provided to patients and to develop the infrastructure of health IT systems.

Industry standards for EHR systems are in need of development and should be adopted so as to allow data to be shared as envisioned by the IOM. Indeed, electronic data storage that employs uniform data standards will enable health care organizations to comply more readily with federal, state, and private reporting requirements, including those that support patient safety and disease surveillance.

To encourage the implementation of EHRs among physicians participating in the Medicare program, the Centers for Medicare and Medicaid Services (CMS) announced that beginning August 2005 it would offer participating physicians—free of charge—a simplified version of EHR software that has been used by the Veterans Administration (VA) for two decades. CMS estimates that by choosing Medicare software, a typical five-physician office practice could save more than $100,000. High start-up costs for purchasing and installing software are frequently cited as a major reason for physician practices' relatively slow adoption of EHRs.

Digitally transforming hospitals, health care services, and physician office practices raises complex issues. IT managers, users, and even IT staff become prophets of the doctrine of unanticipated consequences. Risk management professionals should become familiar with health IT generally, and should prepare thoughtfully for the benefits and risks of electronic technology, whether related to clinical information systems, electronic incident reporting systems, or other health IT applications. Artful risk management professionals will embrace and will benefit from the new information technologies while helping their organizations to set and maintain the standards that govern their use.

This chapter will inform risk management professionals about current and emerging health IT applications, and will look at health IT from three perspectives: 1) ways in which risk management professionals themselves might use IT, 2) ways in which clinical staff might use IT to improve safety and reduce loss, and 3) general risk management issues that are raised as organizations switch to an electronic environment.

············

RISK MANAGEMENT INFORMATION NEEDS

Today's risk management programs require more data, and data from more sources, more frequently. They require creating new loss prevention and control programs for various care settings and liability exposures. To be effective, these programs must be alert to the ever-increasing and changing laws, regulations, clinical practice guidelines, best practices, and evidence-based safety recommendations that ultimately bear on the organization-wide risk management program and its liability exposure. Whatever IT system or programs are used in risk management, the goal should be to turn data into meaningful information that supports the risk management program through effective risk management action.

As health care risk management expands its reach, the number of risk management staff is likely to remain the same, or even decrease in some organizations. Risk management professionals will have to broaden their base of knowledge, understand various health IT applications, and develop new approaches to risk management that foster collaboration with patient safety, quality assurance, performance improvement, legal and regulatory compliance, and other relevant departments and programs within their organizations. As a result, risk management professionals have a need for automated programs and systems that not only capture data from multiple sources, but also produce meaningful and timely reports. Indeed, the failure to adopt new systems might reduce the value—real and perceived—that risk management brings to the organization. Unlike electronic incident reporting systems, manual systems typically are incapable of decreasing time lag, making it difficult to implement a rapid response program. The time lag that occurs when manual systems are used can inhibit timely data analysis and trending, loss control initiatives, and decision making. Ultimately, the use of manual risk management systems might make it impossible to demonstrate reduction in the overall cost of risk.

Health care risk management professionals have many IT needs. The core need is to review the right information at the right time to make the best decisions. Risk management professionals need:

- Tools that automate various risk management processes, such as identifying and analyzing incident and loss information, and performing organizational risk assessments
- A knowledge bank of credible information that underpins risk reduction strategies and helps to promote risk management and patient safety initiatives to others
- Automated ways of gathering the intelligence that will enable a shift from general risk management assessments and evaluations to more focused and in-depth analyses of specific areas of risk that have high payback potential

Information technologies, many with Web-enabled modules, can support these risk management needs. Computer technologies can also help spot problems that were previously unidentifiable and can facilitate efforts to improve the quality and safety of patient care. For example, in performance measurement, automated assessment provides significant advantages over manual review of medical records. Electronic review of EHRs has also been shown to be more accurate, systematic, and efficient than manual review of paper medical records. Automated review systems also eliminate human error caused by fatigue, inattention, difficult-to-read handwriting, buried information, missing data, and the like. Electronic systems have the power to assess archived data quickly, and within minutes, assess data and information that would take weeks or even months to review by non-automated means.

Computer automation is a key to effective risk management. Automated tracking and trending, filing and retrieving information, performing statistical analysis of data, performing risk assessment surveys, electronic claims management, tapping into electronic libraries, and communication with peers through computer listservs, e-mail, and discussion forums are critical tools for today's risk management professional. It can be expected that risk management IT applications will have a significant payoff. Real-time electronic reporting of "near misses," for example, might trigger timely pro-active risk assessment and result in the preventions of losses.

....

RISK MANAGEMENT INFORMATION SYSTEMS

Many health care facilities use some form of risk management information system (RMIS) that automates many aspects of record keeping. Mergers, acquisitions, and joint ventures also have increased the need for RMISs, particularly those with network capabilities that serve multiple sites and locations. These software systems are critical for corporate risk management professionals who have responsibilities for multiple institutions.

RMISs consist of computerized databases which, simply put, are comprehensive collections of information. Risk management data might include incident and occurrence reports, claims tracking and claims administration data (for workers' compensation, professional liability, general liability, directors' and officers' liability, and other claims information), insurance policy information, reserve data, regulatory compliance information, survey reports, patient complaints, litigation management information, and so on. Basic RMISs typically have the capability of data collection and consolidation, data analysis, data reporting, and report circulation, and may permit remote access.

Off-the-shelf and customizable RMISs are available from software vendors or can be developed to meet an organization's specific needs by in-house IT staff. Some insurance carriers, brokers, third-party administrators, and management service organizations also offer specialized RMISs. Regardless of the source of the system that is used, risk management professionals should work closely with IT staff in reviewing or developing software specifications, ongoing support services, data entry and maintenance requirements, Web interfaces, and other key characteristics. Special needs and expectations are best discussed before purchasing software and at the outset of a development project.

Computerized and Web-based incident management systems that provide real-time access to incident data and reports are used in many health care organizations. Web-based systems allow for quick "point and click" entry using standard browser technology at any computer site in the organization. Reporting forms often consist of highly categorized fields using check boxes or drop-down menus. Once a report is entered, the data is immediately available to the organization's management and leadership. Access to information is by authorization and typically varies by job duty: only frontline staff will have the ability to access the reporting form and enter data; department managers might have access to individual and aggregate information on reports filed by that department, and be able to enter or update information; risk management professionals would likely have full access to all reporting information and the analytics.

Paper incident reports may take months and even years to reach the risk management professional's office and get logged into a system. In contrast, online reports facilitate immediate action and investigation, and daily review of reports. The standardization and taxonomy provides better, more accurate data that leads to better analysis. From a security and confidentiality perspective, online reporting permits limitations on who can view, who can print, and who can enter or update data. It also offers better controls on the circulation of reports. System controls also prevent others from deleting or changing data, or "losing" a report.

Interactive Web-based assessment tools are available to help with proactive analysis, often in high-risk or specialized areas. These tools may include questionnaires along with the evidence base that would support the optimal answer. Benchmarking of results may be available if many organizations participate in the assessment program. When assessment results are automated into a computerized database, new benefits arise. A key advantage is the ability to integrate and sort information located in different parts of the overall data collection. This helps to transform risk management data into risk management information. A database system has the capability to retrieve and display records, to extract subsets of data, and to produce formatted reports. Each use, however, must be carefully planned to ensure that it will generate accurate, useful, and effective reports.

Using Information Systems to Generate Reports

When envisioning reports, risk management professionals should consider who should be authorized to receive them, how they will be used, and how often they will be produced. With these facts in mind, they can decide what sources of data should be used and how best to present data (in graphics or in narrative form).

Risk management professionals should consider what factors should be tracked and analyzed. These will vary depending on whether it is an incident reporting, claims management, risk assessment, or other system. The list of elements that can be captured by electronic information systems is endless. The following examples illustrate the types of information that electronic systems typically report:

- Insurance policies and coverage limits
- Newly reported losses or incidents
- Losses or incidents by department or service
- Losses or incidents by date reported
- Losses or incidents by date of occurrence
- Loss costs by accident type or part of body
- Current status of open claims
- Incident frequency by job and location
- Number of employee injuries or patient incidents
- Types of employee injuries or patient incidents
- Lost work time
- Actual medical costs versus average costs
- Most frequent and most expenses causes of loss
- Reserves
- Allegations
- Staff involved in incident or claim
- Patient characteristics
- Names of attorneys
- Names and contact information for witnesses
- Insurance carriers
- Status of the claim
- Actions taken

....

INTEGRATING RISK MANAGEMENT, QUALITY ASSURANCE, AND PATIENT SAFETY

Risk management professionals, patient safety officers, and others involved in quality assurance (QA) should recognize the capabilities of EHR systems to facilitate better and safer patient care, and work together to develop strategies that will take advantage of the technologic capability of EHRs. Interoperable electronic information technology allows different systems to "communicate" with each other. QA information that is captured electronically from routines in daily practice, rather than from reports generated by reviewing medical records, can be referred to risk management and patient safety systems. The transfer of information among risk management, patient safety, and QA systems helps foster effective follow-up on patient safety issues and facilitates proactive risk assessment.

Certain indicators that are tracked for safety and QA purposes should be referred to the RMIS (for example, dental injuries or ocular injuries in the operating room). This information could indicate the need for risk management investigation or for setting up a potential claim file. Conversely, risk management incident trending reports can be incorporated into the QA and patient safety systems. Reports can be coded numerically with selected factors, such as the date, location, individual who assessed the patient, and follow-up information.

....

ELECTRONIC MAIL

The use of electronic mail (e-mail) has burgeoned over the past decade. Few risk management professionals today can envision working without it. The use of e-mail, a means of communication by and between health care providers, patients, health care organizations, and staff, is a revolutionary cultural change. An increasing number of hospitals and physician practices have public Web sites that facilitate direct e-mail communication with staff. Through e-mail, individual providers interact with patients, communicate with pharmacies and hospitals, and consult with colleagues and subspecialty physicians across the globe. A nationwide telephone survey conducted in April 2005 by a marketing information firm and reported in the *Washington Post* on June 7, 2005,[3] showed that about 31 percent of all practicing pediatricians use e-mail to communicate with their patients' parents.

E-mail has many advantages over traditional paper-based mail and voice messaging. E-mail messages can be sent at any time, and recipients can collect their e-mail when they want, from wherever they are. It is easier than writing, printing, proofing, addressing, and stamping a letter. In contrast to voice messages, which typically contain brief contact information, e-mail facilitates communication of detailed messages and makes it easy for recipients to reply to the sender and to forward the message or reply to others. Because of its unique characteristics, e-mail communication between health care providers and patients raises risk management, legal, and regulatory concerns about confidentiality, privacy, and medical record documentation.

For example, although the details of what is communicated by telephone between physicians and patients are rarely recorded and preserved, e-mail communication between the patient and a health care provider can be "saved" electronically and preserved in paper form by sender and recipient alike. Because e-mail can be intercepted, or inadvertently sent to persons not intended to receive it, confidentiality and privacy of e-mail health communication might be jeopardized without appropriate safeguards. The timeliness of replies to e-mail communication requiring a rapid response can be delayed if e-mail systems go down or if messages are delayed by heavy Internet traffic. Written policies and procedures are needed to facilitate compliance with applicable federal and state laws and regulations concerning the privacy, security, and confidentiality of individually identifiable health information communicated by e-mail.

Risk management professionals should participate in drafting and updating their institutions' e-mail policies and procedures, noting guidelines such as the American Medical Association's guidelines for physician-patient e-mail, and applicable federal and state law and regulatory mandates concerning health information privacy and security. Policy should require that e-mail concerning the patient's health care be preserved electronically or printed in hard copy if paper medical records are maintained and made a part of the patient's medical record in accordance with sound documentation and record-keeping practice.

INTERNET- AND WEB-BASED TECHNOLOGY

The Web is rapidly transforming the way clinicians communicate, document, treat, and diagnose. Physicians can get online access from their homes or offices to laboratory and radiology results, pharmaceutical profiles, clinical pathways, and medical references. A system that permits patients with implantable cardiac devices to send clinical information to their physicians over the Internet can result in more timely and efficient monitoring, thus potentially improving patient care. The technology is made up of a handheld monitor that patients hold against their chest to capture electronic signals from the implanted device. The monitor is connected to a small console that resembles an external modem from a personal computer. The console automatically downloads the data from the implanted device and transmits it over a standard telephone line directly to a secure server. The system has two secure Web sites, one for physicians and one for patients, where clinical information can be accessed.

Health care information technology is poised to play a major role in advancing communication of health information between patients and their health care providers. Until recently, the paper medical record was rarely freely shared with patients. Now, large health systems and health maintenance organizations (HMOs) are taking steps to implement EHR systems that will make patient records available to physicians and patients through the Internet.

PERSONAL HEALTH RECORD

Most people who maintain a personal health record (PHR) create paper records, or do so electronically by typing or scanning their personal health information into software applications and storing the information on personal computers. Newer, more sophisticated Web-based services now allow individuals to maintain their health information in online accounts that include e-mail, document sharing, video-conferencing capability, and access to the individual's health information from Internet-connected devices. Some applications give individuals the option of allowing their health care providers and hospital emergency departments access to their electronic PHR, which may include information that is not otherwise readily available, such as end-of-life advance directives. Some systems would also allow providers to enter health care data directly into the PHR. These and similar products are being made available to the public by several entities, such as the medical association-affiliated Medem, and the American Health Information Management Association (AHIMA).

In the near future, technology solutions will allow seamless integration of health information between EHRs and PHRs. Information such as test results could be directly entered into PHRs from EHRs and communication via the Internet and e-mail might become a preferred means of discourse between patient and provider about certain medical conditions. Policies and procedures for dissemination of health information to PHRs will be needed to ensure that clinicians have had the opportunity to review critical test results and confer with patients before results make their way into PHRs.

Although the PHR and EHR may one day be integrated, the PHR will not replace the medical record that must be maintained by health care providers. Risk management professionals should keep up-to-date on developments in this area, as technology-savvy patients begin to use electronic, interoperable PHRs.

ELECTRONIC HEALTH RECORDS AND SYSTEMS

An electronic medical record is generally defined as a longitudinal collection of health information that is made accessible in electronic form to authorized users.[4] In addition to patient information and billing applications, EHR systems may include knowledge and active clinical decision support tools to enhance patient safety, health care quality, and operational efficiency.

Interactive EHR systems can prompt clinicians automatically with reminders about care and can flag potentially adverse outcomes. In place of time-consuming manual reviews of paper medical records, EHR systems can provide automated assessments of performance measurement, such as adherence to clinical guidelines. In a pilot demonstration of a national health information infrastructure, known as eHealth Initiative Healthcare Collaboration Network, participating hospitals provide continuous, real-time electronic data about performance directly to CMS via a secure Internet connection.[5]

EHRs are expected to help provide an effective means of implementing institutional policy and procedures and related accreditation requirements. For example, national patient safety goal 8 of the Joint Commission on Accreditation of Healthcare Organizations (JCAHO)[6] requires accredited organizations to accurately and completely reconcile medications across the continuum of care. Because EHRs store and share information such as medication history, laboratory results, allergies, test results, and other pertinent health data, they support and facilitate patient safety initiatives and facilitate compliance with related policies and procedures.

Innovative comprehensive EHR systems in development in several large health systems may serve as bellwethers for health care organizations nationwide. An EHR system being put into place by Sutter Health, a large California system, will allow affiliated physicians to view comprehensive patient data beginning with an office visit, an emergency department visit, or a hospital admission. Lab test results, medication histories and physician notes will be available as real-time data. Patients will have access to the system using the Internet to schedule physician appointments, view their personal health history, send e-mail to their physicians, and access health information related to their diagnoses. The EHR system will also include numerous patient safety functions, for example, alerts to potential drug interactions and reminders about relevant clinical guidelines.

Few facilities currently employ electronic charting, which typically uses templates for clinician documentation. And although significant advances have been made in voice recognition technology, clinicians in many health care organizations continue to dictate patient information. Many EHR systems store health information that has been dictated and transcribed, often by transcribers in foreign countries who can transmit the transcribed information to providers through the Internet. To ensure legal and regulatory compliance, health care risk management professionals in organizations that outsource transcription of health care information should be aware of the numerous federal and state laws and regulations that apply to their situation. Contracts with transcription vendors should also adequately address related risks.

Health care risk management professionals should champion their organization's transition from paper-based health records to EHR systems while remaining aware of risks to patient safety during the transition. Risk to the quality and safety of patient care can arise during the significant process and cultural changes that occur during transition. For example, whereas laboratory results, x-ray interpretations, and physician progress notes may be available electronically, other vital patient information may remain on paper or be maintained in other media.

Risk management professionals must keep their focus on the end result—safer and better patient care. They can support their organization's transition to EHRs by developing policies and procedures that support the organization's strategic plan for switching to an EHR environment, and by developing policies and procedures pertinent to an electronic environment. AHIMA's practice briefs provide a resource for risk management professionals and others in health care facilities who are switching to the electronic environment.

CLINICAL INFORMATION SYSTEMS AND "SMART" TECHNOLOGIES

Many health information systems have been shown to reduce errors and thereby have a positive effect on quality of care, patient safety initiatives, and medical professional liability. Hospitals and health care organizations are moving incrementally toward the use of electronic information into the clinical aspects of health care delivery. Although risk management professionals are not the primary users of these systems, they should become educated about them and consider their applications to risk management and patient safety programs. Risk management professionals who are equipped with an understanding of clinical information systems can more effectively take steps to identify and reduce risks as facilities evolve from paper-based organizations to integrated digital organizations.

A computerized provider order entry system (CPOE) is a networked system that allows users to electronically enter specific diagnostic orders, such as laboratory tests and radiology exams; medication orders, for which users can maintain an online medication administration record (MAR); nursing orders; and special orders. Data can be accessed from the full range of orders found in a paper-based environment, including medication orders. These systems also provide online clinical decision support and safety alerts. Authorized users have access—from a single workstation or remote location—to clinical data from multiple sources. This data includes patient medical information from workstations within the facility and from physician offices or workstations in physicians' homes. CPOE systems replacing paper-based systems are intended to achieve specific objectives:

- Reduce misinterpretation of handwritten or oral orders
- Eliminate the use of paper documents
- Reduce the number of inputs to generate orders and execute them

- Provide rules-based clinical decision support through embedded clinical guidelines (such as dosage calculations, suggestions for alternate therapy)
- Enhance patient safety by alerting clinicians to certain occurrences, such as an unsafe order (for example, the prescription of a drug to which the patient is allergic, or the prescription of a drug that interacts adversely with another prescribed medication) or the completion of an order (such as notification that laboratory results have been returned)
- Generate a reliable electronic health record

Although hospitals have been slow to adopt the technology, hospitals and health systems in the U.S. are increasingly investing in CPOEs that include hazard alerts for cautions, contraindications, and drug interactions. However, many clinicians who use such systems lack knowledge about the range of patient safety features that exist on their clinical computer systems. A study reported in 2005 in the journal *Quality and Safety in Health Care*[7] discussed the experience of physicians in the United Kingdom where 90 percent of physicians in general practice regularly use advanced computer systems to assist directly in providing patient care. The study showed that only 25 percent of the physicians received formal training in the use of the patient safety features available on their systems, and that many physicians made erroneous assumptions about the safety features' warning functions. The importance of raising clinicians' awareness of patient safety features on their clinical IT systems, and ensuring that appropriate training is available, should be on the agenda of health care risk management professionals in all organizations that have implemented CPOEs, or plan to implement them.

Laboratory information systems are widely used to improve the flow of information inside and outside of clinical laboratories. These systems are designed to order tests, create bench worklists, verify specimens, report results, collate patient demographics with results for reports, and process or transfer billing information. Some systems also integrate with EHR systems.

Automated anesthesia record-keeping systems not only interface with anesthesia gas machines and patient monitoring equipment but also document drug administration, timing, and patient response more accurately and completely than manual recordkeeping. Indeed, the automated record might help to defend against charges of anesthesia professional liability.

Some emergency departments (EDs) use clinical support systems to enhance physician decision-making about whether to admit a patient for a cardiac workup. Artificial intelligence technology estimates the probability of an acute myocardial infarction based on patient history and ECG findings. This technology might help reduce the frequency of inappropriate defensive medicine practices and the frequency and severity of medical professional liability claims that allege failures in diagnosing and treating acute myocardial infarctions.

A number of pharmacy applications help reduce the risk of errors. Examples include automated drug dispensing systems, drug interaction programs, drug allergy warnings, dosage crosschecking, side-effect data, drug and food interaction warnings, and others.

Bar coding, a technology that has been used for years in the retail industry, has the potential for numerous applications in health care. The VA hospital system has been a leader in employing the technology in medication ordering and administration to verify that the right patient gets the correct drug, dose, and route at the correct time. A bar code representing the patient identification number is scanned, and the computer displays the medications that are due. Alerts and pop-up boxes display discrepancies and potential problems. Before administering medications, nurses use retail store-type scanners to compare bar codes embedded in patient identification bracelets against the labels on the medications.

Computer-assisted protocols that are used for antibiotic therapy employ real-time patient data to calculate antibiotic dose, duration of therapy, and cost-effective choices. These systems can pull patient information directly from bedside monitors in intensive care units (ICUs).

Radiology systems are linked to remote viewing units, such as the ICU and off-site physician practices, thereby reducing film retrieval time from a typical twelve hours to less than one minute. All of these applications have the potential to reduce medical professional liability.

Other examples of computerized clinical applications include:

- Automated dispensing systems
- Drug interaction programs
- Triage documentation, discharge instructions, and prescriptions
- Tickler systems for physician office visits and periodic screening examinations
- Patient tracking systems
- Bed tracking systems
- Medical device tracking systems
- Medical equipment control programs
- Health hazard appraisal systems

The list grows daily. Risk management professionals should view computerized clinical applications as potential clinical risk management tools that might help to reduce loss exposures in certain practice settings. At the same time, risk management professionals can champion the adoption of appropriate technologies and encourage the necessary cultural change that must occur as health care organizations change from manual systems to digital technology. Risk management professionals must continue to help develop and maintain policies and procedures that protect the security and confidentiality of electronic data, and that encourage proactive risk assessment to identify risk-prone systems and processes that might benefit from the application of newer computerized health information technology.

Infrastructure Technology

Risk management professionals and their organizations will also need to ensure that there are backups to their electronic health information system so that ongoing operations and patient care are not affected when a system goes down. Redundancy, failover,[8] and disaster-recovery protection features are necessary to avoid downtime that can paralyze an institution, resulting in patient harm and financial loss. Risk management professionals and regulatory compliance officers should work with their organization's IT department to ensure compliance with federal and state laws and regulations addressing the security of electronic health information.

Everything from infusion pumps to magnetic resonance imaging (MRI) scanners is now controlled by computers, thus medical device security should also rank among important risk management, legal, and regulatory compliance concerns. Health care risk management professionals should become familiar with risks that might threaten the security of computer-based medical devices that generate, store, and transmit patient health data, and champion strategies for risk reduction and legal and regulatory compliance. The modernization of medical equipment has seen a proliferation in the number of computer-based devices, which are vulnerable to an increasing amount of viruses and other malicious programs that target computers.

Many medical devices are networked for data exchange or Internet access. Most hospitals currently use technical solutions such as firewalls to isolate the internal hospital network from the outside world. While this usually blocks outside threats, computer viruses could enter a network through an internal device, thereby bypassing the firewall protection. In traditional local area network (LAN) architecture, all of a hospital's devices are connected in a single network, thus allowing a virus that gains access to the LAN to access to all of the devices in a hospital. Because some medical device suppliers do not take an active role in maintaining the security of their devices in the field, health care organizations must be vigilant in ensuring that the device security is regularly updated as it would with any other device on the hospital's network. Health care organizations' IT staff, clinical engineers, and risk management professionals should combine their expertise in a team effort to identify and resolve risks to the security of their institutions' computer-based medical devices. Refer to Exhibit 13.1 for a security checklist for information technologies.

EXHIBIT 13.1   Security Checklist for Information Technologies

- Develop and strictly enforce policies against disclosing or sharing passwords, access codes, key cards, and other means of access to the system.
- Develop policies and procedures for the assignment of passwords, as well as for their deactivation should an employee leave.
- Institute a "time-out" on computer terminals; that is, program terminals should have screens go blank after a certain period (for example, three minutes) of inactivity following the display of a patient record.
- Establish audit trails so that access to each record is tracked by the system.
- Sharply limit access to sensitive records or portions of records (for example, HIV-antibody test results).
- Protect against mass access and extraction of information.
- Educate staff about the importance of privacy and the problems that arise from sharing passwords.
- Ask medical staff members to sign confidentiality statements.
- Hold physicians liable for any entries to a record made by nurses or assistants using the physicians' password.
- Provide 24-hour assistance to authorized users who forget their access codes or to persons who legitimately need one-time access.
- Provide mechanisms for minimizing human error, such as review of input data for accuracy. If bar codes or other programmed codes are used to record clinical observations, there should be a mechanism for visual confirmation or other verification of entries. Document accuracy reviews.
- To the extent possible, limit connections to, and electronic data sharing with, outside computer systems.
- Use disks from reputable software vendors only.
- Obtain antivirus software to protect against computer viruses.
- Require software vendors to indemnify against all damages and costs arising from viruses, bombs, and similar sabotage inserted into the software by the vendor or its agents.
- Explore the feasibility of using optical disk "write once, read many" (WORM) technology; although it is considered antiquated for other industries, it may be ideal for hospitals because records cannot be altered after they are initially recorded in this form.
- Properly maintain hardware, and thoroughly debug and maintain software.
- Include performance standards in any lease or contract with a vendor, as well as guarantees of reliability and ongoing maintenance support.
- Have adequate backup and emergency capability. (For example, frequent backup of databases; off-site as well as on-site computer tape storage; and emergency data processing capability are essential, as is electrical power during power outages.)
- Routinely monitor available security systems and ensure that existing measures are reasonable by current standards.

POINT OF CARE TECHNOLOGY

Current and emerging health information technologies hold the promise of increasing patient safety at the point of care and should become an integral part of risk management programs in health care organizations.

Medical "smart cards" are designed to improve patient care and reduce medical and administrative errors by storing patient data that is accessible at several points of care. The small plastic cards are embedded with microchips that can process information and store numerous pages of a patient's vital health and demographic information, making it easier for patients to interact with the health care system. Smart cards have numerous capabilities. Card readers installed in the emergency department, for example, allow for rapid access to potentially lifesaving information about a patient, such as allergies to medications and chronic medical conditions. Patient information can be updated during physician office visits. Patients can view their medical information and obtain a printed copy of the smart card record. Information stored in the card is encrypted for security purposes, and each card contains a confidential code that is required for decrypting the text. Patients use personal identification numbers to access their information, and unauthorized or questionable use of the smart card automatically deactivates it.

Radio frequency identification (RFID) tags store identifying information and hold promise for various applications in health care, including reducing the risk of elopement by mentally incompetent patients and infant abduction. RFID tags may be attached to patients at the wrist or ankle, and can be used to track patients' whereabouts as they move, for example, from the emergency department to the operating room to the recovery room, and then to a bed on a surgical unit. RFIDs are used for tracking and matching blood for transfusion and tracking inventory. It is estimated that nearly half of U.S. hospitals will employ RFIDs within the next two years.

TELEMEDICINE

Telemedicine is the use of telecommunication technology for medical diagnosis and patient care to sites that are at a distance from the provider. Thus, telemedicine permits providers to provide care without moving the patient. Several technologies are employed in telemedicine. Typically, digital images are transferred from one location to another, and two-way interactive television is used for real-time videoconferencing.

There is a wide range of applications for this technology. Telepathology involves rendering diagnostic opinions on specimens at remote locations. Teleradiology is the electronic transmission of radiological images from one location to another for the purpose of interpretation or consultation. Radiologists who are continents away from the patient can provide "digital readings" of radiology images, transmitting their preliminary interpretations to clinicians in a timelier manner than otherwise could be achieved. The technology also allows clinicians to make virtual house calls to patients in remote locations and permits a surgeon in one location to remotely control a robotic arm for surgery on a patient in another location.

Several hospitals, among them Johns Hopkins Hospital (Baltimore, Maryland), employ robotic technology for making patient rounds within the hospital. Equipped with video camera and microphones, "robo-docs" permit virtual "telerounds" of hospitalized patients by electronically linking a robot to a physician at a remote location, giving the live physician remote presence in the hospital. Viewing a computer monitor, the physician directing the robot that is near the patient, sees and hears what the robot "sees" and "hears." Patients can see the physician's face displayed on a flat screen on the robot's shoulders and can talk with the physician. The system uses the Internet and a wireless network.

Other uses exist and undoubtedly will evolve, as states, such as New Mexico, with its large rural area, establish telemedicine systems and provide funding for telemedicine projects. Although improvements in technology have led to a revitalization of interest in telemedicine, its viability will be shaped by insurance reimbursement policies adopted by public and private payers.

Telemedicine carries a host of risk management, and legal and regulatory issues that must be identified and resolved. One of the first hurdles is the state-based physician licensure system, which runs counter to telemedicine's "virtual" boundaries. The rules for licensure by endorsement and out-of-state consultations vary among the states and pose barriers to development of interstate systems. Risk management professionals should be aware of telemedicine initiatives on the state and national level. A related problem that must be addressed is credentialing of physicians who would need to be granted telemedicine privileges.

Medical professional liability issues for telemedicine practitioners also evolve over time. Telemedicine networks may cross state lines and international boundaries, raising uncertainty about the jurisdiction in which a malpractice suit may be filed and what state or nation's law should be applied. These issues are important for several reasons. For example, different statutes of limitations may apply, and different statutory limitations on the amount of financial compensation that can be awarded to successful plaintiffs. What is the standard of care for a telemedicine practitioner in a particular specialty? Who is legally responsible for the quality of telemedicine equipment? In addition to these legal and risk concerns, measures must be taken to address applicable federal and state laws and regulations affecting the privacy and security of patient health information for information that is electronic and networked to remote locations via modem, telephone lines, satellite, and other communication technology. Refer to Volume III, Chapter 14 on Evolving Risk in Telemedicine for more information on telemedicine.

....

CONCLUSION

The Internet and the application of associated computer and digital technologies in health care will revolutionize the delivery of health care services and the role of the health care risk management professional. Health information technologies will promote collaboration, increase the knowledge base, enhance the quality of health care, and improve patient safety, thus reducing the risk of harm to patients and losses to the organization. Risk management professionals who champion their facilities' transition to an electronic environment will be poised to be key players in ensuring that these changes are in the best interest of the organization and the patients that they serve. Risk management professionals will face many challenges as they adapt health IT risk management functions, collaborate with patient safety and quality assurance to identify the benefits and risks of new technology application, and develop policies and procedures to reduce the risk of harm and ensure legal and regulatory compliance.

Endnotes

1. Institute of Medicine. *Crossing the Quality Chasm: A New Health System for the 21st Century (2001)*. Washington, DC: National Academies' Press, 2001.

2. United States Government Accountability Office (GAO). *Health Information Technology: HHS Is Taking Steps to Develop a National Strategy.* GAO-05–628. Washington, DC: GAO, May 27, 2005.

3. Payne, J. W. "E-Mailed Parents Feel Better." *Washington Post*, June 7, 2005, p. HE 1.

4. United States Government Accountability Office (GAO). *Efforts to Promote Health Information Technology and Legal Barriers to Its Adoption.* GAO-04–991R. Washington, DC: GAO, August 13, 2004.

5. The eHealthInitiative Web Site. [www.ehealthinitiative.org] June 2005.

6. The Joint Commission on Accreditation of Healthcare Organizations Web Site. [www.jcaho.org/accredited+organizations/patient+safety/06_npsg_ie.pdf].

7. Morris, C. J., et al. "Patient Safety Features of Clinical Computer Systems: Questionnaire Survey of GP Views." *Quality and Safety in Health Care*, 14:164–168, 2005.

8. Failover is the capability to switch over automatically to a redundant or standby computer server, system, or network upon the failure or abnormal termination of the previously active server, system, or network. Failover happens without human intervention and generally without warning, unlike switchover. Definition available at (Answers.com) ~ a computer desktop encyclopedia [www.answers.com/topic/failover?method=5&linktext=failover]. Date accessed 12/30/05.

Suggested Readings

The author gratefully acknowledges the many information sources and guidance materials published by ECRI, a non-profit health care research services agency at 5200 Butler Pike, Plymouth Meeting, PA 19452, www.ecri.org, and in particular, the following ECRI publications and programs:

Healthcare Control System. Plymouth Meeting, PA: ECRI.

Health Technology Forecast. Plymouth Meeting, PA: ECRI.

Health Devices. Plymouth Meeting, PA: ECRI.

Health Care Standards Directory Online. Plymouth Meeting, PA: ECRI.

ACCE/ECRI. *Information Security for Biomedical Technology: A HIPAA Compliance Guide*: Plymouth Meeting, PA: ECRI.

Appendix 13.1

⋮ IT GLOSSARY FOR RISK MANAGERS

@ (At)—Separates the specific user ID and domain name of an Internet address.

Access—The ability to use a computer or program to store or retrieve information.

Address—A unique identification assigned to a specific computer. To send e-mail, the sender needs the Internet address. Usually consists of a user ID, the @ symbol, and a domain name, and can be in numbers rather than words.

Anonymous FTP—A public file transfer protocol (FTP) file archive that is made available for Internet users to access.

Application programs—These are designed to carry out specific tasks for the user. They may be purchased from commercial software companies or written by computer staff.

Archie—An Internet search tool used to locate files on anonymous FTP sites.

ASP—An application service provider (ASP) is a company that offers individuals or enterprises access over the Internet to applications and related services that would otherwise have to be located in their own personal or enterprise computers.

ASCII—American Standard Code for Information Interchange is a standard code used in computer telecommunication that allows computers to exchange text-based files.

Bandwidth—The volume of data that a particular transmission channel can carry at once. There are several media for transmission; two types are twisted-pair telephone wires and fiber optics.

BPS—Bits per second. The higher the rate, the more data can be transmitted.

Browser—Software that enables users to move around the World Wide Web to explore Web sites. Examples are Netscape and Internet Explorer.

Bug—An error that occurs in a computer program.

Bulletin board system (BBS)—Software that allows messages to be left on a computer from a remote computer.

Chat—A real-time typed conversation between two or more people over the Internet or a proprietary computer network such as America Online or CompuServe.

.com—A commercial organization's domain designation.

CPR—Computerized patient record.

Database—Entire collection of stored data.

Domain—The name of the computer that is connected to the Internet. Computers are uniquely identified by a series of numbers. The domain name system translates those numbers into a name to which users can relate.

Download—The transfer or capture of data files from a database to the user's computer storage area; to retrieve files from an external computer to one's own computer.

EDP—Electronic data processing; represents the automation of routine manual clerical activity (for example, an association membership list).

.edu—An educational institution's domain designation.

Electronic signature—A feature that allows a physician to sign off on a report through the information system by using a special password, logging off, or other means that do not require signing a hard copy.

EPR—Electronic patient record.

FAQ—Frequently asked questions. A file that contains questions and answers about specific topics.

Field—Specific pieces of data that will be coded as a sequence of characters. Each field is given a name (incident type, incident location, date, shift).

File—A subset of the database that is stored and used as a unit.

FTP—File transfer protocol is a service that supports file transfers between local and remote computers.

Gateway—A hardware and software interface system that links two different types of computer systems, such as a mainframe and a LAN.

Gopher—A search tool that displays information through a system of menus and menu choices.

.gov—A government agency's domain designation.

Hardware—The pieces of equipment used by the system.

Home page—A location on the World Wide Web that identifies an individual or organization, generally used to refer to the first screen at a site. A home page welcomes visitors and points them to other information available at the Web site.

HTML—Hypertext markup language is the standard format for documents on the World Wide Web.

http—Hypertext transfer protocol is used by the World Wide Web for transmitting Web pages and other hypertext-linked files over the Internet.

Hypertext—Text that has contextual links to other related text. For example, if a document uses a term that is defined or explained in depth somewhere else, a hypertext document would include a link from that term to the related text.

Internet—Interconnected collection of computer networks.

IRC—Internet relay chat. Software that allows real-time typed conversations between two or more people over the Internet.

Listserv—A combination of e-mail software and mailing lists. It is commonly used for an electronic newsletter, in which the writer of the newsletter sends it to the listserv, which then transmits it to all the subscribers. Another use for listserv is to facilitate a discussion of a special-interest group. All e-mail sent to the listserv is sent to everyone on the list.

Mailing list—A group discussion distributed through e-mail.

.mil—A military organization's domain designation.

MIS—Management information system. Generally for middle and operating management, an MIS integrates data from several functional areas and produces much of its output on an on-demand basis.

Modem—An electronic device that translates computer signals into a form suitable for long-distance transmission, usually by telephone; modulator/demodulator, the hardware that translates between analog and digital so a digital computer can communicate through an analog telephone line.

.net—An Internet organization's domain designation.

Newsgroup—A discussion group on Usenet. Each newsgroup covers a specific topic. Within a newsgroup, there are initial postings listed by subject and subsequent response postings. Newsgroups are not real-time conversations; the postings are stored and forwarded, and often last for weeks or months.

Node—Any single computer connected to a network.

.org—A not-for-profit organization's domain designation.

Packet—A unit of data sent across a packet-switching network.

Prompt—On-screen instructions.

Protocol—A set of rules governing communication between computers on the Internet.

Record—A collection of related fields describing an entity.

Software—The programs required for the computer to perform desired operations.

Systems software—Software that makes the entire computer system operate sufficiently. It is provided by the manufacturer.

TCP/IP—Transmission Control Protocol/Internet Protocol is the standardized set of computer guidelines that allow different types of machines to talk with each other and exchange information over the Internet.

Telnet—Terminal emulation protocol that allows Internet users to log into a host computer from a remote location using a Telnet program.

Upload—Transfer of information or data files from a user's computer to another computer.

URL—Uniform (universal) resource locator. A unique identifier that points to a specific site on the World Wide Web.

Usenet—A collection of discussion areas (bulletin boards) known as newsgroups on the Internet.

Virus—Software designed to cause damage to computers or files. Viruses generally enter a computer system via files received on floppy disk or over networks.

Web site—An organization's or individual's Web pages, the first of which is called the home page.

14

Health Information Management

Kirk S. Davis
Jane C. McConnell
Elizabeth D. Shaw

The management of patient-specific data and information directly affects the responsibilities of the risk management professional. Health care systems provide a continuum of care which generates many types of data, including inpatient and outpatient health care records, incident reports, quality assurance reports, committee meeting minutes, and medical staff performance reviews. Information in electronic or written form must be handled appropriately to receive protection under the confidentiality provisions and privileges of state and federal law. This protection is necessary because it ensures patient privacy and encourages active peer review and quality improvement.

Over time, the ability to keep information confidential has become a more significant challenge and public concern. This is because of the advances of electronic technology in the health care industry and the linking of many types of patient care facilities, providers, health plans, payors, employers, and vendors through centralized databases such as e-mail and computer-based medical record systems. Technological advances affecting data management also have required additional security safeguards to protect the integrity of patient and health care business data and the inadvertent release of confidential information. In addition, the challenge is increased due to the expanding role and demands of state, federal, and voluntary agencies, and the media, to obtain what health care systems consider confidential information, in their belief that disclosing it will improve patient safety. Until recently, there were only a few federal laws protecting confidentiality, so state regulations predominated. Because state protections could be more than regulations, and because case law in some states was inconsistent with that in others (leaving large gaps in certain states), Congress addressed the need for minimum national health care privacy and security standards through the passage of the Health Insurance Portability and Accountability Act of 1996 (HIPAA).[1] The passage of HIPAA resulted in significant controversy, including several notices of proposed rule-making

355

(NPRM) up until the amended privacy rules were released August 14, 2002. The final rule adopting HIPAA standards was published in the Federal Register on February 20, 2003. It specifies a series of administrative, technical, and physical security procedures to be followed for covered entities to ensure the confidentiality of electronic protected health information. Most entities had to comply by April 15, 2005, but organizations with fewer than fifty people had until April 15, 2006, to comply with the requirements.

Although there are many potential changes under way with regard to privacy and security of confidential information, this chapter focuses on the basic principles for protecting this information and reviews existing state and federal statutes and some aspects of HIPAA, and provides practical advice for risk management professionals. To clarify, historically the term *medical record* was used almost exclusively in reference to data management. HIPAA and new state regulations also use the terms *health information, health care information,* or *individual identifiable health information* to describe types and forms of information associated with confidentiality and privacy protections. Health information referred to in HIPAA relates to a person's physical or mental health, the provision of health care, or the payment of health care. It is information that could identify or be used to identify a person, created by or received from a covered entity, that has been maintained electronically or transmitted by a covered entity. Because the medical record is usually the key document about which risk management professionals are concerned, this chapter will continue to use this term in addition to *protected health information* (PHI) in discussing confidentiality and security concerns. Because the law concerning health care data management continues to evolve, risk management professionals must stay alert to the release of any additional security regulations and Congressional interventions. With the implementation of the privacy rules in 2003, risk management professionals should keep abreast of changes in their respective state laws in response to HIPAA, and ensure that appropriate policies and procedures are developed to comply with the confidentiality and security requirements for the protection of health information.

············

CONTENT AND PURPOSE OF THE MEDICAL RECORD

The medical record is the primary document containing PHI. It usually includes results of physical examinations, a medical history, treatment reports, x-ray reports, physician orders, clinical laboratory reports, consultation reports, anesthesia records, operative reports, signed consent forms, nurses' notes, photographs used specifically for diagnosis and treatment, computer reports and graphs generated during the patient's treatment, and any other diagnostic and treatment related reports. Emergency department (ED) medical records may require additional information to comply with state regulations and the Emergency Medical Treatment and Active Labor Act (EMTALA).[2]

Whether handwritten, typed, or computerized, the medical record must be complete, legible, and accurate. The computerized record can help users of the information network to learn essential information about the patient, enhance completeness and accuracy of information, and make the record immediately available to authorized personnel. Accuracy is enhanced in computerized records because they often automatically record the date and time of each entry and identify the person entering the data.

The medical record serves several purposes. As a repository of information, it is a means of communicating among physicians and other providers involved in the patient's care throughout the health care delivery system. The Joint Commission on Accreditation of Healthcare Organizations (JCAHO) requires that all facilities treating patients maintain adequate medical records "which contain sufficient information to identify the patient, support the diagnoses, justify the treatment, document the course and results, and promote continuity of care among health care providers."[3] Additionally, the medical record is an important business record that may be accessed by authorized personnel not involved in direct patient care, such as physicians engaged in peer review, the billing departments, health plans, HMOs, or health care clearinghouses. Outside the health care system, it is used by government agencies, government-funded organizations, and accreditation bodies to monitor the health care entity and individual provider performance. Medical records also are reviewed by third-party payors for reimbursement and, under certain circumstances, are used for research purposes. From time to time, the medical record and other documents peripherally related to patient care (for example, operative logs and physician peer review records) may be requested by legal counsel, the patient, or the patient's representative. It is generally the most important document available to a health care facility and a practitioner in defending allegations of negligence and ordinarily is admissible as evidence of what transpired in the care of the patient.

This has been a contentious issue in Florida, where voters passed a Constitutional amendment requiring the release of documents about adverse medical incidents. The ballot language for the amendment stated: "Current Florida law restricts information available to patients related to investigations of adverse medical incidents, such as medical malpractice. This amendment would give patients the right to review, upon request, records of health care facilities' or providers' adverse medical incidents, including those which could cause injury or death."[4]

There were several trial court rulings in Florida on whether the amendment was self-executing. A self-executing or self-enacting amendment is one that prescribes all the details necessary for giving it effect without the need for implementing legislation. It was determined that the amendment was not self-executing, and lawmakers created §381.028, Florida Statutes, "Patients' Right-to-Know About Adverse Medical Incidents Act" to implement the amendment. There was no appellate decision regarding whether the amendment is self-executing, so there is no way to know how these courts will rule on this issue in the future.

With medical records as accessible as they are to so many users and for so many purposes, it is essential that users recognize the obligation to keep information confidential. The health care entity or network must have clear policies that comply with federal and state laws, regulations, and credentialing bodies regarding who may make entries in the medical record and how those entries may be corrected and completed to ensure record authenticity. Also necessary are policies on privacy and security measures to prevent tampering or loss, actions to undertake when unauthorized access or use occurs, and stipulations as to how long data is to be retained.[5] Additional privacy protections to be required under HIPAA are briefly mentioned here and discussed in detail in Volume III, Chapter 18 in this series.

Record Authentication

Most state regulations require a signature or other authentication by a health care practitioner to ensure the reliability of the information in the medical record. The JCAHO requires that all entries in the record be dated, authenticated, and that a method be established to identify original authors. Entries can be authenticated by written signature, identifiable initials, electronic signature, or computer key.[6] The Medicare Conditions of

Participation require the person responsible for ordering, providing, or evaluating the service performed to personally authenticate the record.[7]

Because errors in medical record entries are inevitable, in addition to authentication of the record, formal procedures must be followed for making corrections to the record.[8] As a general rule, the person who made the incorrect entry should also correct it. If the correction is significant, a senior person designated by facility policy should review the correction to ensure that it complies with facility guidelines for record amendments. Health care personnel should make only changes that are within their scope of practice, as defined by state licensing and certification laws. A quality control procedure must be in place to ensure compliance with the procedures developed.

Record Retention

The length of time that a medical record is retained is determined by federal or state laws and regulations or, in their absence, by sound administrative policy and medical practice. Record retention is also influenced by the structure of the health care entity and resources available—for example, whether the entity has access to off-site storage facilities, microfilming arrangements, or optical disks.

A few states have acts and regulations that establish general medical record retention requirements. Some states also have specific retention requirements for particular parts of medical records, such as x-rays, or for specific classifications of patients, such as minors, the mentally ill, and the deceased.[9] For example, the Florida Hospital Association has promulgated a compliance standards manual. The Office of the Inspector General's (OIG) Model Compliance Guide for Hospitals indicates that a hospital compliance program should provide for the implementation of a records system. This system should establish policies and procedures regarding the creation, distribution, retention, storage, retrieval, and destruction of documents. The types of documents developed under this system should include all records and documentation, such as clinical and medical records and claims documentation, required by either federal or state law for participating in federal health programs, and all records necessary to confirm the effectiveness of the hospital's compliance process.[10] For example, record retention in regard to research data varies with the type of research and the requirement of the respective funding source. Data managers should consult the Office of Research of the FDA and the Office of Human Subjects Research of the National Institutes of Health for further information.

In considering the development of a record retention policy, it is important to consider the Statute of Limitations under the False Claims Act.[11] This Act states that an action for a false claims violation "may not be brought (1) more than six years after the date on which the violation . . . is committed, or (2) more than three years after the date when facts material to the right of action are known or reasonably should have been known by the official of the United States charged with responsibility to act in the circumstances, but in no event more than ten years after the date on which the violation is committed, whichever occurs last."[12]

Each health care entity should establish its own policy governing medical record retention, with input from the risk management and legal departments. Clearly, medical records should be retained for as long as there is a medical, legal, administrative, or compliance need. Examples of these include records needed for subsequent patient care, medical research, review and evaluation of professional and hospital services, and defense of professional liability claims. Additionally, health care entities should consult state laws that may require a longer retention period for the medical records of minors.

Storage issues make it impractical to retain certain types of medical information. The retention policy should specify the process and retention period for medical information that poses unique record retention problems, such as radiology films, EKG and EEG tracings, slides, videotapes, and fetal monitor strips. For example, a cardiac patient might have several EKG tracings, or a maternity patient might have hours of fetal monitoring strips containing important documentation of the events of the birth. X-rays and scanning technologies such as computed tomography, mammograms, and ultrasound produce medical information in a pictorial rather than written form, which might be difficult or impossible to include in the traditional medical record. Although the physician's reports and interpretations of the tests will certainly be part of the record, they might not be sufficient in defense of a professional liability case. Paper records should ideally be stored together; however, other methods to retain these original films, strips, slides, videotapes, and scans should be used.[13]

Record Destruction

Some states have enacted statutes and regulations that specify the method by which a record may be destroyed after the retention period has concluded, or after the record has been copied into an electronic medium such as microfilm, computer memory, or other machine-readable form. Other states require health care entities to prepare a permanent abstract of the record before destroying it. After the record destruction policy is created, it should be applied uniformly, or the court may allow a jury to infer from the unavailability of the records that the health care entity acted improperly and against its own policies and procedures in keeping essential information in treating the patient.[14]

Access to Medical Records

Although the health care entity or provider is viewed as the owner of the medical record, the record is maintained for the benefit of the patient, who generally is viewed as having proprietary rights to the information. Many states have adopted laws regarding patients' access to their own records. These laws set forth specific guidelines delineating the circumstances under which patients have access to their records, and whether access may be denied. Even in states that do not have a specific statute, it is advisable for a facility to develop a policy that allows patients reasonable access to their medical records.[15] Under HIPAA, individuals are able to obtain access to their PHI. This includes a right to inspect and obtain a copy of their medical records, to request amendments or corrections if there is inaccurate or incorrect information, and to obtain an accounting of the disclosures.

Confidentiality and the Physician/Patient Privilege

The legitimate needs of individuals not involved in a patient's care to have access to the patient's information conflict with the principle that patient information is confidential. There is an ethical and a legal basis for confidentiality of medical information. The ethical principle originates from the concept that an assurance of confidentiality encourages patients to seek needed medical care and to be candid with their physicians about their condition. Confidentiality also is necessary to protect the patient's inherent privacy interest. People who receive medical care are entitled to privacy with regard to their own health care. For instance, an Ohio Supreme Court decision concluded that there is a common law right to privacy and established an independent tort of unauthorized disclosure of medical information based on the physician/patient relationship.[16]

An Iowa case brought the issue of medical privacy to the forefront. The Iowa Supreme Court agreed to hear Planned Parenthood of Greater Iowa's appeal of a lower court ruling that it turn over pregnancy test records requested by local authorities searching for the mother of a newborn found dismembered at a county recycling plant in May 2002. The Iowa Civil Liberties Union and the American Nurses Association filed legal briefs in support of Planned Parenthood. Two months before the Iowa Supreme Court was scheduled to hear the case, the Buena Vista County Attorney withdrew the request to obtain the records because of the time and resources necessary to continue what was believed to be a lengthy legal battle. Subsequently, the Buena Vista District Court Judge vacated the order.[17]

The legal basis for confidentiality derives from the physician-patient privilege, set forth by statute in almost all states. This is one of several relationships recognized as unique by law. Other unique and privileged relationships are attorney-client, husband-wife, and priest-penitent; in all, preservation of confidentiality is viewed as essential to the maintenance of the relationship. The patient has a privilege (right) to refuse to disclose or consent (and to prevent any other person from disclosing, including the physician) confidential communication or records made for the purpose of obtaining medical services, eliciting medical advice, and for medical education research purposes. The physician-patient privilege provides that, absent patient authorization, waiver, or an overriding law or public policy, medical information of a patient is insulated from the process known as discovery, through which parties to a lawsuit normally can compel disclosure of relevant evidence.[18]

Professionals Covered by the Physician-Patient Privilege

In most states, the physician-patient privilege extends beyond physicians to protect the patient's relationship with other health care professionals, such as psychologists and social workers. For example, the U.S. Supreme Court ruled that psychotherapists and social workers who offer counseling generally cannot be forced to provide evidence about their patients. Courts also have interpreted the physician-patient privilege to protect information provided by a patient to employed nurses, physician assistants, and other professionals working for a physician. However, in the absence of a statute, there generally is no privilege on the information provided by a patient to a nurse who has acted independently.[19] Risk management professionals should check the law of their jurisdiction to ascertain which health care professionals are specifically covered by the privilege.

Information Covered by the Physician/Patient Privilege

To be privileged, patient information must satisfy certain criteria. For example:

- It must have been communicated or created in the context of the physician-patient relationship.
- It must have been given with the expectation that it remain confidential.
- It must be necessary for the diagnosis and treatment of the patient.

Once the privilege is determined to exist, it extends beyond oral communications between physician and patient to cover written entries in the patient's record. Also included are x-rays, cardiograph strips, lab results, patient photographs, and other past or future health information on a patient's physical or mental condition that is kept by the individual provider or health care entity.[20] However, other information, such as the patient's name and address and the fact that the patient is receiving medical treatment, is not privileged because that information is not necessary for the patient's diagnosis and treatment.[21]

Assertion of the Physician-Patient Privilege

The physician-patient privilege belongs to the patient because it exists for the patient's benefit. Frequently, however, the patient is not available and does not even have knowledge that records concerning treatment have been requested. In such a case, the privilege must be asserted on the patient's behalf by the physician or the entity where the patient received treatment.[22] A patient claiming negligence in the performance of a particular procedure might seek a judicial order allowing discovery of the records of other patients who underwent similar surgeries. In those situations, the administrator should raise the issue of privilege for these patients' records.[23] If records are released, the court may order names and other identifying details to be removed from copies of the records.

Waiver of the Physician-Patient Privilege

Unlike assertion of the physician-patient privilege, a waiver of the privilege may be made only by the patient or, in cases of incompetency, infancy, or death, by the patient's legal representative. Waiver may be either express or implicit. Obviously, a patient may expressly waive the privilege by authorizing the provider to release information to a third party, such as an attorney. Under HIPAA, to ensure voluntary authorization to release the minimum amount of PHI necessary, the form must state what information is to be disclosed and the purpose of the disclosure. When a health care provider receives a letter from an attorney requesting copies of a patient's medical record, the records custodian confirms that the letter is accompanied by an authorization from the patient allowing release of the records to the requesting attorney, or that the request otherwise complies with state law on release of records.

Implicit waiver of the privilege occurs when patients bring personal injury actions concerning medical conditions for which they were treated, or otherwise disclose or consent to disclose significant parts of the communications previously made to treating physicians. In this instance, the patients have placed information about their medical condition at issue, so they may no longer claim the privilege.[24]

Risk management professionals sometimes must decide whether a patient who has not yet commenced a lawsuit but has performed some affirmative act, such as sending an "attorney request letter," has waived the privilege and thereby has entitled the physician or the hospital to turn over the patient's medical records to its liability insurance carrier. Courts have held that where a physician has a reasonable basis for believing that a claim of medical negligence will be made, the physician and the insurer are entitled to investigate and prepare for an anticipated lawsuit, justifying disclosure of the medical records to the attorney and the insurer.[25]

In some instances, defense counsel in a medical professional liability action may seek information on a plaintiff's medical condition that is not the subject of the suit. For example, to impeach the credibility of the plaintiff's claim about a lasting physical injury, the defense might wish to show that the plaintiff has received psychiatric treatment.[26] In birth injury cases, the defense frequently seeks discovery about the medical condition of the infant's siblings and about other pre-natal and labor and delivery records of the mother in an effort to prove a genetic cause for the infant's condition.[27] Court decisions vary from jurisdiction to jurisdiction on whether the privilege waiver extends to other conditions, and, if so, how information can be obtained from treating physicians who are not parties in the suit.

Courts generally permit liberal discovery of records of subsequent treatment by physicians applicable to the condition that is the subject of the litigation or is demonstrably related to it. However, even if the defendant is permitted to obtain access to information from the plaintiff's non-party treating physicians, courts are divided as to whether the plaintiff's condition can be discussed with those physicians in the absence of plaintiff's attorney (ex parte), or whether they must go through formal discovery proceedings.[28] Most courts have held, even though there has been a waiver of the physician-patient privilege, that the defendant must use formal discovery methods.[29]

RELEASE OF CONFIDENTIAL INFORMATION WITHOUT PATIENT CONSENT

The right of confidentiality and the physician-patient privilege are never absolute. Certain interests of society outweigh the physician's duty to maintain confidentiality of patient records, even when there has been no waiver or authorization. For instance, most states have laws mandating physicians and hospitals to report communicable diseases, incidence of cancer, cases of suspected child abuse or neglect, gunshot or knife wounds, physician misconduct, and incidents of adverse patient care.[30] The statute or regulation mandating disclosure usually contains a confidentiality provision restricting the ability of the public to gain access to that information.[31] Under HIPAA, covered entities can use or disclose PHI without authorization for treatment, payment, health care operations, and national priority activities.[32] With regard to business associates, covered entities can release PHI only if satisfactory assurance is obtained that the business associate will safeguard this information. However, the final modifications of HIPAA clarified that a breach by the business associates is not considered a breach by the covered entity.[33]

Physician Duty to Third Persons in Psychiatric Cases

One of the most difficult areas concerning unauthorized disclosure of privileged patient information arises in psychiatric cases. The guarantee of confidentiality is especially important in the patient-psychiatrist relationship. Statutes in many states require institutions to implement special procedures to prevent any disclosure of mental health records. HIPAA also contains such protections.[34] At the same time, situations might arise in which psychiatrists and other mental health professionals treating a potentially violent patient might find a conflict between their fiduciary obligation to maintain confidentiality and their countervailing duty to disclose that a third party might be a potential victim of their patient's violent acts.

First set forth in the landmark case of *Tarasoff v. Regents of the University of California*,[35] a judicial doctrine was developed that has been codified in most states: When a patient is determined to be a danger to others, the treating psychiatrist or therapist has a responsibility to disclose the danger to the extent necessary to protect potential victims.[36] Some state courts have held that the endangered third party must be specifically identified, whereas others have held that a general threat is a sufficient basis for breaching the patient's confidentiality. Before developing a policy for the institution or advising affiliated mental health professionals about disclosure to endangered third parties, the risk management professional should review any applicable state statutes and consult with legal counsel.

Records of Alcohol and Drug Abuse Patients

Special federal rules exist regarding confidentiality of information on patients treated or referred for treatment of alcohol and drug abuse.[37] In general, the regulations prohibit any disclosure or release of patient information, whether recorded or not, that would identify the patient as a substance abuser. The regulations were amended in 1987 in an attempt to make them clearer and to narrow their application with respect to general care hospitals. Under the amendments, a general medical facility is not subject to the regulations unless it has either a distinct substance abuse program or specialized personnel whose primary function is treatment, diagnosis, or referral for treatment of substance abuse patients. Regardless, the rules apply only to that special program or unit unless the hospital elects to place the entire facility under the regulations. Therefore, in a situation where a patient who is a substance abuser is being treated for a medical problem other than substance abuse in the general part of the hospital, information on that patient will not be covered by the regulations. On the other hand, the records of a patient who is in a substance abuse program are protected, and that patient's records may not be released or transferred, even to another department of the hospital, without a special consent. The regulations require that patients be given a written summary of the confidentiality regulations.

Under the regulations, information may be released with the patient's authorization if the authorization is in writing and contains all of the following elements:

- Name of the program
- Name of the proposed recipient of the information
- Name of the patient
- Purpose or need for the disclosure
- Extent and nature of the information to be disclosed
- Signature of the patient or of the person authorized to give consent if the patient is a minor, incompetent, or deceased
- Date on which the authorization is signed
- A statement that the authorization is subject to revocation at any time
- Date, event, or condition on which the authorization will expire if not revoked before that time

Each disclosure made with the patient's written authorization must be accompanied by a specific written statement, set forth in the regulations, prohibiting redisclosure.

The regulations permit disclosure without patient authorization if the disclosure is to medical personnel to meet any individual's bona fide medical emergency, or to qualified personnel for research, audit, or program evaluation. They also permit disclosure for certain specified purposes, pursuant to a court order, after the court has made a finding that (1) "good cause" exists, (2) the information is not otherwise available to the requesting party, and (3) the public interest in disclosure outweighs the potential harm to the patient. The person requesting court-ordered disclosure has the burden of demonstrating its necessity. A subpoena or similar legal document then must be issued to compel disclosure.

If a hospital receives a request for disclosure of patient information that does not comply with the regulations, it must respond with a non-committal answer that will not reveal that a specific patient has been diagnosed or is being treated for substance abuse. If the request is for treatment information on a patient known to be a substance abuser, the hospital should respond either with the non-committal answer or by sending a copy of the regulations and an attached statement that they restrict disclosure of substance abuse records. It is permissible, however, for a hospital to state that a specific person is not, and never has been, a patient of the program if that is the case.[38]

Medical Records Containing HIV- or AIDS-Related Information

Because discrimination against an individual might result from disseminating information regarding the individual's HIV status, such information is highly confidential. States have enacted different laws addressing the confidentiality of HIV test results and treatment records. Most states make available anonymous HIV testing, but also establish non-anonymous, but confidential, testing programs under which public health officials have access, under specific conditions, to the names of those testing positive.[39]

Risk management professionals must review the laws in their states and develop written policies that ensure that hospital procedures regarding disclosure conform to the applicable statute. In the absence of such a statute, it might be advisable to model the hospital's policy after the federal drug and alcohol rules, so that no HIV or AIDS information is released without patient authorization or a court order.[40]

Release of Patient Information to Law Enforcement Agencies

Risk management professionals frequently ask how they should respond to subpoenas and other requests for patient information received from law enforcement officers, including police officers, district attorneys, and grand juries. In general, without a specific statute compelling disclosure, law enforcement officers have no authority to examine a patient's medical records. This means that the results (for example, blood alcohol levels on a patient brought into the ED) should not be disclosed to the police unless required by statute.[41] Subpoenas and other legal processes issued by law enforcement agencies also should be carefully scrutinized, in consultation with the health care facility's attorney, before releasing privileged information. HIPAA contains a specific provision for use and disclosure of PHI for law enforcement purposes without the authorization of the individual. These purposes relate to a legitimate law enforcement inquiry, for identifying a suspect or victim, or national security activities and health care fraud.[42]

Research Programs

Risk management professionals play an important role in biomedical research by ensuring that Institutional Review Boards (IRB) maintain patient safety during clinical trials through the establishment of appropriate safeguards. These safeguards include protocol review procedures, an adequate informed consent process, database tracking systems, regular monitoring, and interpretation of data with prompt reporting of adverse events.

In accordance with HIPAA, IRBs must protect the privacy of the participants and maintain the confidentiality of the research data. Authorizations for the use and disclosure of such information are required for certain types of research programs. Further information regarding the contents, circumstances, and risks involved with Clinical Research and IRBs is discussed in Volume II, Chapter 5 of this series.

....

RELEASE OF PATIENT INFORMATION IN CIVIL LITIGATION

After a lawsuit is initiated, both sides engage in "discovery," whereby they gain access to factual information about the dispute in the control of either their adversary or persons who are not parties to the suit. Whether this information will later be "admissible" in a trial is a separate inquiry.

With respect to parties to the lawsuit, discovery of documents is initiated by serving a notice specifying with reasonable particularity the documents sought to be reviewed, and the time, place, and manner of inspection. Document discovery from non-parties (for example, the hospital where a patient was treated when only the patient's private physician has been sued) also is authorized but is more cumbersome. Usually, this involves a two-step process: serving a discovery notice on all other parties to the lawsuit, and then serving a subpoena or court order on the non-party in possession of the documents.

Remember that despite its official-looking appearance, a subpoena is rarely issued by the court itself. A subpoena may be issued by a clerk or a judge, administrative agencies, an arbitrator or referee, any member of a board or commission, and, in criminal cases, a prosecutor. In civil litigation, subpoenas are issued frequently by the attorney of record of any party to an action. Under the procedural law of most jurisdictions, an attorney, as an officer of the court, has the power to issue such a directive without the court's specific authorization. Therefore, risk management professionals should carefully scrutinize all subpoenas, including those signed by a judge, and should challenge the propriety of the subpoena in appropriate circumstances when privileged material is requested. In most jurisdictions, it is the health care entity's responsibility to assert the physician-patient privilege on behalf of a patient who is not a party to the lawsuit. In addition, many other records maintained by the hospital may be privileged and not subject to discovery by way of a subpoena or other court order.

As custodians of their patients' medical records, health care entities frequently receive subpoenas for records in the context of litigation not involving allegations of medical professional liability. For example, when an accident victim sues another party to the accident, hospital medical records contain information necessary to further litigation. Such records may be subpoenaed by one or both of the parties to the lawsuit.

As a practical matter, a risk management professional who believes that a subpoena is requesting privileged materials should contact the attorney issuing the subpoena and request that it be modified or withdrawn. If that is not successful, an application to the court, called a "motion to quash" or a "motion for a protective order," is the appropriate and proper method to test the subpoena.[43]

....

DISSEMINATION OF INFORMATION TO INTERNAL OR EXTERNAL REVIEW ORGANIZATIONS

Patient authorization is not a prerequisite to dissemination of information to either internal or external review organizations. However, it should not be assumed that all review agencies have the automatic right to demand immediate access to patient records without producing subpoenas. The generally accepted rule is that authorization or consent is not required for:

- Use of a medical record for automated data processing of designated information
- Use in activities concerned with the monitoring and evaluation of the quality and appropriateness of patient care
- Departmental review of work performance
- Official surveys for compliance with accreditation, regulatory, and licensing standards
- Research programs approved by the entities IRBs

Increasingly, official federal and state agencies such as health departments, attorney general offices, the Centers for Medicare and Medicaid Services (CMS), and the Drug Enforcement Agency, and also professional review organizations (PROs) are accessing patient records for many purposes, such as compliance, fraud allegations, and quality-of-care outcomes. These agencies are bound to maintain confidentiality of the information that they review and usually are permitted access to the patient's medical records.

Usually, such agencies make confidential all information reviewed or generated (other than general summaries or aggregate statistical data) that explicitly or implicitly identifies an individual patient, practitioner, or reviewer. Increasingly, the laws and regulations are amended to contain exceptions to total non-disclosure, and the risk management professional should consult with counsel about how to proceed when dealing with a special situation or quasi-governmental agency such as a PRO. It is suggested that health care entities have specific confidentiality policies and that they educate their staff accordingly. In fact, some may require certain members of their staff to sign an agreement that they will maintain confidentiality of this information and records. There is at least one case where an employee was terminated for violation of a hospital's confidentiality policy.[44] Additionally, some states have statutes that impose criminal or civil penalties on people for unlawful disclosure of medical information.[45]

Risk Management Information System

Risk management information systems (RMIS) are well established in many health care organizations. An RMIS allows the input of clinical data for more efficient analysis and reporting of claims information. Today, there are national databases available for benchmarking claims statistics and developing strategies to reduce medical error. Hospitals can compare their statistics with those of similar organizations to better evaluate their performance. An RMIS provides risk management professionals with the technological tools necessary to report results in a meaningful manner. Further information regarding RMIS is discussed in Volume III, Chapter 15 of this series.

Medical Error Reporting

Ever since the release of the 1999 Institute of Medicine (IOM) report, *To Err is Human: Building a Safer Health System,* which estimated that medical errors kill 44,000 to 98,000 hospital patients each year, patient safety has become a national concern.[46] First, the JCAHO adopted Patient Safety Standards, effective July 1, 2001, which requires hospitals to tell patients when a medical error has occurred, or risk losing their accreditation.[47] Then, the Senate introduced legislation known as the Patient Safety and Quality

Improvement Act (PSQIA) which would develop a voluntary reporting system of medical errors to private Patient Safety Organizations (PSO). The PSOs would then provide recommendations for corrective measures.[48] This legislation has been proposed and has undergone several changes over the past several years. The Patient Safety and Quality Improvement Act of 2005 would amend title IX of the Public Health Service Act to provide for the improvement of patient safety and to reduce the incidence of events that adversely effect patient safety. This legislation was signed into law by President George W. Bush on July 29, 2005.[49] The data collected by these organizations would become part of a national database created by the Department of Health and Human Services (DHHS). This new law would establish legal protections for information reported voluntarily for the purposes of quality improvement and patient safety, and would impose civil money penalties for violations of these protections.

To encourage hospitals to report patient safety data, the PSQIA establishes a statutory privilege for patient safety data. Improved legal protections are necessary because many state peer review protections are inadequate and the data could be subpoenaed in court and administrative proceedings.

PSQIA defines patient safety data broadly to include reports, statements, and quality improvement processes that are collected, developed, or reported by a provider to a patient safety organization. The privilege created by the PSQIA, however, would not apply to data that have been developed and exist separately from the process by which the provider collects or develops information for reporting to a patient safety organization, such as a patient's medical record.

In accordance with JCAHO's Patient Safety Standards, and because no federal legislation had been passed, several states had enacted laws requiring the same. For example, in Florida, the law states "an appropriately trained person designated by each licensed facility shall inform each patient, or an individual identified pursuant to s. 765.401(1), in person about adverse incidents that result in serious harm to the patient. Notification of outcomes of care that result in harm to the patient under this section shall not constitute an acknowledgment or admission of liability, nor can it be introduced as evidence."[50]

Similarly, Massachusetts, Montana, North Carolina, Ohio, Oklahoma, Oregon, South Dakota, and Wyoming have also enacted legislation that protects "statements, affirmations, gestures or conduct expressing apology, sympathy, commensuration condolence, compassion, or a general sense of benevolence."[51]

At a presentation at the Annual Meeting of the American Health Lawyers Association, it was reported that patients and families want three things when an adverse outcome occurs: (1) an apology; (2) an explanation; and (3) an assurance.[52] Presenters suggested using the anagram, STAR (adapted from a talk delivered at The Johns Hopkins Hospital in 2003 by The Honorable Howard Chasnow, retired Judge from Maryland's Court of Appeals) to remember the steps to take in a disclosure discussion.

S – Sympathize and apologize

T – Tell what happened

A – Assure what changes have been or will be made

R – Remain available and accessible

Risk management professionals should be cognizant of their state's law regarding patient safety and whether apologies are admissible as evidence. Further information regarding patient safety is discussed in Volume II, Chapter 1 of this series.

Sentinel Event Reporting

Hospitals have an affirmative duty to report certain sentinel events to specific regulatory agencies. A sentinel event is defined as "an unexpected occurrence involving death or serious physical or psychological injury, or the risk thereof. Such events are called 'sentinel' because they signal the need for immediate investigation and response."[53] The JCAHO requires hospitals to investigate sentinel events, which result in death or serious injury, through a root cause analysis process. A root cause analysis is a method to determine the cause of an unexpected adverse incident. Hospitals are encouraged, but not required, to self-report these events, along with the root cause analysis and corrective action plan, to the JCAHO.[54] These internal data are generally protected under the state's peer review privilege; however, there is concern that the privilege is waived once the data are reported to an outside agency and the outside agency may use these data in generating its report. Once the agency includes the data in its report, the protection is lost unless the state's law specifically provides for the continued protection of the data.

A New Jersey case has proven this concern to be a very real one. A New Jersey trial court ruled that Meadowlands Hospital Medical Center had to provide the plaintiff in a medical professional liability or wrongful death case with the root cause analysis created by the hospital in relation to its sentinel event policy.[55] The trial court pointed out that the definition of sentinel event was much broader than the scope of what would have been protected under peer review. It is advisable that risk management professionals review their existing sentinel event policies and confirm that the content is consistent with applicable state laws affording peer review privilege. Unfortunately, there is considerable variation in the evidentiary protection for root cause analysis under federal and state law, so hospitals and health care providers might be subject to liability based on the disclosure of the analysis if the disclosure is not considered privileged. Risk management professionals must take proactive steps to minimize the risk of reports becoming discoverable and admissible in medical professional liability claims.

With the improved legal protections proposed by the PSQIA, the volume of reports and the opportunities for improving patient safety should expand substantially. Risk management professionals should stay alert to similar proposed changes in state laws and seek adequate data protection.

FDA Reporting

Hospitals are required to report certain adverse events related to medical devices to the Food and Drug Administration (FDA). Suspected medical device-related deaths must be reported to both the FDA and the manufacturer, if known, and serious injuries to the manufacturer or to the FDA, if the manufacturer is unknown. These reports must be submitted on the MedWatch 3500A Mandatory Reporting Form. The risk management professional is responsible for the compilation of the data, report submission, and securing the device.

CONFIDENTIALITY OF BUSINESS AND OTHER RECORDS

A health care facility's business records may contain several different kinds of documents, including incident reports and reports of hospital and medical staff committees. Incident reports usually are generated following any event that is inconsistent with routine operation of a facility or an adverse event. They provide the facility with the information necessary to determine what happened and how it could possibly be avoided in the future.

Most states have adopted legislation that protects clinical information generated as part of a hospital's quality assurance (QA) activities from discovery or admission into evidence. This includes the incident report and peer review documents generated to review a physician's performance.[56]

Incident Reports

Incident reports can be a source of incriminating evidence if they are discoverable. Consequently, the discoverability of incident reports has been litigated in many states. If they are protected, protection usually depends on state QA and peer review statutes, or statutes creating an attorney-client or insurer-insured privilege.

In many states, incident reports that describe occurrences or incidents where the hospital has an expectation that it will be sued may be protected under the attorney-client privilege, the attorney work product doctrine, or a similar qualified immunity accorded to reports made to an insurer by an insured in anticipation of, or preparation for, litigation.[57] However, with respect to minor incidents that happen very frequently in the hospital, such as patient falls or medication errors, routinely prepared incident reports are more in the nature of accident reports maintained in the ordinary course of business. In most states, such reports are discoverable even if they ultimately are used in connection with litigation of a claim. Discoverability generally will turn on whether the accident report has a "mixed purpose;" it will be protected only if it was prepared exclusively in anticipation of litigation, not if it was prepared also for hospital administrative purposes.[58] In a state with a more comprehensive QA statute, incident reports involving serious occurrences that were prepared both in anticipation of litigation and as part of the hospital's effort to evaluate and improve the quality of health care should be protected.[59]

Incident reports should be labeled and treated as confidential and their distribution limited. The risk management professional should conduct in-service programs on how to write such a report. Incident reports should contain only a summary of objective facts and should avoid subjective analysis, conclusion, or finger-pointing. They should be addressed to the hospital's lawyer or insurance carrier, if appropriate, by state statutes. Depending on the breadth of state law, the risk management professional may consider forwarding a copy of the report to the QA committee.[60]

Even in a state with broad protection, a court may find that the privilege is not absolute and, upon a showing of "exceptional necessity" or "extraordinary circumstances," a plaintiff will be permitted to obtain incident reports generated by the hospital's internal risk management program, and also related peer review committee documents.[61]

Credentials Files

The JCAHO requires a process for delineating clinical privileges and for reappointment to the medical staff and reappraisal of such clinical privileges. Collection and review of information regarding credentials are required by most state statutes and the Federal Health Care Quality Improvement Act (HCQIA).

Regardless of the extent of protection from discovery accorded to credentials files, they should by maintained with an appreciation that they might be accessed by a wide variety of third parties, including physicians who have been denied privileges, the JCAHO, and state and federal regulatory organizations. In addition, there are cases in which medical professional liability plaintiffs who were treated by private attending physicians have asserted a separate cause of action for negligent credentialing against the hospital. As part of a claim of corporate liability, many have sought discovery of credentialing files. It is unclear at this time how many states will recognize this cause of action, but even in those states that currently grant protection from discovery to credentials files, it cannot be guaranteed that such existing qualified protections will be maintained.[62]

Ironically, regardless of any statutory protection that might exist if a hospital is sued for negligent credentialing, it might find itself in a situation in which the only defense is with the very documents it is seeking to protect. In those states where the statute granting protection does not specifically allow the hospital to use those documents in its defense, some lawyers advise the hospital never to voluntarily disclose peer review or credentialing documents. Selective disclosure might end up being detrimental in a subsequent case because of the legal precedent.

Some hospitals choose to place relatively mundane information in individual credentials files and "reference" by code the more sensitive information that is located elsewhere in the hospital, such as risk management case files, the QA files, or the offices of individual clinical department chairs. Only at the time of credentials review is the information brought together for the credentials committee's consideration.

Other hospitals maintain a bifurcated system in which sensitive qualitative information is kept in credentials files, including information obtained from other institutions, information regarding the physician's history of medical professional liability claims and professional misconduct, and information regarding the physician's delivery of medical care obtained through the hospital's QA process. In contrast, the physician's separately maintained personnel file contains objective factual information, such as educational qualifications, date of licensure, salary, and title, but does not include any evaluation comments. The majority of discovery requests can then be satisfied by producing only the personnel file, and the hospital can reserve its confidential arguments for the more sensitive credentials files.

Release of Information to the National Practitioner Data Bank

The Federal HCQIA, passed in 1986, established the National Practitioner Data Bank (NPDB), which contains a centralized source of information on physicians, dentists, and other licensed health care professionals. The act requires that each person or entity, including an insurance company, that makes a medical professional liability payment under an insurance policy, self-insurance, or otherwise for the benefit of a physician, dentist, or other health practitioner in settlement of, or in satisfaction in whole or in part of, a written claim or judgment against such physician, dentist, or other health care practitioner must report this information to the NPDB and the appropriate state licensing board(s). It also requires (following due process procedures) that: (1) state medical and dental boards report disciplinary actions taken against the license of a physician or dentist, (2) hospitals and other health care entities report their professional review actions that adversely affect a physician's or dentist's appointment or clinical privileges, and (3) medical and dental societies report adverse membership actions based on professional competence or conduct.[63] In addition, hospitals must request information directly from the NPDB on each physician, dentist, or health care practitioner they are considering for appointment, and at least every two years, on those on their medical staff to whom they have granted clinical privileges previously.

Although there is great political pressure to make this information more available to the public, in general the information reported will be considered confidential and may not be disclosed. However, it will be disclosed to the physician or practitioner involved, and to a hospital or health care entity that needs information concerning a physician, dentist, or other health care practitioner who either is on its medical staff or has clinical privileges, or is entering an employment or affiliation relationship with it. With respect to medical professional liability cases, a plaintiff's attorney may obtain confidential information on a specific physician, dentist, or health care practitioner named in the action or claim upon a showing that the hospital did not, as part of its credentialing and appointment process, obtain information on the individual involved from the NPDB. The plaintiff's attorney also must agree that the information will be used solely for that specific litigation. Failure to adhere to the confidentiality provision and its use solely for the purpose requested could result in a $11,000 penalty.

············

HEALTH CARE INTEGRITY AND PROTECTION DATA BANK

Included in HIPAA was the creation of another national data bank to contain information on certain final adverse actions taken against health care providers, suppliers, and practitioners. This bank is called the Healthcare Integrity and Protection Data Bank (HIPDB), and its purpose is to foster quality health care and help stem health care fraud and abuse. The information to the data bank will be reported by state and federal law enforcement organizations; state and federal agencies responsible for licensing or certifying any type of health care practitioner, provider, or supplier; federal agencies that administer or provide payment for health care; and private health plans. The information that they are to report includes:

- Civil judgments, with the exception of medical professional liability judgments, against health care providers, suppliers, and practitioners in federal or state courts related to the delivery of a health care item or service
- Federal or state criminal convictions against health care providers, suppliers, and practitioners related to the delivery of health care items or service
- Actions by federal or state agencies responsible for the licensing and certification of health care providers, suppliers, and practitioners
- Exclusion of health care providers, suppliers, and practitioners from participation in federal or state health care programs

Information reported to this data bank is confidential. Access to HIPDB is also strictly limited by statute; the general public, and health care entities, other than private health plans, do not have access. Where managed care organizations once asked the hospital to provide credentialing information on a physician, it now may be necessary for the hospital to ask the managed care organization for such information. To avoid overlap and confusion, a single NPDB-HIPDB Integrated Querying and Reporting Service will be used to report and query both data banks on the Internet. The statute provides that only the government agencies and private health plans required to report to the data bank will be authorized to obtain data bank information. However, subjects of reports may obtain access to their reports. Information may be requested for privileging and employment information, professional review, licensing, certification or registration, fraud and abuse investigation, certification to participate in a government program, and civil and administrative actions.[64]

Although hospitals and other health care entities do not currently have access to HIPDB, they do have access to, and are required to check, the OIG List of Excluded Individuals or Providers so as to verify that new, temporary and existing employees, independent contractors, and vendors are not excluded from participation in federal health care programs. The OIG posts a list of providers excluded from federal health care programs on its Web site [exclusions.oig.hhs.gov]. The site is searchable by name, specialty, city, state, ZIP code, or sanction type for any excluded individuals or entities, including registered nurses, licensed practical nurses, and certified nurse assistants.

Peer Review Privilege

In some states, the so-called peer review privilege is quite narrow, protecting only those proceedings in which physicians review the quality of medical care delivered. More recently, as part of comprehensive tort reform legislation in a large number of states, the privilege has been extended to include all the professional committees, such as credentials, utilization review, and QA. It also covers other documents maintained in connection with programs to monitor and improve the quality of care, regardless of whether they are related to a specific committee performing a medical review function.[65]

Courts generally have recognized, even in the absence of statute, that a guarantee of confidentiality and protection from discovery is necessary to promote an important state interest in effective peer review proceedings. Only a few courts have given greater deference to a plaintiff's need for all relevant information to prove a case.[66] Some medical professional liability plaintiffs' attorneys have argued that the proceedings and records of peer review committees, physician credentials files, and other QA documents contain relevant evidence about a physician's general qualifications, and information about the particular case in suit. Sometimes attorneys try to circumvent the privilege related to those documents by arguing that the applicable statute should be construed to cover only a very narrow category of documents and information. The issue most often arises in lawsuits alleging medical professional liability by physicians for whom the hospital may have vicarious liability, such as ED physicians. With greater frequency, however, it is being raised as part of a claim of corporate negligence on the part of the hospital for negligently credentialing the treating physician.[67] This issue also has extended to discrimination cases. The 4th U.S. Circuit Court of Appeals ruled that a North Carolina hospital had to turn over twenty years of peer review records to a physician who sued the hospital for discrimination.[68] The court held that the need to obtain probative evidence in an action for discrimination outweighed the interest to promote candor in the peer review process.

It is important to emphasize that even in states with a relatively broad privilege, the applicable statute frequently protects only the review process itself. The statute may cover discussions at committee meetings, and records and documents specifically created for a committee, but may not protect documents otherwise available from non-protected sources, such as accident reports made in the ordinary course of business, some patient record information, personnel records, and other administrative records of the hospital, even if they are necessary to the committee's deliberations. In addition, actions taken as a result of the committee's deliberations, such as curtailment of a physician's privileges or other disciplinary action, may not be privileged.[69]

A very significant exception, incorporated into almost every statute, is that the prohibition against discovery does not apply to any statements made by a person at the meeting who subsequently is a party to an action concerning the subject matter reviewed at that meeting.[70] Therefore, if a physician whose practice is being reviewed participates in the meeting, any statements that physician makes may be discoverable in a subsequent medical professional liability action against the physician and the hospital.

Because of questionable protection for certain types of information and documents, the policy concerning peer review materials prepared outside a committee must indicate that they were created to further the work of a committee whose records are privileged under the statute.[71] Some risk management professionals stamp each such document with a statement that the document has been prepared at the request of a peer review or QA committee and is confidential under the relevant statute.

Other practical suggestions to maximize protection include controlling distribution of and access to peer review committee records; distributing and collecting minutes at the meeting rather than mailing them; destroying all copies except the original; prohibiting names of patients and physicians from being recorded in minutes; and inserting provisions in medical staff bylaws that recognize the confidentiality of peer review activities and prohibit unauthorized or voluntary disclosure of peer review information.[72]

The scope of activities, the types of committees, and the specific information and documents that are protected vary widely from state to state. Before establishing the hospital's procedures for generating and maintaining records in this area, it is important to become familiar with case law, statutes, and regulations of the state. The entity's bylaws and its QA and risk management plans and practices should be developed to maximize the protection from discovery available in the jurisdiction. In addition, the risk management professional, in coordination with legal counsel, should develop systems for reviewing all discovery requests for each type of information to avoid inadvertently releasing a document that might be privileged.

Attorney-Client Privilege

If the state has a very narrow peer review privilege, as mentioned previously, another privilege that might be available to protect committee minutes and other sensitive documents is the attorney-client privilege. The precise limits of the attorney-client privilege and the extent of protection from discovery afforded to an attorney's work product vary by jurisdiction. In general, however, where legal advice is sought from a lawyer, the confidential communications between client and attorney relating to that advice are protected from disclosure, unless the client waives the privilege.[73] Therefore, when a committee discusses a patient care incident and a strong possibility exists that the hospital will be sued, it might be advisable to have outside legal counsel in attendance. The drawback to relying solely on in-house counsel in those circumstances is that some courts have found that in-house counsels function in a dual capacity as administrator and attorney, rendering communication with them not privileged.[74] With outside counsel present, it might be possible to argue that the issues were discussed in anticipation of litigation and are protected from discovery under the attorney-client privilege. If the lawyer keeps the minutes of the meeting and also writes an advisory memo about the committee's deliberations to hospital administration, which contains the lawyer's advice and opinions on the matter, those records probably would be protected by the privilege.

ELECTRONIC RECORDS

Computerization is increasing the volume and sophistication of patient information and the complexities of the records that contain that information. New technology makes it possible to collect, store, and analyze worldwide bases of information at a relatively low cost. However, although the principles of medical record-keeping have remained the same in the electronic format, computerization has brought with it additional problems.

The advantages of computerized medical records include enhanced patient care brought about by instant access to records by a variety of health care professionals and the creation of legible and complete records that are difficult to lose or destroy. However, the disadvantages include potential review of confidential records by unauthorized users, authentication and accuracy issues, lack of durability of the storage media, and a lack of clear, uniform legislation protecting the records.

The Health Privacy Project working group outlined its eleven best principles for health privacy. The 1999 report discussed non-identifiable information; privacy protections for the data; right of access; notice; safeguards; authorization; organizational policies; research; law enforcement; discrimination; and remedies.[75] HIPAA is designed to protect the privacy of the information, whether oral or written, not just the specific record. While DHHS may not have the authority to protect all medical records, including paper records, HIPAA attempts to broaden its scope of application. If the information has been maintained or transmitted electronically, then DHHS intends to apply the privacy standard to the source record and to subsequent electronically generated records.[76]

Other criticisms and disadvantages of electronic records include that HIPAA does not allow DHHS to issue standards for records that are maintained by other insurers or by employers for workers' compensation purposes. HIPAA does not establish appropriate restrictions on the use of redisclosure of such information by likely recipients such as researchers; life insurance issuers; marketing firms; or administrative, legal, and accounting services. DHHS also lacks the authority to provide Americans the right to take action in court when their medical information is used inappropriately, a critical consumer protection that only Congress can provide.

The eHealth Initiative (EHI), a group of non-profit health care organizations, released guidelines which establish a framework to the facilitate the transmission of health information technology (HIT) to physician practices in the United States. The new guidelines, *Parallel Pathways for Quality Health Care*, focus on three categories: (1) quality capabilities; (2) HIT capabilities within the physician practice; and (3) health information exchange capabilities in communities across the country.[77] It is believed that these guidelines will help physicians remove barriers that prevent them from implementing HIT in their practices.

A survey by the Centers for Disease Control and Prevention (CDC) reported that fewer than one-third of the nation's hospitals and emergency departments and only 17 percent of physician offices used electric medical records.[78] The CDC study noted the biggest barriers that health care providers face in adopting electronic medical records are the time and personnel necessary to switch.

DHHS Secretary Michael O. Leavitt announced on June 9, 2005, that DHHS is launching a national strategy to have electronic medical records for most Americans within ten years. Leavitt said, "the national strategy for achieving interoperability of digital health information is for federal agencies, who pay for more than one-third of all health care in the country, to work with private sector health care providers and employers in developing and adopting an architecture, standards, and certification process. Electronic health records and other information technology would reduce medical errors, minimize paperwork hassles, decrease costs, and improve care."[79]

The cornerstone of the effort will be a commission called the American Health Information Community (AHIC), a private-public collaboration to be formed under the Federal

Advisory Committee Act, Leavitt said. It is expected that AHIC would remove the barriers faced by providers to implement electronic medical records.

Six weeks later, CMS reported that it planned to announce that it would give physicians low-cost electronic health record system software. The program began in August 2005, and the software is a version of a well-proven electronic health record system called Vista, which has been used by the Department of Veterans Affairs. Physicians would pay a "token" charge of approximately $37 and an additional licensing fee of $10 or so for use of the American Medical Association codes. Along with the software, physicians will receive a list of companies trained to install and maintain the system. CMS officials noted that "an office with five doctors could save more than $100,000 by choosing the Medicare software rather than buying software from a private company."[80]

In a recent news release, the FDA reported that it is "reexamining 21 C.F.R. Part 11, the landmark regulation that made electronic records and signatures as valid as paper records and handwritten signatures."[81] The FDA decided to review the regulation because of concerns that some interpretations might unnecessarily restrict the use of technology and significantly increase the costs of compliance to technical controls such as validation, audit trails, and record retention.

Legal Requirements

Many states permit hospitals and health care facilities to have fully computerized patient records; however, these states carefully regulate how those electronic records are kept. For example, a California statute requires that licensed health care providers that use electronic record-keeping systems for patient records comply with additional requirements, unless hard copy versions of patient records also are retained.[82] Some of those requirements include use of an off-site backup storage system, an image mechanism able to copy signature documents, and a mechanism to ensure that once a record is input it is unalterable.[83] Additional requirements include development and implementation of policies and procedures to outline safeguards against unauthorized access to electronically stored patient health records, including authentication by electronic signature keys.[84] The 2005 JCAHO Accreditation Manual for Hospital Standards has an entire section dedicated to management of information. The standards focus on organization-wide information planning and management processes. The standards attempt to provide guidance as to:

- Ensuring timely and easy access to complete information throughout the hospital
- Improving data accuracy
- Balancing requirements of security (the protection of data from intentional or unintentional destruction, modification, or disclosure, and ease of access)
- Using the aggregate (combination of standardized data and information) and comparative data to pursue opportunities for improvement
- Redesigning information-related processes to improve efficiency
- Increasing collaboration and information sharing to enhance patient care

Electronic medical records necessarily include electronic signature standards, and DHHS has issued a proposed rule regarding these.[85] In electronic signatures, there should be an attribute affixed to an electronic document to bind it to a particular entity. An electronic signature secures the user authentication, supplying proof of the claimed entity at the time the signature is generated. It creates the logical manifestation of a signature that will include the possibility for multiple parties to sign a document and have the order of application recognized and proven. It further supplies additional information such as a time stamp and signature purpose specific to that user. The electronic signature also ensures the integrity of the signed document to enable the transportability of data, interoperability, independent verifiability, and continuity of signature capability. Verifying a signature on the document substantiates the integrity of the document and its associated attributes and verifies the identity of the signer. The standard for an electronic signature is based on cryptographic methods that use a set of rules and parameters so that the identity of the signer and the integrity of the data can be verified.

In addition to the JCAHO standards, individual states are promulgating requirements for hospitals and other facilities that must be met for electronic authentication of medical record entries to be permitted. For example, some states require that medical records be dated and authenticated and their authors identified. Entries may be confirmed by written signature or initials, rubber stamp, or computer "signatures" (or sequence of keys). Any practitioners who use a rubber stamp or computer signature to authenticate entries sign a statement that they alone will use it. A stamp or computer signature authorized for one person is not used by anyone else.[86] Each state law should be reviewed, particularly with the continuing changes being promulgated within the JCAHO standards and the new HIPAA.

System and Data Security

With electronic collection, storage, and analysis of data comes increased access. Several problems, including those of confidentiality and security, arise as a result. Unfortunately, no security system in general use today can withstand the efforts of a skilled computer expert who is determined to break into a system.

The standard of computer security legally required for computerized patient records is not always clear. It is clear, however, that computer and data security for computerized patient records must be, at a minimum, reasonable.[87] Whether security is reasonable depends on several factors. The American Health Information Management Association (AHIMA) has created the following criteria to consider when determining the reasonableness of security:

- The state of commercially available computer technology
- The affordability of security technology, procedures, and techniques
- The likelihood of failure of security and the risk that such a failure could be caused intentionally
- The magnitude of harm that could result if security fails, is inadequate, or is breached
- Known and reasonably anticipated threats to security
- Standards promulgated by nationally recognized standard-setting organizations and professional associations in the fields of health information, health care informatics, and computer security[88]

Security Threat Technologies

Even insurance companies, managed care companies, pharmaceutical firms, physicians, and outside ancillary health care providers dialing in from their computers pose a threat to data security because they might inadvertently access unauthorized information. Finally, the addition and integration of new medical record technology into an existing medical record-keeping system can threaten the security of data, because such integration often requires exposure of data so that systems specialists can make sure that the integrated system is working properly. Fortunately, the computer security technology that previously was available only in the movies is with us today.

Passwords often are used as a security measure to ensure data confidentiality because they are based on something a user knows. However, problems can occur, including cracking, sharing passwords, and simply forgetting the appropriate password, particularly if it is changed on a routine basis. Because of the problems with passwords, some institutions have begun to protect their documents by using biometrics technology. Biometrics permit entry based on some characteristic of a user, for example, fingerprints, voice patterns, hand geometry, retinal patterns, and facial recognition.[89] The advantages of this type of technology include that this information is difficult to crack and is not easily shared. The disadvantages include false acceptance and individuals' hesitancy to subject themselves to this technology.

Tokens provide another form of data security. These may include credit cards or calculator-sized devices that generate passwords.[90] There are some problems with tokens; one major disadvantage is cost, particularly for large organizations where employee turnover is constant and tokens are easily lost.

Less costly ways of improving data security include the use of software that renders computer terminals inactive after a certain timeframe and logs out certain users or otherwise prohibits their access. In addition, certain systems make their users go through multiple levels of authentication, and others have one set of computers as a boundary between the end product and the outside world. Finally, data can be encrypted—that is, scrambled in such a way as to be unintelligible to anyone without the appropriate information to unscramble them.

Medical information should be made available only to those with the need to know. Therefore, it is essential that the accountability of the people who have access to sensitive information be ensured. Risk management issues that need to be addressed to ensure data accountability include:

- Establishing written policies for employees to maintain security and confidentiality and discipline violators
- Tracking of user activities as to the time and nature of modifications made to the data
- Auditing to reflect the logging-in on the system
- Intrusion detection, which flags undesired behavior
- Provision of a mechanism for users to validate that information they receive electronically came from the person who claims to have sent it
- Digital signatures that may use encryption technology

Protection of Confidentiality with Vendors and Data Clearinghouses

Health information system contracts are complex.[91] In a typical vendor form contract, such as medical record copy services, medical record transcription services, and claims adjudication services, the only restriction on the vendor's use or disclosure of patient and provider data is that no patient will be identified by name. Such a restriction is inadequate to protect patient confidentiality in an environment where combining and cross-matching data are possible and inferences are available for determining the identity of record subjects. In fact, in the current environment, there is no certain protection of patient confidentiality in data disclosed by the vendor, unless the data are aggregated into cells of sufficient minimum size that the probability of anyone identifying a patient whose data are included in the cell approaches zero.

A provider should agree to permit vendor use of its data only if the agreement includes detailed confidentiality obligations applicable to the vendor, its agents, employees, and subcontractors. In addition, the agreement should protect patient identifiable data, any information identified as proprietary information of the provider and its affiliates, and practitioner- or provider-identified data. The agreement also should include detailed procedures and protocols that the vendor must follow when handling the provider's data.[92]

Contracts with clearinghouses and other third parties handling unencrypted data also should include protections such as clear delineation of ownership rights in the data and detailed provisions stating the extent to which the clearinghouse or third party may disclose or distribute data to others. The contract should contain a clear statement of the purpose(s) for which the third party is being granted access to the data. Such provisions may be important in preventing third-party access to data, even pursuant to subpoena. For example, if the third party has access to data for purposes of performing peer review or utilization review, a privilege may apply in some states.

Detailed data quality standards, delineation of procedures for maintaining data quality, and provisions for auditing data quality also should be included in a contract with a vendor or other third party. As a part of maintaining quality standards, it is important to require the third party to comply with the provider's security requirements if the third party will be granted remote access to the provider's patient information system.

Because a third party presumably will have several employees reviewing confidential data, it is necessary that all employees, agents, and subcontractors of the third party sign confidentiality agreements before being given access to those data. These confidentiality agreements should contain clear definitions of the information to be held in confidence. It is particularly important that the agreements be signed by anyone who will have access to patient-identifiable information in unencrypted form. However, the provider also may wish to protect as confidential any proprietary information of the provider and its affiliates and any information that identifies the provider or an affiliate or a practitioner.

In addition, the contract should provide for remedies for breach of confidentiality obligations, including injunctive relief. Provisions limiting the third party's liability for breach should be avoided, if possible. The contract should anticipate protections on data security after termination of the relationship with the third party. A provision stating that confidentiality obligations survive termination of the agreement and requiring the third party to return all copies of the provider's data upon termination should be included. Finally, the contract should include provisions requiring that the third party indemnify the health care provider for any actions brought against the provider as a result of the third party's breach of confidentiality obligations.[93]

There also must be a real concern for patient rights regarding record disclosure between entities. This issue becomes even more troublesome when confidential information such as HIV status, mental health treatment, and alcohol or drug abuse treatment is discussed.

Electronic Incident Reporting Systems

Electronic incident reporting systems greatly enhance the risk management professional's ability to manage and report data. These systems are generally simple to use and can be interfaced with the electronic medical record. This interface allows the risk management professional to review the incident report and access the patient's medical record without ever leaving the office. Data is stored in database management systems and can be reported in many different categories, including but not limited to, the type of incident, location of incident, severity of injury, and personnel involved. Many systems have the capability to design customized reports to meet the needs of individual hospitals. In seconds, a risk management professional could generate a report of how many falls occurred in a particular month, on a particular floor, identify whether the patient was restrained, and determine the severity of the injury.

Systems provide for varying levels of security access: (1) basic access for personnel to enter an account of the incident and witnesses to enter statements; (2) next-level access for department managers to view the initial report, witness statements, and enter the results of their investigation; and (3) the highest level of security access for risk management professionals to review all information entered, enter their analysis on restricted screens, file probable claims, and run reports. Unlike paper forms that can be altered, misplaced, or destroyed, electronic systems can better maintain the integrity of the data because once the information is filed, it cannot be altered. If a documentation error occurs, an addendum would need to be filed to clarify any misstatement because the original statement would remain intact. Electronic incident reporting systems provide for more effective tracking and trending of data and improved accuracy of reports through the elimination of lost paper incident reports.

Scanning of Medical Records

Because of the high cost of storage, lack of adequate storage area, and the need to access records quickly, many health care organizations have begun scanning medical records. Unfortunately, the scanning process can be very cumbersome if the scanner speed is too slow. The speed of scanners can range from one minute to fifteen minutes to scan one record. If the scanning capability is too slow, a growing backlog of records can occur and records can be misplaced. High-speed scanners can perform other functions such as automatically indexing records, which saves personnel time and costs.

Once the record is scanned, the paper record is generally destroyed. Risk management professionals should be cognizant of the quality of the scanned medical records, because the scanned record would then be the only record available to be used as evidence in any future litigation. Risk management professionals should be familiar with their respective state laws regarding what constitutes an "original" record. Whether or not a record is an original is especially important during litigation. The best evidence rule is based on the premise that, when the contents of a writing are at issue, the best evidence of the contents is the original document. Rule 1001(3) of the Federal Rules of Evidence provides that if data are stored in a computer or similar device, any printout or other output readable by sight, shown to reflect the data accurately, is an "original."[94] The evidentiary rules of some jurisdictions follow the Federal Rules of Evidence, and provide that computer-generated documents shall be regarded as originals, therefore computer printouts stored on tape or disk may be admissible into evidence. Hospitals could be liable for spoilage of evidence if the hospitals are negligent in the protection and maintenance of the medical records.

············

USE OF E-MAIL

Increasingly, risk management professionals are using e-mail via intranet or the Internet to communicate with hospital personnel, claims departments, and defense attorneys. Many hospitals have developed intranets to connect all the hospital personnel onto one secure network. This intranet allows the hospital to narrowly prescribe access. When e-mailing outside of the intranet, the risks of interception of the information increase because the Internet is an open network of millions of computers with minimal security.

The benefits of electronic communication include speed, convenience, low cost, informality, efficiency for group communication, and the ability to attach documents, which reduces copying and postage costs. However, risk management professionals need to be aware of the risks of using electronic communication for incident-related information. A detailed discussion of the risks is included in Chapter 13 on Information Technology and Risk Management.

The most significant risks of using e-mail are: (1) PHI might be improperly disclosed, resulting in a breach of confidentiality and privacy; (2) e-mail of privileged information might result in a loss of privilege protection; and (3) e-mail can be used as evidence in litigation.

As discussed in the section on Security Threat Technologies, there are e-mail security products available which can solve the problems associated with standard e-mail by "encrypting" the mail so that the message is put into a "secret code" which can be read only by the intended recipient. Risk management professionals should discuss these options with their information technology departments.

In addition, risk management professionals should include a disclaimer with each e-mail message that lets the recipient know that the e-mail message contains privileged and confidential information and that if the e-mail is inadvertently sent to an unintended recipient, the recipient should not read, copy, or forward the e-mail. The recipient should notify the sender by reply e-mail that the e-mail was received and delete the e-mail from the recipient's records.

············

MOTIVATIONS FOR ADDRESSING SECURITY IN HEALTH CARE SYSTEMS

There are many reasons that motivate an organization to address security in its health information systems, such as legislative requirements, regulations by accrediting organizations, and litigation by individuals who are harmed because their sensitive private medical information is improperly shared.

The legal requirements for maintaining the security of health care records (whether in electronic or paper form) are based on a complex mix of federal and state regulations.[95] A portion of HIPAA's provisions directs the development and implementation of uniform national standards for the secure electronic transmission of health information.

A series of definitions demonstrates the expansiveness of HIPAA. Health information—that is, information created or received by a health care provider, health plan, public health authority, employer, life insurer, school, university, or health care clearinghouse—relates to an individual's past, future, or present physical or mental health or condition, receipt of health care, or payment for such health care. DHHS adopted standard "data elements" and "code sets" for the electronic encoding of health information. These standard data elements and code sets must work for all financial and administrative transactions involving health claims, enrollment and eligibility, referrals, and authorizations, and for first reports of injury and coordination of benefits. These data cannot permit the disclosure of trade secrets or confidential information, and must reduce the administrative costs of providing and paying for health care. Each of the organizations that are covered will be assigned a unique health identifier.

DHHS issued an NPRM proposing the security standard called for in HIPAA on August 12, 1998. The security standard was effective April 21, 2005. Succinctly, the security standard consists of requirements that a health care entity must address to safeguard the integrity, confidentiality, and availability of electronic data. Additionally, the standard describes the features that must be implemented to satisfy the rule. There are four security standard categories:

- Administrative procedures
- Physical safeguards
- Technical security services
- Technical security mechanisms

Failure to use these standards results in penalties unless the organization has reasonable cause.

HIPAA also stipulates specific health data privacy requirements to maintain "reasonable and appropriate" safeguards for the integrity and confidentiality of health information. Any "reasonably anticipated" threats to the security or integrity of individually identifiable health information and unauthorized use or disclosure of that material must be prevented.

Specific security provisions must consider: (1) the technical capabilities of health information record systems, (2) security measure costs, (3) personnel training, (4) audit trails for computerized record systems, and (5) the needs and capabilities of small and rural health care providers. Penalties for breach of privacy where there is knowing procurement or disclosure of individually identifiable health information include a $50,000 fine and a one-year prison sentence. If this information is used through false pretenses, the fine increases to $100,000 and the prison term to five years. If there is an intent, transfer, or use of the information for commercial advantage, personal gain, or malicious harm, the fine increases to $250,000, and the prison term extends to ten years. Ultimately, the most stringent requirements, whether state or federal, to protect privacy rights are mandated to be followed.

In a surprise move, the Department of Justice (DOJ) severely limited the government's ability to prosecute individuals for criminal violations of HIPAA. A recent authoritative ruling by the DOJ notes that employees of a covered entity are not automatically covered by HIPAA and may not be subject to its criminal sanctions.[96] This ruling appears to directly contradict *U.S. v. Gibson*, Plea Agreement, No. CR04–0374-RSM, the first criminal conviction for HIPAA violation.[97] In this case, Gibson, a health care employee, stole a patient's protected health information to fraudulently obtain credit cards. He pleaded guilty to wrongful disclosure of individually identifiable health information for economic gain and was sentenced to sixteen months in prison.

The DOJ ruling clarified that individuals who violate HIPAA could still face penalties under state laws or other federal laws, including, but limited to, those laws that address identity theft, aiding and abetting, conspiracy, and also as a result of civil lawsuits filed by patients. Because this ruling is binding on the executive branch of the federal government, but not on judges, it will be interesting to see how this ruling affects future HIPAA enforcement efforts.

HIPAA regulations outline many compliance requirements. They are discussed in detail in Volume III, Chapter 18 of this series.

....

CONCLUSION

Advances in computer technology, combined with advances in health care, have created complex legal and ethical considerations for all health care providers and entities. With the increase in the electronic storage and transmission of health care information, the legal framework within which confidentiality, security, patient care, and other critical issues are addressed will change. Furthermore, as the health care marketplace continues to evolve, greater demands will be placed on hospitals, health systems, health plans, and other providers for access to confidential patient and peer review information. To be effective, mechanisms to protect confidentiality and security of health care information must be a part of a complete security package. This includes well-thought-out security policies and procedures, security training, and security management and maintenance. A comprehensive security management program is a significant undertaking but is well worth the investment of required resources and, under future federal regulations, might be required.

Endnotes

1. P.L. 104–191, 110 Stat. 1936 [herein after HIPAA], § 264 (a).

2. Conner, C. "Medical Records." *Hospital Law Manual.* Vol. 3. Gaithersburg, Md.: Aspen, 2005.

3. Joint Commission on Accreditation of Healthcare Organizations (JCAHO). "Management of Information." Comprehensive Accreditation Manual. Oakbrook Terrace, Ill.: JCAHO, 2005.

4. [www.votesmartflorida.org/voterguide.asp#amend7]. See, § 381.028, Fla. Stat., 2005.

5. Conner, *op. cit.* pp. 14,31,34–35.

6. JCAHO, Standard 6.10, 2005.

7. 42 C.F.R. §482.24 (c). See, Security and Electronic Signature Standards, 63 Fed. Reg. 43241 (1998) (to be codified at 45 C.F.R. Part 142) (Proposed Aug. 12, 1998).

8. Conner, *op.cit.,* p. 34.

9. In states that have adopted the Uniform Preservation of Private Business Records Act, a three-year preservation requirement applies to the medical records maintained by private hospitals, even though the act does not specifically address medical records.

10. For example, documentation that employees were adequately trained; reports from the hospital's hotline including the nature and results of any investigation that was conducted; modifications to the compliance program; self-disclosure; and the result of the hospital's auditing and monitoring efforts. Further, Medicare's Conditions of Participation Requirement states that hospital records regarding Medicare claims be retained for a minimum of five years. (42 C.F.R. § 482.24 [b][1] and HCFA Hospital Manual §413 [C][12–90]).

11. 31 U.S.C. 3731 (b).

12. The suggested retention schedule was compiled from information in the Code of Federal Regulations, basic IRS regulations, corporate records retention manuals, Healthcare Financial Management Association reference materials, the Medicare Hospital Manual

(Publication 10), the College of American Pathologists, Joint Commission on Accreditation of Healthcare Organizations, Florida's General Records Schedule (GS-4) for Public Hospitals, Health Care Facilities, and Medical Providers, and state laws.

13. Conner, *op. cit.,* pp. 9–12.

14. *Ibid.*

15. The Uniform Health Care Information Act of 1985 has been adopted in Montana and Washington, but many states have passed legislation that accomplishes the same objective. See, for example, Colo Rev. Stat. Tit. 25–1–801, 2005; 735 Ill. Comp. Stat. Ann.5/8–2001, 2005. In states without a statute, courts sometimes will find a common-law right of access.

16. *Biddle v. Warren General Hospital,* 715 N.E. 2d 518 (Ohio 1999). In the case of *Weld v. CVS Pharmacy, Inc.,* (1999 WL 494114 [Mass. Super. Ct.]), Massachusetts's Superior Court regarding the marketing of pharmacy information held that there was a common-law right of privacy. *Cossette v. Minnesota Power & Light,* 188 F.3d 964 (8th Cir. 1999). Here the Eighth Circuit Court of Appeals determined that the Americans with Disabilities Act (ADA) created its own set of privacy restrictions for medical information, and that these protections were not limited to "disabled" people but would apply to any employee or other person potentially covered by the ADA. States differ as to whether there is a legal, as opposed to a moral or ethical, "right to privacy." Under a variety of legal theories, most states protect some type of privacy interest. Some state courts have held that breach of the duty of confidentiality is a tort and that a cause of action for breach of confidentiality might exist in circumstances where there has been extrajudicial disclosure of confidential information, or in cases such as custody disputes where the plaintiff's physical condition is not in issue. See generally, Annotation, Physician's tort liability for unauthorized disclosure of confidential information about patients (48 ALR 4th 668, 1985). A medical provider that reveals privileged information by mailing patient's medical records in lieu of attending a deposition as required by a subpoena may be sued in tort for breach of the fiduciary duty of confidentiality. State *ex rel. Crowden v Dandurand,* 970 S.W. 2d 340 (Mo. 1998). Expert affidavit submitted by patient in medical professional liability action against psychologist was adequate despite contention that expert's opinion was premised on violation of professional ethical standard, which could not alone serve as basis for the action; expert did not merely opine that psychologist's alleged disclosure of confidential information violated ethical standard, and expert specifically stated that disclosure was deviation from "standard of care" of psychologist, although such statement was followed by reference to ethical rule. OCGA § 9–11–9.1 *Bala v. Powers Ferry Psychological Associates,* 225 Ga. App. 843, 491 S.E. 2d 380 (1997), cert. denied (Sept. 4, 1997). A medical professional liability claim may be based on the unauthorized disclosure of confidential information. G.S. § 8–53. *Jones v. Asheville Radiological Group, P.A.,* 129 N.C. App. 449, 500 S.E. 2d 740 (1998), related reference, 506 S.E.2d 254 (N.C. 1998). *Horne v. Patton,* 287 So.2d 824, 1973 (physician disclosed confidential information to plaintiff's employer); *MacDonald v. Clinger,* 84 AD 2d 482, 446 NYS 2d 801, 1982 (psychiatrist revealed confidential information to patient's wife). Probably a more logical basis for finding liability is that, as part of an implied contract between physician and patient, the physician agrees not to release information about the patient without the patient's consent. *Hammonds v. Aetna Casualty and Surety Co.,* 243 F. Supp. 793, ND OH, 1965. Suits against practitioners for invasion of privacy typically allege an unwarranted exploitation of the patient's personality or a publication about the patient's private affairs that would cause outrage, mental suffering, shame, or humiliation. See, for example, *Barber v. Time, Inc.,* 348 Mo. 1199, 159 SW 2d 291. That type of action might be brought when a photograph or description of the patient is published without permission. As to whether there is a constitutional right of privacy, although not explicitly stated anywhere

in the Constitution, the Supreme Court has held that there is a fundamental right of privacy emanating from various provisions in the Constitution that limit the extent to which the government may interfere with an individual's privacy. See, for example, *Griswold v. Connecticut,* 381 US 479, 1965; In re Search Warrant, 810 F.2d 57, 3d Cir. cert. denied, 107 S.Ct. 3233, 1987 (patients have a privacy interest under the Constitution in their medical records in the possession of their physicians; however, the protection afforded by the right to privacy is not absolute and must be balanced against the legitimate interests of the state in securing the information contained therein).

17. Mack, P. "Judge Drops Pregnancy Records Request." [www.ktiv.com/News/NewsDetail64.cfm?Id=26,4769]. Oct. 23, 2002.

18. The four traditional criteria for a privileged communication are: (1) it originates in confidence that it will not be disclosed; (2) the element of confidentiality is essential to the full maintenance of the relationship between the parties; (3) the relationship is one that the community thinks ought to be fostered; and (4) the injury to the relationship that would occur from the disclosure would be greater than the benefit gained by the aid-giver to the litigation. 8 Wigmore, Evidence §2285 at 527, McNaughton rev., 1961.

19. See *Jaffee v. Redmond,* 518 U.S. 1 (1996). See also 8 Wigmore, Evidence §2380. *Hinzman v. State,* 53 Ark. App. 256; 922 S.W.2d 725 (1996). Because psychologist notified patient that findings from their session would be reported to the prosecuting attorney's office, communications were not confidential and therefore not subject to psychologist-patient privilege. *Halacy v. Steen,* 670 A.2d 1371 (1996). When assailant agreed that his pre-sentence investigation report from a related criminal proceeding could be released to a particular third party, he did not waive his psychologist-patient privilege over those reports as to other third parties. Me. R. Evid. 503 (physician and psychotherapist-patient privilege).

20. Annotation, physician-patient privilege as extending to patients' medical or hospital records, 10 ALR 4th 552, 1981. Hospital records are included within physician-patient privilege. VAMS §491.060(5). *State ex rel. C.J.V. v. Jamison,* 973 S.W.2d 183 (Mo. Ct. App. E.D. 1998). Personal injury plaintiff waived physician-patient privilege in her medical records insofar as they concerned medical condition at issue under pleadings. *State ex rel. Jones v. Syler,* 936 S.W.2d 805 (MO. 1997). Patient was entitled to obtain dates on which his physician had obtained medical treatment in six months prior to and sixty days following patient's surgery, where patient alleged that physician was suffering from disability or illness that limited his ability to perform surgery, patient sufficiently showed through physician's admissions to patient regarding his own medical condition that physician's physical condition was in controversy and physician-patient privilege did not protect dates on which physician received treatment. *Klein v. Levin,* 242 A.D.2d 682, 662 NYS 2d 793 (2d Dep't 1997). Probationer could not have reasonably expected that his communications with psychologist would be privileged and could not claim psychologist-patient privilege, and thus trial court abused its discretion in denying motion in negligence supervision suit against city on behalf of child raped by probationer to compel discovery, where municipal court had ordered probationer to participate in treatment as condition of continued probation and probationer signed consent form for release of information to probation officer. West's RCWA 18.83.110 *Hertog v. City of Seattle,* 88 WA App., 41, 943 P 2d 1153 (Div. 1 1997). Patient records and files were indispensable to insurer's defense in action by insured, a physician, under disability insurance policy; insurer was entitled to records from insured's medical practice to determine whether he was unable to perform substantial and material duties of his job, and insured could not hide behind Ohio's statutory physician-patient privilege to impair insurer's ability to defend itself. Ohio R. C. §2317.02 *Varghese v. Royal Maccabees Life Ins. Co.,* 181 FRD 359 (S. D. Ohio 1998). Defendant was not entitled to production of

witness's confidential drug treatment records, to show extent of witness's addiction and payments made to clinic by witness, who defendant claimed was perpetrator of charged robbery; because information was available through other means, defendant's need for information did not outweigh statutory emphasis on keeping treatment records confidential. Public Health Service Act, §543, as amended, 42 USC §290dd-2. *U.S. v. Obele,* 136 F3d 1414, (10th Cir. 1998), cert. denied, 119 S. Ct. 197 (U.S. 1998).

21. See, for example, *Payne v. Howard,* 75 FRD 465, DDC, 1977 (court permitted plaintiff to discover the names and addresses of patients of plaintiff's physician who had received similar treatment so that plaintiff could contact them and determine whether they would be willing to waive the statutory privilege attaching to their records); *Hirsh v. Catholic Medical Center,* 91 AD 2d 1033, 458 NYS 2d 625, (2nd Dept., 1983) (disclosure of the name of a nonparty patient who may have witnessed an occurrence would not violate the privilege). Contra, *Schecket v. Kesten,* 126 NW 2d 718, MI, 1964 (names of non-party patients are protected by physician-patient privilege and are not subject to discovery); *N.O. v. Callahan,* 110 FRD 637, D. MA, 1986 (plaintiffs complaining of inadequate state psychiatric facilities could tour facilities but could not videotape other patients without their consent).

22. See, for example, *Tucson Medical Center Inc. v. Rowles,* 21 AZ App. 424, 520 P.2d 518, 523, 1974. ("Our decision . . . that hospital records are covered by the physician-patient privilege where neither the patient nor his physician are parties to the proceedings. To hold otherwise would deprive a patient of the confidentiality granted him by [the statute] simply because neither the patient nor his physician are parties to the proceeding." The court then reviewed the record in camera to ascertain if there was any relevant non-privileged information and denied access.)

23. See, for example, *Ziegler v. Superior Court of the County of Pima,* 134 AZ 390, 656 P.2d 1251, AZ Ct. App., 1982. Other courts have rejected this approach because of the perceived danger that the non-litigant patient's identity would not remain confidential. *Parkson v. Central Du Page Hospital,* 105 IL App.3d 850, 435 NE 2d 140, 1982.

24. *In re Lifschutz,* 85 CA Rptr. 829, 467 P.2d 557, 1970, quoting *San Francisco v. Superior Court,* 37 CA 2d 227, 232, 231 P.2d 26, 1951; *Hoenig v. Wesohal,* 52 NY 2d 605, 439 NYS 2d 831, 1981 (by commencing personal injury action, plaintiff waived any privilege she previously had and was required to produce reports of treating physicians).

25. *Hammonds v. Aetna Casualty and Surety Co.,* supra note 16; *Rea v. Pardo,* 132 AD 2d 442, 552 NYS 2d 393, 4th Dept., 1987.

26. See, for example, *Friedlander v. Morales,* 70 AD 2d 501, 415 NYS 2d 831, 1st Dept., 1979 (court permitted defendant to discover records of plaintiffs treating psychiatrist in case where plaintiff alleged defendant's medical professional liability caused serious physical and emotional injury). However, courts will not allow so-called blunderbuss notices for discovery. Although waiver of the physician-patient privilege has occurred, its scope is limited and does not permit discovery information involving unrelated illnesses and treatments.

27. See, for example, *Williams v. Roosevelt Hospital,* 66 NY 2d 391, 497 NYS 2d 348, 1985. (Infant plaintiff alleged Erb's palsy and brain damage caused by cephalopelvic disproportion and defendant's failure to perform caesarean. Court ruled mother could not refuse to answer questions during her deposition concerning condition of plaintiff's siblings and mother's obstetrical history, although court did not decide, in this case, whether defendant also could gain access to actual medical records of plaintiff's siblings and mother.)

28. Most jurisdictions disapprove of ex parte interviews. See generally, Annotation, Discovery: right to ex parte interview with injured party's treating physician. 50 ALR 4th

714, 1986; see also, *Petrillo v. Syntex Laboratories Inc.,* 148 IL App.3d 581, 102 IL Dec. 172, 499 NE 2d 952, 1986 (court held patient's implied consent, in filing suit, was only to release medical information relevant to suit; *Anker v. Brodnitz,* 98 Misc.2d 148, 413 NYS 2d 582, 1979, aff'd, 73 AD 2d 589, 422 NYS 2d 887, 2nd Dept., 1979 (court prohibited private interviews with treating physicians during the pre-trial discovery phase absent patient's express consent or a court order). But see *Nielson v. John G. Appison, MD, PC,* 138 Misc.2d 74, 524 NYS 2d 161, trial term, 1988 (limiting this prohibition to the pre-trial discovery stage of litigation and permitting defendants to privately interview plaintiff's treating physicians in anticipation of presenting them for testimony at trial). No court, however, has permitted recovery against a physician for breach of confidentiality under facts such as these.

29. Cases permitting ex parte interviews include: *Doe v. Eli Lilly & Co.,* 99 FRD 126, DDC, 1983; *Langdon v. Champion,* 745 P.2d 1371 AK, 1987; *Coqdell v. Brown,* 531 A.2d 1379, NJ Super. L., 1987; *Moses v. McWilliams,* 549 A.2d 950, 959. PA Super., 1988 (interpreted a statutory exception to the privilege for "civil matters brought by the patient" to apply to ex parte disclosures by physicians, court noted "ex parte interviews are less costly and easier to schedule than depositions, are conducive to candor and spontaneity, are a cost-efficient method of eliminating non-essential witnesses . . . and allow both parties to confer with the treating physicians").

30. For examples of mandatory reporting statutes, see, for example, CA Penal Code §11160, 2005 (injury caused by deadly weapon); 325 Ill. Comp. Stat. Ann.5/4, 2005 (child abuse); Conn. Gen. Stat. §19a-215, 2005 (communicable diseases); Minn. Stat. Ann. §144.34, 2005 (occupational diseases, including poisoning from lead, phosphorus, carbon monoxide, and so on).

31. The Federal Freedom of Information Act (FOIA), 5 USC §552, sets forth a general rule of disclosure for records in the possession of the executive branch. The statute contains an exception for "personnel and medical files and similar files the disclosure of which would constitute a clearly unwarranted invasion of personal privacy," 5 U.S.C. 552(b)(6). State freedom of information laws contain similar exclusions.

32. 45 C.F.R. § 164.512, Uses and Disclosures Permitted without Individual Authorization.

33. 67 Fed. Reg. 53,236 (2002).

34. 45 C.F.R. § 164.508(a)(2), Exception for Psychotherapy Notes.

35. In *Tarasoff,* the victim of the therapist's patient was clearly identified. Subsequently, in *Thompson v. County of Alameda,* 167 CA Rptr. 70, 27 CA 3d 741, 614 R2d 728, 1980, the California Supreme Court held that the duty to warn depends on and arises from the existence of a prior threat to a specific identifiable victim. A few courts have gone beyond *Tarasoff* to hold that psychotherapists also will be liable for their patients' violent acts against persons who are not identifiable in advance but are "foreseeable victims." In those cases, liability arises where the therapist or psychiatric facility negligently releases a potentially dangerous patient who subsequently harms a third party. See, for example, *Leverett v. State,* 61 OH App.2d 35, 399 NE 2d 106, 1978 ("A hospital may be held liable for the negligent release of a mental patient only when the hospital, in exercising medical judgment, knew or should have known that the patient, upon his release, would be very likely to cause harm to himself or others.").

36. See, for example, 740 Ill. Comp. Stat. Ann.110/1, et seq., 2005, which requires that confidential records and communications be disclosed "when, and to the extent, a therapist, in his sole discretion, determines that such disclosure is necessary to initiate or continue civil commitment proceedings or to otherwise protect against a clear imminent risk of serious physical or mental injury or death to the patient or another." Like most statutes, this one allows, but does not require, a psychiatrist to warn.

37. 42 C.F.R. Subchapter A, Part 2.

38. For an excellent article on the amendments to the alcohol and drug abuse regulations, see: Kramer, D. V. "Confidentiality of Patient Alcohol and Drug Abuse Information." *Kentucky Hospitals,* Spring 1988.

39. George Washington University, Intergovernmental Health Policy Project, State AIDS Policy Center, State AIDS Reports, #7, Feb.–Mar. 1989, p. 1.

40. Discovery was allowed in *Belle Bonfils Memorial Blood Center v. Denver District Court,* 763 P.2d 1003, solo. 1988; *Tarrant County Hospital District v. Hughes,* 734 SW 2d 675, TX App. 1987, cert. denied, 484 U.S. 1065, 108 S.Ct. 1027, 1988. Discovery was denied in *Rasmussen v. South Florida Blood Service, Inc.,* 500 So.2d 533, 1987; *Krygier v. Airweld,* 137 Misc.2d 306, 520 NYS 2d 475, 1987.

41. *State v. Copeland,* 680 SW 2d 327, MO App., 1984. A few medical record confidentiality statutes authorize disclosure of medical records information without patient authorization or a subpoena when necessary to cooperate with law enforcement agencies.

42. 45 C.F.R. § 164.512 (f), Disclosure for Law Enforcement Purposes.

43. See, also, 45 C.F.R. § 164.510(e), Uses and Disclosure for Judicial and Administrative Proceedings. Interestingly, a physician-patient privilege may not be asserted to quash a subpoena ad testificandum on the theory that a witness cannot assert the privilege in advance of the questions being asked. However, the witness can refuse to answer a question seeking privileged material, in which case the questioner could ask a court to determine if the privilege has been raised appropriately and, if not, to order an answer.

44. *Tehven v. Job Service North Dakota and St. Luke's Hospital,* 488 NW 2d 48, (N.D. 1992).

45. See, also, 45 C.F.R. § 164.510(b), Uses and Disclosure for Public Health Activities and 164.512(d), Use and Disclosure for Health Oversight Activities. Tenn. Code Ann. §68–11–311, 2005.

46. LeGros, N. C. "The New JCAHO Standards on Disclosure of Unanticipated Outcomes," *Health Law Digest,* 29(12), 2001, 3–11.

47. *Ibid.*

48. "Senate Medical Errors Bill Introduced," *Health Lawyers News,* 6(7), 2002, p. 10; and See, also, Congressional Budget Office. *Cost Estimate of S. 544, The Patient Safety and Quality Improvement Act of 2005.* [www.cbo.gov/showdoc.cfm?index=6234&sequence=0] March 31, 2005.

49. See full text of S. 544, *The Patient Safety and Quality Improvement Act of 2005.* [www.theorator.com/bills109/s544.html]; and see Zwillich, T. "Patient Safety System Becomes Law: Bush Signs Law Creating First National Reporting System," [my.webmd.com/content/Article/109/109267.htm?z=1728_00000_1000_tn_04] July 29, 2005.

50. § 395.1051, Fla. Stat. 2004.

51. Kidwell, R. P., and Smith, M. L. "Proactive Malpractice: Disclosing and Resolving Adverse Outcomes." Paper presented at the Annual Meeting, American Health Lawyers Association AHLA San Diego, CA., June 26–29, 2005; See, Appendix A: Cal Evid Code § 1160, 2005; 13–25–135. C.R.S., 2004; Fla. Stat. § 395.1051, 2004; Md. Court and Judicial Proceedings Code Ann. § 10–920, 2004; ALM GL ch. 233, § 23D, 2005; H.R. 24 59th Leg., (Mont. 2005); NRS § 439.855, 2004; NJ. Stat. § 26:2H-12.25, 2005; N.C. Gen Stat. § 8C-1, Rule 413, 2005; ORC Ann. 2317.43, 2005; 63 Okl. St. § 1–1708.1H, 2004; ORS § 677.082, 2003; 40 P.S. § 1303.308, 2004; H.R. 1148 8th Leg., (S.D. 2005); Ten., Evid. Rule 409.1, 2004; Tex. Civ. Prac. & Rem. Code § 18.061, 2004; Rev. Code Wash. (ARCW) § 5.66.010, 2004; Wyo. Stat. § 1–1–130, 2004.

52. *Ibid.*

53. Sentinel Event Glossary of Terms. (available at: [www.jcaho.org/accredited+ organizations/sentinel+event/glossary.htm]).

54. Mulholland, D. "Unanticipated Consequences of Unanticipated Outcomes Disclosures," *Journal of Health Law,* 35(2), 2002, 211–226.

55. *Reyes v. Meadowlands Hospital Medical Center,* 355 NJ Super 226, 809 A2d 875 (NJ Super. L. Apr. 12, 2001).

56. For examples of peer review statutes, see: Arizona Rev. Stat. Ann. §36–445.01A, West, 2005; Cal Evid Code §1157, 2005; §§ 381.028, 395.0193, 395.0197 and §766.101, Fla.Stat., 2004. 735 Ill. Comp. Stat. Ann.5/8–2101, 2005; NY CLS Public Health §2805-m, 1996; *Bayfront Medical Center, Inc. v. State Agency for Healthcare Administration,* 741 So. 2d 1226 (Fla. 2d DCA 1999), where the appellate court ruled that the Medical Center's report of the results of a peer review investigation, as contrasted to the actual records of the investigative procedures of the peer review panel, was not privileged from disclosure to the state agency reviewing the Medical Center's risk management procedures. Without a statute, courts have refused to create a privilege. *Davison v. St. Paul Fire and Marine Ins. Co.,* 75 WI.2d 190, 248 NW 2d 433, 1977 (declining to apply retroactively a subsequently enacted statute granting protection from discovery in medical professional liability cases and rejecting argument in favor of a common-law peer review privilege).

57. For a discussion of the attorney-client privilege, the insured-insurer privilege, and the work product doctrine, see generally, Jones, Evidence §19: 18–19, 1972. *Hickman v. Taylor,* 329 US 495, 1957, remains the seminal case on the question of protection afforded to attorney work product. Some states, such as Florida, specifically provide that incident reports required under a hospital's risk management program "shall be considered to be part of the workpapers of the attorney defending the establishment in litigation relating thereto . . ." making them subject to discovery only upon a showing of undue hardship. §395.0197, Fla. Stat., 2004, Fla. R. Civ. P 1.280(b)(2). Without a privilege, an incident report would represent a contemporaneous statement of fact generated in response to a specific event and would not be protected.

58. *Sims v. Knollwood Park Hospital,* 511 So.2d 154, (AL, 1987) (patient who fractured hip when she fell in hospital may discover incident report about the fall because it is not work product protected by the attorney-client privilege; the mere possibility of eventual litigation is not enough to protect the report); but see *Enke v. Anderson,* 733 SW 2d 462, MO App., 1987 (incident report was still entitled to the more limited protection available to materials prepared for litigation under the attorney work product doctrine). See also *Shaffer v. Rogers,* 362 NW 2d 552, IA, 1985 (routine internal investigation report was protected even though it might serve a variety of possible future uses; its primary purpose was in anticipation of litigation).

59. See, for example, Mass. Ann. Laws, Ch. 111 §205(b), 2005, which provides protection for incident reports as records necessary to comply with risk management and QA programs; *Gallagher v. Detroit-Macomb Hospital Association,* 171 MI App. 761, 431 NW2d 90, 1988 (discovery of an incident report about a patient's fall from bed not permitted; report came within statutory protection afforded to records prepared for hospital quality-of-care data collection purposes; hospital administrator for legal affairs had testified that incident reports on unusual occurrences were routinely forwarded to internal safety and QA committees).

60. Conner, C., *op. cit.,* pp. 108–11.

61. For example, Florida allows discovery of materials protected as work product "upon a showing that the party seeking discovery has need of the material in preparation of his

case and that he is unable without undue hardship to obtain the substantial equivalent of the materials by other means." Rule 1.280, Florida Rules of Civil Procedure. But, in application, this is a difficult standard for a plaintiff to meet. *Bay Medical Center v. Sapp,* 535 So.2d 308, FL App. 1st DCA, 1988 (where plaintiff was not entitled to production of incident reports in absence of required showing of undue hardship and inability to obtain substantially equivalent materials by other means).

62. Many statutes specifically state that the privilege does not apply to proceedings in which a health care provider contests denial or status of staff privileges or authorization to practice. See, for example, Cal. Evid Code §1157 (c), 2005; Kan. Stat Ann. §65–4915, 2005; La.Rev. Stat. Ann. §§13:3715.3, 2005; 735 Ill. Comp. Stat. Ann.5/8–2101, 2005. Case law is divided on this question. See, for example, *Roseville Community Hospital v. Superior Court,* 70 CA App. 3d 809, 139 CA Rptr. 170, 1977 (statements made by individuals at a committee meeting of hospital's medical staff were discoverable by persons whose requests for staff privileges were denied); contra, *Parkview Memorial Hospital v. Pepple,* 483 NE 2d 469, IN App., 1985 (Indiana's peer review confidentiality law applies to civil actions brought by physicians challenging private hospitals' decisions concerning staff privileges in addition to medical professional liability cases).

63. 42 U.S.C. §11111.

64. 45 C.F.R. Part 61 Governing the Healthcare Integrity and Protection Data Bank.

65. Conner, C., *op. cit.,* pp. 102–108.

66. See, for example, *Humana Hospital Desert Valley v. Superior Court County of Maricopa,* 154 AZ 396, 742 P.2d 1382, 1386, AZ App., 1987 ("If this court were to eliminate the peer review privilege, it would negate an important state interest. . . . The confidentiality of peer review committee proceedings is essential to achieve complete investigation and review of medical care. These deliberations would terminate if they were subject to the discovery process."). See also *Willing v. St. Joseph Hospital,* 176 Ill. App. 3d 737, 531 NE 2d 824, IL App. 1st Dist., 1988; *Caroll v. Nunez,* 137 AD 2d 911, 524 NYS 2d 578, NY AD 3d Dept., 1988. See generally, Annotation, Discovery of hospitals' internal records or communications as to qualifications or evaluations of physicians. 81ALR 3d 944, 1977; Cunco, M.K. "Disclosure versus Confidentiality of Hospital Peer Review Committee Records." *Medical Trial Technique Quarterly,* Fall 1984, pp. 172–83; Goldberg, B.A. "The Peer Review Privilege: A Law in Search of a Valid Policy," *American Journal of Law and Medicine,* 10(151), 1984. Under Florida law, no public policy reasons barred disability insurer from obtaining discovery of insured physicians' peer review materials in suit to recover disability benefits; insurer made a sufficient showing of exceptional necessity or extraordinary circumstances to justify production of the small portions of the hospital applications possibly stating that the physician suffered from no physical or mental limitations impairing ability to practice medicine. *Toyos v. Northwestern Mut. Life Ins. Co.,* 1 F. Supp. 2d 1462 (S.D. Fla. 1998). Provision of Nurse Practice Act allowing claims for retaliatory acts relating to peer review committees did not include within its definition of "peer review" the evaluation of a licensed vocational nurse; such a nurse was not a proper subject for "peer review." Vernos' Ann. Texas Civ. St. art 4525b, §6 *Clark v. Texas Home Health, Inc.,* 971 SW2d 435 (Tex.1998) State statutes prohibiting disclosure of physician peer review procedure were inapplicable to a medical professional liability action brought under the Federal Tort Claims Act. 28 USC §2671 et seq.: NY McKinney's CPLR 4504; *Syposs v. U.S.,* 179 FRD 406 (WDNY 1998) Letter from doctor, allegedly a letter of reference to third party containing a confidential assessment of physicians' professional competence, generated at request of hospital's credentialing committee for use in determining whether permanent privileges should be extended to physician, could be privileged from discovery under Medical Studies Act in medical professional liability litigation

between patient and physician and hospital, as granting or limiting staff privileges could constitute internal quality control. SHA 737 ILCS 5/8–2101, 8–2102. *Stricklin v. Becan,* 293 IL App. 3d 886, 689 NE 2d 328 (4th Dist. 1997) Statutory peer review privilege did not apply to physicians' action against hospital seeking damages for actions of its peer review committee that restricted his staff privileges, such that privilege did not preclude discovery of hospital's peer review committee records, even those documents regarding matters unrelated to the physician. VAMS §537.035 State ex rel. *Health Midwest Development Group, Inc. v. Daugherty,* 965 S.W. 2d 841 (Mo. 1998), reh'g denied (Apr. 21, 1998).

67. In cases alleging corporate negligence of hospitals, most decisions appear to protect against disclosure of peer review records. See, for example, *Terre Haute Regional Hospital, Inc. v. Basden,* 524 NE 2d 1306, IN App., 1988; *Humana Hospital Desert Valley v. Superior Court,* supra; *Shelton v. Morehead Memorial Hospital,* 318 NC 76, 347 SE 2d 824, 1986; *Snell v. Superior Court,* 158 CA App.3d 44, 204 CA Rptr. 200, 1984; *Somer v. Johnson,* 704 F.2d 1473, 11th Cir., 1983; contra, *Byork v. Carmer,* 109 App. Div.2d 1087, 487 NYS 2d 226, 1985; *Greenwood v. Wierdsma,* 741 P.2d 1079, WY,1987.

68. *Virmani v. Novant Health.,* Inc., 259 F. 3d 284 (4th Cir. 2001).

69. See, for example, *Willing v. St. Joseph Hospital,* 176 IL App.3d 737, 531 NE 2d 824, IL App. 1st Dist., 1988 (Interpreting the Illinois Medical Studies Act, the court stated, "Records and documents are protected under the Act if they are utilized as part of the peer review process and not as a result or consequence thereof. . . . the privilege will be accorded only after each document is scrutinized in light of the Act's purpose."); *Byork v. Carmer* (upholding but limiting state's peer review statute to the records of the proceedings of peer review committees and not protecting knowledge gained from other sources); *Harris Hospital v. Schattman,* 734 SW 2d 759, TX App., 1987 (holding that non-discoverable records include only those documents generated by committee, but not communications between hospital and physician); *Humana Hospital v. Superior Court,* supra, note 46 (evidence possessed by credentials committee that was not otherwise privileged could be discovered, although credentials committee files themselves were protected); *Richter v. Diamond,* 108 IL 2d 265, 483 NE 2d 1256, 1985 (statutory privilege applies to the peer review process but is not accorded to the imposition of restrictions that may result from the process).

70. See, for example, Cal. Evid. Code §1157 (c), 2005: The prohibition relating to discovery of testimony does not apply to the statements made by any person in attendance at . . . a meeting of any of those committees who is a party to an action or proceeding the subject matter of which was reviewed at that meeting; *Carroll v. Nunez,* 137 AD 2d 911, 524 NYS 2d 578, 1988 (in motion for protective order, court held that plaintiff was not entitled to physician's personnel folder or copies of complaints made against him for performing unnecessary surgery, but was to be furnished with any statement made by physician at the hospital's peer review committee proceedings regarding the subject matter of the suit).

71. *Jordon v. Court of Appeals,* 701 SW 2d 644, TX 1985 (privilege protects documents prepared by, or at direction of, hospital committee for committee purposes; does not apply to documents that have been created without committee impetus and purpose).

72. For suggestions on how to protect peer review records, see Fishman, L. W. "Confidentiality of Medical and Peer Review Records." Paper presented at National Health Lawyers Association, 1988.

73. 8 Wigmore, Evidence, §2292, McNaughton rev., 1961.

74. The attorney-client privilege, especially in the corporate context, only protects disclosure of communications; it does not protect disclosure of the underlying facts by

those who communicated with the attorney. The application of the privilege is determined on a case-by-case basis. An analysis of this concept can be found in *Upjohn Co. v. United States*, 449 U.S. 383, 1981. Additionally, the Florida Supreme Court has established set criteria to judge whether a corporation's communications are protected by the attorney-client privilege: (1) the communication would not have been made but for the contemplation of legal services; (2) the employee making the communication did so at the direction of a corporate superior; (3) the superior made the request of the employee as part of the corporation's effort to secure legal advice or services; (4) the content of the communication relates to the legal services being rendered, and the subject matter of the communication is within the scope of the employee's duty; and (5) the communication is not disseminated beyond those persons who, because of the corporate structure, need to know its contents. *Southern Bell Telephone and Telegraph Co. v. Deason*, 632 So.2d 1377, (FL 1994). These and similar cases should be consulted for in-depth discussions of these issues.

75. Lo, B. *Best Principles for Health Privacy*, Georgetown, Va.: The Health Privacy Project Working Group, Georgetown University, July 1999.

76. 45 C.F.R. §164.505.

77. BNA's Health Reporter, 14(22), June 2, 2005, p. 749. "eHealth Initiative Announces New Guidelines for Implementing Electronic Health Records." See full text, available at: [www.ehealthinitiative.org/assets/documents/ParallelPathway5–25–052PM.doc].

78. BNA's Health Reporter, 14(11), March 17, 2005, p. 364. "CDC Study Describes Limited Adoption Of Electronic Records by Health Sector." See full text, available at: [pubs.bna.com/ip/BNA/hlr.nsf/is/a0b0p5g4t6].

79. BNA's Health Reporter, 14(23), June 9, 2005, p. 785. "HHS Chief Announces the Creation of Panel to Prepare for Electronic Health Records." See full text, available at: [pubs.bna.com/ip/BNA/hlr.nsf/is/a0b0y1m3d1].

80. Kolata, G. "U.S. Will Offer Doctors Free Electronic Records System." available at: [www.nytimes.com/2005/07/21/health/21records.html?hp&ex=1122004800&en=30f428a18089ce33&ei=5094&partner=homepage]. Jul. 21, 2005; and BNA's Health Reporter, 14(30), July 28, 2005, p. 1015. "CMS to Offer Physicians Low-Cost Electronic Health Record Software Soon." See full text, available at: [pubs.bna.com/ip/BNA/hlr.nsf/is/a0b1d8t9g9].

81. Master Control, Inc. "21 CFR 11: Risks of Noncompliance White Paper," Unpublished, 2005. Available at: [www.mastercontrol.com/PDF/lit/part11risk.pdf].

82. Cal. Health & Safety Code, §123149, 2005.

83. *Ibid.*

84. *Ibid.*

85. 63 Fed. Reg. 43,241 (1998).

86. JCAHO, Standard 6.10, 2005.

87. *Estate of Behringer v. Medical Center at Princeton*, 249 NJ Super. 597, 592 A.2d 1251, 1991 (finding defendant hospital negligent for failure to take reasonable steps to maintain confidentiality of a patient's medical records).

88. American Health Information Management Association. "Model Language for Health Information Legislation on Creation, Authentication, and Retention of Computer-Based Patient Records." Unpublished, 1995 (available at: [www.netreach.net/~wmanning/ahima.htm]).

89. "One system that uses the iris of the eye for identification because it has more unique physical characteristics than fingerprints claims annual fate of 1 in 131,158." Excerpt taken from "ATMs May Make Eye Contact," *St. Petersburg Times*, May 28, 1996, p. 8A.

90. Although tokens traditionally have been implemented as hardware devices, software-only versions of tokens have recently been developed.

91. For a checklist of contractual items to address, see *Health Information Systems and Electronic Medical Records Practice Guide,* Washington, D.C.: American Health Lawyers Association, 1997.

92. For example, an electronic medical records contract uses language indicating that the vendor will abide by all laws and regulations on confidentiality that are now, or may become, applicable to the records. Ensure that the vendor warrants and represents that it will not use any data it obtains in any form.

93. All system usage, including e-mail, must have stated employee regulations. These regulations include a warning that no employee who communicates through the system should expect that communication to be private. Further, it should be stated that the system is to be used only for business purposes and that its misuse will result in termination. Moreover, it should be stated that information access is limited without proper authorization; no personal disks can be used, no files can be copied, and violation of the policies will result in discipline.

94. Fed. Rules Evid. 1001(3).

95. See the Electronic Privacy Information Center [www.epic.org] and the Privacy Page [www.privacy.org].

96. Department of Justice. Office of legal Counsel. Memorandum for Alex M. Azar, II, General Counsel, Department of Health and Human Services and Timothy J. Coleman, Senior Counsel to the Deputy Attorney General, from Steven G. Bradbury, Principal Deputy Assistant Attorney General *Re: Scope of Criminal Enforcement Under 42 U.S.C. § 1320d-6* (June 1, 2005).

97. See full text of plea agreement, available at: [www.usdoj.gov/usao/waw/press_room/2004/aug/pdf_files/cr04_0374rsm_plea.pdf].

Suggested Readings

American Bar Association. *Health Care Facility Records: Confidentiality, Computerization and Security.* Chicago, Ill.: Forum on Health Law of the American Bar Association, 1995.

Blair, J. S. *Overview of Standards Related to the Emerging Health Care Information Infrastructure.* Schaumburg, Ill.: The Computer-Based Patient Record Institute, Inc., 1995.

Daniels, A. R. "Confidentiality of Medical Records." Presentation for the National Health Lawyers Association, Chicago, Ill., June 1994.

Electronic Medical Records: Effective Risk Management after HIPAA. Annual Conference and Exhibition of American Society for Healthcare Risk Management, Chicago, Ill., October 3–6, 1999, presented by Adele A. Waller.

Florida Healthcare Risk Management Basics. Florida Society for Healthcare Risk Management, 2004–05.

Guidelines for Establishing Information Security Policies at Organizations Using Computer-Based Patient Record Systems. Schaumburg, Ill.: The Computer-Based Patient Record Institute, Inc., 1995.

Guidelines for Information Security Education Programs at Organizations Using Computer-Based Patient Record Systems. Schaumburg, Ill.: The Computer-Based Patient Record Institute, Inc., 1995.

Jones, R. T. "Computerized Medical Records: A 'Practical Guide' for Avoiding the Legal Hazards of the Computerized Hospital Record." *LegaLetter. Florida Hospital Association,* June 19, 1995.

Kidwell, R. P., and Smith, M. L. "Proactive Malpractice: Disclosing and Resolving Adverse Outcomes." Paper presented at the Annual Meeting, American Health Lawyers Association AHLA San Diego, CA., June 26–29, 2005.

Waller, A. A., B. M. Broccolo, and D. K. Fulton, "The Electronic Medical Record." Paper presented at the 16th Annual Meeting and Education Conference, American Society for Healthcare Risk Management of the American Hospital Association, November 3, 1994.

15

Introduction to Risk Financing

Dominic A. Colaizzo

Chinese merchants were among the earliest known business people to use risk financing in the conduct of trade and commerce. Merchants who shipped their goods on the Yangtze River could never be sure that their goods would arrive safely at the trading centers downriver. It was not unusual for a merchant boat to sink, losing both the boat and its cargo because some sections of the river were treacherous and difficult to navigate. To avoid total loss, merchants would coordinate their shipping activities and distribute their cargo among several ships. If a boat and its cargo were destroyed during its voyage, then an individual merchant suffered only a partial loss instead of a disastrous total loss. By pooling their interests, these merchants had greater assurance that all would not be lost.

In the late 1600s, individuals interested in investing or financially participating in shipping and trade ventures would gather at Lloyd's Coffee House in London. Notices of trade voyages would be posted that identified the type of ship, its cargo, destination, crew, and captain. Individuals would write their names under these notices with the amount of liability that they would assume in the event of a loss at sea. Each underwriter pledged his personal assets to cover his percentage of the loss in return for a premium for taking the risk. When the notice or slip was fully subscribed, the contract was complete.

Throughout history, close-knit communities have practiced risk financing in an informal way by pooling their resources. In central Pennsylvania, Amish tradition provided for the entire community to help rebuild a barn or house devastated by fire or storm. In return for each member's pledge and resources to participate in the rebuilding effort, the risk of disaster was transferred and distributed to everyone in the community.

In recent years, health care institutions have faced aggressive audits and investigations of their billing practices under the Medicare program by the Centers for Medicare and Medicaid Services (CMS, formerly known as the Health Care Financing Administration) and the Office of the Inspector General (OIG). As billing practices were found to be in non-compliance with the government's interpretation of the reimbursement regulations, many providers were (and still are) faced with the repayment of large amounts to Medicare plus fines and penalties. Providers, for the most part, never anticipated or funded for these business losses, which have had a material negative effect on the financial solvency of their institutions. Traditional insurance for such losses is, for the most part, unavailable. To finance these payments, some providers entered into contracts with insurers that indemnified the provider for the full loss in the year of payment in return for a full repayment of the insurance proceeds, plus the insurer's expenses, over a designated time period. Although this transaction had all the characteristics of a loan, it was structured as an insurance transaction, allowing the provider to spread the financial impact of this loss over several years.

In the examples mentioned, the Chinese, English, and Amish entrepreneurs, and health care executives all used some form of risk financing to deal with the potential for financial loss associated with adverse events. The basics of risk financing for a trip down the Yangtze River or to address Medicare fraud and abuse are essentially the same, including some or all of the following:

- The need to anticipate the risks of the group's operations
- A plan or means to financially deal with a loss if it occurred
- The pooling of resources to finance risk
- Transferring risk to others
- Spreading the risk among others with similar risks
- Risk retention
- Written contracts to substantiate financing arrangements in the event of a loss
- Identifying the simplest, least expensive, and most creative way to finance loss without jeopardizing the financial integrity of their operations
- The motivation to prevent the loss in the first place

Today, risk financing is viewed as a complicated subject involving legal contracts, sophisticated accounting, and a myriad of government regulations. All sorts of risk financing structures are available: an indemnification clause in a contract; an insurance policy that transfers the risk for a given exposure for a given price; the use of a captive insurance company for self-insurance; or a risk securitization plan that uses corporate bonds triggered by pre-established loss criteria. The types of exposures and losses faced by health care institutions for which a planned approach of risk financing is needed are also numerous and complex. Examples include the slip and fall in the parking lot, failure to properly diagnose a patient's condition, water damage to facilities as a result of severe weather, employee injuries while at work, a reduction of an institution's financial assets as a result of poor investment performance, the loss of key management individuals to the competition, the business risks of capitated reimbursement, Medicare fraud and abuse, and most recently, acts of terrorism.

This chapter will introduce you to the concepts of risk financing within the overall context of the risk management process. It will establish the principles and foundation for structuring and implementing the various risk financing techniques. Further discussion on this topic can be found in Chapter 16 on Insurance: Basic Principles and Coverages in this volume, and in Volume III, Chapter 4 on Risk Financing Techniques. You will gain an appreciation of the importance of risk financing and a framework for a successful program.

....

RISK FINANCING IN THE CONTEXT OF THE OVERALL RISK MANAGEMENT PROCESS

The risk management process involves two major areas that are intricately tied to each other—the identification and analysis of exposures and treating the exposures through some form of risk management technique. Figure 15.1 delineates the structure of this process and its key elements.

If we cannot treat these exposures in a manner that significantly eliminates the potential for loss through loss control, we must plan for their treatment through some form of risk financing.

The focus of this chapter is on the risk financing techniques and methods for generating funds to finance loss that risk control could not avoid. In some cases, the potential for loss was not identified or anticipated to allow for risk treatment. As Figure 15.1 depicts, risk can be financed through risk retention or transfer to an outside party.

The decision to use a specific method to treat your organization's risk should be based upon cost efficiency, financial stability and security, and the control over program administration that each method affords your organization.

....

RISK RETENTION

Risk retention techniques can vary from the unplanned payment of a loss from operating funds to a more planned approach such as the use of a captive insurance company. Basically, there are four methods employed by organizations for the financing of loss through retention.

Use of Available Cash

Losses can be paid out of available cash from operations. Neither loss reserves nor funds have been established or designated for these payments. For example, institutions typically pay the deductible for an automobile or property loss out of available operating cash. These deductible payments typically are treated as unplanned expenditures from operations.

From a risk financing perspective, this technique is acceptable for losses that are small in nature and infrequent in occurrence. However, this is not an acceptable technique for financing medical professional liability exposures that typically are significant and frequent for most health care organizations. Unplanned or unfunded payments for this exposure could materially affect the financial stability of the organization at any given time.

The Establishment of Loss Reserves—Recognizing and Potentially Funding the Liability in Advance

A loss reserve can be established for the potential liability of payment for losses. The reserve is typically based on expected losses and is treated as an accounting entry that identifies the potential liability on the organization's financial statements. Cash, securities, or other liquid assets can be earmarked to fund this liability. This technique recognizes that a potential for loss exists. It can go as far as setting aside assets to fund these potential losses. This is the significant difference from the first technique described.

FIGURE 15.1 Risk Management Process Structure

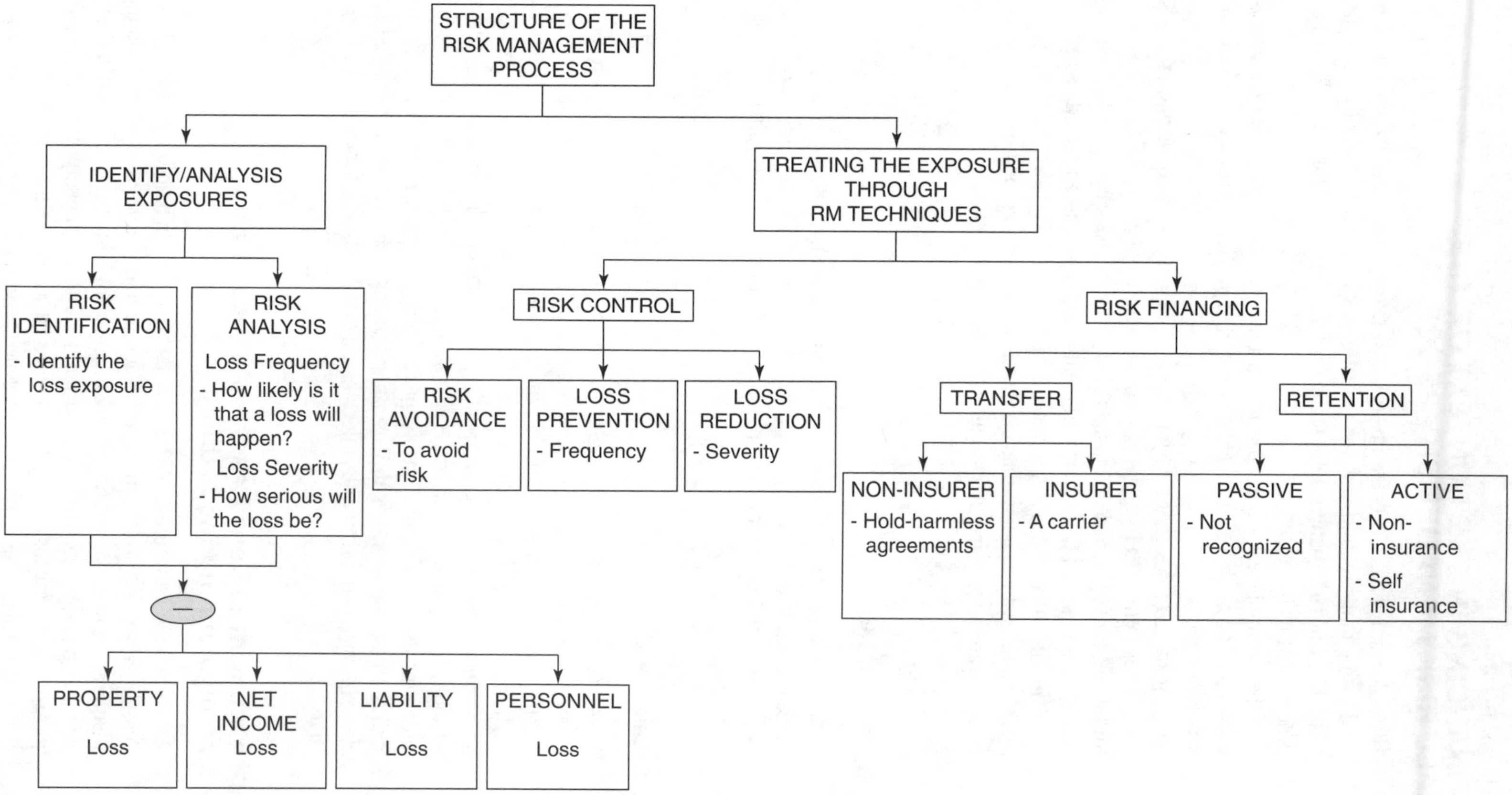

An example of the use of this technique is the treatment of the tail liability that an organization has when it uses a claims-made insurance policy for its professional liability exposures. Accounting standards for health care providers require them to "book" or account for the liability they have for claims incurred but not reported (IBNR) at the end of each accounting year. An accounting entry is made on the financial statements to reflect the liability for this IBNR. This liability may or may not be funded, depending upon the philosophy or resources of the organization.

Use of Borrowed Funds

Borrowed funds can be used to pay for losses when they become payable. For the traditional health care provider, this method is inefficient, because it reduces the ability of the organization to borrow funds for more appropriate purchases. Moreover, the cost of unplanned borrowing typically is more inefficient and expensive. The use of borrowed funds to pay for losses is essentially a means of borrowing time. Ultimately, the institution must pay for the loss with its own earnings or other resources.

Formal Self-Insurance Techniques

Formalized methods of self-insurance can be used when an organization finances its losses through a planned strategy. The most typical forms of self-insurance that health care institutions use today are the self-insurance trust or some form of a captive insurance company.

Self-Insurance Trust   A trust is a funding vehicle that, in simplest terms, is a bank account administered by an independent third party (trustee). The funds are designated for the sole and restricted purpose of paying losses. The trustee administers the trust through a formalized agreement and a statement of coverage that outlines the type and limits of loss to be paid. Funding in the trust typically is established at levels determined by an actuarial study and operated in accordance with Medicare requirements. From an accounting perspective, the trust's assets and liabilities are recognized on the financial statements and a description of the liabilities and funding are generally disclosed in a footnote to those statements. Both profit and not-for-profit entities can establish trusts.

Because a trust is not an insurance vehicle, it is strictly limited to the funding purposes for which it was established. For not-for-profit entities, a trust typically cannot be used for its for-profit subsidiaries. Also, a trust lacks the flexibility to accommodate regulated lines of insurance and cannot accommodate the risks of third parties (those entities or individuals outside the parent's economic family). Such activities would be considered the conduct of insurance and would be subject to state insurance regulations or would jeopardize the parent's not-for-profit status.

The trust was once the most common vehicle for self-insurance of the primary professional and general liability exposures of a health care provider. Over time, trusts were replaced by captive insurance companies because these vehicles are more flexible in accommodating the various exposures and risk financing needs that a health care institution faces in today's environment. Recent hard market conditions for professional liability are once again elevating this risk financing option for consideration, especially for smaller not-for-profit providers whose financial resources are limited and whose risk financing priorities are not driven by the need to accommodate other lines of coverage or the risks of third parties. Many providers are now combining the use of the trust and captive to take advantage of the benefits that each vehicle has to offer.

Captive Insurance Company   A captive is a closely held insurance company whose insurance business is primarily supplied by and controlled by its owners, and in which the original insureds are the principal beneficiaries. Simply stated, a captive is a corporation for which the product is the payment of losses and the revenue is premium payments. Because a captive is an insurance vehicle and can be structured in many ways, it has great flexibility to accommodate the numerous and varied risk financing needs of organizations such as third-party businesses, for-profit entities, and multiple lines of coverage. It is a more formalized method of self-insurance in that it has separate financial statements and is regulated in the domicile in which it is established. This vehicle elevates the risk management function in an organization as its separate financial statements are scrutinized by board members typically drawn from the senior ranks of management and the parent's board. Because of a captive's visibility, there is a greater emphasis on controlling losses, the primary driver of costs for any program.

The form, structure, and ownership of captives can be established in different ways and combinations to meet the ownership, control, and coverage goals of their insureds. A more detailed discussion of these is presented in later chapters.

Note that the use of captive insurance companies, trusts, and other forms of self-insurance (often referred to as the alternative risk transfer [ART] marketplace) has grown significantly in recent years. According to AM Best, ART now comprises over 50 percent of the commercial insurance marketplace in the United States. For health care institutions, this percentage is much higher because of the nature and volatility of the risks that must be dealt with in the context of a limited standard insurance marketplace. For financing of all types of risk, ART can no longer be referred to as the "alternative," as it has become a standard approach by which institutional insureds finance their risks.

Risk Transfer

When an outside third party pays for losses when they occur, some form of risk transfer agreement is used. The most common method of risk transfer is the purchase of commercial insurance. Risk transfer also can be accomplished through non-insurance techniques, such as the use of an indemnification provision in a contract. Indemnification is the process by which one is restored or reimbursed to the extent of the loss ("made whole again").

Insurance is a contractual relationship that exists when one party (the insurer) for consideration (premium) agrees to reimburse or pay for another party's (insured) fortuitous loss caused by a predefined event (peril). Risk is shifted to others and spread among many parties. In general terms, covering the risks of unrelated parties by a company owned by multiple owners will constitute insurance.

From a practical view, insurance will nearly always involve some form of risk retention on a planned or unplanned basis. The use of a deductible would be an example of a planned retention. Denial of coverage as a result of an adverse policy coverage interpretation by the commercial insurer would certainly be an unplanned retention. The insurance policy, therefore, should never be viewed as a "complete" transfer of risk.

There are many forms and types of insurance that are generally classified in four areas as defined and illustrated in Table 15.1. Chapter 16 will provide a more detailed discussion of these coverages. Remember the principles and practices of these coverages as you apply them effectively in a risk financing program.

The other method of risk transfer, the use of indemnification provisions in a contract, can be an effective tool to lower the overall cost of risk. A hold-harmless agreement is an agreement between two or more parties that defines an obligation or duty resting on one party to make good the liability, loss, or damage that the other party has incurred or may

TABLE 15.1   Types of Insurance

Type of Insurance	Definition	Examples
First Party	Provides coverage for the insured's own property or person. Is intended to indemnify and restore the insured to the same financial position that they had prior to the loss.	Fire/Property Business Interruption Boiler & Machinery Builders Risk Flood Earthquake Crime HMO/Capitation Stop Loss
Third-Party/Liability Insurance	Provides coverage to a party other than the insured. Coverage is intended to indemnify the third party for loss or injury caused by the insured. Involves three parties: 1. The insured who caused the harm or damage; 2. The party who is harmed; and 3. The insurer.	Professional Liability General Liability (Premises liability) Excess/Umbrella Liability Employers Liability Auto Liability Director's & Officer's Liability Management Errors & Omissions Environmental Impairment
Health and Welfare Insurance (Benefits)	Provides coverage for an insured's employees. Coverage is intended to indemnify the employee by restoring his or her health and earnings to the level they maintained prior to the loss.	Workers' Compensation Health Benefits Long-Term Disability Short-Term Disability Dental Vision Life
Financial Guarantees (Surety/Bonds)	Provides a guarantee that specific obligations of a contract or performance will be fulfilled. These differ from traditional insurance in that assets are pledged for the full amount of risk transferred.	Surety/Bonds Public Official Bonds Judicial Bonds Contract/Performance Bonds License & Permit Bonds

incur. Hold-harmless indemnification provisions can vary significantly. A common type of mutual indemnification clause may read as follows:

> Provider agrees to indemnify and hold harmless the managed care organization (MCO) against any negligent act or claim made with respect to items or services provided by Provider under this Agreement to the extent that the negligent act or claim is attributable to any person or activity for which Provider is solely responsible or which arises in connection with the use or maintenance of property, equipment, or facilities under the direction or control of Provider. MCO agrees to indemnify and hold harmless Provider against any negligent act or claim made with respect to items or services provided under this Agreement to the extent that the negligent act or claim is attributable to any person or activity for which MCO is solely responsible or otherwise arises from duties or obligations that are solely the responsibility of MCO under this Agreement.

This clause states that each of the parties to the agreement will be responsible for indemnifying the other party for loss caused due to their negligence. This method of risk transfer is practical in certain situations such as the execution of construction or supply contracts, but not in others, such as for the professional liability risks of providing care to patients. Patients are unlikely to sign a hold-harmless agreement before agreeing to be admitted to the hospital for care. Consent-to-treat agreements that patients are asked to sign before surgery or other invasive treatment are not intended to transfer risk but to authorize the particular treatment being proposed.

As with any risk financing technique, indemnification provisions need to be evaluated for the cost efficiency, financial security, and control that they afford in the risk transfer process. Therefore, these agreements need to be supported by the financial resources of the contracting party or some form of insurance or surety. They also need to be written or supported in such a way as to clearly define each party's rights and obligations in the event of a loss. In any event, given the legal uncertainties in enforcing hold-harmless agreements, they should never be relied upon exclusively to accomplish risk transfer. Refer to Chapter 12 on Contract Review for a more detailed discussion of the use of contracts in transferring risk.

Risk Retention versus Risk Transfer

The decision whether to transfer rather than retain risk will depend upon many factors, including:

- The size and type of the organization and its operations
- Financial strength and resources of the organization
- Type of risk to be treated
- Risk-taking philosophy
- An organization's future goals and objectives
- The overall effectiveness of the risk management and loss control programs

Risk financing can be viewed as a continuum (see Figure 15.2) between total risk transfer to total retention. The figure provides a framework of the cost efficiency and cost certainty that each technique provides. Total risk transfer through insurance will fix costs

FIGURE 15.2   Risk Financing Continuum

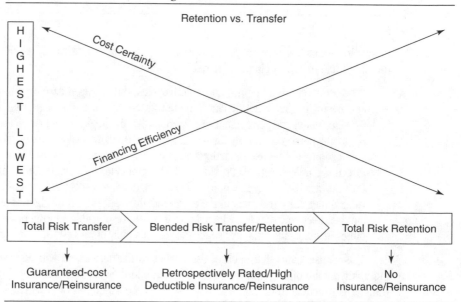

with certainty, but cost efficiencies are sacrificed as a result of the insurance cariers' company's charges for taking on the full risk. The opposite is true for self-insurance of total exposures.

As an example, if you purchased insurance for the first dollar of loss for your professional liability exposures, your financing costs for a given period of time would be fixed, providing you with the highest level of cost certainty. Theoretically, it could also be the most costly approach as your premium would include:

- The insurance company's profit and overhead
- Estimate of the losses to be paid under the policy
- Charges for use of its policy form and the administration of the insurance program such as claims handling, loss control, and other policy services
- Reinsurance
- A charge for the "risk" it is assuming for this exposure
- Charges to reflect adverse loss development of other insureds and hard market conditions

Because the insurance company is taking the risk, it will want to retain control over most or all major decisions involving the coverage. This might be the best risk financing technique for a small organization with limited assets and resources in which maximum cost certainty is important for financial well-being. It might also be a better technique for financing miscellaneous exposures for which the frequency or severity of loss cannot be reasonably predicted. These exposures can usually be insured at a "reasonable" price.

At the other end of the continuum, you could choose to retain all the risk for your professional liability exposures through some method of self-insurance. The cost of financing the risk would be most uncertain and would vary significantly with the frequency and severity of losses. Your cost efficiency would be at a high level because you would not pay an insurer for profit, overhead, and program service administration charges, and because you would retain control over all aspects of the risk-financing program. This approach might make sense for very large organizations that have the resources to manage all aspects of their risk management programs in an effective manner, and have sufficient assets to accommodate the volatility of loss payments without impairing the financial strength of the organization.

Typically, risk managers use a combination of risk transfer and retention for professional liability exposures, whereby the predicable layer of loss is retained while the unpredictable, catastrophic loss is transferred. This approach strikes a balance between cost efficiency and certainty. By retaining the predictable loss layer, insurance company profit and overhead and other charges are minimized. Transferring the unpredictable, more volatile catastrophic losses to an insurer at a "reasonable" premium prevents significant swings in overall program costs and promotes financial stability over the long term, a key objective of any well-run organization. Program control is also balanced in a more effective and appropriate manner between your organization and the insurer.

As you chose between risk transfer and retention, consider the following guidance:

- The risk-taking philosophy of your organization affects the goals of the risk financing program. Define the risk you are willing to take versus what you can afford. Senior management needs to be involved in establishing the philosophy.
- Self-insure the predictable layer of loss where possible. To do otherwise would be trading dollars with an insurer with a loss of control over your program.

- Transfer the unpredictable or catastrophic layers of potential loss at limits sufficient to protect the assets of your organization. Excess coverage at sufficient limits is usually available at reasonable prices. Self-insuring this exposure to loss would be risking a lot to save a little.

- If you retain risk, you should have an effective risk management program in place to control or minimize loss. Sound risk information, loss control, claims handling, and litigation management systems are prerequisites. You also need to involve senior management and all "your" insureds in the process. An effective program will also make your organization an attractive risk for insurance purposes as you purchase coverage for catastrophic exposures. Keep in mind that risk retention through some form of self-insurance is not a cure for poor loss experience.

- Always take a long-term review of your risk transfer versus retention strategy. In a soft marketplace, you might be able to purchase insurance at a cost that is lower than expected losses. What effect does this have on your long-term costs and control over the program? Will the purchase of insurance take focus away from loss control efforts?

- Be prudent and conservative in funding for your self-insurance program. You can always fund less in the future if your loss experience develops better than expected. You always need a buffer to accommodate adverse loss experience in any program.

- When purchasing insurance, know your carrier better than it knows itself. Make sure it has the financial security, stable management, and policy services to be a good partner. Investigate its track record for paying claims and honoring its commitments. Do you have a relationship with your insurer to resolve gray areas of coverage?

- Choose your risk financing consultants, brokers, actuaries, legal advisers, defense counsel, and auditors carefully. They need to be your partners and advocates in safeguarding your organization's assets and reputation. They not only have to be qualified through education and experience, but also need the integrity to have your total interest at heart. Make sure they can work together as a team to make your program as effective as possible. Refer to Chapter 13 in Volume III of this series for more information on request for proposals.

············

CONCLUSION

The risk financing of losses that occur despite your best risk control efforts may be from the unstructured payment of loss from operating funds, from the application of the indemnification provision of a contract, or financed under the structured terms of a formal captive insurance company. The best and most effective method for your organization will depend upon many factors including the type of risk, its predictability for loss, the financial effect on your organization, your risk-taking philosophy, the sophistication of your risk management program, the degree of control you desire over program services, and the availability and affordability of insurance coverages.

As a risk management professional, it is your responsibility to guide your organization in making the best choice in meeting the overall mission and objectives of the organization. A sound risk financing program is important in protecting the assets of your organization and ultimately its reputation and ability to serve its customers and patients.

Suggested Readings

AM Best Review Magazine.

Elliot, Michael W. *Risk Financing,* (1st ed.). Insurance Institute of America, 2000.

Captive Insurance Company Reports, published monthly by International Risk Management Institute, Inc.

The Hold Harmless Agreement. Cincinnati, OH: The National Underwriter Co., 1987.

Krauss, G. E. *Essentials of Property and Casualty Insurance: A Complete Guide to the Pennsylvania Licensure* (11th ed.), 2002.

Rejda, G., and Elliott, M. *Insurance Perspectives.* American Institute for Chartered Property Casualty Underwriters, 1994.

16

Insurance: Basic Principles and Coverages

Kimberly Willis
Judy Hart

This chapter presents insurance principles and practices that apply to the health care industry. There are two main themes in this chapter. One theme will discuss the basic concepts of insurance and how it is purchased and regulated, and the second will review the major types of insurance purchased by health care organizations.

The most common method of transferring or financing risk is to purchase insurance. Unfortunately, many individuals charged with health care risk management duties and assigned responsibility for the purchase of insurance have limited knowledge of its nuances. Many health care risk management professionals are seeking an insurance product that is a comprehensive and cost-effective method of transferring unwanted risk to an insurer. This dictates a need to understand the nature of insurance, how to read an insurance policy, understand traditional coverages applicable to health care, and an ability to determine when changes are necessary. Insurance alone cannot prevent risk, but it can provide financial security against loss.

DEFINITION OF INSURANCE

Barry Smith defines insurance as "a system by which a risk is transferred by a person, business, or organization to an insurance company, which reimburses the insured for covered losses and provides for sharing of costs or losses among all insureds. Risk, transfer, and sharing are vital elements of insurance."[1] Risk, or the possibility of loss, creates the need for insurance. An organization can retain risk or transfer its risk to another organization. Risk is commonly transferred to an insurance company. By accepting and sharing in the risk of many organizations, the insurance company can statistically calculate the likelihood that losses will or will not occur. It can also calculate their likely severity. This calculation results in a premium that is then charged back to the organization wishing to transfer its risk. If the method of premium calculation is sound, the insurer should be able to pay the claims that are incurred and still earn a profit.

An insurance policy is a legal contract that creates obligations for both the insured (the individual organization wishing to transfer risk) and the insurer (the insurance company accepting the risk). Under this contract, the insurer promises to pay certain amounts if defined events take place. For example, the insuring agreement of a medical professional liability policy obligates the insurer to pay on behalf of the insured sums that the insured shall become legally obligated to pay as damages for the rendering or failure to render professional health care services. This obligation is modified by various other clauses, coverage terms, exclusions, and definitions in the insurance contract. An insured's obligations vary but most frequently it is required to pay a premium, report claims or likely losses in a speedy manner, and minimize the likelihood for loss. Insured losses must usually be fortuitous events—sudden and accidental. Intentional acts that result in loss are generally not covered by the insurance contract.

Although insurance contracts vary, they usually contain four standard elements: the declarations page, insuring agreement, conditions of the policy, and exclusions.

The declarations page identifies the named insured and describes the property or activity to be insured. Components of the page include the policy number, coverage inception and expiration dates, retroactive date, insured address, policy limit, applicable deductibles, insurer, and premium. The declarations page may also identify the various forms or endorsements to be attached to the policy.

The insuring agreement states the insurer's obligations under the terms of the contract. In general, the insuring agreement is often broadly stated, but later narrowed based on additional wording elsewhere in the policy. The insuring agreement contains conditional promises to pay. For example, if the policy states that the insurer will pay sums related to the rendering or failure to render "professional services," the meaning of professional services is defined elsewhere in the policy. If the claim does not fall within this definition, it will not be covered. When interpreting the policy, the insured should remember that the insuring agreement is subject to the declarations, conditions, exclusions, and definitions contained elsewhere in the policy.

The conditions of the policy spell out many of the obligations of the insured and the insurer. Examples of important conditions include:

- The insured's obligation to provide prompt notice of loss
- The insured's obligation to cooperate with the insurer in investigation and settlement of loss
- The insured's obligation to pay the premium in a timely manner
- The conditions under which the policy may be canceled or non-renewed
- The insurer's right to inspect the premises
- The coverage territory of the policy
- The applicability of limits, deductibles, and defense expenses

Failure of an insured to adhere to the policy's conditions could result in the insurer's refusal to honor a claim.

Exclusions refer to policy provisions that eliminate or minimize coverage that the insurer does not intend to provide. Exclusions are usually identified in a specific section of the policy; however, additional exclusions may be dispersed throughout the insurance contract. In some cases, exclusions are added by endorsement(s) attached to the main policy form. Although exclusions appear punitive, they might not be. In some cases, an exclusion may be added to eliminate the potential for duplicate coverage or coverage not needed by a typical insured. Under other circumstances, an insurer may add an exclusion for its own benefit. Such is the case when the carrier is trying to limit risks it considers undesirable, a morale hazard, or outside its reinsurance arrangements. Typical exclusions include intentional acts, war, pollution or nuclear energy, terrorism, mold, and criminal acts. Many liability policies also exclude or minimize coverage provided for sexual misconduct, anti-trust, punitive damages, and discrimination.

Insureds should work closely with the broker, agent, consultant, or carrier to make certain their insurance policy(ies) provide comprehensive, cost-effective, and financially secure transfer of risk.

How Insurance is Regulated

Insurance is a highly regulated industry. Most regulation is mandated at the state level. The rules and regulations vary by state. Nearly all states give their insurance departments the power to regulate rates, to license insurers and insurance company representatives, to approve policy forms, and to respond to consumer complaints.

Insurance brokers and agents must be licensed in their state(s) of operation. This usually involves a state examination and continuing education requirements.

Most insurance carriers must apply and financially qualify in every state in which they wish to solicit or conduct business. Once a carrier is approved by the state, it is considered admitted. As an admitted insurer, the carrier must obey all state laws regulating the operation of an insurance company. In addition, it must file its current policy forms, any changes in forms, and any premium rate increases or decreases with the state for approval by the insurance department. Most states have established guaranty funds to protect insureds from the insolvency of admitted carriers. These funds typically are financed by assessments against those insurers.

For various reasons, some carriers operate as non-admitted or surplus lines carriers in a state. These companies are exempt from rigorous state regulations. Neither their premium rates nor the contents of their policies are subject to regulation and review. Because these carriers are exempt from various state regulations, they are not allowed to participate in the guaranty fund. Most states require that insureds who purchase coverage from a surplus lines carrier pay taxes or other fees on the premium. These taxes are usually in addition to the annual premium quoted by the carrier.

Insurance Company Financial Security

The financial stability of an insurance carrier should be a key consideration in an insured's decision to transfer risk. If an admitted carrier fails, its insureds may have access to the state guaranty fund. Unfortunately, the protection offered by these funds is limited. Not all state funds cover all policies or claims. For example, some guaranty funds exclude medical professional liability policies. Others limit the time in which a claim can be reported to the fund. The duration may be shorter than the time provided under the original insurance policy. In some cases, the limits of liability provided by the fund are lower than the limits the defunct insurance carrier provided. For example, the fund may pay 33 cents on each dollar of the policy limit, or it may provide only a $100,000 limit. Under this scenario, the insured is responsible for the remainder of any claim.

It is critical that insureds carefully evaluate the financial position of their insurance carriers. To assist insureds and others with this evaluation, a rating system has been developed to categorize the financial condition of carriers. The most frequently cited rating resource for insurance companies is A.M. Best (Best). Best performs a comprehensive quantitative and qualitative analysis of the company's balance sheet strength, operating performance, and business profile.

Financial Strength and Size

Best's reviews include an evaluation of (1) the company's spread of risk exposures; (2) appropriateness of reinsurance; (3) quality and diversification of assets; (4) adequacy of loss reserves; (5) adequacy of surplus; (6) capital structure; (7) management experience; (8) market presence; and (9) policyholders' confidence. These tests primarily focus on (1) profitability, (2) leverage and capitalization, and (3) liquidity. Each carrier's financial performance is examined and more than 100 financial tests are performed. Based on the ratios, A.M. Best assigns a value from "A++" (superior) to "F" (in liquidation).

Companies that receive a letter rating from Best are further evaluated as to their financial size (FSC) and placed in a size class category. Policy holder surplus plus other conditional or technical reserve funds are the basis for this rating. The rating is expressed in roman numerals from the smallest financial size category of Class "I" to the highest Class of "XV." Most insured will purchase insurance coverage from insurers that they feel can best provide adequate limits to cover their risk.

An insured can obtain an insurer's A.M. Best rating by asking their insurance carrier, agent, or broker for a copy of the current report. In addition, A.M. Best manuals are usually available at large public or university libraries. For more information on A.M. Best go to [www.ambest.com/ratings/pcbirpreface.pdf]. Other sources for financial information are Standard and Poor's and Moody's rating agencies.

Health care risk management professionals should inquire as to the financial rating of their current and past insurance carriers. Health care medical professional liability is a long-tail exposure. Although some claims are reported promptly and paid quickly, other claims might not be known or paid until several years in the future. When the policy is purchased, a carrier may be financially sound but over time, the carrier's financial strength could weaken to the point of insolvency.

How Insurance is Purchased

Most health care risk management professionals gain access to the commercial insurance market by using an insurance broker or independent agent.

Traditionally, brokers are independent insurance professionals who represent the insurance buyer to the insurance company. In this role, they participate in the evaluation of risk potential, gathering of exposure and loss information, presentation of the data to the insurance community, negotiation of coverage terms and premium pricing, and evaluation of quotations. Brokers may also provide assistance in loss mitigation, with alternative means of financing risk. Historically, agents have legally and contractually represented the interest of the insurance carrier, not the insured. An agent may represent one or many insurance carriers. In practice, the line between a broker and agent has blurred. Both act as facilitators for the evaluation and purchase of insurance.

Brokers and agents are often compensated on a commission basis. The amount of commission varies by line of coverage and carrier. Brokers are frequently willing to accept compensation on a flat fee basis. This removes any bias the broker might have regarding its commission level with a particular carrier. Some brokers are willing to work on a fee plus incentive basis. Regardless of the method of compensation, your broker or agent should be willing to openly discuss and disclose all methods of compensation received from placing coverage.

Drafting Coverage Specifications

Risk management professionals often have the responsibility of securing cost-efficient, comprehensive insurance coverage. This is not an easy task. The process should begin at least six months before policy inception. The first step is an evaluation of exposures and the insurance products available to cover the exposures. Once the exposure(s) to be transferred are identified, an application for coverage is prepared. This application is often called an underwriting submission. The submission serves as a tool to present your organization's business strategies, risk exposures, and insurance desires to the insurance marketplace.

Some carriers will allow the insured to develop its own application for coverage. Others require that the submission be prepared based on a standard format developed by the carrier. The submission is then submitted to the carrier's underwriting department. A quotation is developed. The insured, the broker or agent, and the insurer then negotiate through coverage terms, services, and pricing considerations. Upon agreement the coverage is bound. Components of the underwriting submission frequently include:

- A description of operations and organizational chart
- Listing of named insureds and additional insureds
- Retroactive dates (if the coverage is on a claims-made basis)
- Location listing
- Current and historical exposure information
- Currently valued historical loss experience (five to twenty years of loss experience)
- Large loss detail for any claim over $100,000
- Signed application (as requested by the carrier)
- Current annual report or other financial statements
- Description of risk management department procedures including loss prevention, quality improvement, patient safety initiatives, and claims management
- Current actuarial report
- Trust, captive, or underlying coverage document
- JCAHO or other accreditation report
- Description of desired coverage—limits, deductible, coverage extensions, underlying coverages, pricing guidelines, policy period, key coverage terms, or services

Identifying the carriers who are interested in assuming your risk is the next step. Since 2000, various carriers have been liquidated, and others have voluntarily left the market. Some carriers have refocused their health care initiatives, and new entrants have entered the marketplace. Key criteria to consider when selecting a carrier include:

- Does the purchase of this policy support the short-term or long-term objectives of the health care organization and risk management department?
- Is the insurance carrier financially secure? What is its financial rating according to A.M. Best or other rating organizations?

- Is the carrier knowledgeable in health care operations?
- Is the carrier flexible?
- Is the pricing competitive?
- How will future pricing be affected by your organization's favorable or unfavorable loss experience?
- How will future pricing be affected by losses within the health care industry or outside of the health care industry?
- Is the carrier capable of meeting the claims administration, loss prevention, clinical risk management, risk management information systems (RMIS), and educational needs of your facility?
- How long has this carrier been offering this type of coverage? What is its past history in the marketplace? Is it a long-term option?
- What is the carrier's claims handling philosophy? Will it allow input from your organization?
- Who does the carrier use for legal counsel?

Once quotations are received, they must be analyzed for price, terms, services, and other qualitative issues. Insurance policies vary in terms and conditions, but key coverage considerations should include:

- Is the quotation based on complete and accurate exposure and loss information? If the information is not complete, could the pricing change based on outstanding data?
- What are the limits of the policy? How do they apply?
- Is there a deductible or retention and how does it apply?
- Does the policy include a co-insurance provision?
- What is the policy period, effective date, and expiration date of coverage?
- What is the premium? Is there a minimum premium? Is the premium flat, assessable, or auditable?
- Is coverage claims-made or occurrence?
- If coverage is claims-made, what is the retroactive date?
- What is the intent of coverage? Has the carrier released sample forms and endorsements?
- What are the key exclusions? Are these common? Can they be amended?
- Who is covered by the policy—organizations in addition to individuals?
- What is the coverage territory?
- What is the procedure for reporting claims?
- What is the definition of a claim?
- What is the timeframe within which claims must be reported? Is there a prescribed format for reporting? Who must report claims?
- Does the application become a warranty to the policy?
- How are defense costs handled? Are they included within the limit or retention or exclusive outside of the limit or retention?
- Are there provisions for adding or deleting exposures during the policy period?
- Under what circumstances can the insured and insurer cancel or non-renew the policy?

Once coverage has been bound, the broker or carrier will issue a binder of insurance evidencing that coverage was purchased. Once the actual policy is issued, the binder is no longer needed. It also might be helpful to have your broker or agent prepare an insurance summary. This tool emphasizes key components of your insurance policy. The summary will often include a description of the type of policy purchased, policy numbers, policy period, limits of coverage, deductibles, premiums, a coverage overview, and major exclusions.

Another helpful tool that is often prepared by your broker or agent is a schedule of insurance. This schedule is a condensed version of all insurance coverage placed, and is used as a quick reference or guide. Many risk management professionals have this schedule readily available as a reference to answer questions The schedule of insurance generally covers much of the same material as in a policy summary, except that the coverage overview and narrative description of policy type is not included and all lines of coverage are included.

The Hard and Soft Market

The insurance industry is cyclical. It is characterized by periods of low premium, flexible terms, and generous capacity followed by periods fraught with escalating premiums, strict underwriting procedures, and limited availability of coverage. The periods of flexible pricing and terms are known as "soft" markets. Once pricing and terms become more limited, the market is considered to be in a "hard" cycle. The last soft market started in the late 1980s and lasted until 2000–2001. The cycles usually last five to seven years, so the latest soft market was unexpectedly long. Although no one can predict a turn in the market or the best position to take in a hard market, certain considerations should be evaluated. These include:

- What is the overall business strategy of the carrier?
- Has it historically been committed to the health care industry?
- Is it committed to your organization?
- How has the carrier reacted to other pricing cycles?
- What is the financial status of the carrier?
- What is the carrier's loss ratio for similar accounts? Is the exposure profitable for the carrier?
- Does it make sense to put all the organization's exposures with one carrier and hope that the economies of scale prove beneficial, or is it better to disperse the exposures throughout the marketplace and create numerous relationships?

The potential for a hard market also dictates that a health care organization reevaluate its current risk-financing program. Analysis should include:

- Review of limits purchased: Are they enough? Should they be reduced, increased, or restructured?
- Review of retentions: Should the retentions be restructured?
- Should the organization continue to transfer this risk? Could the risk be better managed by the use of an alternative risk financing vehicle or retention of the risk?
- Review of the organization's risk and claims management programs: Are they in order?

Throughout the course of their professional careers, risk management professionals will have to deal with hard markets. Because of this certainty, health care risk management professionals should constantly be reviewing their risk financing vehicles for short-term and long-term benefits. They must also evaluate the best method and technique for presenting their risk to the insurance marketplace. Without proper planning, coverage might not be available at any cost. A hard market cycle dictates that the risk management professional:

- Consider alternative program structures. This might include considering higher deductibles, purchasing lower limits, going without coverage, and establishing a captive or trust in addition to other finite risk vehicles.

- Start the process of securing coverage six months before inception of the policy. This will allow time for adequate planning, preparation of the submission, presentation of the risk, and evaluation of alternatives.

- Develop a timeline for each viable alternative. Identify critical dates.

- Engage senior management in the process. In a hard market, senior management might find its insurance budget woefully inadequate. Premiums could escalate.

- Rely on experts to assist in the process. Consultants or knowledgeable health care brokers can provide assistance as to the marketplace and presenting the risk, but actuaries, accountants, legal firms, clinical risk specialists, claims specialists, and other experts may be needed if your organization is considering increasing retentions significantly through the use of a trust, captive, or other alternative financing arrangements.

- Recognize that underwriters view certain risk areas more or less favorably. For example, certain carriers are comfortable with physician exposures, whereas others are not, and prefer to focus primarily on hospital exposures.

- Present the risk in a way that appeals to the carrier. Each carrier's appetite for risk is different. Research each carrier's senior management and risk philosophy. Present your risk in a way that differentiates it in the marketplace. Be concise. Minimize the difficult areas of your risk picture and maximize the positives. Present a complete and accurate loss picture and identify steps that have been taken to reduce the likelihood of future occurrences.

A Discussion of Claims-Made versus Occurrence Policies

Certain health care related policies are often written on a claims-made basis. Examples include directors' and officers' liability and managed care errors and omissions. Other policies are offered on an occurrence basis. Automobile, property, and workers' compensation are usually written on an occurrence form. Still other coverages, such as medical professional liability, are commonly written on either a claims-made or occurrence basis.

An occurrence policy covers an insured for incidents that occur while the policy is in effect, regardless of when the incident is reported to the insurer. Unlike claims-made, there is no need for an insured to obtain an additional policy endorsement or extension when the insured wishes to move to a new insurer. The date the claim or incident is filed has no effect on the applicable policy period. The date that the claim occurred determines the applicable policy period.

A claims-made policy covers an insured for incidents that both occur and are reported to the insurer while the policy is in force. This method of tracking claims can be burdensome because claims or incidents might occur during one policy period but are not reported until after the policy period has ended. If this happens, coverage might not apply for the claim. This potential gap in coverage can be minimized through the maintenance of an original retroactive date (nose) or the purchase of an extended reporting period (tail).

For coverage under a claims-made policy to apply, the incident or claim must have occurred after the retroactive date of the policy. The retroactive date is usually the first date that the insured purchased claims-made coverage. Under most circumstances, the retroactive date should be maintained on all subsequent policies.

For example, assume a physician purchases a first claims-made policy on July 1, 2001, from XYZ Insurance. The policy will cover those claims that are incurred and reported from July 1, 2001, to June 30, 2002. Because this is the first claims-made policy the physician has purchased, it will have a July 1, 2001, retroactive date. Now assume that three years pass and the physician has maintained claims-made coverage with XYZ for the entire three-year period. In addition, the original retroactive date of July 1, 2001, has been maintained. Unknown to the physician, an incident occurred on August 1, 2001, but was not known to the physician until the current policy period (July 1, 2003, to June 30, 2004). Even though the claim occurred on August 1, 2001, it will be paid under the current claims-made policy rather than the original July 1, 2001, to June 30, 2002, policy. This is because the physician has maintained the retroactive date of July 1, 2001, on the current policy. The current policy covers those claims incurred and reported for the current policy period (July 1, 2003, through June 30, 2004) and that occurred subsequent to July 1, 2001, and reported during the current policy period. The current policy, however, would not cover any claim that occurred previous to the retroactive date of July 1, 2001, or any claim reported in a previous policy period. If the physician failed to maintain the July 1, 2001, retroactive date, the claim would not have been covered by either the July 1, 2001, to June 30, 2002, policy (in place at the time of the event) or the July 1, 2003, to June 30, 2004, policy (in place at the time of the report) In contrast, if the physician had purchased occurrence coverage, the claim would have been paid under the July 1, 2001, to June 30, 2002, occurrence policy.

Nose

Under a claims-made form, the nose is the period of time between an insured's retroactive date and the current policy period. In the example above, the nose is the period July 1, 2001, through June 30, 2003. The policy will respond to claims that have been incurred during the period July 1, 2001, through June 30, 2003, but are not reported until the July 1, 2003, to June 30, 2004, policy year. In addition, the July 1, 2003, to June 30, 2004, policy will also provide protection for those claims incurred and reported during the July 1, 2003, to June 30, 2004, policy year.

Tail

A tail is also known as an extended reporting period (ERP). Various scenarios create the need for an ERP, but the most common scenario is when an insured changes carriers. The ERP essentially converts a claims-made policy to an occurrence policy by extending coverage to all claims that arise from care rendered during the policy period (and nose period, if applicable), regardless of when the claim is reported.

ERPs can be limited in time and in the limits of liability that they offer. An unlimited time for the extended reporting period is preferred, but some carriers limit the ERP to twelve months, thirty-six months, or some other limited period of time. The limits of liability purchased with an ERP also can vary. They can simply be an extension of the policy limits remaining and available from the last or expiring policy period, a new set of limits identical to the limits on the expiring policy, or some other negotiated limit. Remember that the limits of liability for the ERP are available for the payment of claims only if the limits have not been exhausted by payment of previous claims. Should the limits be exhausted through the payment of reported claims, many carriers will allow the insured to purchase an additional set of limits for a premium. This is called "reinstating the limits."

The carrier will charge an additional premium for the ERP. The additional premium is 100 percent to 200 percent of the annual premium for the current policy period. During a soft-market cycle, carriers might be more willing to offer this extension at a more reasonable price. An ERP can be purchased from the expiring carrier or the new carrier. Generally, using the new carrier is the more cost-effective option.

An additional item to consider when purchasing claims-made coverage is the definition of a claim. Most claims-made policies define a claim as "a suit or an incident likely to result in a lawsuit." This allows the insured to report incidents which it feels could give rise to a lawsuit and have any subsequent lawsuits covered under the current policy regardless of when the claim is made. This definition minimizes the likelihood of a gap in coverage. Some policies, however, define a claim as only a written demand for compensation or a filed lawsuit. Care must be taken when moving from one claims-made insurance carrier to another. Even if the new carrier agrees to maintain the insured's original retroactive date, it is possible for a gap in coverage to result if each carrier defines a claim in different terms.

How Much Should We Purchase?

Health care risk management professionals often question the appropriate amount of insurance coverage to purchase. This question is not easily answered. Guidelines are provided by reviewing the limits historically purchased by the organization, the loss history of the organization, analysis of the regulatory and legal climate, evaluation of exposures created by the organization's business strategies, and benchmarking these factors against other similar organizations. Included in this analysis is a review of what limits are being purchased and of risk retained through a deductible or self-insured retention.

Limits of Liability

The policy limits of liability state the maximum obligation of the insurer. Limits are frequently quoted on a per occurrence and annual aggregate basis. For example, coverage might be purchased to provide $1 million per claim with a $3-million annual aggregate. These limits are commonly represented as $1 million to $3 million. Under this scenario, the most the carrier will pay is $1 million for a claim during the policy year. In addition, the most the carrier will pay for all claims in the policy year is $3 million regardless of the number of claims filed.

How defense cost will be treated is a key coverage condition. Defense cost can be inclusive or exclusive. Inclusive defense cost means that the costs to defend the case are part of the limits of liability (included) and erode the limits as costs are paid. This treatment diminishes the limits available (amount of money) to pay for any subsequent awards, judgments, or settlements. Under these circumstances the maximum amount of money the carrier will pay out on behalf of the insured is $1 million. This is the less desirable method. Defense costs that are exclusive do not erode the limits of liability and are paid in addition to the available limits remaining on the policy. It is preferable to have defense costs outside of the policy limits. Under these circumstances, the carrier will pay up to $1 million plus all defense costs.

The treatment of defense cost also has a direct effect on premium calculation. Policies that offer defense cost inclusive of the limits of liability are generally less expensive than policies where defense cost are exclusive or in addition to the limits. Limits of liability for policies that provide for inclusive defense cost will erode faster than policies with defense cost excluded. Once the insurer has paid out the limits of liability on a defense-included policy, its responsibility ends. Coverage for policies with defense cost exclusive or outside the limits of liability will have a higher premium cost because the possibility exists that they will pay out more money. The insurer who writes coverage with defense cost excluded could pay out not only the limits of liability but also the cost of defense for each claim. It becomes understandable that the insurer would charge more for policies that offer defense cost exclusive of the limits of liability.

In addition to per claim and aggregate limits, some policies contain sub-limits. A sub-limit caps the most the policy will pay for a particular peril. This limit is usually within the limits provided by the policy. The sub-limit is seldom in addition to the policy limit.

Deductibles or self-insured retentions (SIR) state the amounts the insured has agreed to retain. Deductibles or SIRs may apply to each claim, each occurrence, or in aggregate for all losses for the policy period. Both serve to reduce premiums. Under a deductible, claims handling usually remains within the authority and responsibility of the insurance carrier. The actual limit provided by the policy is usually the per claim limit minus the deductible. Thus, if the policy contains a $1 million limit and a $100,000 deductible, the most the policy will actually pay is $900,000. In most cases, the insurer will pay the total cost of the claim and request reimbursement from the insured for the insured's deductible. In contrast, if the policy includes a SIR, the policy will pay the full limit described excess of the insured's SIR. The SIR obligates the insured to pay the first $100,000, then the carrier will pay up to $1 million. SIRs usually allow the insured influence or control over the claims administration process.

....

SPECIFIC TYPES OF INSURANCE FOR THE HEALTH CARE INDUSTRY

Several broad categories of insurance are offered by the insurance industry. These types of coverage are categorized by the kinds of loss that they insure against. The most common types of coverage relating to losses inherent in the health care industry are *first-party* coverage, *third-party* or *liability coverage, health and welfare* insurance, and *financial guarantees* provided by carriers in various forms of bonds such as surety bonds.

First-Party Insurance

First-party insurance provides financial reimbursement as the result of damage or destruction to the insured's own property. This type of insurance is also called "direct damage" coverage.

A significant exposure faced by a health care organization is direct damage to property it owns, operates, controls or is under the obligation to insure for physical loss or damage, and the loss of income should all or a portion of its property be unusable as the result of a loss. Such losses can result from fire and lightning, windstorm, hail, explosion, smoke, impact from aircraft and vehicles, objects falling from aircraft, strike, riot, civil commotion, vandalism, theft or attempted theft, sprinkler leakage, or collapse of buildings and other perils.

The common risk treatment for property losses is the purchase of commercial insurance. Property insurance for health care organizations has traditionally been readily available in the insurance market because of the positive nature of health care industry property risks. Most health care property is classified as highly protected risk (HPR) meaning that the risk is adequately protected and that management has a proactive attitude toward loss avoidance and life safety. Health care property risks are considered well below the national average.

The property insurance marketplace for health care risks is cyclical, based on the overall insurance market cycle and on natural and man-made events that can have a catastrophic affect on the industry. The four hurricanes to hit the State of Florida in 2004 resulted in an estimated loss of more than $20 billion, becoming the second-largest catastrophic property loss in history. The devastating impact of hurricane Katrina in 2005 is still to be determined. The estimates to date are catastrophic both in terms of dollars and people. The magnitude of 9/11 losses affected every insurance product and the risk appetite of every insurance carrier. Those effects are still being felt in the industry, particularly in the availability of terrorism insurance. Total losses from 9/11 are estimated to be in the neighborhood of $50 billion, the costliest disaster in U.S. history. In spite of that, the health care property market has not been severely affected by the loss of capacity. Adequate capacity remains available in the market at attractive terms, however; certain catastrophic exposures in high-risk areas are more difficult to place. In certain coastal areas, coverage can be acquired only through the purchase of government-sponsored insurance programs such as the National Flood Program, and catastrophic wind pools formed in some coastal states.

Many property carriers provide loss prevention services to their policyholders. These value-added services can assist the risk management professional in maintaining the status of the current facilities, and can provide input on new construction. Generally these carriers provide inspections and recommendations on an ongoing basis. The benefits of complying with the insurers' recommendations should be measured against the cost of compliance.

The majority of property policies available to the health care industry are "comprehensive" in form. A single policy can incorporate coverages such as:

- Physical damage to real and business personal property
- Time element coverage
- Boiler and machinery
- Transit coverage
- Automatic builders risk protection
- Fine arts coverage
- Valuable papers and records
- Electronic data processing (EDP)
- Accounts receivable

Property policies specify the exact property and business personal property to be covered, the dollar amount of coverage afforded, and the types of loss covered under the policy. Property insurance may protect any covered person or organization that has an "insurable interest" in the property.

Property coverage can be written on an actual cash value (ACV) basis or replacement cost basis. Actual cash value is the replacement value of the property, at the time and place of the loss or damage, minus deductions for depreciation. Under a replacement cost basis, claim payments will be based on the cost to repair or replace the property without any deduction for depreciation. Because this preferred option requires that the insured carry enough coverage to replace damaged or destroyed property, it is very important to determine the correct property limit. Most replacement cost policies contain a "co-insurance" provision. This provision requires the insured to carry insurance equal to a specified percentage of the replacement cost of the value of the property covered. If the amount of coverage is inadequate, a coinsurance penalty is assessed at the time of loss. This may result in reimbursement for loss that is less than the replacement cost or cost to repair.

Named Peril versus All Risk Coverage

Insurance to protect against direct damage losses can be purchased on a named peril or "all risk basis." Under a named peril policy, only losses that fall under the specific perils named in the policy are covered. The burden is on the insured to prove that there has been a loss. The preferred form of coverage is the all risk form. Its broad, blanket-insuring agreement covers all loss unless specifically excluded. In the all risk form, the burden of proof is on the insurance carrier to prove that a loss is not covered.

Even with comprehensive all risk forms, several perils are difficult to insure or are uninsurable. These include earthquake, landslide, mudflow, subsidence, flood, nuclear reaction or contamination, volcanic eruption, war and terrorism, intentional losses, normal expected wear and tear, and business perils such as marketing and political risk.

Where significant exposure exists for perils such as earthquake, wind, and flood, carriers may provide sub-limits of coverage, or exclude coverage all together. In such instances, excess or wrap-around coverage can be provided by purchasing a difference in conditions (DIC) policy. In these policies, the definition of earthquake includes landslide, quake, and other similar movements. The definition of flood includes surface water, tidal or seismic sea wave, rising or overflowing of any body of water, and seepage or influx of water from natural underground sources into basements or other floors.

Time Element Coverage

In addition to direct damage losses, a health care organization faces the peril of losing revenues as a result of an insured loss. Coverage for this kind of loss is provided by consequential loss or time element insurance.

Major wind damage, fire, or flood could result in either a partial or total shutdown of a hospital's operation. During the shutdown, revenues generated by those operations are lost and there would probably be additional expenses in attempting to continue as nearly as possible the normal conduct of business. Business interruption, a time-element coverage, pays for the loss of earnings and continuing expenses resulting from a covered loss. These expenses can include ordinary payroll if included in the limit determination. It will also reimburse the insured for extra expenses incurred to keep a facility operating while repairs are being made or to mitigate further damage. These "extra-ordinary" expenses are those considered above and beyond the insured's ordinary expenses of operation from the time ordinary operations are interrupted to the time ordinary operations are resumed. Examples include the expense of transferring patients to another facility, or the loss of income as the result of closing the emergency room or operating room while repairs are being made.

Time element claims are some of the most difficult claims to adjust. Potential disputes relating to lost revenue and expenses can be avoided by providing the insurance carrier with a completed business interruption worksheet each year. The completed worksheet will identify continuing expenses and loss of income that the insured will experience if an insured claim results in a total or partial facility closure.

This coverage can provide a contribution clause that operates much like a coinsurance clause. To ensure that the limit of coverage applicable to the risk meets the policy's requirements, limits should be reviewed annually with the insurance carrier or broker. The deductible for this form of insurance is typically stated as a specified number of hours or days following the actual loss.

Boiler and Machinery

Boiler and machinery insurance provides insurance for mechanical and electrical breakdown of equipment and can extend to cover such exposures as ammonia contamination, hazardous substances spoilage, water damage, and the drying out of electrical equipment. Equipment covered can extend to pressure vessels, refrigeration equipment, heating and air-conditioning systems, and pumps and compressors. It covers owned property and resulting damage to other property, including property in "your care, custody, and control for which you are liable." Accidents to boilers and machinery are, in most instances, directly related to the energy inherent in their operations such as heat, pressure, electrical energy, centrifugal force, and reciprocating motion.

Standard property policies cover losses to boilers and machinery, and to other property, when caused by perils insured against in the policy. However, these forms do not cover damage to boilers and machinery or anything else when the loss is caused by uninsured or excluded perils. These might include explosions or other sudden breakdowns in the boilers and machinery. Where such losses are excluded, a separate boiler and machinery policy is necessary. Many of the newer "comprehensive" property policies have limited boiler and machinery exclusions, eliminating the need to carry separate coverage.

Builder's Risk

Property risk associated with new construction is typically covered under a "builder's risk" policy. Buildings under construction face unique hazards. Building materials on the premises are subject to theft or destruction. Because fire protection systems, such as sprinkler systems, might not be fully installed and operational, the risk characteristics for a loss are modified.

A builder's risk policy may be issued to cover the interest of the building owner, the interest of the contractor, or the owner and the contractor jointly as their interests may appear. A separate builder's risk policy may be provided by the contractor, or purchased by the health care organization. Under a comprehensive policy form, automatic builder's risk coverage is generally extended to construction on any existing premises. Coverage can be added to cover exposure at an off-site location, subject to carrier notification and acceptance.

Electronic Data Processing (EDP) and Media Coverage

Electronic data processing equipment is subject to loss from all the perils to which other equipment is exposed, such as fire, windstorm, and so on, and is sensitive to perils that have little effect on other property. These include dust, temperature, and humidity changes that can affect the equipment enough to result in an actual loss. Recorded media data are vulnerable to the same losses including magnetic storms. They can also be lost, stolen, erased, or tampered with.

In addition to direct loss, the temporary loss of data processing facilities could result in a serious interruption to the organization. The extra expense coverage in an EDP policy could reimburse for equipment rental or use of time-sharing facilities, additional payroll, temporary office equipment, or temporary help.

Separate EDP policies, or an EDP extension on a standard property policy, provide protection for the added risks associated with these exposures. Standard property policies pay for the loss of media but not the loss of information. EDP coverage will pay for replacement of information displayed on cards, disks, drums, or tapes.

Commercial Crime Insurance and Employee Dishonesty

Crime insurance covers two broad categories of risk—crimes committed by outsiders and crimes committed by employees. Because crime-related losses are not typically covered under property insurance policies, crime insurance is an important coverage in a health care organization's insurance portfolio.

Crime insurance can cover money and securities against burglary, robbery, theft, destruction, disappearance, and employee dishonesty.

Crime insurance also covers property other than money and securities against loss due to specified crime perils such as burglary, robbery, theft, computer fraud, extortion, and employee dishonesty. Crime coverage also extends to loss as the result of property damaged, but not stolen by burglars or robbers.

Probably the most significant financial risk for health care providers is employee dishonesty. This can include embezzlement, the theft of drugs or other hospital supplies, or the alteration of financial records for personal gain. Along with the rapid growth in technology has come a new opportunity for criminal loss. Computer fraud is at an all-time high and is rapidly increasing. Computer crime includes electronic theft of money and securities, embezzlement, fraud, or erased or modified information.

Third-Party Insurance

Third-party insurance provides coverage to pay on behalf of the insured or reimburse the insured for bodily injury, personal injury, or property damage loss due to negligence caused by an insured. It involves three parties—the party who is harmed, the insurer, and the insured party who caused the harm or damage. Unlike first-party coverage, the named insured is never a direct recipient of the payment for loss responded to by a liability policy. The most common third-party coverages applicable to a health care organization are:

- Medical professional liability
- General liability (premises liability, personal injury, products or completed operations, independent contractor's liability, and contractual liability)
- Umbrella excess liability
- Employment practices liability
- Automobile liability
- Director's and officer's liability
- Miscellaneous errors and omissions, including managed care errors and omissions

- Environmental impairment liability
- Fiduciary liability
- Heliport and non-owned aircraft liability

Medical Professional Liability

Medical professional liability insurance provides coverage for claims arising from the rendering or failure to render medical, surgical, dental, x-ray or other imaging or nursing service or treatment, or the furnishing of food or beverages in connection therewith; furnishing or dispensing of drugs or medical, dental, or surgical supplies or appliances; postmortem handling of human bodies and service by any persons as members of a formal accreditation, standards review, or similar professional board or committee, as a person charged with executing the directives of such board or committee.

The named insured should be broad enough to cover all corporate entities, the insureds' interest in joint ventures, the board of directors or trustees, members of committees, employees, students, volunteer workers, and members of religious congregations acting at the request or behest of the named insured. If interns, residents, fellows, or employed or contracted physicians and surgeons are to be covered for their personal interest, basic policy wording requires modification. The basic policy form should also be reviewed to ensure that physicians are covered for administrative responsibilities without a requirement to specifically extend the coverage to include that exposure. Coverage extended to employees that include physicians and surgeons typically extends to negligent acts occurring within the scope of their duties on behalf of the named insured. Even though there are several insureds covered under the policy, the limit of liability applicable to each medical incident applies on a per medical incident or per occurrence basis. The aggregate limit on the policy is the maximum amount of losses to be paid in any particular year.

Health care entity employees, particularly nurses, frequently ask the risk management professional whether they should carry their own insurance. In responding to that question, the risk management professional should inform employees who and what the entity's policy covers. The risk management professional should also review the other insurance provision of the organization's medical professional liability policy to see how the coverage would respond if an employee carries individual coverage. In some instances, the policy would be excess over and above the employee's personal insurance. In other instances, the policy would contribute to the claim proportionately with the employee's carrier based on the limits carried on each policy. The entity's policy usually will cover employees for negligent acts and omissions within the scope of their employment. Coverage would not extend to a second job, or moonlighting activities. If those activities exist, a separate policy should be purchased. Additionally, the risk management professional should remind employees that, although the entity's policy protects them from costs of defense and indemnity, they will have no decision-making authority over how their defense is conducted—something they may have with their own policy.

Most hospital bylaws require all voluntary attending physicians to carry their own medical professional liability coverage at stated minimum limits. If the physician and health care entity are found to be negligent, the entity may be held financially liable for the inadequacy of the physician's limits under the theory of joint and several liability. Where physicians have challenged the entity's ability to impose minimum insurance requirements as a condition of staff membership, the courts have said the entity may do so if the requirement is not applied arbitrarily or capriciously.

Medical professional liability insurance is considered a "specialty coverage." Most carriers have developed customized policy forms, many of which differ in terms and conditions. It is critical that the risk management professional performs a thorough evaluation and comparison of coverage terms and conditions in selecting a medical professional liability carrier. A broker, agent, or insurance company representative can be very helpful in this process. In addition to the product itself, most carriers provide a portfolio of risk management services that are available to assist the risk management professional in meeting their risk management objectives. These services should be evaluated based on their perceived effectiveness and need on the part of the risk management professional.

Two forms of medical professional liability coverage are available in the industry—claims-made and occurrence. In purchasing this coverage, it is critical that the risk management professional be knowledgeable about the differences in the forms ensuring that all claims—those reported and those that have occurred but are not yet reported—are covered by a single or by continuous policies. (Please refer to the section called claims-made versus occurrence policies elsewhere in this chapter.)

The delivery of health care services in an integrated setting has presented additional exposures that the health care risk management professional must address. Basic medical professional liability policies need to be reviewed to ensure that they extend coverage to new exposures. Some of these are:

- Miscellaneous errors and omissions (E&O) coverage, such as data processing E&O, employed attorney's E&O, hospital or physician management E&O
- Contractual liability as it relates to professional liability assumed on behalf of others if liability would not have been present in the absence of the agreement
- Utilization management and review—particularly as it relates to liability assumed on behalf of a Health Maintenance Organization
- Marketing, advertising, Internet exposures
- Confidentiality issues
- Credentialing of physicians and allied health care providers for others
- Antitrust or restraint of trade
- Third-party claims administration and claims management for others
- Enterprise liability and vicarious liability for all aspects of delivery in an integrated network
- Coverage for day care centers, special health care events and volunteer activities
- Architects or design-build legal liability
- Telemedicine and the associated licensing issues
- Medicare billing errors and Medicare fraud and abuse issues

Commercial General Liability

Most medical professional liability policies cover all injury to patients on or about the premises for the purpose of receiving medical treatment. A health care provider is subject to third-party claims from members of the public other than patients for injury as the result of negligence in connection with the nonmedical aspects of its premises. This would include nonmedical related contractual obligations, injury to visitors, product liability, independent contractors' liability, advertising liability and personal injury allegations such as libel, slander, false arrest, or defamation of character.

Commercial general liability protects the named insured against financial loss resulting from liability to third parties arising out of the premises owned or occupied, acts of independent contractors hired, products sold that leave the premises, and liability assumed under contract, subject to the exclusions in the policy. Coverage applies to bodily injury, property damage, and personal injury allegations.

The same insurer that provides the medical professional liability coverage to the health care entity usually provides general liability coverage. Those two types of protection frequently are combined in a single policy, avoiding a "gray" area as to what is a professional versus a general liability claim. Where coverage is purchased separately, the general liability carrier will include an amendment excluding injury to patients. This limitation will typically read:

> Coverage is excluded for bodily injury to any person who is in your building, or on your premises for the purpose of receiving any type of medical evaluation, care, or treatment.

In some instances the coverage can be modified with the following additional language ". . . except for injuries caused by windstorm or fire, including any injury from smoke, fumes, or panic, earthquake, lightning, or explosion." This extension of coverage provides the risk management professional additional protection in the event of a catastrophic loss injuring patients in addition to visitors.

Additional commercial general liability exposures can exist for organizations providing child care centers. These exposures may include corporal punishment, sexual molestation, or failure to maintain sanitary conditions resulting in the spread of disease.

In addition, many health care entities are affiliated with academic universities that require special protection for claims that might arise out of an educational setting. Examples of those claims are failure to educate, wrongful suspension from a program, or inadequate supervision. Commercial general liability policies should be reviewed to make certain that coverage is included for these exposures, or a separate policy must be purchased.

The risk management professional is challenged to stay informed about the health care entity's activities, to ensure that the policy is broad enough to cover new ventures and operations. Common areas of concern are increased advertising including e-marketing, environmental impairment or hazardous waste disposal exposure, asbestos removal, and the general liability exposures applicable to patient-owned premises in home health operations.

Managed Care E&O Coverage

The emergence of managed care has significantly increased the need to purchase managed care E&O coverage. Managed care entities such as preferred provider organizations (PPO), management service organizations (MSO), physician-hospital organizations (PHO), health maintenance organizations (HMO), independent practice associations (IPA), and foundations have presented new exposures for health care risk management professionals to address. As stated earlier, a medical professional liability policy responds to bodily injury allegations as the result of the delivery or the failure to deliver medical services. However, it may not respond to allegations for "wrongful acts" in the design and administration of a managed care plan. These allegations may allege economic loss, not bodily injury.

Allegations of negligence against managed care organizations may include:

- Improper design or administration of cost control systems
- Physician incentive agreements

- Breach of patient confidentiality
- Employee Retirement Income Security Act of 1974 (ERISA) violations
- Anti-trust
- Economic credentialing
- Denial of benefits or services
- Failure to refer, delay in referral
- Discrimination
- Violation of state insurance regulations
- Invasion of privacy
- Insolvency or bankruptcy

The insurance industry has responded to this risk with separate managed care E&O policy forms. Some forms will include coverage for the administrative risk associated with managed care and extend to provide direct medical professional liability coverage for employed providers. Other forms are intended to cover the administrative risk associated with managed care and provide vicarious liability coverage for the organization facilitating the delivery of health care services. The typical insuring agreement of these policies covers damages because of personal injury in the performance of professional services, including but not limited to utilization review, peer review, claims processing, enrollment, and marketing of services.

Managed care E&O policy forms contain several exclusions or coverage limitations applicable to the risk associated with managed care contracting and health care delivery. It is important the risk management professional review these restrictions to have a clear understanding of what portion of the risk is insurable and what portion cannot be covered by insurance.

Excess Umbrella Liability

Catastrophic losses can have a major effect on the bottom line of a health care entity, threatening its long-term financial viability. Excess umbrella liability coverage can be purchased to provide additional coverage after the first layer—the primary layer—of liability coverage has been exhausted. The primary layer is typically considered a minimum $1 million per claim and $3-million annual aggregate. The excess policy picks up over and above the primary limits afforded per claim, and if so written will drop down to effect coverage in the event of aggregate exhaustion of the underlying coverage. Umbrella excess liability coverage is a comprehensive form of excess liability coverage, providing coverage excess of several third-party exposures such as medical professional liability, commercial general liability, automobile liability, employer's liability, non-owned aircraft, and heliport liability. It can normally be extended to cover managed care E&O.

To maintain concurrency (avoiding gaps in coverage), primary and excess insurance policies should maintain the same effective date. If the coverage is claims-made, policies should also maintain the same retroactive date. In addition, it is important that the primary and umbrella excess medical professional and commercial general liability coverage be written on concurrent coverage forms. If the primary is claims-made, the excess coverage should be written on a claims-made form to avoid gaps and overlaps in coverage. If the primary is written or self-funded on an occurrence basis, the excess should be maintained on an occurrence basis. If primary coverage is afforded on an occurrence basis and the excess coverage is written on a claims-made basis, it is necessary for the risk management professional to maintain two sets of loss data, one on an occurrence basis as required by the primary carrier and one on a claims-made basis to meet the requirements of the claims-made excess carrier.

As with primary medical professional liability policies, all umbrella excess liability carriers have customized policy forms. Most of these forms are "stand-alone" in nature, and do not necessarily follow the form of the primary policies, or self-insured documents that they sit over. It is important that the risk management professional conducts a thorough evaluation of policy forms to make certain that continuity of coverage exists.

Although there has been little increase in the frequency of losses in the past few years, loss severity has continued to increase. In view of this, it is important that the risk management professional continually review the limits of liability insurance purchased, making certain that the assets of the organization are adequately protected.

Automobile Liability

Health care entities are exposed to liability as the result of owned or leased automobiles, and non-owned and hired automobiles. In addition, automobile exposures can exist from the operation of parking garages, including valet parking. A commercial automobile policy protects against loss arising out of the ownership, maintenance, or use of automobiles and their equipment. It extends to vehicles "you own, hire or borrow, and those you do not own but may be responsible for," such as the personal car of an employee used in a home health operation. Coverage provided for vehicles not owned is excess over any coverage the owner may have.

Uninsured motorists (UM) coverage and personal injury protection (PIP) is also included subject to limits required by each state. This covers bodily injury in most states. Repairs for physical damage to the vehicle caused by an uninsured driver will not be covered. The policy should provide automatic coverage for newly acquired or leased vehicles, including those used for emergency or patient transport. Automobile physical damage—comprehensive and collision coverage—should be considered for owned and long-term leased vehicles.

Insurers determine rates for automobile coverage based on loss experience, territory of operation, location of the vehicle while garaged, and type and use of the vehicle. Loss prevention activities such as safe driver programs and insurance requirements for individuals using their personal vehicles on behalf of the organization are taken into consideration in the final pricing determination.

The risk associated with employees using their personal vehicles associated with home health organizations has materialized into a major exposure for many health care risk management professionals. In some instances, automobile carriers are adding premium surcharges to accounts with this exposure. It is important that health care organizations maintain liability insurance requirements for all individuals using their personal vehicles in business at an adequate level of liability coverage. Certificates of insurance should be required and maintained on a current basis for all drivers. It is also recommended that each driver participate in a safe driving course at least every two years. Updated motor vehicle records (MVRs) should be obtained on each driver annually.

Garage Liability Exposure

Some health care organizations provide valet parking for emergency room patients and visiting family members. Two significant exposures are created by this service. A third-party liability exposure develops when hospital employees operate the vehicles. The hospital can also be held responsible for damage to patient vehicles while parked in hospital-owned or -operated parking garages. While difficult to quantify, this ultimate exposure can be determined by the maximum value of all vehicles parked in the garage. Protection for this risk can be found in both the automobile and commercial general liability policy. The risk management professional should review commercial general liability and automobile policies before purchasing a separate garage liability policy.

Most general liability policies respond to garage operations as the result of damages such as a parking garage entrance arm malfunction that causes damage to a third-party vehicle. It also responds to injury due to the "existence" exposure of the premises, such as a visitor slip and fall in the parking garage. An automobile policy can protect the insured for the ownership, maintenance, and use of *any* vehicle. A garagekeeper's legal liability policy provides coverage for physical damage (comprehensive and collision) for automobiles in the care, custody, and control of the insured. The basic coverage in this form applies to damages for which an insured is legally liable. The policy can be endorsed to provide "goodwill" coverage providing reimbursement for damages where there is a question of legal negligence. This can be used as a public relations tool for the risk management professional. The coverage can be modified to respond on either a primary or excess basis. If written on a primary basis, coverage for damage to the third-party vehicle is provided automatically regardless of any other insurance. Coverage on an excess basis only applies excess of the owner's automobile coverage.

The risk management professional can take several steps to reduce the probability of loss. Garage security and a system to provide vehicle key protection should minimize vandalism and theft. A driver-recruiting program, including MVR verification for all employees driving third-party automobiles, may reduce exposures. Outsourcing the garage operations to a third party by contract will shift the majority of the exposure to the garage management company.

Directors' and Officers' (D&O) Liability

Decisions made by directors, officers, trustees, and other key executives have a significant effect on the financial health and daily operations of a health care entity. It is essential that they have the freedom to make wise, responsible, and sometimes difficult decisions without risk to their personal assets.

The board delegates authority to conduct affairs on a day-to-day basis to the administrative and medical staff officers. However, the board is ultimately responsible for the establishment and maintenance of appropriate standards relating to all activities associated with the delivery of health care services. This governance responsibility cannot be delegated. The purpose of D&O insurance is to protect directors, officers, trustees, and key executives in the event of personal liability litigation, or to insure the health care entity itself from its obligation to provide indemnity from such litigation.

Staff-related issues are becoming a more significant exposure for directors and officers, who are being held increasingly accountable for medical staff decisions related to staff credentialing and privileging. In making these decisions, they may be accused of lack of due process or interference with a person's right to practice a profession. What were once routine denials of staff privileges can now give rise to anti-trust allegations with charges of restraint of trade by denying an individual the right to practice a profession, or by favoring one group of competing interests over another.

Statutory immunity laws have been enacted in several states that grant immunity from personal liability to directors of not-for-profit health care facilities. However, this relief does not guarantee immunity from being sued. Also, state laws provide no protection from legal actions under federal statutes involving for example, anti-trust, discrimination, and environmental protection.

Changes in the health care industry have opened new areas of risk for health care executives. Integrated delivery networks are engaged in joint ventures with physicians, private enterprises, or other health care providers. These alliances hold a strong potential for antitrust allegations from excluded providers or suppliers who claim that a cooperative arrangement restricts their ability to compete in the community. Heightened competition for patients, managed care contracts, and other revenue sources present a restraint of trade exposure.

Mergers, acquisitions, and divestiture activities among hospitals and physicians is another area of concern. Companies involved in these ventures experience a significantly heightened frequency and severity of D&O claims.

Another source of exposure is third-party contractual relationships. As health care organizations increasingly take advantage of opportunities to deliver care on an outpatient basis, it is often difficult to maintain the same quality standards across their owned and managed facilities and their off-site delivery facilities, such as surgi-centers and home health operations.

There are several ways to manage this risk. Most organizations purchase directors' and officers' liability insurance, including employment practices liability insurance coverage from the commercial insurance market. Others are now assuming this risk in their alternative risk financing vehicles, such as a captive insurance company.

The directors' and officers' liability policy, typically written on a claims-made form, pays on behalf of the organization all losses for which the organization grants indemnification to the insured persons and for which the insured persons have become legally obligated to pay on account of any claim for a *wrongful act*. A wrongful act means any error, misstatement, misleading statement, act, omission, neglect, or breach of duty.

Directors' and officers' liability insurance policies typically have three distinct insuring agreements. The first agreement pays on behalf of the individual insureds' claims for wrongful acts, which are non-indemnifiable events under the organization's bylaws indemnification agreement. The second reimburses the entity for wrongful acts on the part of individual insureds who can be indemnified under the corporate bylaws. These insuring agreements are considered "Individual" coverage (Part A) and "Corporate Reimbursement" (Part B). "Entity" coverage (Part C) can be purchased to provide coverage for the entity if it is held legally responsible for wrongful acts covered in the individual coverage sections of the policy.

Employment Practices Liability (EPL)

Employment practices liability coverage can be included in the D&O policy by endorsement or purchased as a separate policy. The risk management professional should evaluate this risk and determine if a combined D&O approach is appropriate, or if separate coverage should be purchased.

The EPL policy is designed to reimburse an organization for alleged negligence in the selection and hiring of employees and other employment issues associated with all current health care personnel. Recent legislative changes and increased public awareness have expanded liability risk for employment related claims, making it easier to file claims and secure greater compensation. Some of these exposures are discrimination, sexual harassment, hostile work environment, wrongful termination, and violation of the American with Disabilities Act (ADA).

Fiduciary Liability

The need for insurance protection for individuals who exercise management or administrative responsibilities for employee benefit plans was redefined by the Employee Retirement Income Security Act of 1974 (ERISA).

ERISA defines the principal responsibilities for individuals who are fiduciaries of employee benefit plans while making the fiduciaries personally responsible for their actions. Employers with more than twenty-five employees are subject to ERISA with limited exceptions. Two of these exceptions are plans providing government-sponsored benefits (including Medicare) and some plans sponsored by religious affiliated organizations.

Every plan subject to ERISA must have a written plan document that defines the benefits provided, to eligible participants, their vesting rights, and how claims will be handled. In addition, the plan document must identify by name the individuals responsible for the management of the plan. An annual update to plan participants is required.

Fiduciaries are defined by ERISA as individuals named as fiduciaries in the plan documents, and any other persons or organizations responsible for administering benefits or claims or collecting or handling funds relating to the plan. Fiduciary liability insurance covers the alleged breach of a fiduciary's responsibility under common law or ERISA for directors and administrators of the plans.

Employee Benefit Legal Insurance

In addition to management responsibilities, individuals with duties relating to the administration of employee benefit plans can create situations in which they or their employees might become liable for misadministration of an employee benefit program.

Administrative risk arising from workers' compensation, social security, unemployment compensation, or statutorily required non-occupational disability benefit programs exists even though they do not fall under the ERISA regulations.

Insurance protection against this administrative risk is called employee benefit liability. This coverage is usually endorsed on to a commercial general liability policy.

Environmental Impairment Liability

There is an increased awareness and concern among insureds over the extent of potential liabilities related to the transfer of properties that might be contaminated.

Exposures include the particularly serious cases of gradual pollution that can occur in the course of normal operations of a hospital entity and liability for sudden and accidental exposure. Impairment is considered to be in place when substances (shock, noise, pressure, radiation, gases, vapors, heat, or other phenomena such as light) propagate or spread through soil, air, or water. Examples in the hospital environment include underground storage tanks, hazardous waste incinerators, or radioactive, hazardous, medical, pathological, and infectious wastes.

Since 1973, most commercial general liability policies have excluded contamination and pollution except when sudden and accidental. This exclusion created a gap in basic liability coverage that very few insurers have filled, even under specialty coverage or in the excess and surplus lines marketplace. Certain specialty underwriters, however, have developed environmental impairment liability coverage, which insures liability for environmental impairment, including clean-up costs. "Sudden and accidental" contamination or pollution is excluded unless the insured cannot obtain the coverage under the commercial general liability policy.

Aviation Coverage—Non-Owned Aircraft and Heliport Coverage

Many health care facilities have landing sites available for helicopter landings. A separate heliport liability policy should be purchased if such a site is designated as a helipad for use by life-flight operators or other emergency helicopter landings. The exposures associated with this risk depend on the hospital's role in the operation and use of the heliport premises along with any contractual obligation it assumes as the result of its operation.

Heliport liability policies cover bodily injury and physical damage arising out of the use, ownership, or operation of a helipad including slips and falls that occur during the loading and unloading of patients, bodily injury to bystanders, and property damage to the property of others. Operation and use of the helipad is excluded from a commercial general liability policy.

Non-owned aircraft liability policies cover bodily injury and property damage caused by an "accident" involving a non-owned helicopter or an accident involving a non-owned aircraft for which the organization is responsible.

The frequency of air travel by employees and health care executives should be evaluated to determine the need for this type of coverage. Claims have been made against corporate entities arising out of their sponsorship of meetings wherein employees were victims in commercial air disasters or in chartered aircraft crashes. Risk management professionals should also evaluate the adequacy of insurance provided by charter companies and helicopter services.

Health and Welfare Insurance-Employee Benefit Insurance

Although most employee benefit insurance plans are coordinated by human resources departments, it is important for risk management professionals to be familiar with the types of plans provided by their employers. Some risk management professionals may have responsibility for coordinating such programs, or be involved in the decision making process for carrier selection. These coverages can include long- and short-term disability, life, health, accident, dental, and vision insurance.

Workers' Compensation

All states create a statutory obligation on the part of employers to provide compensation to employees for injuries arising out of, and in the course of, their employment. All employers are subject to the applicable workers' compensation laws of the states in which they operate and under appropriate circumstances to federal statutes. Failure to comply with these laws can result in fines and penalties, one of which is statutory removal of the employer's defense to suit by employees alleging injury as a result of their work. Workers' compensation insurance is a pure form of no-fault insurance. Adherence to the workers' compensation statute is governed by each state's division of workers' compensation.

Employers who fall under the workers' compensation statutes are required to purchase insurance, qualify as a self-insured, or reject the act, which is permissible in some states. Workers' compensation insurance provides statutory benefit coverage with virtually unlimited medical benefits to work accident victims. It also replaces a portion of lost wages defined as indemnity payments. Employer's liability, part of the standard workers' compensation policy, protects employers from suits brought by injured employees to recover monetary damages separate and distinct from claims for statutory benefits. Employer's liability claims can arise from:

- Employees who reject the act (which is possible in some states)
- Injuries not covered by the act (questionable claims relating to scope of employment)
- Suits by a spouse for loss of consortium or companionship
- Suit by a third party that has been held liable for the injury and seeks reimbursement from the employer.

The premium for workers' compensation insurance is based on the application of rates established on a state-by-state basis to employee remuneration. The rates are based on classifications determined by the risk associated with the responsibilities of the employee. Individual claims history is used to modify the ultimate premium based on experience rating models for each classification of employee. Risk management professionals should work closely with the human resources and employee health departments in identifying, measuring, and addressing workers' compensation risks.

Financial Guarantees

Surety bonds are frequently required to comply with laws associated with several health care exposures. In a surety contract, one party (the surety) agrees to be bound, along with the principal, to a third party in the same agreement. The surety and the principal on the bond become the promisor to a third-party promisee. The third party would be able to collect the obligation from the surety, if the principal cannot meet the financial responsibility. If the surety is called upon to meet the obligations under the bond, it attempts to collect the obligation (seek reimbursement) from the principal. This is the major difference in financial guarantee insurance versus other insurance contracts.

Health care organizations are required to post surety bonds to comply with laws in a number of areas. They include but are not limited to:

- Patients' valuables
- Durable medical equipment
- Home health bonds
- Liquor bonds
- Residents funds bonds
- Performance and payment bonds for construction projects
- License bonds.
- Various court bonds such as appeal bonds
- Notary bonds
- Pharmacy bonds

Provider Stop-Loss Coverage

Provider stop-loss coverage may be needed by those organizations that have agreed in advance to bear financial risk for the provision of health care services under full or partial capitated managed care contracts. Provider stop-loss coverage reimburses a health care provider, subject to daily limitations and co-insurance requirements, for losses in excess of a stipulated amount per member per year.

There are two avenues for the risk management professional to consider in purchasing such coverage. Some managed care organizations are willing to include a certain amount of stop-loss protection in the provider's capitated agreement. The coverage can also be purchased from the commercial insurance industry.

Risk management professionals should evaluate both options to ensure that the avenue selected provides maximum protection for the financial performance of their organizations. (Refer to Chapter 2 in Volume III of this series on Managed Care.)

···········
CONCLUSION

Insurance is only one of the many tools available to the health care risk management professional to manage the financial aspects of risk. The risk management professional's primary insurance responsibility is to identify the organization's risk exposures and determine whether the transfer of risk to an insurance company is the appropriate method of treatment of that risk. Using insurance products for risk treatment requires the risk management professional to develop a level of insurance knowledge and a good working relationship with agents or brokers and with the insurance industry. The risk management professional's role should also include the preparation of statistical risk data including rating data and up-to-date historical loss data for use by the carriers in determining the appropriate premium. The risk management professional should also be familiar with the resources external to the organization such as brokers, agents, and consultants, who are available to help place coverage, the analysis of carriers, and the proposals submitted by those carriers.

Endnote

1. Smith, B. D. *How Insurance Works: An Introduction to Property and Liability Insurance*. Malvern, PA: Insurance Institute of America, 1984, p. 4.

References

Best's Insurance Reports: Oldwick, NJ: A. M. Best, Updated annually.

Head, G. L., M. W. Elliot, and J. D. Blinn. *Essentials of Risk Financing,* 3rd ed. Vol. I Malvern, PA: Insurance Institute of America, 1996.

MacDonald, M. G., K. C. Meyer, and B. Essig B. *Health Care Law: A Practical Guide*. New York City: Mathew Bender, 1987.

Malecki, D. S., R. C. Horn, E. A. Wiening, and J. H. Donaldson. *Commercial Liability Risk Management and Insurance*. 2nd ed. Vol. II, Malvern, PA: American Institute for Property and Liability Underwriters, 1986.

Rodda, W. H., J. S. Trieschmann, E. A. Wiening, and B. A. Hedges. *Commercial Property Risk Management and Insurance*. 3rd ed. Vol. I, Malvern, PA: American Institute for Property and Liability Underwriters, 1988.

Smith, B. D. J. S. Trieschmann, and E. A. Wiening. *Property and Liability Insurance Principles*. 2nd Ed, Malvern, PA: Insurance Institute of America 1994.

Troyer, G. and S. Salman. *Handbook of Health Care Risk Management*, Rockville, MD: Aspen, 1986.

17

Organizational Staffing

Mary Lynn Curran

This chapter introduces health care risk management professionals to the challenges posed by organizational staffing in the changing health care workforce environment and how these issues affect liability exposure. Risk management professionals, including managers who have been assigned responsibility for risk management duties in any health care organization (hospital, nursing home, home health agency, physician practice, ambulatory or outpatient setting, retirement community, pharmacy, laser center, and so on) must be able to understand how the challenged workforce affects the organization's liability exposures and how to act to protect the organization. Also, this chapter addresses staffing techniques to consider when the risk management department is affected by reorganization, cutbacks, or risk management staff shortages. Several tools and strategies are offered for creative staffing in the risk management department.

U.S. HEALTH CARE WORKFORCE

The following are facts about the health care workforce.[1]

- Health services is the largest industry in the country, with more than 12.9 million jobs: 12.5 million jobs for the wage and salary workers; 382,000 jobs for the self-employed.

- Approximately 16 percent of all wage and salary jobs created between 2002 and 2012, or 3.5 million jobs, will be in health services—more than in any other industry.

The author and editor recognize the late Dorothy Bazan for her important and insightful contribution to this chapter and exhibits. Ms. Bazan died unexpectedly in 2002. We appreciate the timelessness of her contribution and how it helps to keep her memory meaningful and real.

- Ten out of twenty occupations projected to grow at the fastest pace are concentrated in health services.

- Most health care jobs require less than four years of college education; however, the health diagnosing and treating practitioners are among the most educated workers.

- More than 518,000 establishments make up the health services industry, representing a variety in size, structure, and staffing needs.

- Three-fourths of all private health services establishments are offices of physicians or dentists and other health care practitioners.

- Hospitals constitute less than 2 percent of all private health services establishments, yet employ 41 percent of all workers. When combined with government hospitals, the proportion rises to 45 percent of all workers in the industry. Nursing and residential care facilities employ the next largest group of workers, with 11 percent of all health care workers.

The health care industry is viewed in nine segments by the U.S. government:[2]

1. *Hospitals.* Hospitals provide complete medical care, ranging from diagnostic services to surgery to continuous nursing care. Some hospitals specialize in treatment of the mentally ill, cancer patients, or children. Hospital-based care may be on an inpatient or outpatient basis. There are approximately 5,000 hospitals in the country, each employing workers with a variety of educational and training backgrounds and requirements for the job. Hospital human resources departments report having more than 100 job descriptions to manage in the service area alone. About one in four hospital workers is a registered nurse. Some hospitals provide specialty care, such as psychiatric, pediatric, and cardiac services, all of which require specially trained workers. Many hospitals also provide long-term care and home health care services, thus providing a continuum of services that extend beyond hospital walls. These organizations need a broader mix of workers with varied educational, licensure, certification, and training backgrounds.

2. *Nursing and residential care facilities.* Nursing facilities provide inpatient nursing and rehabilitation care to patients who need continuous care, but not in a hospital setting. Nursing aides provide the vast majority of direct care in these settings. Residential care facilities provide around-the-clock social and personal care to children, the elderly, and others who have limited ability to care for themselves. Workers care for residents of assisted-living facilities, alcohol and drug rehabilitation centers, group homes, and halfway houses. Nursing and medical care, however, is not the main focus of establishments providing residential care, as it is in nursing care facilities.

3. *Offices of physicians, including osteopaths.* These are typically physicians' offices and include small, independent one- or two-physician practices, and large-group practices where physicians and all staff are employees of the clinic.

4. *Home health care services.* Skilled nursing or medical care is provided in the home setting to the elderly or disabled. These services call for nursing and home health aides. They compose one of the fastest growing industries in the United States.

5. *Offices of dentists.* One of every five health service establishments counted by the U.S. government is a dentist's office. Most employ only a few workers who provide general and specialty dental care.

6. *Offices of other health practitioners.* This segment includes offices of chiropractors, optometrists, and podiatrists, in addition to occupational and physical therapists, psychologists, audiologists, speech and language pathologists, dietitians, and other

miscellaneous health practitioners. Hospitals and nursing facilities may contract out for these services. Also included in this segment are alternative-medicine practitioners such as acupuncturists, homeopaths, hypnotherapists, and naturopaths.

7. *Outpatient care centers.* Among the diverse establishments in this group are kidney dialysis centers, outpatient mental health and substance abuse centers, health maintenance organization medical centers, and freestanding ambulatory surgical and emergency centers.

8. *Other ambulatory health care services.* Included in this relatively small industry segment are ambulance services, blood and organ banks, and other miscellaneous ambulatory health care services, such as pacemaker monitoring services and smoking cessation programs.

9. *Medical and diagnostic laboratories.* Medical laboratories provide analytic or diagnostic services to medical professionals, or directly to patients based on a physician's order. Workers analyze blood, take X-rays and computerized tomography scans, or perform other clinical tests. Medical and diagnostic laboratories provide the fewest number of jobs in health services.

An experienced risk management professional knows that lack of training and experience for health care workers are common factors in patient injury and liability exposure. In the current workforce environment, there is generally a significant shortage of health care workers, especially qualified workers such as nurses and pharmacists, to fill positions with highly technical and intricate job requirements. Thus, a risk management professional must be aware of the organization's staffing status, staffing philosophy, and plans for remedying staff shortages. In addition, the risk management professional plays a key role in supporting the individuals within the organization who have staffing decisions by demonstrating the risk costs associated with making poor staffing choices.

············
BACKGROUND

The current health care workforce environment faces a serious shortage of qualified staff in significant clinical areas.[3] Added to this challenge, we now see mandatory staffing per patient requirements, mandatory work hours, and other staffing regulations posed by the federal government, accrediting agencies, and some states. The staff shortages and mandated staff ratios offer strong arguments in the public debate as consumers and purchasers of health care services demand—publicly and legally—that their health care be provided without harm in a safe environment. Risk management professionals know well the litigious recourse that patients may take when injured. Any suggestion that staffing is not adequate or that credentials of staff are questionable certainly complicates the defense of a claim alleging negligent care.

Shortage in the workforce takes several forms including increased job vacancy rates due to absenteeism, turnover, and retirement, a tightness of the labor market, and difficulty in filling positions.

In a report issued by the United States Department of Labor, Bureau of Labor Statistics in 2002–2003, five of the top thirty fields projecting the largest growth rate over the next ten years are in health care:[4]

1. Registered nurses: 40-percent growth needed to meet the needs of the population projected for 2020

2. Nursing aides, orderlies, and attendants: 24-percent growth needed

3. Home health aides: 47-percent growth needed

4. Personal and home care aides: 62-percent growth needed

5. Medical assistants: 57-percent growth needed

These projections apply to all health care settings, from acute care hospitals to the patient's home. The growth of an aging population as the baby boomers reach retirement and the expansion of longevity are key drivers in this phenomenon.

JCAHO

The Joint Commission on Accreditation of Healthcare Organizations (JCAHO) has established standards that require organizations to strategically monitor staffing. The original standards appeared July 1, 2002. The revised standard, called the Staffing Effectiveness Standard, became effective July 1, 2005.[5] These new standards require accredited hospital, long-term care, and assisted living organizations to collect data per units or divisions in hospitals, and per populations or settings for long-term care and assisted living facilities. The standard also requires input from clinical staff in the selection of the areas of focus and the indicators to be measured. The standard directs organizations to focus on nurse staffing (direct care providers in assisted living facilities) in the human resource indicators. Other care providers may be included as the health care organization sees fit. The newly revised standard incorporates the performance measures of the National Quality Forum.[6]

STUDIES ON STAFFING IN RELATION TO PATIENT INJURIES

Many reports critical to health care organizations have been published that point to staffing levels as critical factors in addressing patient safety issues. Two significant studies follow:

The 1999 landmark study by the Institute of Medicine (IOM) report found that up to 98,000 Americans die every year from preventable medical errors in hospitals.[7] The number of annual deaths in the United States due to medical error has since been estimated to be even higher.[8] The National Patient Safety Foundation (NPSF) was formed as a result of the IOM study. Funded by the American Medical Association, CNA HealthPro Insurance Company, and 3M Company, the NPSF delved into measuring the problem and finding appropriate solutions. In addition, the Leap Frog Initiative was begun, formed as a group of health care purchasers representing Fortune 500 companies. In response to the IOM study, they established initiatives to raise the level of patient care quality in hospitals and all health care organizations. One of these initiatives involves staffing intensive care units with physicians credentialed in critical care medicine.

Another study, "Hospital Nurse Staffing and Patient Mortality, Nurse Burnout and Job Dissatisfaction," was reported in *The Journal of the American Medical Association* (JAMA) in October 2002.[9] This study demonstrated a high correlation of nurse-to-patient staffing ratios to untoward deaths of patients, and factored in job-related burnout and job dissatisfaction. This study indicates that when a nurse is responsible to care for more than four patients, for each additional surgical patient over four, the risk of an untoward death increases by 7 percent. In hospitals with the lowest nurse staffing levels, defined as eight patients per nurse, patients have a 31-percent greater risk of dying than those in hospitals with four patients per nurse. According to this study, on a national scale, staffing differences of this magnitude could result in 20,000 unnecessary deaths each year.

These and other similar studies point to staffing and credentialing as key factors that affect patient safety. Considering the nursing shortage reported in a Health and Human Services report,[10] however, improving staffing ratios is very difficult. Consider these facts published by the Division of Nursing within the Bureau of Health Professions.[11]

- One hundred and twenty-six thousand nursing positions are unfilled in hospitals across the country.
- Fifty-six percent of hospitals report using agency or traveling nurses, at great expense, to fill vacancies.
- On average, nurses work eight and a half weeks of overtime per year.
- By 2020, it is estimated that there will be 400,000 fewer nurses available to provide care.
- Ninety-nine percent of long-term care organizations lack sufficient nurse staffing to provide even the most basic nursing care.
- There are roughly 21,000 fewer nursing students today than in 1995.
- Nursing schools turned away over 5,000 qualified baccalaureate program applicants in 2001 because of faculty shortages.
- In the state of Georgia alone, a quarter of the state's nursing school faculty will retire over the next four years.
- The average age of a working registered nurse, now 43.25 years old, is increasing more compared to other workforces in the country.
- Organizations that are better able to retain their nurses fare better on quality measures. Low turnover hospitals—at rates under 12 percent—had lower adjusted mortality scores and low severity-adjusted lengths of stay, as compared to hospitals with turnover rates that exceeded 22 percent.
- Staffing levels have been a factor in 24 percent of the 1,609 sentinel events reported to the Joint Commission over a five-year period.
- If recent trends go unchecked, the nation's nursing shortage would continue to worsen significantly over the next two decades. In 2000 the shortage was estimated at 6 percent; by 2020, it is expected to reach 29 percent.

STAFF TURNOVER

Turnover rate may be defined differently by organization segment. The risk management professional should have an understanding of how the organization defines turnover in each staff category so that reports of adequate or short staffing episodes are understood.

The costs associated with turnover, such as time spent in managing, recruiting, replacing, and training a new employee, and the associated lost productivity, are frequently estimated as a multiple of the employee's salary. Consequently, the turnover rate in each segment and sub-segment of a health care organization is a significant indicator for the management and reputation of an organization.

From a risk management perspective, high turnover equates to high-risk exposure. Staff members are unfamiliar with the culture of the organization. Loyalties might be in question when the staff is focused more on surviving than on paying attention to the customer or the patient. All of these describe an organization vulnerable to patient safety issues and liability exposure.

············

PHYSICIAN STAFFING

During the 1990s, some felt that the managed care approach would decrease the need for physician specialists and for hospital beds. The concept of managed care promised to care for individuals and families from birth to death, and to prevent illness and maintain health. The ideal system would involve primary care physicians in preventing illness and maintaining health, and therefore would require fewer specialists. Consequently, several physician specialty societies responded by decreasing the number of residencies available for their specialty. Physician specialties such as gastroenterology, anesthesiology, and dermatology decreased the open residency training slots, as it was expected that the primary care physicians would reduce the need for these specialist services.

While managed care was growing, reimbursement systems to hospitals, physicians, and other organizations were undergoing change or projected to undergo change, resulting in less revenue to the providers.

Meanwhile, technology improved. Studies were published that described how several procedures conducted on a preventative basis could save lives and treatment costs associated with some diseases. For example, colonoscopies are now recommended for adults over 50 years old to rule out cancer. The demand for colonoscopies, performed by gastroenterologists, has increased so much that waiting times for appointments are measured in months.

············

RISK MANAGEMENT ISSUES RELATED TO ORGANIZATIONAL STAFFING

Given the sobering outlook on the state of the health care workforce, the risk management professional is well advised to stay current on the organization's human resource issues. Factors that affect an organization's ability to fill and retain jobs at any level include:

- Geographic location and job market
- Economic situation
- Comparative pay scale for different job categories
- Complementary or co-paid benefits
- Organization's reputation or philosophy of care and its work environment

Each one of these factors can override the other. For example, a good candidate with experience and an unblemished history might select an organization with a poor reputation when offered an attractive salary and benefit package. The economy and the challenge in finding qualified candidates may drive the decision. In addition, candidates might seek organizations with poor reputations based upon proximity to their homes or because a candidate's background might be blemished.

In protecting the organization and promoting patient safety, the risk management professional can play a significant role in several staffing activities:

1. Provide orientation to new staff members on the incident reporting system. Reinforce the chain of command policy and procedures, disclosure policy, preservation of evidence procedures, documentation guidance, informed consent issues, and management of sentinel events.

2. Reinforce the mission statement and current safety goals to new staff members, including physicians, residents, and medical students.

3. Meet new staff members and introduce them to the organization's risk management efforts, giving it a face to recognize. This personal contact will encourage reporting procedures and convey the sense of importance placed on patient safety and risk management in the organization.

4. Provide an overview of the organization's safety program, prevention of workplace violence, prevention of injuries, and various programs to assist employees with problems and issues.

5. Present data to clinical departments regarding significant events and claims where staffing issues where identified. Data, properly collected and analyzed, can provide compelling information to managers who make budgetary decisions based on many factors, including risk avoidance and cost-benefit analysis.

6. The JCAHO sentinel alert program, where specific events are reported to the Joint Commission, offers a template for analyzing the root causes involved in a significant or sentinel event. These can include breakdowns in communication, problems with patient assessment processes, continuum of care issues, orientation and training of staff, timely availability of critical patient information, staffing inadequacies, and availability of physician specialists. Each one of these root causes implies a staffing problem, be it understaffing, wrong qualifications, or lack of training or orientation. Risk management should be aware and informed in root cause analysis of significant problems. The evidence of the data in comparison with dollars paid out in claims and defense can be powerful information to encourage management to change and improve staffing plans. For non-JCAHO accredited organizations, this process holds invaluable information and processes.

7. The incident report or quality report system (whatever method the organization uses to report events documenting injury to patients, customers, visitors, or staff members, in addition to near-misses) is the key communicator of facts, which later can be analyzed, trended, and tracked for reoccurrence. The data from this system, combined with staffing plans and actual work schedules, enable an organization to piece together its own story on how staffing affects safety and risk management issues. Thus, the risk management professional and staffing director(s) should collaborate on reports to management and possibly to the board on a regular basis.

Other staffing issues with strong risk management implications include:

- *Transfer procedures.* When staffing is not meeting planned levels, does the organization have a sound process for diverting new patients or to transfer in-patients out to other facilities?

- *Staffing plans.* Are they realistic and in sync with available staff? For example, if satellite pharmacies are planned to care for critical or off-site areas, will there be available licensed personnel to staff them, given the national shortage of pharmacists?

- *Staff ratios.* Although JCAHO does not provide specific ratios, some states do. California has established minimum staffing ratios affecting hospitals and long-term care departments.[12] Certain specialty nursing organizations stipulate ratios of registered nurses or licensed nurses to patients. To fall below these ratios can be a liability exposure if identified as a causal factor of a patient's injury. Special circumstances might be explainable by a health care organization, but patterns of unacceptable staffing can provide damaging evidence in defending a case alleging medical negligence. Patterns of understaffing are generally admissible evidence. If the organization cannot care for patients within the nurse-to-patient ratios established by external professional and regulatory organizations, the organization should consider rerouting admissions, delaying elective admissions, or transferring patients. The argument that the problem was temporary or rectified by bringing in supplemental staff is acceptable unless a pattern is evident. When the risk management professional identifies a pattern of staffing problems resulting in injury or claims, a management report on how often and how much this situation has cost the organization can be a compelling argument for change.

- *Agency use.* Temporary agencies are frequently used during times of "short staff." The risk management professional should be aware, if not directly involved, in the selection of these business partners. Are they conducting background checks, references, license and certificate verification, and competency testing? Even though the organization remains responsible for conducting primary source criminal background and verification of credentials, the agency can assist with initial screening. And very important, what is the arrangement for the agency personnel as far as insurance, such as workers' compensation and professional liability? Ideally, the agency provides these coverages, but this is not always the case as personnel might be independent contractors. The agreement or contract should stipulate insurance coverages and indemnification of loss. Should the organization have its own pool of personnel, the organization is assumed to provide the needed insurance coverages; however, this too should be in writing between the organization and the pool personnel.

Minimum staff ratios have been established in nursing homes by the Centers for Medicare and Medicaid Services (CMS). These statistics tell an organization what is expected as far as time spent in direct patient care per twenty-four hours and are expressed in nursing hours per patient load. This data per nursing facility is now available online. It reports the national and state-specific thresholds. The Web site also reports on specific nursing homes and how they compare statewide and nationally.[13]

Regarding chain of command procedures, during times of staffing shortages or using alternate staffing techniques (agency personnel, staffing pools), the chain of command procedure should be revisited with directors and managers who can, in turn, review it with staff. A faulty chain of command, or failure to use an existing chain of command policy, are components in many reported patient injuries and a significant factor when preparing to defend a litigated claim.

SHORTAGE OF PHARMACISTS

There is a significant shortage of licensed pharmacists across the nation. The reasons for this shortage include:

- Demand has grown because of an aging population that requires more pharmaceuticals.
- The growing number of medications available to treat serious illnesses and chronic maladies increases demand on those qualified to dispense them.
- Expanded health care coverage offering medication benefits adds 10 to 20 percent paper workload for pharmacists.
- Pharmacists may be lured away from not-for-profit facilities to the commercial sector.

- The role of the hospital pharmacist has expanded to assist with decisions in several clinical areas, such as intensive care units, surgical suites, and neonatal units.

- Pharmacists are entering PharmD programs for the doctoral credentials needed to counsel patients and advise physicians, thus creating a shortage in the general pharmacy arena.

- There is strong competition for pharmacists trained at the residency or fellowship level. Schools of pharmacy, managed care organizations, pharmaceutical corporations, and hospitals all compete for highly trained pharmacists, resulting in sector shortages for schools and hospitals less able to offer competitive salaries.

In 2004, the average vacancy rate for pharmacists was 5 percent, which is an improvement compared to 8.9 percent in 2000.[14] Improved incentives and pay scales have helped to retain pharmacists in health care organizations during the last few years. Recruiting new pharmacy managers and directors is still a challenge.

Most pharmacies rely on the assistance of pharmacy technicians, who assist pharmacists by performing duties that do not require the professional judgment of the licensed pharmacist. Technicians may be trained on the job or by completing a formal program provided at a community school. Technicians may be certified by taking the Certified Pharmacy Technician (CPhT) exam, which is offered by the Pharmacy Technician Certification Board. Many commercial pharmacies require pharmacy techs to earn this credential within a certain time period after their hire date. Because there is no national standard requiring certification, the risk management professional should explore the percentage of certification in the organization and encourage the requirement of certification to demonstrate competency in pharmacy technicians.

Following are additional risk management issues related to the pharmacist shortage.

- The pharmacy staff plan and schedule should reflect an appropriate ratio of pharmacists, certified technicians, and non-certified technicians.

- If pharmacy services are provided by an independent contractor organization instead of the pharmacy staff, the risk management professional should assure that the contract requires appropriate stipulated services, such as pharmacist to pharmacy technicians ratio; supervision of pharmacy technicians; cooperative reporting of significant incidents; participation in monitoring of sentinel events; cooperation with quality assurance efforts such as eliminating medication errors; and inclusion of adequate insurance coverage limits commensurate with the services that the contracted pharmacy corporation provides.

- Pharmacy services for long-term care and home services should include teaching and competency testing services as part of the agreement. Also, a shared stewardship for eliminating medication errors should be part of the agreement, which would include a flow of information between the nursing staff and the pharmacy staff as they cooperate in this important effort.

....

RESIDENTS IN TRAINING

The Accreditation Council for Graduate Medical Education (ACGME), the accrediting agency for the 7,800 physician residency programs in the United States established new standards on residents' work hours as of July 1, 2003.[15] Traditionally, residents across the country had been expected to work up to 130 hours a week depending on their program and sponsoring hospital. A landmark medical professional liability case, *Libby Zion vs. Cornell Medical Center,* brought to light the issue of overworked, undersupervised resident physicians. New York established maximum work hour rules for residents at that time, but in a later study found that the rules were not followed. The new standards set by ACGME include:

- No resident will work more than eighty hours per week averaged over four weeks.
- Moonlighting done in the sponsoring organization counts toward the weekly limit.
- One day in seven the residents must be free from all patient care and educational obligations, averaged over four weeks.
- In-house calls limited to no more than once every three nights, averaged over four weeks.

The underlying reasons for these requirements are the safety of the patients who are treated by residents, as well as the safety of the physicians-in-training. Not surprisingly, the Institute of Medicine (IOM) report was frequently referenced in the ongoing debate over residents' duty hours.

The risk management professional in a teaching institution, whether there is one residency program or multiple programs, must work with the medical education department to ensure that the organization operates within these rules. In New York, where state laws were enacted in 1987 to govern maximum work hours by residents, a study conducted ten years later revealed that at least 37 percent of residents were required to work more hours than the rules allowed. Most New York hospitals were found to be in violation.[16] A main reason is that residents fill many roles—surgical assistants, phlebotomists, historians, intravenous technicians, hospitalists—and at the same time provide a continuum of care.

Teaching hospitals have long relied on residents as critical staff members. To replace one resident's role might require several other staff members and the redesign of job duties and job descriptions. In other words, a teaching hospital with many residency programs will need to be creative to meet the new rules. Monitoring the residents' schedules and time worked is another necessary challenge. Risk management professionals can anticipate that plaintiffs will request these records in a case involving a resident's care, when misjudgment, fatigue, or lack of supervision are alleged. The duty hours and associated rules are monitored by ACGME through various means, including:[17]

- Confidential Internet resident surveys
- Interviews with program directors, staff, and residents during accreditation site visits
- ACGME Monitoring Committee assessment of local resident review committees and how they apply the accreditation standards
- Education of residents, program directors, and other audiences about resident duty hours

....

STAFFING THE RISK MANAGEMENT FUNCTION

To this point, the chapter has identified issues and influences that affect the organization's ability to supply properly trained patient care providers and support staff. The next section of the chapter will focus on how to staff the risk management function on an ongoing basis.

Risk management departments are not immune to cutbacks in staff. Thus, the risk management professional must be prepared to face the reality of accomplishing normal department functions with potentially fewer resources. To prepare for this possibility, one approach is to develop a creative staffing plan that enables the department to survive the inevitable disruptions caused by reductions in staff. The plan's primary purpose is to create new resources for the department. This can be accomplished in three separate but related ways:

1. *Internal transfer:* Shifting selected department functions to other departments
2. *Internal resource utilization:* Assigning underused personnel to other departments to perform specific functions
3. *External resources:* Covering selected functions through outsourcing

The degree to which the staffing plan succeeds will depend on the risk management professional's creativity in developing additional resources and on the plan's soundness and practicality. A simple plan that is well executed and managed should enable the risk management professional to build and maintain a successful risk management team.

············
DEVELOPING A CREATIVE STAFFING PLAN

Five major steps are involved in developing a creative staffing plan:

1. Assessing the full range of current functions
2. Evaluating options for internal and external transfer of functions
3. Determining a new staffing plan after functions are transferred
4. Establishing processes to manage the external resources effectively
5. Developing monitors to assess the plan's effectiveness and make changes as necessary

The following section examines each of these steps in detail.

Step 1. Assessing the Full Range of Current Functions

The first step in designing and planning a creative staffing plan is to thoroughly assess the full range of functions currently performed by the risk management department. To ensure that the listing is complete, the risk management professional should make every effort to separate the functions that are accomplished from the job positions to which they are assigned. A good technique for this process is to conduct a department-wide brainstorming session. Such a session can enable the manager to capture undocumented functions that otherwise might be overlooked. Moreover, by involving staff in this process, it increases the likelihood that they will support the plan should it become necessary to implement it. This process should include thoroughly documenting each function's specific elements. Defining all the elements will help ensure that a vital responsibility is not inadvertently overlooked if it becomes necessary to shift it to someone outside the department.

After all the functions are listed, the manager must pare them down to a workable set. This can be done through consolidation of overlapping or parallel functions into clearly understandable categories. The creative staffing prioritization model in Exhibit 17.1 provides an example of the types of categories that might be included. The left-hand

EXHIBIT 17.1   Range of Alternatives for Moving the Function or Position

This is a sample model of a tool for use in developing and displaying the organization's priorities for moving functions outside the risk management department. To use it, the risk management professional follows four basic steps:

1. List all functions or positions to be evaluated and prioritized
2. Determine and list the appropriate alternatives for the organization
3. List the top three priorities for each function being evaluated
4. Review the process with the management team to obtain input

FUNCTION OR POSITION	INTERNAL SOURCES				EXTERNAL SOURCES			
	Permanent Assignment	Project Assignment	Short-Term Assignment	Limited-Function Employee	Permanent Contractual	Contractual By Project	Outside Consultant	Vendors as Prepaid Service
Loss Control and Management								
Department Manager	1				2		3	
Legal Counsel		3			2	1		
OSHA Training	2		3					1
Fire & Safety surveys	1		2					
Regulatory Compliance		1	2				3	
SMDA		1		2				3
Medical Staff Credentialing		1	2		3			
Staff Education						2		3
Policy/Procedure Review			2	1			3	
ADA Compliance			2	1		3		
Disaster Control Training		1				2		3
Risk Finance								
Contract Review/Negotiations	1		3			2		
Premium Audit		1		2		3		
Broker Selection	1	2			3			
Insurance Purchasing	1	2			3			
Insurance Application Processing			1	2		3		
Risk Analysis	2			1	3			
Claims Administration								
Medical Record Liaison				1			2	3
Variance Report Tracking		2		1			3	
Claims Analysis		2		1	3			
MSC Attendance	1	3					2	
Legal File Maintenance	1				3		2	
Staff Education (Reporting)		1				3	2	
Loss Ratio						2	1	3

side of the model includes the three major categories of loss control and management, risk finance, and claims administration. Although these categories can be tailored to meet the needs of the institution, the model works best when the number of categories is limited to three or four major areas.

A side benefit of this process is identifying the strengths and weaknesses of the current staffing plan. This can stem from considering staff expertise, cost of managing the exposure, and amount of time allocated to particular projects or risk functions. Particular attention should be paid to the amount of department involvement in the management of risk financing, claims, and loss control activities. Involvement in each of these activities is paramount to the risk management program's success and should not be minimized without due consideration.

Step 2. Evaluating Options for Internal and External Transfers of Functions

This second step in the planning process requires the most creativity. During this step, the risk management professional must think beyond today's operations to identify all potential resources, both internal and external, that could be part of the final plan. Two essential resources should be considered:

Other People or Departments within the Organization Could Provide Key Services   This would typically be found on a part-time basis only. The model in Exhibit 17.1 offers an example of a tool the risk management professional can use to both prepare and present alternatives in a clear and easily understood manner. In this model, a priority of one (1) means that a function is best accomplished by that alternative. A priority of two (2) would be assigned to the next best alternative, and so on. The model provides a tool to help the risk management professional consider prioritizing and treating a variety of risks.

Many risk management projects might require short-term staffing, which an internal personnel pool could supply. Staff may be put on limited duty for several reasons, such as pregnancy, health situations, or workers' compensation rehabilitation periods. The number of risk management tasks that can be assigned to "newly created staff" is limited only by the risk management professional's imagination and ability to create new staffing opportunities. The following examples illustrate just a few of these opportunities:

- Home office workers: Data collection, off-site auditing, and preparation of meeting materials
- Workers' compensation or limited-work persons: Updating policy and procedures, trending of data, assignment to various committee meetings, and research
- Americans with Disabilities Act: Policy and procedure review, development of loss and trending information, auditing, credentialing functions, and committee assignment
- Physical therapists: Ergonomics, staff education, safety committee assignments, and health and exercise programs
- Safety and security staff: Staff education, assignment to various committees that contribute to the risk data collection process

Outsourcing   Risk management professionals must not only analyze functions that can be outsourced, but also what resources are required to monitor and manage the outsourced functions. Ideas of functions that could be considered for outsourcing include:

- Pre-accreditation survey for a specific department
- OSHA education for a high-risk employee group
- Pre-construction survey and building compliance

- Staff development and education
- Third-party administration of claims
- Contract review and negotiations

The following are some of the resources available to the risk management team and examples of how they may be used for outsourcing:

- *Risk consultants:* Provide focus or full-facility surveys; address targeted risk concerns; present or supplement educational programs; or help to develop and implement a risk management program.

- *Insurance brokers:* Provide assistance in the proper and accurate completion of insurance applications; promote updating the organization's insurable interests inventory; evaluate the scope and limits adequacy of the organization's insurance program.

- *Insurance companies:* Provide on-site risk management surveys or educational consultations via conference call or Web-based seminars to address immediate risk concerns. (The various professionals available include nurses, industrial hygienists, safety engineers, workers' compensation case managers, and ergonomic technicians.)

- *Disaster planning personnel:* Involving local community disaster planning resources, state agencies, city agencies (fire department, emergency medical technicians, rescue units) can expand and improve the disaster planning process. Benefits to the risk program will include on-site education for staff, updating of current fire and evacuation safety issues, and enhanced communication with community-based disaster planning personnel.

- *Law firms:* Communicate updates on changes in the law, provide education programs on preventing liability claims (including medical staff and the board), and attend meetings requiring legal input.

- *Third-party adjusters* (TPAs): Assist the organization in managing claims files and participate in mandatory settlement conferences.

An important aspect of outsourcing is the cost-benefit analysis. Risk management professionals should help their organizations determine whether it would cost more to hire an outside contractor to perform specific functions than it would to provide it with employed staff. Outsourcing then becomes an ongoing process of measuring this cost and benefit, to justify whether it still makes fiscal sense.

Step 3. Determining a New Staffing Plan After Functions Are Transferred

During this step, the risk management professional makes the difficult decisions on which functions or positions to eliminate or transfer in light of cutbacks. Unfortunately, because such decisions are specific to a department and an institution and involve personnel issues, there are no set guidelines to follow. However, the practical basis for making such decisions and for communicating the rationale behind them can be found in the creative staffing model.

After identifying the functions to be transferred, the model should be revised and the changes documented. This enables the risk management professional to monitor the effectiveness of the new model. For example, if a function is outsourced, the employee currently performing that function should be able to take on other responsibilities or will be transferred to another assignment within the organization.

Step 4. Establishing Processes to Manage External Resources

The risk management professional must redesign the staffing program to keep it effective, because the personnel who accomplish the functions will not all be reporting within the traditional department structure. However, by adapting a few basic processes to the new situation, the risk management professional can ensure a manageable situation. For example, the risk management professional should have the following in place:

- A policy for assignment within the risk department
- A credentialing process for all candidates (internal and external) (Exhibit 17.2)
- An orientation for all staff members (Exhibit 17.3)
- A mandatory confidentiality statement
- A project-tracking mechanism to effectively evaluate the progress, needs, and expectations of the various assignments (Exhibit 17.4)

EXHIBIT 17.2   Risk Management Department Credentialing Checklist

Name: _____ Area of expertise: _____

Position: _____

Project: _____

Qualifications required:

Degree requirements:

Years of experience:

Experience level:

Certification:

Confidentiality statement:

Curriculum vitae:

License(s):

OSHA training:

The applicant/consultant _____ received OSHA training on _____ at _____. A certificate of completion is attached.

The applicant/consultant will require OSHA training prior to any assignment at _____.
Upon completion, the certificate of completion must be included in the credentialing file.

References:
1.
2.
3.

References submitted by candidate: Yes ____ No ____ Date _____

Permission to contact references: Yes ____ No ____ Date _____

References returned:
1. _____ Date _____ Reviewed _____
2. _____ Date _____ Reviewed _____
3. _____ Date _____ Reviewed _____

EXHIBIT 17.3   Risk Management Department Orientation

Name: _____ Date: _____

Project: _____ Site: _____

Consultant   Yes _____   No _____

Employee   Yes _____   No _____

Date _____   Department _____ Initials (department head) _____

Identification badge _____   Computer introduction _____

Physical plant tour _____   Human relations _____

Keys _____   OSHA education _____

Key personnel (introductions) _____   Confidentiality _____

Computer/security clearance _____   Policy and procedures _____

Job description _____   Organizational chart _____

General safety _____   Committee assignments _____

Project summary _____

RM dept _____

Date _____   Committee _____   Location _____

EXHIBIT 17.4   Risk Management Department Project Summary

Project: _____ Site location _____

Goal: _____ Estimated start date: _____

Estimated completion date: _____

Reports to: _____

Phone nos. _____   (cell) _____

Fax: _____

Pager: _____

Personnel assigned to: _____   Project _____

1. Name _____ Dept. _____ Tel. _____ Fax _____

2. Name _____ Dept. _____ Tel. _____ Fax _____

Committee attendance required: Yes _____   No _____

1. Committee _____ Scheduled date/time _____ Location _____

2. Committee _____ Scheduled date/time _____ Location _____

Project progress report requirements

Forward all progress report to: _____

Due by _____ day of each week/month

Progress reports to include:
1. Summary of activity
2. Goals attained in previous week/month
3. Projected new goals for upcoming week/month
4. Detailed expense/budget report to date
5. Explanation of overbudget items
6. Expected completion date

The creative staffing plan must include a mechanism to ensure that properly qualified personnel are assigned to manage specific risk functions. Monitoring of the various internal and outsourced staff projects is critical to the risk management program's success. Therefore, it is strongly suggested that some of these tools and processes be used for all risk management projects, whether the person involved is internal or external, temporary or permanent. For example, the risk management department project summary example shown in Exhibit 17.4 could be used as the one common tracking and management tool for most of the department's projects. The format should be tailored to the institutional circumstances, but the concept of using consistent tools for documenting projects in a common format is essential when working with diverse and changing personnel.

Step 5. Developing Monitors to Assess Staffing Plan Effectiveness

The final step in the process is to create a mechanism for monitoring and displaying the results of the overall department after the new structure is in place. By determining in advance what results are expected, the risk management professional can design the reporting tools needed to monitor whether the expectations for the new structure are being met.

A good deal of time and effort will be required to jointly develop a reasonable and easily measured performance status (metric) for each individual component. However, the investment will pay off handsomely in ease of monitoring and reporting the current status.

Exhibit 17.5 is an example of a monitoring tool that can be used for this purpose. Its organization and format are drawn from the creative staffing model (Exhibit 17.1) developed previously so that the two correlate. This same summary sheet can be used for reporting outside the department so that the organization's management is informed of the effect of the restructuring and the department's progress in maintaining or improving on the previous level of service provided.

This summary presentation will permit the risk management professional to continually monitor and display the status of the individual assignments, and will quickly reveal any need to reallocate resources.

••••••••••••

RISK MANAGEMENT OUTSOURCING IMPLICATIONS

Using the model or grid shown in Exhibit 17.1, the risk management professional can measure and weigh the importance of selected risk management outsourced responsibilities. The risk management professional needs to be aware of potential risk management concerns that might arise, not only within the specific outsourced risk function, but also those concerns that arise from the engagement of a specific consultant.

Outsourcing to a risk management consultant has its own risks. Before engaging, these issues should be reviewed:

- Has credentials and references—If the consultant will be subcontracting a portion of the services promised, the subcontractor's credentials and references should also be reviewed
- Has ability to complete project within a given timeline
- Has expertise in health care risk management consulting

EXHIBIT 17.5   Sample Monitor Tool for Risk Management Function

This is a sample model of a tool for use in monitoring the organization's performance after moving some functions outside the risk management department. To use it, the risk management professional follows three basic steps:

1. List all functions or positions to be monitored
2. Determine an appropriate progress measure (metric) for each item to be tracked and display the plan status (ahead, on plan, behind plan)
3. Review the progress and the process with the individuals on a regular basis

Departmental Summary
See individual project-tracking sheets for detailed data

Function	INDIVIDUAL ASSIGNED & SOURCE			MEASUREMENT & PLAN PROGRESS			
	Individual/ Organization	Internal Resource	External Resource	Measurement (Metric)	Ahead of Plan	On Plan	Behind Plan
Loss Control and Management							
Legal Counsel	Marques, Shawn & Little		X	% or Response Deemed Timely		X	
OSHA Training	M. Robinson		X	% of Training Completed		X	
Fire & Safety Surveys	Vacant			Not Available			XXX
Regulatory Compliance	J. Jones	X		% of Required Audits Completed		X	
SMDA	Vacant			Not Available			XXX
Medical Staff Credentialing	S. Glover	X		% of Staff with Complete Records			X
Staff Education	N. McNew	X		% of Required Training Completed	X		
ADA Compliance	J. Sherz	X		# of Outstanding Issues		X	
Disaster Control Training	ADC, Inc.	X		% of Required Training Completed		X	
Risk Finance							
Contract Review Negotiations							
Premium Audit							
Insurance Application Processing							
Variance Report Tracking							
Claims Analysis							
MSC Attendance							
Legal File Maintenance							

- Avoids extraneous services that might not be of value to your entity
- Provides professionally acceptable work product, written or data management
- Has literacy in risk management information system (RMIS) and computer applications

- Has ability to communicate with a wide range of professionals
- Complies with HIPAA Business Associate Agreement

....

DUE DILIGENCE

It is usually wise to engage the human resources and legal departments before signing a contract for outsourcing services. They offer invaluable insight and will assist in eliminating risk associated with a poorly drafted contract. Also, be sure to have the agreement signed by one authorized to bind your organization by contract—usually an officer of the company.

Because of the sensitivity and confidentiality of the information to which the consultant will be privy, in addition to the above information requested, it is suggested as part of the background check that a detailed work history be obtained to determine if the following might be of concern:

- Fraudulent financial practices
- Failed prior fiduciary relationships
- Criminal record
- Failure to timely complete contract
- Lack of knowledge concerning insurance products, coverages, or exclusions
- Inability to understand various computer programs and related software platform functions for creating a data management system
- Fraudulent disclosure of completion of particular education or certification programs
- Political sensitivity to the culture, style, and needs of the organization
- Conflicts of interest, where they may have a financial interest in any vendors they recommend for additional services

....

THE CONSULTANT AGREEMENT

The service agreement should be reviewed by legal counsel and by human resources. The agreement is the document by which the consultant's results will be evaluated and compensation paid. Basic contract requirements are listed in Chapter 12 (of this volume), and at a minimum should include:

- Scope of the project
- Timeline for completion
- Account team and biographical sketches of team members
- Compensation
- Service standards
- Cancellation clauses
- Confidentiality statements
- Evaluation criteria

. . . .

CONCLUSION

The role of the risk management professional is ever-challenging. With each new law, regulation, and professional guideline comes the responsibility to weigh the risks and exposures and to plan for implementation. Every organization in which health care is provided, and in which therefore liability exposures exist, needs to address its method of staffing. Although risk management professionals might not be the experts in these areas, asking the right questions and working to foster the right approach can significantly improve the risk position of the organization. Specifically, it can greatly assist senior management with decisions on staffing ratios, residents' work hours, and provision for temporary staffing. In addition, when staff reductions affect the risk management department itself, the manager with an organized creative staffing plan will be equipped to cope with the changes and contribute to the cost-saving goals of the institution while still maintaining a level of control over the department's vital risk management functions. By using the creative staffing model, the risk management professional can develop and communicate a plan that will accommodate various levels of staffing cutbacks depending on the circumstances of the institution. Once functions are transferred outside the department, the risk management professional needs to put processes in place to manage them despite the absence of direct control. The need to thoroughly document qualifications, project status, personnel training, and other aspects of the creative staffing program will increase with the reduction in staffing. To best manage the processes, the risk management professional should develop and use tools that make managing and documenting the program consistent and easy. Regardless of whether cutbacks occur, creation of a creative staffing plan helps the manager assess the risk management program's current strengths and weaknesses, and is thus a worthwhile endeavor.

Endnotes

1. U.S. Department of Labor, Bureau of Labor Statistics, *Career Guide to Industries* (2003–2004).

2. *Ibid.*

3. "Hospital Nurse Staffing and Patient Mortality, Nurse Burnout, and Job Dissatisfaction," *Journal of the American Medical Association*, October 23–30, 2002.

4. U.S. Department of Labor, Bureau of Labor Statistics, *Career Guide to Industries* (2002–2003).

5. Joint Commission Perspectives, February 2005, Publication of the Joint Commission on Accreditation of Healthcare Organizations.

6. *Ibid.*

7. Kohn, L. T., Corrigan, J. M., and Donaldson, M. S., Eds., *To Err is Human: Building a Safer Health System*. Washington D.C.: National Academy Press, 1999.

8. Journal of American Medical Association 2005, May 18, 293 (19) 2384, Five Years After To Err Is Human.

9. "Hospital Nurse Staffing and Patient Mortality, Nurse Burnout, and Job Dissatisfaction," *Journal of the American Medical Association*, October 23–30, 2002.

10. Projected Supply, Demand, and Shorted of Registered Nurses: 2000–2020, Department of Health and Human Services http://usgovinfo.about.com/library/weekly/

11. "Bureau of Health Professions Health Work Force Reports," National Sample Survey of Registered Nurses, February 2002 http://bhpr.hrsa.gov/healthworkforce/reports/rnsurvey/default.htm

12. California Healthcare Association, www.calhealth.org
13. Centers for Medicare and Medicaid Services, cms.hhs.gov/medicaid/reports
14. American Society of Health-System Pharmacists (ASHP) Study, May 2003, www.ashp.org/practicemanager/staffsurvey2003.pdf
15. Accreditation Council for Graduate Medical Education, [www.acgme.org/website/newsroom].
16. American College of Surgeons, November Bulletin, 2002.
17. American Council for Graduate Medical Education, Resident Duty Hours Standards [www.acgme.org/newsroom].

18

Emergency Management

Michael L. Rawson
Harlan Y. Hammond

INTRODUCTION

It is Monday morning and as you answer the phone in your Nashville office you are told that the first floor of your flagship hospital in Houston is under three feet of water, thanks to tropical storm Dorothy and the resulting flooding. Your day has just begun, however, as the next call brings news that your system's long-term care center in Little Rock has been without water and sewer service for six hours due to Dorothy, with little hope that services will be restored soon. As you turn on the Weather Channel you note that Dorothy is heading northeast, and has remained stronger than was forecast by weather experts. Three additional facilities in your system are directly in its path, including the office building where you currently sit. You reach for your system emergency response plan wondering what direction it offers for this type of emergency.

Health care facilities (HCFs) face many scenarios that might require an emergency response. Some are internal conditions limited to the HCF itself, which are typically man-made. Examples include bomb threats, terrorism, hostage situations, release of hazardous materials, loss of medical gases, fires, loss of utilities, or communication system failures. Others faced are external to the HCF, which can damage or destroy the infrastructure of the area around the HCF. Weather disasters, landslides, floods, earthquakes, volcanic eruptions, infectious diseases, accidents involving mass transit, structural collapses, explosions, chemical spills, civil disobedience, and war are examples of external conditions that may require an emergency response.[1] Both internal and external conditions can create mass casualties, and also can put the ongoing operations of the HCF in question. Since September 11, 2001, much has been published on emergency management and more is being learned each day as scenarios are examined and re-examined. This chapter will address key basic elements of emergency management but will not cover all possibilities and contingencies in depth.

The goal is to offer sufficient information for HCF risk management professionals to assess whether their emergency management plan is comprehensive, yet flexible enough to address any number of emergencies, regardless of type, size, or scope.

Besides not wanting to be caught unprepared when an emergency happens, there are other reasons for keeping response plans current. The HCF's commitment to comply with federal, state, community, and regulatory requirements for responding to emergencies offers a compelling motivation to maintain an effective, up-to-date plan. The guidelines, requirements, and recommendations of organizations such as the Occupational Safety & Health Administration (OSHA), the Joint Commission on Accreditation of Healthcare Organizations (JCAHO), the National Fire Protection Agency (NFPA), the Environmental Protection Agency (EPA), and others add complexity to designing an appropriate plan. Beyond compliance, however, is the risk management responsibility to prepare the HCF to manage and recover from emergencies that do occur. Clearly, this presents a risk management opportunity at its fullest.

··········

THE STEPS OF EMERGENCY MANAGEMENT

The foundation for preparing a workable plan is understanding what steps are involved in emergency management. There are several variations on how to describe these steps, but all seem to fit into the following four categories:[2]

Prevention   Establish robust internal reporting systems to enable information about key risks to flow freely upward. Take warnings seriously. Foster a management culture that is open to hearing bad news and knows how to respond to it.

Preparation   Maintain an effective emergency response plan that addresses all key functions of response and recovery. Rehearse the plan. Ensure that management understands how their roles may differ when the emergency plan is activated.

Implementation and Response   Know how to activate the emergency response plan and how to recognize the differing roles that people will assume when responding to the emergency. Ensure the readiness of your public information officer to manage media relations.

Recovery   Get the HCF operational as quickly as possible. Initiate and manage the process of financial recovery. Minimize the effects on the workforce, which can be severe and long lasting.

Attention to each of these steps, regardless of the size or configuration of the health care organization, can result in a plan that will provide a valued resource at the moment it is most needed. A more in-depth discussion on these steps follows.

··········

PREVENTION

The best prevention starts with an assessment and understanding of the types of risk inherent in HCFs that make them susceptible to emergency situations. The Vulnerability Analysis Chart[3] shown in Exhibit 18.1 can help assist HCFs to identify where to focus

EXHIBIT 18.1   Vulnerability Analysis Chart

TYPE OF EMERGENCY	Probability	Human Impact	Property Impact	Business Impact	Internal Resources	External Resources	Total
	High 5 ←→ 1 Low	High Impact 5 ←→ 1 Low Impact			Weak Resources 5 ←→ 1 Strong Resources		

The lower the score, the better.

preventive efforts to maximize the benefits from the resources invested. "Prevention is the cornerstone of public and occupational health."[4] By evaluating vulnerabilities and taking appropriate preventative action, loss can be minimized in an emergency. A framework for prevention planning is shown later in this chapter.

Design and Location

The location of the HCF has a direct relationship to its vulnerability to loss. Most HCFs cannot change locations easily; so, mitigating vulnerabilities by implementing appropriate architectural design elements becomes critical. A few examples follow on how these two aspects work together.

Earthquake   Unless your HCF was constructed after the most recent seismic code was enacted, your facility most likely was built to a lower (albeit approved at the time) construction standard, which might make it more susceptible to an earthquake. The costs of retrofitting a building to bring it into compliance with a higher seismic code are significant and often not affordable. Even so, each addition, upgrade, rehabilitation, or replacement to current standards will help the HCF survive an earthquake while meeting the goal of compliance with current building codes. Architects can advise how best to incorporate current seismic standards into any construction plans. Property insurers can also be helpful in identifying what can be done to mitigate the potential damage to the physical plant, short of replacing the HCF outright.

Another design element to consider is having sufficient space to store vital earthquake supplies, including food, water, drugs, and other medical supplies; for those at the HCF when an earthquake strikes or who might seek shelter after the earthquake.

Flood   The location of your HCF may make it vulnerable to flood. Again, assuming it is not feasible to change location, the incorporation of design elements to prevent or mitigate loss should be considered such as: (1) traffic water flow away from the HCF using drainage channels, earth or concrete aqua ducts and barriers, or other means; (2) use sandbags in strategic locations to divert water flow. Keep equipment and materials on hand with the appropriate procedures in place to facilitate the sandbag operation; and (3) consider where expensive equipment and supplies can be housed within your facility to protect them from potential water damage, such as moving them to a higher floor in the facility. The insurance company providing your flood damage coverage will also have loss prevention techniques to share.

Biological Terrorism   The Centers for Disease Control and Prevention's National Institute for Occupational Safety and Health (NIOSH) (www.cdc.gov) offers resource materials on protecting facilities from chemical, biological, and radiological attacks. There are no guarantees to prevent terrorist attacks; however, there are steps to minimize their effect. The NIOSH recommendations are multifaceted. They suggest starting with the simple step of *knowing your building*. This includes knowing the condition of your mechanical equipment, what filtration systems are in place and how well they work, whether the HVAC system responds to manual fire alarms, how the HVAC system is controlled, how air flows though the building, where the outdoor air louvers are located, and whether the roof is accessible from adjacent structures or landscaping, among other items. You can protect the outdoor air intakes where airborne agents can be introduced into your facility by relocating them, redesigning them to minimize public accessibility (the higher on the building the better), or by establishing a security zone around the intakes. These steps, when accompanied by appropriate security surveillance (adding security lighting, surveillance cameras, and additional security officer patrols of the area), could deter harmful activity or detect its potential earlier to minimize resulting harm.[5]

Training

Preventive efforts will be meaningless unless human resources are available and trained to implement the right steps at the right time. For example, if HCF staff is trained to recognize and respond to clinical symptoms from the introduction of biological agents introduced into the air system, lives can be saved. Training should include the steps necessary to not only protect themselves, but also their patients from the harmful effects of those agents. Training on how to initiate the HCFs emergency response plan in case of an attack is critical. A training tool[6] developed to keep track of training is shown in Exhibit 18.2.

Participate with Local Emergency Planning Councils

Some mistakenly believe that a local hospital or HCF should take the lead in responding to community emergencies, when in reality the response is led by community leaders in a coordinated effort. Active participation by the HCF with Local Emergency Planning Councils (LEPCs) can help to define the appropriate boundaries for the HCF's emergency

EXHIBIT 18.2   Training Drills and Exercises Schedule

	January	February	March	April	May	June	July	August	September	October	November	December
MANAGEMENT ORIENTATION/ REVIEW												
EMPLOYEE ORIENTATION/ REVIEW												
CONTRACTOR ORIENTATION/ REVIEW												
COMMUNITY/MEDIA ORIENTATION/ REVIEW												
MANAGEMENT TABLETOP EXERCISE												
RESPONSE TEAM TABLETOP EXERCISE												
WALKTHROUGH DRILL												
FUNCTIONAL DRILLS												
EVACUATION DRILL												
FULL-SCALE EXERCISE												

Source: FEMA. Emergency Management Guide for Business and Industry a Step-by Step Approach to Emergency Planning, Response and Recovery for Companies of all Sizes, Training Drills and Exercises, Appendix p. 67.

response plan. By knowing what community resources will be available in an emergency, the HCF can avoid duplicating resources and focus its efforts on providing necessary assistance. Identifying what role each organization will play in a complementary response effort will avoid unnecessary competition and duplication. More information on working with LEPCs will be addressed later in the chapter.

Seek Priority from Essential Service Providers

To ensure the continuation of essential services such as electricity, water, gas, oil, phone, garbage, and sewer for an HCF requires the ongoing commitment by local service providers in advance of the emergency. This commitment will necessitate an understanding by the service providers of the nature and types of emergency scenarios that can occur in HCFs, along with the HCF's role. HCFs should discuss and explain their need to be a priority when emergency service is needed. With this understanding and up-front commitment by local service providers, HCFs are being proactive in mitigating future loss. Essential service providers should be invited to visit the HCF as often as needed to become familiar with how utility services are configured and where main switches and other key components are located. Keep the relationship between the HCF and the service providers strong and productive so as to promote a quick and willing response when it becomes needed.

Review Your Facility's Insurance

A good start to prevent financial loss to the organization is to review what insurance is in place and identify coverage gaps that exist pertaining to key vulnerabilities. If there are gaps in the insurance coverage, identify whether those gaps can be closed and at what price.

A local emergency could affect several types of insurance carried by the HCF, such as those noted here:

- **Property and Business Interruption.** These policies are most often written on the "all risk" form, which covers all physical damage perils other than those specifically excluded. Although the burden is on the insurance company to prove that the peril is *not* covered, there have been several terrorism-related clauses added back to the core policy: electronic data processing, decontamination expenses, service interruption, ordinance or law coverage, civil authority, ingress and egress coverage, terrorism, and contingent business interruption. Typically a sub-limit, or a coverage amount less than that provided for other claims under the policy, applies to these provisions. Other exclusions that can relate to terrorism are: nuclear reaction or nuclear radiation, hostile or warlike action in time of peace or war, dishonest acts, and pollution.[7] It is important to review this coverage with the broker or insurance representative to learn the extent to which the policy contains sub-limits and exclusions and what can be done to address any gaps they might create. Refer to Chapter 16 for more information on Insurance: Basics Principles and Coverage.

- **Directors' & Officers' Liability.** If the directors or officers are sued alleging negligence in overseeing the HCF's efforts to appropriately prepare for and respond to an emergency, this coverage would apply. A key issue would be to what extent the limits available to the directors or officers are eroded by other covered losses, such as D&O entity losses, employment practices liability, or fiduciary liability. Clearly, each HCF should procure limits sufficient to cover probable losses in all risk categories covered by the policy.

- **General, Professional, and Auto Liability.** Each of these insurance coverages likely contain exclusions specific to certain catastrophic exposures. In our current environment, though, one might see a suit claiming an omission on the part of the HCF to appropriately plan for an emergency and that lack of preparedness resulted in injury or death. Depending on policy language, legal fees may or may not be covered and reimbursed to the HCF.

- **Workers' Compensation.** In the September 11, 2001, World Trade Center attack, this coverage was very high profile. With so many people killed, injured, or emotionally scarred, the total loss to carriers was catastrophic.[8] Claims under this program are of three major types for those who witnessed and survived the disaster: (1) Physical-mental, which typically involve a physical injury that precipitates a mental disability;

(2) mental-physical, which involve mental stress that causes a physical disability; and (3) mental-mental, which involve psychiatric neuroses alleged to have developed without physical trauma.[9]

- **Aviation.** Resulting from the September 11, 2001, terrorist attacks, terrorism exclusions in aviation policies have become commonplace. In some cases, however, limits for terrorism can still be purchased for an additional premium.

Any gaps in the HCF's insurance coverage should be discussed with senior management. Part of this discussion should include options to cure the gap in coverage including the terms, conditions and cost. All discussions regarding gaps in coverage (including decisions not to implement recommendations to cure gaps found), should be documented and preserved and revisited at time of coverage renewal, or if the HCF's vulnerability to loss increases or decreases during the year. Part of this documentation should be the rationale behind the decision to implement or not implement recommendations presented. To assist in this process the risk management professional should prepare a cost-benefit analysis of the recommendation. This analysis will highlight possible reasons for not implementing an alternative including high cost, limited coverage, reduced markets, or restrictive language.

Risk management professionals should also have a thorough understanding of the conditions contained in each insurance policy, such as reporting requirements (what to report, to whom, how, and when). This will avoid having a claim denied on the basis of a reporting technicality.

. . . .

PLANNING AND PREPARATION

It has been said that emergency planners "should plan for the worst and hope for the best." Planning for the worst implies that planners review, evaluate, and develop contingencies for all possible emergencies. However, planning based upon worst-case assumptions frequently results in written plans that are lengthy, detailed, cumbersome, and costly to produce and maintain. Lengthy plans are seldom read and rarely understood.

In this section, information, suggestions, and resources will be provided to allow planners to write emergency management plans that are easily read, quickly understood, and rapidly implemented.

Emergency Management Planning

HCF leaders must assume accountability for ensuring that emergency management plans are developed, written, and communicated to the organization. They should assign the development of the plan to a person or persons familiar with the facility and the organization, and who possess appropriate writing and communication skills. Once written, the plan should be reviewed, accepted, and approved by the organizational leaders including executive leadership, board of directors, and the medical staff.

The plan writer must have access to a committee that represents departments critical to the success of the plan, such as the emergency department, nursing, medical staff, security, and those who are familiar with the building, operations, and the environment. The plan will be accepted more quickly if the key stakeholders have had the opportunity to provide input during its development.

Hazard Vulnerability Analysis

An "All Risk" hazard vulnerability analysis should be performed using available HCF and community resources. Emergency preparedness plans are unique, mainly because each HCF is in a specific community or neighborhood. A good plan for one HCF may be inadequate elsewhere. At a minimum, the plan should be:

- Updated annually or whenever environmental or staffing changes make it necessary
- Communicated to all managers and employees
- Tested and evaluated

The American Society for Healthcare Engineering (ASHE) has developed an effective tool for conducting a hazard vulnerability analysis, shown in Exhibit 18.3, which is also available at www.ashe.org.[10]

Community Planning

Health care facilities must participate in community planning efforts. The JCAHO, under the Environment of Care Standard, EC 4.10,[11] requires JCAHO-accredited organizations to use and coordinate with community emergency planning and management agencies when developing and testing their plans. In addition, the Centers for Medicare and Medicaid Services (CMS) require community coordination under 42 CFR 482:55(b) (2).[12] To help meet the regulatory and accreditation standards and guidelines, each HCF should be represented on the Local Emergency Planning Council (LEPC). Participating in the LEPC allows the facility to understand community expectations and to prepare for hazards and events identified by community and state agencies.

HCFs have traditionally prepared for a variety of disasters. Past events experienced by the HCF often dictate the direction of planning efforts. California prepares for earthquakes, Florida for hurricanes, and Montana for snowstorms. JCAHO now requires planning based on a "hazard vulnerability analysis" performed by the HCF.[13] This analysis will certainly include many of the emergencies currently identified, but might also reveal others that should be evaluated. The ASHE tool in Exhibit 18.3 can assist in this effort; while its use is not *required* by JCAHO, the tool and methodology meets JCAHO requirements. Regardless of the form or tool used, HCFs should include in their analysis the elements of probability, risk and preparedness.

The analysis must include natural, technological and human events, and internal and external vulnerabilities and risks. Once prioritized, the facility can then focus its efforts on the hazards with the highest probability of an occurrence and the most costly in terms of financial impact.

Emergency planners are challenged to consider a variety of emergencies including the threat of a bioterrorism attack. The CDC and local health departments have established reporting criteria and systems to assist in the early detection of such an attack. Refer to the NIOSH recommendations mentioned earlier in this chapter on how buildings can be protected from a bioterrorism attack.[14] Insurance companies can assist by bringing experts in to help review and strengthen the planning process.

Community Resources

The importance of HCF participation in the LEPC cannot be overemphasized. HCF leaders should appoint a person or persons to represent the HCF on the LEPC. This appointment

EXHIBIT 18.3   Hazard Vulnerability Analysis

INSTRUCTIONS:

Evaluate every potential event in each of the three categories of probability, risk, and preparedness. Add additional events as necessary.

Issues to consider for probability include, but are not limited to:

1. Known risk
2. Historical data
3. Manufacturer/vendor statistics

Issues to consider for risk include, but are not limited to:

1. Threat to life and/or health
2. Disruption of services
3. Damage/failure possibilities
4. Loss of community trust
5. Financial impact
6. Legal issues

Issues to consider for preparedness include, but are not limited to:

1. Status of current plans
2. Training status
3. Insurance
4. Availability of back-up systems
5. Community resources

Multiply the ratings for each event in the area of probability, risk, and preparedness. The total values, in descending order, will represent the events most in need of organization focus and resources for emergency planning. Determine a value below which no action is necessary. Acceptance of risk is at the discretion of the organization.

EVENT	PROBABILITY				RISK						PREPAREDNESS			TOTAL
	HIGH	MED	LOW	NONE	LIFE THREAT	HEALTH/ SAFETY	HIGH DISRUPTION	MOD DISRUPTION	LOW DISRUPTION		POOR	FAIR	GOOD	
SCORE	3	2	1	0	5	4	3	2	1		3	2	1	
NATURAL EVENTS														
Hurricane														
Tornado														
Severe Thunderstorm														
Snow Fall														

(Continued)

©2000 American Society for Healthcare Engineering

Developed by SBM Consulting, Ltd.

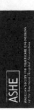
CONSULTING, LTD.

EXHIBIT 18.3   Hazard Vulnerability Analysis *(Continued)*

EVENT	PROBABILITY				RISK						PREPAREDNESS			TOTAL
	HIGH	MED	LOW	NONE	LIFE THREAT	HEALTH/ SAFETY	HIGH DISRUPTION	MOD DISRUPTION	LOW DISRUPTION		POOR	FAIR	GOOD	
SCORE	3	2	1	0	5	4	3	2	1		3	2	1	
NATURAL EVENTS														
Blizzard														
Ice Storm														
Earthquake														
Tidal Wave														
Temperature Extremes														
Drought														
Flood, External														
Wild Fire														
Landslide														
Volcano														
Epidemic														
TECHNOLOGICAL EVENTS														
Electrical Failure														
Generator Failure														
Transportation Failure														
Fuel Shortage														

©2000 American Society for Healthcare Engineering

Developed by SBM Consulting, Ltd.

SBM CONSULTING, LTD.

Natural Gas Failure									
Water Failure									
Sewer Failure									
Steam Failure									
Fire Alarm Failure									
Communications Failure									
Medical Gas Failure									
Medical Vacuum Failure									
HVAC Failure									
Information Systems Failure									
Fire, Internal									
Flood, Internal									
Hazmat Exposure, Internal									
Unavailability of Supplies									
Structural Damage									
HUMAN EVENTS									
Mass Casualty Incident (trauma)									
Mass Casualty Incident (medical)									
Mass Casualty Incident (hazmat)									

(Continued)

Developed by SBM Consulting, Ltd.

EXHIBIT 18.3   Hazard Vulnerability Analysis *(Continued)*

EVENT	PROBABILITY				RISK						PREPAREDNESS			TOTAL
	HIGH	MED	LOW	NONE	LIFE THREAT	HEALTH/ SAFETY	HIGH DISRUPTION	MOD DISRUPTION	LOW DISRUPTION		POOR	FAIR	GOOD	
SCORE	3	2	1	0	5	4	3	2	1		3	2	1	
HUMAN EVENTS														
Hazmat Exposure, External														
Terrorism, Chemical														
Terrorism, Biological														
VIP Situation														
Infant Abduction														
Hostage Situation														
Civil Disturbance														
Labor Action														
Forensic Admission														
Bomb Threat														

Reprinted with permission from the American Society for Healthcare Engineering of the American Hospital Association, Hazard Vulnerability Analysis, February 21, 2001, written by Susan B. McLaughlin, MBA, CHSP, MT(CASP) SC, Pages 10–13.

©2000 American Society for Healthcare Engineering

Developed by SBM Consulting, Ltd.

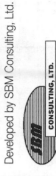
CONSULTING, LTD.

should be documented in the minutes and annual report of the Environment of Care Committee (safety committee). The HCF representative to the LEPC should report regularly to the Environment of Care Committee and other committees as needed on LEPC developments.

Typically, LEPCs are called together and chaired by a government official. On occasion, the HCF leader may be asked to chair the LEPC. This may require significant political sensitivity, as the HCF may be one of several competing HCFs participating on the LEPC. Whether in a leadership role or simply as an active participant, it will be key to the LEPC's success for the HCF leader to provide active input regarding what resources and capabilities the HCF has available to respond to a community emergency. In return, the HCF understands community expectations for its services, and what community resources will be available to the HCF in time of an emergency. It also provides a forum for alerting community leaders if expectations for the HCF exceed its capability.

Community planning should include coordination between the health care facility and community resources such as:

- Emergency medical services
- Public safety agencies, such as law enforcement and fire
- Utilities (electric, gas, propane, telephone, cellular telephone, water, sewer, and garbage collection)
- Suppliers (food, medical supplies, office supplies, and so on)
- Contractors (maintenance, housekeeping, food service, and so on)

Agreement to restore essential services temporarily lost by the HCF was mentioned earlier in the chapter. For example, many cellular phone companies will routinely restrict or limit service to subscribers during an emergency to allow public service agencies to communicate. Has the HCF been designated as on a priority basis as a public service customer? What phones are designated for priority service, meaning that they will not be turned off or given limited or restricted service on the network during an emergency?

A valuable community resource often overlooked is the amateur radio operators' network. Amateur radio operators are often members of volunteer emergency communication groups. One group organized in many communities is the Amateur Radio Emergency Services (ARES). ARES is dedicated to amateur radio as it pertains to disaster services. When phone service is interrupted by a disaster, amateur radios have the ability and means to communicate. HCF emergency planners should contact local amateur radio operating groups for assistance in establishing emergency communication networks between HCFs, public safety officers, and the community.

Other Resources

Other community, governmental, and private resources exist to help public and private organizations succeed with emergency management. Consider contacting:

- Local, county, and state Department of Health
- Local building departments and inspectors
- Federal Agencies including Federal Emergency Management Agency (FEMA), Centers for Disease Control and Prevention (CDC), US Army Corps of Engineers, and so on
- Insurance companies
- Risk management consulting firms

These organizations have valuable information that can assist in organizing an effective and comprehensive plan.

Incident Command System

JCAHO, governmental regulatory agencies, and other standard or code writing organizations require (or recommend) that HCFs create written plans to address different emergencies. Refer to Exhibit 18.4. Emergencies ranging from single-car accidents to large-scale disasters or terrorist activity require cooperation among several agencies, other HCFs, and health care providers.

Considering the number of hospitals, agencies, and organizations potentially involved in an event, a standard and common emergency management system was needed. This has resulted in adoption of the Incident Command System (ICS) by regulatory agencies and public response organizations alike.

ICS was originally developed by an interagency workgroup known as FIRESCOPE (Firefighting Resources of California Organized for Potential Emergencies) after several large wildfires in the early 1970s demonstrated the need for interagency cooperation. Since then, FEMA, NFPA, state, and local public safety agencies have adopted ICS as a standard.

NFPA 99 *Standard for Healthcare Facilities* states: "The emergency management committee shall model the emergency management plan on the incident command system (ICS) in coordination with local emergency response agencies."[15]

Although initially developed to respond to major wildfires, ICS principles apply to any emergency or mass casualty event. Emergencies occur without advance notice, develop rapidly, and grow in size and complexity. Often several agencies and organizations respond simultaneously, each with its own specialty or responsibility.

These and other factors make ICS an effective health care management tool useful in response to an emergency event. In 1991, Orange County, California, used ICS principles to develop the Hospital Emergency Incident Command System (HEICS). HEICS is the joint property of the State of California Emergency Medical Services Authority and the San Mateo

---

EXHIBIT 18.4   Emergency Management Planning—Standards and Regulations

When developing an emergency management plan HCFs must take into account the requirements imposed by JCAHO and the Environmental Protection Agency (EPA). The Occupational Safety and Health Administration (OSHA) regulations and National Fire Protection Association (NFPA) codes and standards must also be taken into account, as well as the Centers for Disease Control and Prevention (CDC) Strategic Plan for Preparedness and Response to biological and chemical terrorism. The American Institute of Architects (AIA) has also issued certain guidelines for design and construction of facilities in location where there is a recognized potential for certain natural disasters. These requirement include:

A. JCAHO Standards (Environment of Care (EC)[1]
    1. Provide processes to:
        a. Initiate a plan.
        b. Integrate the HCF's role with community-wide emergency response agencies, including who is in charge.
        c. Notify external authorities.
        d. Notify, identify, and assign personnel during emergencies.
        e. Manage the following:
            i. Patients, staff, and staff and family support activities
            ii. Logistics of critical supplies
            iii. Security
            iv. Interaction with media

(Continued)

EXHIBIT 18.4   Emergency Management Planning—Standards and Regulations *(Continued)*

    f. Evacuate entire HCF.

    g. Establish alternative care sites, including processes to:

       i. Manage patient necessities

       ii. Track patients

       iii. Communicate between HCF and alternate site

       iv. Transport patients, personnel, and equipment

    h. Continue or reestablish operations after a disaster.

  2. Identify

    a. Alternative means of providing essential building utilities, including electricity, water, ventilation fuel, medical gas, and vacuum systems

    b. Back internal and external communications systems

    c. Nuclear, chemical, and biological decontamination facilities

    d. Alternate roles and responsibilities for personnel (such as non-clinical staff) during emergencies, including a command structure consistent with that used by the community (for example, an incident command system)

  3. Establish

    a. Education and training of personnel, including biannual drills

    b. Performance monitoring of personnel knowledge

    c. Annual plan evaluation

B. Environmental Protection Agency (EPA) Requirements

    EPA's Emergency Planning and Community Right-to-Know Act[2] relates to the release of hazardous substances, including biological and other disease-causing agents, which cause an emergency.

  1. Each state must establish an Emergency Response Commission.

  2. States divide into local emergency planning committees (LEPCs).

  3. Hospitals designated by the LEPC to handle victims of a hazardous substance emergency must have an emergency response plan.

C. Occupational Safety and Health Administration (OSHA) Requirement

    OSHA requires HCFs to prepare plans to deal with certain man-made disasters, including hazardous-substance emergencies, ethylene oxide releases, and fires. Plans must address, at a minimum, emergency escape procedures, procedures for employees who stay to perform critical operations, and procedures to account for all employees after an emergency.[3]

D. Centers for Disease Control and Prevention (CDC)

    CDC's Bioterrorism Preparedness and Response Program coordinates implementation of the national preparedness and response plan for biological and chemical terrorism.[4] HCFs must coordinate with state and local public health agencies to ensure they are properly coordinating their own efforts with the national plan.

E. National Fire Protection Association (NFPA), American Institute of Architects (AIA)

    The NFPA health care facilities standard states that HCFs should have a total program for responding to any disaster that could reasonably occur.[5]

    AIA provides facility planning and design guidelines for disasters, whether they are natural, nuclear, biological, or chemical. The guidelines require:

  1. Wind- and earthquake-resistant designs

  2. Suitable location for new facilities

  3. Adequate storage capacity, or a function program contingency plan, to ensure a day's supply of the following:

    a. Food

    b. Sterile supplies

    c. Pharmacy supplies

    d. Linens

    e. Water for sanitation

  4. Emergency radio communication system that operates independently of the facility

---

[1] Joint Commission on Accreditation of Healthcare Organizations. "Emergency Preparedness Management Plan." In: Comprehensive Accreditation Manual for Hospitals. Oakbrook Terrace, Ill.: JCAHO, 2001, EC 1.4.

[2] 42 U.S.C. 11001 et seq.

[3] 29 C.F.R. 1910.38.

[4] Centers for Disease Control and Prevention. "Biological and Chemical Terrorism: Strategic Plan for Preparedness and Response." MMWER, April 21, 2000, 49(RR-4).

[5] National Fire Protection Association. Standard for Healthcare Facilities. Quincy, Mass.: NFPA, 2000.

County Health Services Agency Emergency Medical Services, but is available free of charge to health care facilities. It may be downloaded from their Web site at [www.emsa.cahwnet.gov]. Also available is a smaller version, called the Medical Aid Station Incident Command System (MASICS), for freestanding clinics and medical complexes.

Many HCFs and organizations have taken the basic ICS system and adapted it to the health care emergency response environment. Although HEICS is the standard, other examples may be found in the reference section of this chapter.

ICS Organization in Health Care Facilities

The ICS command structure uses the existing HCF organization to establish five major functions: (1) command, (2) operations, (3) planning, (4) logistics, and (5) finance and administration.

These functions, or elements within each function, can flex to apply effectively to a minor emergency or manage response to a major disaster. While the HCF can adapt the ICS organization to meet its specific needs, several duties are common to each function and should be identifiable in all emergency responses.

Command   The Command function is the hub of the ICS. It determines where the Incident Command is located. It provides direction, order, and control of the organization when the ICS becomes active. Because information flows into the ICS from multiple sources, the Incident Commander should have advisors designated to help formulate responses to issues brought to the ICS for resolution. These advisors may include the Safety or Security Officer, Public Information Officer, Liaison Officer, and others as needed.

Planning   The Planning function is responsible to gather and report information about the event, establish a labor pool, provide staff support services, and monitor recovery-planning activities. The planning function typically is a record keeper, providing an accurate account of activities and responses.

Operations   The Operations function coordinates all patient care activities, directs emergency care operations, and supports evacuation procedures under the direction of the medical control officer.

Logistics   The Logistics function supports facility operations by managing the utility systems and securing and distributing supplies needed for patient care operations. It coordinates meeting transportation requirements, oversees food service operations, and implements damage control activities as needed.

Finance and Administrative   The Finance and Administrative function provides financial resources for response needs, tracks expenses, charges for cost recovery, and coordinates activities for liability control and claims management.

Large-scale events usually require that each function, be established as a separate entity. Each of the five functions can be subdivided into several smaller sections as needed. During a small event, not all functions or sections may be needed. One person may manage a number of functions or sections, whereas in a large-scale disaster all functions or sections will require one or more people.

Ideally, the CEO will assume the role as incident commander. Realistically, the CEO is often away from the facility when an emergency occurs. In the CEO's absence, the administrator on call, nursing supervisor, or another designated leader must temporarily assume ICS leadership. Upon arrival, the CEO should assume the Incident Commander role. This order of leadership should be documented in the written plan. All persons who might assume the Incident Commander role must be regularly trained on the basics of incident command, and must be familiar with the location and contents of the written plan.

The effectiveness of ICS is most frequently demonstrated by its ability to expand and contract based on the level of emergency and the number of resources required. Physicians and nurses are needed to treat patients; administrative and clerical personnel may be used in several functions as the emergency develops. Security personnel are generally kept in a staff position reporting to the Incident Commander, and not used to fill ICS positions. This allows the security manager and officers to fulfill their role in building security, crowd control, and so on.

Emergency Operations Center (EOC)

The EOC serves as the centralized management center for emergency operations. This is where ICS activities are coordinated and disseminated. Regardless of size, every facility should designate an EOC where decision makers can gather during an emergency.

The EOC should be located in an area of the HCF not likely to be involved in the incident, but near enough to allow efficient communication with those responding to the emergency. An alternate location should be identified in the event the primary location is not available.

Each facility must determine its requirements for an EOC based on the ICS functions needed and the number of people involved. The EOC should be equipped with communication equipment, reference materials, activity logs, and tools necessary to respond quickly and appropriately to an emergency.

Operational Issues

Planning for emergency events requires considering operational issues beyond the basic care and treatment of patients and the safety of patients, employees, and visitors. The emergency planner should consider the following points:

Employee Support   Employees are the HCF's most valuable assets. Employees will respond more effectively if they know that their families are safe during the emergency. Health care facilities should write procedures to help employees contact and verify the well-being of family members. This process should include employees who are working at the time of the emergency and those called back to the HCF to assist.

Solutions include using on-site day care facilities to support families of employees. Arrangements might also be made in neighboring churches, schools, offices, or public facilities to gather employee family members. Employees called back to work might feel more inclined to respond if they know their family is welcome where health care, food, and shelter are available. Consider also how employees will communicate with their families to learn of their status and needs, assuming telephone communication is interrupted or limited due to increased patient care needs. Beyond employees, it is important to consider the families of physicians and volunteers. The ability to retain and call in essential patient care providers and support personnel may depend on the effectiveness of planning in this area.

Consider special services and accommodations the HCF could provide for employees and their families during an emergency, including:

- Cash advances
- Salary continuation
- Flexible or reduced work hours
- Crisis counseling
- Care packages (including clothing, food, and personal items)

It is essential that all employees are accounted for when an emergency strikes, especially if there is damage to the HCF or if evacuation becomes necessary. Having a predetermined place to meet can help with this responsibility. Holding individual department leaders accountable to determine the location and well-being of each employee is essential. If there are employee injuries, they should be handled appropriately and compassionately by benefits and workers' compensation teams. If there are employee deaths, plan for surviving family members to be supported by HCF leaders, and assign responsibility for working with the employee's family in submitting appropriate claims for death benefits.

Mutual Aid Agreements   To avoid confusion and conflict in an emergency, establish mutual aid agreements with local responders, HCFs, and businesses. These agreements should define or identify:

- Type of assistance available
- The chain of command for activating the agreement
- Communication procedures

Include these agencies and facilities in training exercises whenever possible.

Security   Emergency planners must consider the role of security during the event. Planning must include procedures for facility security, staffing, and resource allocation. Examples of specific areas where additional planning might be needed include:

- How will you "lock down" the facility with limited security resources available to lock the doors and monitor entrances?
- What effect will increased security have on your operations? Is it more difficult for employees, physicians, and visitors to access your HCF? How will it affect vendors who deliver essential supplies and materials? When limitations are put into place that change the daily routine, can you implement effective communication and directional signage to help minimize the inconvenience?
- If you close or evacuate buildings, how do you protect against vandalism?
- What staff is available to assist in crowd control, media activity, and vehicle and traffic control?
- Are employees and volunteers trained to perform security related duties? Have you planned for increased security staffing for ongoing operations during emergencies?

Service Reduction   Planners must consider what services the facility will continue to operate during an emergency. A multi-vehicle traffic accident will not limit range of services, but a major earthquake might overwhelm the facility due to structural damage or increased activity in the emergency room. Questions of whether day-care centers, physician offices, clinics, and so on will continue to operate, and who will make the decision to temporarily close specific sites, must be considered as plans are written.

Training Training is vital to the success of any emergency planning effort. Do employees, physicians, and volunteers understand their individual and department responsibilities once an emergency is declared? How is staff trained regarding their responsibilities? When is the training conducted and at what frequency? How are program and plan changes communicated to staff, physicians, and volunteers? Is your training program documented?

Integrated Delivery Systems Integrated delivery systems (IDSs) have a distinct opportunity to manage an emergency by shifting resources from one HCF to another. Aid in recovery can be promoted within the health system. Staff, supplies, and equipment can be moved to aid the facility most affected by the emergency. Following the Northridge, California, earthquake on January 17, 1994, staff at the central office of one IDS was heard to say, "We didn't know what to do or how to help, even though we knew one of our hospitals had been hit hard." In this case, resources were available but not organized in a manner sufficient to offer the hospital in crisis any assistance.

Multi-hospital systems should evaluate communication plans and identify how resources, including personnel, can be adjusted and relocated during times of emergency.

Drills and Practice Events

The plan, if not tested before a real emergency occurs, is of little use. Regulatory agencies require HCFs to periodically test and evaluate their emergency management plans. These requirements specify that each health care organization conduct an emergency preparedness drill twice each year. Currently, JCAHO specifies no less than four months and no more than eight months between drills.[16] JCAHO further requires that one drill annually involve the influx of real or simulated patients.

Tabletop drills are an effective tool and can help to evaluate planning effectiveness at minimal expense and inconvenience to the HCF staff. Tabletop drills can be organized using previous emergencies the HCF has experienced. Participants are given a designated scenario and then discuss how they and their teams will respond. Additional suggestions and options are given to each participant as the discussion takes place to provide them with more understanding of how their response affects other members of the emergency response team and the overall recovery success of the HCF. Under JCAHO standards, tabletop drills do not fulfill the requirement for a biannual drill.

Evaluation As soon as possible after the drill, incident commanders, observers, and other HCF leaders should meet and evaluate the drill or actual event looking for both successes and failures. Hospital leaders and others involved in the drill should be asked for observations and recommendations. Community responders (EMTs, police, fire department, and so on) should be involved in the critique.

Disaster drills should use observers familiar with the organization's plan and should be able to evaluate response accordingly. Observers should be briefed before the drill and provided with a checklist to help organize observations.

Good, Bad, and Ugly An effective critique will identify good, bad, and ugly circumstances or events. Those identified as "bad" and "ugly" should have a corresponding corrective action plan developed, completion date established, and responsible individuals identified. Corrective actions should be reviewed during the next drill to ensure that they have been implemented effectively. It is important to document the drill, the critique, and the resultant corrective actions. If it is not documented, change will seldom result.

A Job Well Done   In our haste to get through a drill, we often fail to recognize efforts of staff, physicians, and volunteers. Congratulate participants for a job well done. Health care workers are famous for expending extraordinary efforts in the most demanding circumstances, and yet often receive little credit for such efforts. "Well done" and "thank you" go far to build support for the HCF's emergency response efforts.

....

IMPLEMENTATION AND RESPONSE

HCFs, clinics, and physician offices are routinely confronted by events that many might classify as disasters. Due to training and planning, most events involving multiple patients come and go as part of a normal day's work. Nevertheless, most health care workers know that the potential for a major event involving significant numbers of patients and damage to the HCF is very real—not if, but when!

Planning and training must establish the foundation upon which each worker can offer a meaningful response. Although the plan cannot possibly anticipate or answer all potential emergency events, it does give the assurance that a plan exists with a starting point and a way to expand to meet unexpected circumstances that arise.

Command and Control

Typically, the Incident Commander (IC) will be the senior management person available. As additional personnel arrive, command will transfer based on who has primary authority for overall control of the incident. At transfer of command, the outgoing IC must give the incoming IC a full briefing and notify all staff of the change in command. As incidents grow, the IC may delegate authority for performing certain activities to others, as required. When expansion is required, the IC will establish the other staff positions as needed.

Safety

The IC's first priority is always the safety of patients, staff, and the public. Effective communication processes are essential to fulfill this priority. Early in the emergency management process, the IC should identify an individual to handle communications to both internal and external audiences.

Internal   Maintain a continual flow of updated information to:

- Medical staff
- Managers and employees
- Trustees, governing boards, and volunteers

External   To exercise media and community leadership:

- Identify one available spokesperson.
- Determine where your media briefing area will be.

- Encourage rapid approval of press releases through the command center. If you do not have the information requested or cannot answer a question—say so. You can always get back to them later with what has been requested. In a rush to provide information, do not let accuracy suffer. Inaccuracy and mixed messages can create misunderstandings that are difficult to correct.
- Conduct regular briefings.
- Coordinate with government agencies and organizations.
- Test media plans in practice drills.

RECOVERY

Much of our planning time and effort is spent organizing how to respond to the event. Planners must also consider how the organization will recover from the emergency event. As plans are written consider the following issues:

- Who will inspect your HCF to determine whether it is structurally sound and safe to occupy? Who will inspect incoming utilities systems to ensure their safety? Local building inspectors can be very helpful in developing a plan for your HCF on what to check and who to involve.
- Who will make the decision to close the incident command center? Who will take the logs and notes created and summarize the event to facilitate future improvement and media interaction?
- How will the financial impact of the event be documented? Is the finance department ready with a system to track the costs associated with providing emergency patient care? How will you prepare evidence to assert a business interruption claim? How will you document repairs made to your facility to assert a property damage claim? Should you have a third-party consultant retained to help with asserting insurance and governmental claims?
- How will the organization help its employees recover? Will additional counseling resources be brought in to help with the emotional trauma and grieving some will experience? Will senior management provide continued updates on how the HCF is recovering to promote a feeling of job security among employees? Will recognition be given for the extraordinary efforts made by staff? Will staff members who have worked for extended hours have time off to rest and recover?
- If the HCF must be closed in whole or in part while repairs are made, how will management keep staff informed of progress? When ready to reopen, will the HCF have the labor pool needed to initiate operations? Does the business interruption policy provide salary continuation to keep essential staff paid during the HCF reconstruction?
- Is the public relations team prepared to keep media appraised on recovery progress?

Naturally, returning the HCF to its usual and customary service level is the objective, but this cannot be accomplished without addressing key safety, human resource, and financial issues.

CONCLUSION

By carefully addressing prevention, preparation, implementation, and response and recovery (the four steps of emergency management), the HCF will be better prepared to initiate an effective response to and recovery from an emergency. The challenge is to make this a dynamic process. Perhaps a rally cry of "Remember 9/11!" or "Remember the hurricanes of 2005" will help to remind us that emergencies happen throughout the world, and that we cannot lose our focus of being ready to respond. Develop and document the plan, train employees and leaders, rehearse it, and change it to incorporate what is learned along the way. Keep the plan as simple and flexible as possible, ensuring that everyone knows their respective role to enable a successful response. By staying ready, our HCFs will be safe places for patients and employees, and they will be able to provide essential patient care in the face of emergencies. When tropical storm Dorothy approaches, we won't be left wondering what to do, but can instead follow the steps identified in our plan to respond appropriately.

Endnotes

1. ECRI Healthcare Hazard Control Analysis, Emergency Preparedness Management: Overview, February 2002.
2. Bremer, L. Paul III, "Crisis Management,"*Directors & Boards*, Winter 2002, p.16.
3. Emergency Management Guide for Business and Industry, A Step-by Step Approach to Emergency Planning, Response and Recovery for Companies of all Sizes, Vulnerability Analysis Chart appendix p. 66, FEMA 141/October 1993, FEMA Guide can be accessed at (www.fema.gov/pdf/library/bizndst.pdf) last accessed December 21, 2005.
4. Department of Health and Human Services, Centers for Disease Control and Prevention, National Institute for Occupational Safety and Health, "Protecting Building Environments from Airborne Chemical, Biological, or Radiological Attacks," Foreword, p. 6, May 2002.
5. Phillips, D. S. "Healthcare Insurance I"ssues and Terrorism," *HealthLine*, Aon Healthcare Alliance, Nashville, TN, Volume IX, No. 1, May 2002, pp. 3–6.
6. "Emergency Management Guide for Business and Industry, A Step-by Step Approach to Emergency Planning, Response and Recovery for Companies of all Sizes," *FEMA 141*, October 1993. Training Drills and Exercises, Appendix, p. 67.
7. Phillips, *op. cit.*
8. Phillips, *op. cit.*
9. Phillips, *op. cit.*
10. McLaughlin, S. B., "Hazardous Vulnerability Analysis," Reprinted with permission from the American Society for Healthcare Engineering of the American Hospital Association, February 21, 2001, pp. 1–13.
11. Comprehensive Accreditation Manual, for Hospitals (CAMH) , Joint Commission on Accreditation of Healthcare Organizations, Oakbrook, IL, JCAHO, 2005 EC 4.10.
12. Department of Health and Human Services, Centers for Disease Control and Prevention.
13. CAMH, 2005 EC 4.10.
14. Department of Health and Human Services, Centers for Disease Control and Prevention.
15. National Fire Protection Association, NFPA 99, 12.2.3.2, Standard for Healthcare Facilities, Battermarch, MA. 2005.
16. JCAHO.

Web Sites

As of 12/21/05, we noted that a word search for Disaster Planning resulted in 43,900,000 site references, and Emergency Response and Emergency Management showing 95,200,000 and 133,000,000 site references, respectively. Clearly there is much information available on the Web. While our ability to offer a complete review of these materials is clearly impractical, a few helpful sites are noted below. All have the prefix of http://.

[www.drii.org]—DRI International—Professional practices for business continuity planners.

[www.fema.org]—Federal Emergency Management Agency—Education, training and planning materials.

[www.fmglobal.com/library/rmStrategies/emergOrg.html]—Creating a disaster plan.

[www.ccep.ca/cceppubl.html]—Canadian Centre for Emergency Preparedness.

[www.er1.com]—ER One—National prototype for the next-generation emergency.

[www.bioterrorism.slu.edu]—Center for the Study of Bioterrorism.

[www.hazmatforhealthcare.org]—HAZMAT for Healthcare, a method for hospitals to handle hazardous materials emergencies, including internal spills and contaminated patients.

[www.osha.gov/dts/osta/oshasoft/index.html]—OSHA eTools and Electronic Products for Compliance Assistance.

[www.ares.org]—Amateur Radio Emergency Services.

19

Occupational Safety, Health, and Environmental Impairment: A Brief Overview

John C. West

ealth care facilities are subject to intense levels of regulation as a result of both federal and state legislation regarding occupational safety and health and environmental impairment. However, legislation is rarely self-enacting or clear enough to allow for concrete interpretation in day-to-day practice. As a result, administrative agencies[1] typically use the legislation as a springboard for enacting rules and regulations to implement the legislature's intent in passing the statute. It is often informative to understand the processes by which administrative agencies perform their work, to appreciate the full effects of legislation.

As noted above, many agencies on both the state and federal level have rules and regulations that affect the operation of health care facilities. This discussion will focus on the agencies that have jurisdiction over worker safety and health and environmental impairment. However, the processes by which these agencies accomplish their missions are, overall, similar to the ways in which other agencies accomplish their missions.

This chapter will also provide an overview of the safety and health concerns commonly found in health care entities. For greater detail on any of these concerns, the reader is referred to Volume III, Chapter 5 in this series.

ADMINISTRATIVE PROCEDURE ACT

There are specific processes for rulemaking and the enforcement of regulations. If the rules are promulgated at the federal level, the Administrative Procedure Act[2] (APA) governs the process. If the rulemaking is performed by state agencies, the process may vary according to state law, but it often follows the federal procedures. This chapter will use the federal approach as a model.

The APA was born out of the explosive growth of administrative agencies in the latter half of the nineteenth century and the early part of the twentieth century, but was given particular impetus by the growth of administrative agencies during President Roosevelt's New Deal years.[3] By and large, it was felt that administrative agencies were becoming a fourth branch of government, and their internal workings were largely unregulated.

Rulemaking Processes

The rulemaking process is largely governed by the APA. On certain occasions, agencies may decide to publish an advance notice of proposed rulemaking, especially in situations where the rule may be complex and the agency would like public comment before enacting the final rule. This aspect of the procedure is not required by the APA.

The APA requires an agency to publish a general notice of proposed rulemaking in the Federal Register, unless another form of notice can be given. The agency then allows for public comment, which can normally be in writing or at a public hearing. The public also has the right to access the rulemaking record to determine the basis for the proposed rule. The agency is required to consider the public's comments before publishing its final rule. The comment period may vary, depending on the nature of the rule, but cannot be less than thirty days.[4]

The final rule must also be published in the Federal Register. The agency normally addresses all of the comments received and discusses their effect on the proposed final rule. Sometimes, final rules are remarkably similar to the proposed rule, but, occasionally, there are marked changes. On rare occasions, agencies may withdraw proposed rules altogether after considering the public comments. The agency must give an effective date for the final rule, which can range from months to years, but cannot be less than thirty days.[5]

Adjudicatory Process

Once the rules have been promulgated, the administrative agency will normally be charged with the task of enforcing the rules. It may do this by permit approval or by adjudicative procedures, such as inspections and the assessment of fines and penalties. Adjudicative processes can be formal or informal. Formal processes involve hearings, a written record, and a final decision by an arbiter (ultimately the secretary of the department) within the agency,[6] which is then subject to judicial review by the courts. Informal adjudicative procedures may involve inspections and negotiations to resolve disputed issues.

Hearings may be held for the purposes of adjudicating matters arising under the regulations that have been promulgated. These are often very similar to a judicial process, with specifications for notice, an opportunity to be heard, the submission of evidence, a written record or transcript, and a final decision.[7] The hearing is normally before an employee of the agency, and levels of appeal may be available within the agency. The decision of the agency is subject to judicial review by a court.

Judicial review can be founded on any number of objections to the rule or the enforcement of the rule. For example, the decision of the agency might have been arbitrary or capricious, or it might have been unsupported by the record. It is sometimes argued that the rule exceeds the statutory authority granted to the agency by the enabling legislation. It is also sometimes argued that the proposed rule did not give adequate notice of the provisions of the final rule to allow for effective public comment.[8]

ADMINISTRATIVE ENFORCEMENT

Not all administrative agencies have enforcement powers. For example, neither the National Institute of Occupational Safety and Health (NIOSH) nor the Centers for Disease Control and Prevention (CDC) have enforcement powers. Their missions are to perform research and to educate the public and relevant industries. The Occupational Safety and Health Administration (OSHA) and the Environmental Protection Agency (EPA), on the other hand, have enforcement powers that include fines and penalties. This discussion will focus on the enforcement techniques employed by OSHA, because OSHA's enforcement techniques should be a major concern for health care entities.

Enforcement Process

OSHA has programs by which entities, industries, or associations can work cooperatively with it and remove some of the threat of enforcement action. OSHA's Voluntary Protection Program (VPP) allows entities to enter into a participation agreement and then, after a rigorous on-site evaluation if the entity qualifies, it can be admitted into the VPP.[9] If an employer participates in a VPP, the employer may be exempted from programmed inspections.

It is also possible to enter into a collaborative agreement with OSHA through its Strategic Partnership Program. In this program, an industry, association, or entity works with OSHA to solve a particular safety or health issue. OSHA acts as a technical resource and facilitator. It is also possible to bring in other interested parties, such as trade unions, insurance companies, or local or state governments. The idea is to create a synergy that any of the participants, working alone, may not have been able to achieve.[10]

For entities that do not participate in the voluntary programs above, the inspection and enforcement process is as follows.

Pre-Inspection Processes   Pre-inspection processes are outlined in the OSHA Field Inspection Reference Manual CPL 2.103.[11] Inspections can be unprogrammed (following reports or complaints of imminent dangers) or programmed (in industries with known high hazard activities). Inspections follow a priority schedule, as follows: reports of imminent danger; investigations of fatalities or catastrophes; follow-up inspections of serious violations; investigation of complaints or referrals that are not felt to be serious; and programmed inspections. Unless a complainant allows it, disclosure of the identity of a complainant is prohibited. Under exigent circumstances, an inspector may obtain an inspection warrant or an administrative subpoena before making an inspection. Unless specifically authorized to do so, an inspector may not give advance notice of an inspection.[12]

Inspection Procedures   Inspections, as noted previously, can be unprogrammed or programmed. In either case, they fall into one of two categories: comprehensive (a complete inspection of all of the high-hazard areas of the establishment) or partial (limited to certain potentially high-hazard areas or operations at the establishment).[13]

The employer has the right to refuse admittance when the inspector appears on the premises. If the employer refuses admittance, the inspector must get an inspection warrant to enter the premises. There are exceptions to this rule, however. If the circumstances are exigent, for example, if there is a known high-hazard condition or operation on the premises that places employees at risk of harm, the inspector may enter without a warrant. There is also no need for a warrant if the operations are in plain view (the operations can be viewed from a public way or other areas off the employer's premises). The employer always has the right to require a warrant; the employer's consent to an inspection merely acts as waiver of the requirement that the inspector obtain a warrant. Additionally, the consent of one employer on a multi-employer worksite (as where a construction contractor is performing renovations within a hospital) operates as valid consent for entry for the inspector. If a warrant is obtained, the inspection must be in accordance with the provisions of the warrant.[14]

OSHA inspectors are also permitted to obtain administrative subpoenas for the production of records, documents, or testimony to complete an inspection. Documents that may be sought could include illness and injury records, exposure records, the written hazard communication program, the lockout-tagout program, or other records relevant to the employer's safety and health program.[15]

An inspection generally follows a set format. OSHA encourages the inspector and the facility to have an opening conference in which the inspector, the employer, and employees may participate. The inspector may be accompanied on the inspection by "walk-around representatives," who may be designated by the employer or employees (for example, union representatives or members of a safety committee). The inspector may collect samples (for example, air samples), take measurements, such as for noise levels, or take photographs while inspecting the premises. Inspectors also have the right to interview employees in private, which may include interviews off the employer's premises. OSHA encourages inspectors to provide advice on the abatement of hazards during the inspection.[16]

Post-Inspection Procedures   There are specific procedures that must be followed after an inspection. If the inspector recommends that a citation be issued, the inspector must prescribe an abatement period, which must be a reasonable amount of time, but which does not usually exceed thirty days for safety violations. Abatement periods may be longer for health violations, because these might require structural changes to the workplace. The employer may contest either the issuance of the citation, the length of the abatement period, or both. A notice of contest must be filed within fifteen days of the receipt of the citation. The running of the abatement period is stayed during the period of a pending contest.[17]

Employers may use several techniques to reduce the risk presented by the hazard. The most desirable abatement technique is to use engineering controls, which remove the hazard from the environment. These can be in the form of substitution, isolation, ventilation, or equipment modification, among others. Administrative controls constitute the second tier of abatement controls. These involve reducing exposure to the hazard through manipulation of the work schedule (for example, limiting the amount of time that someone can be in a high-noise environment). Work practice controls involve changes in the manner by which the work is performed, such as improvements in sanitation and hygiene practices. These should be implemented in the foregoing priority, if feasible. OSHA considers an abatement control "feasible" if it "can be accomplished by the employer." Personal protective equipment (PPE) is not considered an abatement procedure, because its use does not reduce the risk of exposure to the hazard. PPE may be used only if there is no feasible abatement control.[18]

Citations are issued in the same manner as other forms of legal process. Certified mail, return receipt requested, is preferred, but hand delivery is allowed. OSHA encourages a signed receipt for a citation whenever possible. As with other forms of legal process, entities must have a process in place to receive and handle citations in a timely manner.[19]

OSHA has authority to assess penalties for violations of its standards. For serious violations, the penalty may be up to $7,000. For willful violations, the penalty may not be more than $70,000 or less than $5,000. Penalties may be adjusted based on the gravity of the violation, on the good faith of the employer, on the employer's history and experience with respect to violations, and on the size of the business (certain reductions are available if the employer employs 250 or fewer employees).[20]

Penalties may also be imposed for failure to maintain reporting or recordkeeping systems. For example, the employer may be cited for failing to maintain and post the OSHA logs that all employers are required to maintain. The employer may also be cited for failing to verbally report any occupationally related employee death or the hospitalization of three or more employees within eight hours of an occurrence. Compared to some of the other penalties, these penalties are somewhat nominal.[21]

OSHA also has the power to impose criminal penalties. Criminal penalties may be imposed for the willful violation of a standard, rule, or order that causes the death of an employee. Criminal penalties can also be imposed for giving unauthorized advance notification of an inspection or for giving false information to an inspector. Obviously, criminal penalties may also be imposed for killing, assaulting, or hampering an inspector.[22]

The employer may request an informal conference following the inspection. This will normally be performed within the fifteen-day period for providing the notice of contest. The informal conference requires the participation of an OSHA Area Director. Area Directors have the authority to enter into settlement agreements with employers. If the matter is not resolved at this level, the notice of contest is forwarded to the Occupational Safety and Health Review Commission (OSHRC) for adjudication.[23] If the parties are not satisfied with the decision of the OSHRC, the matter can be appealed to federal court.

EPA's Enforcement Powers   The U.S. EPA has detailed its enforcement policies, procedures, and practices, all of which are a matter of public record. The structure of the EPA's enforcement practices is not markedly different than OSHA's, but the enforcement plan does differ in its details.[24]

············

SPECIFIC OCCUPATIONAL SAFETY AND HEALTH ISSUES

The primary regulatory agency with jurisdiction over occupational safety and health matters is, as noted previously, OSHA. OSHA has authority to promulgate standards pursuant to the Occupational Safety and Health Act of 1970,[25] which has a general duty clause that requires that each employer shall furnish to each employee a job and a workplace that are free from recognized hazards that are causing or are likely to cause death or serious physical harm to employees.[26] OSHA has full regulatory authority to enforce its standards and regulations.

NIOSH, on the other hand, has no regulatory authority. It is an agency dedicated to research and education. Unlike OSHA, which is part of the Department of Labor, NIOSH is a branch of the CDC within the Department of Health and Human Services.[27] NIOSH publishes the results of research and literature searches. Those publications often consist of recommendations to OSHA that a standard be developed to regulate exposure to a substance, or abate the hazards associated with a given operation. These recommendations do not have the force of law, and OSHA must go through the rulemaking process to enforce them. Sometimes these recommendations are taken up rapidly by OSHA, but in other cases they might remain in the recommendation state for years.[28]

The CDC plays something of a tangential role in occupational safety and health, somewhat similar to that of NIOSH. OSHA has not hesitated to incorporate many of the guidance documents that the CDC has published on such topics as the prevention of transmission of bloodborne pathogens,[29] or the prevention of transmission of tuberculosis.[30] The CDC's guidance has had a great impact in health care in preventing transmission of nosocomial infection, and in the adoption of public health measures and availability of immunizations.[31]

The U.S. EPA has inspection and enforcement powers regarding air pollution, water pollution, solid waste disposal, hazardous waste disposal, clean-up of contaminated hazardous waste dump sites, and many other matters. The EPA has allowed the states to provide most of the regulation of medical or infectious waste.[32] Most of its regulations deal with environmental impairment, but the EPA does provide guidance on some matters that involve occupational safety and health. For example, the EPA regulates exposure to asbestos during renovation or demolition.[33] It also provides guidance materials on indoor air quality and remediation of mold.[34]

Specific Issues Regulated by OSHA

OSHA regulates several specific substances and practices. As noted previously, the general duty clause in the OSHA Act requires that each employer shall furnish employment and a place of employment that are free from recognized hazards that are causing or are likely to cause death or serious physical harm to employees; but this does not really give OSHA free rein to cite an employer for any hazardous condition. OSHA still must go through the rulemaking process to set standards. The substances or practices listed below include the areas of health care operations for which OSHA has set standards. These include:

- Acetone[35]
- Alcohol, Ethyl (widely used)[36]
- Alcohol, Isopropyl (widely used)[37]
- Alcohol, Methyl (methanol or wood alcohol; used in laboratories)[38]
- Asbestos (formerly used in insulation)[39]
- Benzene (sometimes encountered in laboratories)[40]
- Bloodborne Pathogens (HIV, Hepatitis B, Hepatitis C, and so on)[41]
- Cadmium (sometimes used in radiology or plant operations)[42]
- Confined space entry[43]
- Ethylene Oxide (used in central processing and central sterile)[44]
- Formaldehyde (used in the laboratory, surgery, and morgue)[45]
- Hazard Communications (employee "right to know")[46]
- Hazardous Waste Operations and Emergency Response (HAZWOPER) (spill training)[47]

- Hydrogen Peroxide (used in central processing and central sterile)[48]
- Laboratory Standard (hazard communications in the laboratory)[49]
- Lead (used in radiology and plant operations)[50]
- Lockout-Tagout rule (control of hazardous energy)[51]
- Mercury (used in various kinds of instruments and devices)[52]
- Methyl Methacrylate (a component of bone cement)[53]
- Noise (encountered in equipment areas near boilers and generators)[54]
- Personal protective equipment (PPE)[55]
- Toluene (used in laboratories)[56]
- Tuberculosis exposure (can occur in any clinical area)[57]
- Xylene (used in laboratories)[58]

The foregoing constitutes the areas for which OSHA has promulgated primary standards that are somewhat unique to health care operations. There are certainly other standards, primarily for safety, that can be applied to health care, especially to non-clinical operations. These include standards that regulate such things as walking and working surfaces,[59] wooden ladders,[60] metal ladders,[61] and welding,[62] to name a few. These standards have wide applicability to any industry and are too numerous to mention in a treatise of this sort.

Other Health Hazards Not Specifically Regulated by OSHA

Once outside the realm of OSHA regulation, trying to determine all safety and health hazards faced by health care workers becomes less straightforward. Some are known hazards, some are suspected hazards, and there are some that could be hazards, but we simply do not know enough about them at this time to determine that.

These issues include, but are not limited to:

- Compressed gases (used in surgery and laboratory)[63]
- Ergonomics and musculoskeletal disorders (an issue anywhere that lifting and transferring occurs)[64]
- Extremely low-frequency electric and magnetic fields (exist wherever electricity is present)[65]
- Flammable liquids (fire hazards due to bulk storage)
- Glutaraldehyde (used for cold sterilization of certain equipment, such as endoscopes)[66]
- Hazardous drugs, such as chemotherapeutic drugs and so on[67]
- Indoor air quality[68]
- Lasers (optical hazards)[69]
- Laser or electrocautery plume (smoke from surgical procedures)[70]
- Latex sensitivity (present in materials made from natural rubber)[71]
- Mold and fungus (an issue whenever materials can get, and stay, wet)[72]
- Radiation[73]
- Video display terminals[74]

- Waste anesthetic gases (WAG) (for example, nitrous oxide)[75]
- Workplace violence[76]

OSHA has not promulgated standards on these issues, so they should not be the subject of an OSHA inspection. However, the risks associated with some of these substances or conditions are real, and employers would be well advised to manage the risks to the extent that it is feasible to do so.

Specific Issues Regulated by EPA

The EPA tends, as a general rule, to regulate materials and activities outside of buildings. For example, although OSHA regulates ethylene oxide exposure to employees inside a building, EPA regulates its discharge into the atmosphere. OSHA is very much concerned about protection of human health at the individual level. The EPA is also concerned about the protection of human health, but it is more concerned about protection of populations by controlling environmental contamination.

The primary statutes by which EPA has been given the authority to regulate environmental impairment are as follows:

Resource Conservation and Recovery Act[77]   The Resource Conservation and Recovery Act (RCRA) gives the EPA the authority to regulate the dumping of solid and hazardous waste. It also provides the EPA with the authority to regulate underground storage tanks (UST). It should be noted that the RCRA applies to currently active sites, but not to abandoned sites.

Comprehensive Environmental Response, Compensation and Liability Act[78]   The Comprehensive Environmental Response, Compensation and Liability Act (CERCLA) is also known by the popular title of Superfund. It imposes liability on landowners and past landowners of contaminated waste sites for the costs of cleaning up the site. A current landowner can be liable for the costs of cleaning up a Superfund site unless the landowner can show that it did not dump materials on the site, that all dumping on the site has ceased, and that it took the land without knowledge of past dumping practices (the "innocent landowner" defense). Whenever land that has ever been used for commercial purposes is acquired, it is extremely important that an environmental assessment for past contamination be performed.

Clean Air Act[79]   The Clean Air Act was originally passed in 1970 and has been amended since then. It gives the EPA the power to implement the National Ambient Air Quality standards to address air pollution. The EPA regulates medical waste incineration under the Clean Air Act.

Toxic Substances Control Act[80]   The Toxic Substances Control Act (TSCA) gives the EPA the authority to track and control the toxic or potentially toxic chemicals used by industry.

Some of the specific areas that are regulated by the EPA that are or should be of concern to health care organizations include the following:

- Above-ground storage tanks[81]
- Asbestos release (during renovation or demolition)[82]

- Disposal of hazardous waste (any waste that readily ignites, is corrosive, is reactive, or is toxic)[83]
- Medical waste incineration[84]
- Superfund liability for environment contamination[85]
- USTs (at least 10 percent of tank volume is below ground)[86]

The EPA also has the power to regulate medical waste under RCRA, but has largely delegated the regulation of this material to the states.[87]

....

CONCLUSION

As noted in the beginning of this chapter, this discussion is merely meant as an overview of this topic. If more detail is required, please refer to the chapter entitled "Occupational and Environmental Risk Exposures for Health Care Facilities" found in Volume III, Chapter 5 of this series.

Occupational safety and health can be a significant issue for health care entities. The failure to manage this risk can lead to increased workers' compensation costs, dissatisfaction among workers, property damage, and the potential for administrative fines and penalties. Managing these risks appropriately can lead to improved productivity, improved morale, and improved community relations.

Environmental impairment claims can be enormously expensive if not managed appropriately. For example, if a contaminant gets into sources of groundwater, it can take millions of dollars, or generations, for the hazard to be abated. Environmental impairment is important because this is the only planet that we have.

Finally, violations of any of the administrative regulations do not just carry fines and penalties. There are also potential criminal penalties that can be imposed. In today's environment, with CEOs going to jail for accounting and other sins, this is not an exposure to be taken lightly.

Endnotes

1. For the purposes of this chapter, the term "administrative agency" will include departments of the federal executive branch of government, such as the Department of Health and Human Services, and subordinate agencies, such as the Food and Drug Administration or the Centers for Disease Prevention and Control. It also includes any non-judicial governmental unit with the power to determine private rights and obligations by rulemaking or adjudication.
2. 5 U.S.C. §551, *et seq.*
3. Shepard, G., "Fierce Compromise: The Administrative Procedure Emerges From New Deal Politics" *90 Northwestern University Law Review* 1557 (1996).
4. 5 U.S.C. §553.
5. *Ibid.*
6. 5 U.S.C. §556.
7. 5 U.S.C. §556; 5 U.S.C. §554.
8. Shepard, *op. cit.*
9. More information is available on the OSHA Web site at [www.osha.gov/dcsp/vpp/index.html] (accessed June 21, 2005).

Risk Management Handbook for Health Care Organizations

10. More information is available on the OSHA Web site at [www.osha.gov/dcsp/partnerships/index.html] (accessed June 21, 2005).

11. Available at [www.osha.gov/Firm_osha_toc/Firm_toc_by_sect.html] (accessed June 21, 2005).

12. OSHA Field Inspection Reference Manual, Chapter I, available at [www.osha.gov/Firm_osha_data/100005.html] (accessed June 21, 2005).

13. OSHA Field Inspection Reference Manual, Chapter II, available at [www.osha.gov/Firm_osha_data/100006.html] (accessed June 21, 2005).

14. *Ibid.*

15. *Ibid.*

16. *Ibid.*

17. OSHA Field Inspection Reference Manual, Chapter IV, available at [www.osha.gov/Firm_osha_data/100008.html] (accessed June 21, 2005).

18. *Ibid.*

19. *Ibid.*

20. *Ibid.*

21. *Ibid.*

22. *Ibid.*

23. *Ibid.*

24. For more detail, visit the enforcement section of the EPA's Web site at [www.epa.gov/ebtpages/complianceenforcement.html] (accessed June 23, 2005).

25. 29 U.S.C. §651, *et seq.*

26. 29 U.S.C. §654(a)(1).

27. More information is available on the NIOSH Web site at [www.cdc.gov/niosh] (accessed June 21, 2005).

28. For example, the NIOSH publication on waste anesthetic gases (NIOSH, "Criteria for a Recommended Standard . . . Occupational Exposure to Waste Anesthetic Gases and Vapors." (NIOSH Pub. 77-140) (1977)) was published in 1977 and OSHA has never promulgated a standard for any of these gases.

29. CDC, "Practice Recommendations for Health-Care Facilities Implementing the U.S. Public Health Service Guidelines for Management of Occupational Exposures to Bloodborne Pathogens" (2001) (available at [www.phppo.cdc.gov/cdcRecommends/showarticle.asp?a_artid=1306++++&TopNum=50&CallPg=Adv] (accessed August 17, 2005).

30. CDC, "Guidelines for Preventing the Transmission of Mycobacterium tuberculosis in Health-Care Facilities (1994) (available at [www.phppo.cdc.gov/cdcRecommends/showarticle.asp?a_artid=M0035909&TopNum=50&CallPg=Adv] (accessed August 17, 2005).

31. For more information on the CDC, visit its Web site at [www.cdc.gov] (accessed June 22, 2005).

32. Information on state programs for dealing with medical waste can be accessed on the U.S. EPA Web site at [www.epa.gov/epaoswer/osw/stateweb.htm] (accessed June 25, 2005).

33. See, e.g., EPA, "Managing Asbestos in Place: A Building Owner's Guide to Operations and Maintenance Programs for Asbestos-Containing Materials" (Pub No. 20T-2003). (1990); and EPA, "Guidance for Controlling Asbestos-Containing Materials in Buildings" (Pub. No. 560/5-85-024). (1985) (both available at [www.epa.gov/asbestos/buildings.html] (accessed July 14, 2005).

34. For more information on the EPA, visit its Web site at [www.epa.gov] (accessed June 22, 2005).

35. 29 CFR §1910.1000, Table Z-1.

36. *Ibid.*

37. *Ibid.*

38. *Ibid.*

39. General Industry Standard: 29 CFR §1910.1001; Construction Standard: 29 CFR 1926.1101.

40. 29 CFR §1910.1028.

41. 29 CFR §1910.1030.

42. 29 CFR §1910.1027.

43. 29 CFR §1910.146.

44. 29 CFR §1910.1047.

45. 29 CFR §1910.1048.

46. 29 CFR §1910.1200.

47. 29 CFR §1910.120.

48. 29 CFR §1910.1000, Table Z-1.

49. 29 CFR §1910.1450.

50. 29 CFR §1910.1025.

51. 29 CFR §1910.147.

52. 29 CFR §1910.1000, Table Z-1.

53. *Ibid.*

54. 29 CFR §1910.95.

55. 29 CFR §1910.132.

56. 29 CFR §1910.1000, Table Z-2.

57. 29 CFR §1910.134 (respiratory protection).

58. 29 CFR §1910.1000, Table Z-2.

59. 29 CFR §1910.22.

60. 29 CFR §1910.25.

61. 29 CFR §1910.26.

62. 29 CFR §1910.251, *et seq*.

63. OSHA, "Safety and Health Topics: Compressed Gas and Equipment," available at [www.osha.gov/SLTC/compressedgasequipment/index.html] (accessed June 23, 2005).

64. OSHA, "Safety and Health Topics: Ergonomics," available at [www.osha.gov/SLTC/ergonomics/index.html] (accessed June 23, 2005); see also Proposed OSHA Ergonomic Standard, 64 Fed. Reg. 65768 (November 22, 1999).

65. OSHA, "Safety and Health Topics: Extremely Low Frequency (ELF) Fields," available at [www.osha.gov/SLTC/elfradiation/index.html] (accessed June 23, 2005).

66. NIOSH, "Glutaraldehyde: Occupational Hazards in Hospitals," (NIOSH Pub. No. 2001–115) (May 2001) available at [www.cdc.gov/niosh/2001-115.html] (accessed June 23, 2005).

67. OSHA Technical Manual, Section IV, Chapter 2, "Controlling Exposure to Hazardous Drugs," available at [www.osha.gov/dts/osta/otm/otm_vi/otm_vi_2.html] (accessed June 23, 2005).

68. EPA, "The Inside Story: A Guide to Indoor Air Quality," EPA Document # 402-K-93-007 (April 1995) available at [www.epa.gov/iaq/pubs/insidest.html] (accessed June 23, 2005).

69. OSHA, "Safety and Health Topics: Laser Hazards," available at [www.osha.gov/SLTC/laserhazards/index.html] (accessed June 23, 2005).

70. OSHA, "Safety and Health Topics: Laser/Electrosurgery Plume," available at [www.osha.gov/SLTC/laserelectrosurgeryplume/index.html] (accessed June 23, 2005).

71. OSHA, "Safety and Health Topics: Latex Allergy," available at [www.osha.gov/SLTC/latexallergy/index.html] (accessed June 23, 2005), NIOSH, "NIOSH Alert: Preventing Allergic Reactions to Natural Rubber Latex in the Workplace," NIOSH Pub. No. 97-135, available at [www.cdc.gov/niosh/latexalt.html] (accessed June 23, 2005).

72. Center for Indoor Environments, University of Connecticut, "Guidance for Clinicians on the Recognition and Management of Health Effects Related to Mold Exposure and Moisture Indoors" (September 30, 2004), available at [oehc.uchc.edu/clinser/MOLD%20GUIDE.pdf] (accessed June 23, 2005); EPA, "Mold Remediation in Schools and Commercial Buildings," available at [www.epa.gov/mold/mold_remediation.html] (accessed June 23, 2005).

73. OSHA, "Safety and Health Topics: Ionizing Radiation," available at [www.osha.gov/SLTC/radiationionizing/index.html] (accessed June 23, 2005).

74. OSHA, "Working Safely With Video Display Terminals," (OSHA Pub. 3092) (1997), available at [www.osha.gov/Publications/videoDisplay/videoDisplay.html] (accessed June 23, 2005).

75. NIOSH, "Criteria for a Recommended Standard: Occupational Exposure to Waste Anesthetic Gases and Vapors," (NIOSH Pub. 77-140) (1977)), available at [www.cdc.gov/niosh/77-140.html] (accessed June 23, 2005); OSHA, "Safety and Health Topics: Waste Anesthetic Gases," available at [www.osha.gov/SLTC/wasteanestheticgases/index.html] (accessed June 23, 2005).

76. OSHA, "Safety and Health Topics: Workplace Violence," available at [www.osha.gov/SLTC/workplaceviolence/index.html] (accessed June 23, 2005); OSHA, "Guidelines for Preventing Workplace Violence for Health Care and Social Service Workers" OSHA Publication 3148 (2003), available at [www.osha.gov/OshDoc/data_General_Facts/factsheet-workplace-violence.pdf] (accessed June 23, 2005).

77. 42 U.S.C. §6901, *et seq.*

78. 42 U.S.C. §9601, *et seq.*

79. 42 U.S.C. §7401, *et seq.*

80. 15 U.S.C. §2601, *et seq.*

81. For more information on the regulation of aboveground storage tanks, visit the U.S. EPA Web site at [www.epa.gov/OUST/cmplastc/asts.htm] (accessed June 20, 2005).

82. EPA, "Managing Asbestos in Place: A Building Owner's Guide to Operations and Maintenance Programs for Asbestos-Containing Materials" (Pub No. 20T-2003). (1990); and EPA, "Guidance for Controlling Asbestos-Containing Materials in Buildings" (Pub. No. 560/5-85-024). (1985) both available at [www.epa.gov/asbestos/buildings.html] (accessed July 14, 2005).

83. For more information on hazardous waste disposal, visit the EPA Web site at [www.epa.gov/epaoswer/hazwaste/id/index.htm] (accessed June 20, 2005).

84. More information on medical waste incineration is available on the EPA Web site at [www.epa.gov/ttn/chief/ap42/ch02/final/c02s03.pdf] (accessed June 21, 2005).

85. More information on CERCLA and Superfund liability is available on the EPA Web site at [www.epa.gov/superfund/action/law/cercla.htm] (accessed June 20, 2005).

86. For more information on the regulation of underground storage tanks, visit the U.S. EPA Web site at [www.epa.gov/swerust1/pubs/index.htm] (accessed June 20, 2005).

87. For links to the various state programs, please visit [www.epa.gov/epaoswer/osw/stateweb.htm] (accessed June 21, 2005).

20

Early Warning Systems for the Identification of Organizational Risk

Roberta Carroll

The effectiveness of a risk management program is commensurate with the organization's ability to identify and analyze its risk exposure. Risk management professionals use a five-step decision-making process developed by the Insurance Institute of America[1] and supported by the American Society for Healthcare Risk Management.[2] This is the foundation for health care risk management programs. It has as its first step identifying and analyzing an organization's exposure to loss. This is the starting point from which all risk initiatives emanate.

The principles of risk identification and analysis can be used in all care settings and with all programs regardless of scope or size. All care settings, from an acute care hospital, home health agency, skilled nursing facility, and ambulatory surgery center to a physician group practice, find that early identification and analysis is pivotal to risk management program success.

Program scope can vary within the same type of care settings. One health care risk management program is just that: one health care risk management program. Factors on which program scope might be based include:

- Services—Services offered are prioritized by the frequency and severity of losses or are known to be problematic in the industry. For example, most risk management professionals promote patient safety in obstetrical practices even if there have been no medical professional liability lawsuits. On the other hand, if the organization does not have a labor and delivery unit, the only aspect of obstetrical risk of concern for the risk management professional is whether or not the emergency department manages laboring patients properly under EMTALA. For more information about emergency

The author would like to thank William McDonough for his previous work on Risk Identification Systems in the 4th edition of the Risk Management Handbook for Health Care Organizations.

department obstetrical risk and EMTALA please refer to Chapter 10 in Volume II of this series.

- Locale—Several states have statutes that require the implementation of a risk management program. For example, Florida requires risk management programs in hospitals,[3] long-term care facilities,[4] and HMOs.[5] One component of these programs is the development and implementation of an incident reporting system.
- Skill, expertise, and interest of the risk management professional.
- Organizational environment and culture—Organizations that are caring, trusting, and open to process change have more robust and effective risk management programs than those organizations that do not embrace those attributes.

Regardless of the setting or scope, all risk management programs must identify and analyze exposure to loss. This is the premise on which this chapter is written.

....

SYSTEMS AND PROCESSES FOR THE EARLY IDENTIFICATION OF AN ORGANIZATION'S EXPOSURE TO LOSS

Tactical initiatives that help an organization identify risk may be thought of as "early warning systems." The risk management professional is often best positioned to implement such systems when they are based on a comprehensive assessment of organizational risk.

Health care risk management programs employ many such initiatives to identify in a timely manner those events, activities, initiatives, practices, systems, and processes that can threaten or actually do create or contribute to loss. One example is the inclusion of *near misses* or *close calls* in the reporting system of many health care organizations. In this chapter, *near misses* and *close calls* are included in the definition of an incident.

Getting Started—Risk Identification

If an organization does not identify real, threatened, or perceived exposure to loss, the organization will be unable to implement risk control techniques necessary to eliminate the exposure, minimize the loss, or implement financing measures to pay for losses that do occur despite best efforts. Because all other activities stem from this first step in the risk management process, it is a critical component of all risk management programs.

Assessment of organizational risk is a logical first step in program development and a useful process when evaluating the effectiveness of current programs. Identifying risk across an organization's structure or on an enterprise-wide basis in what is now termed *enterprise risk management* allows the risk management professional to:

- *Identify all risk confronting the organization regardless of organizational setting*—Risk management professionals need not act alone in this process. It is wise to engage others who have knowledge of the risk inherent in areas under their supervision. This is particularly true where the risk management professional might lack technical expertise and need the assistance of subject matter experts.
- *Identify and analyze the relationship among risks*—What is the synergistic relationship among risks? For example, consider how risks associated with human capital (personnel risk) such as staffing shortages, fatigue, low morale, turnover, and intimidation can increase the possibility of medical errors. Identifying risk across the

organization's continuum of care will allow the risk management professional to better understand the relationship that exists among risks.

- *Understand organizational dynamics and its effect on culture and the environment.*
- *Corroborate the organization's mission, vision, and strategy.*
- *Understand the organization's structure and identify lines of business, units, divisions, and programs*—Engaging staff in identifying risk in their areas of responsibility allows the risk management professional to facilitate and partake in the assessment process and empower the staff to follow through with any recommendations. Such an approach also produces the most relevant solutions. Given the opportunity to contribute, staff who work daily in specific units or divisions are best suited to identify areas of weakness and risk and can offer meaningful and sustainable solutions.
- *Educate senior leadership in understanding the risk exposure of the organization*—Risk management professionals are perfectly positioned to see risk from an organization-wide perspective—the "big picture." This understanding will support the offering of educational initiatives to the board of directors, medical staff leadership, and administrative leadership on risk issues that affect mission, vision, and strategy.
- *Garner support necessary to develop and implement future solutions.*
- *Build credibility and promote collaboration for risk management activities.*

Risk management professionals do not act alone. They engage all members of the organization in identifying and analyzing exposure to loss.

Knowledge of the organization is critical to the success of risk management programs. The consequences of not thoroughly understanding the organization can threaten and weaken a risk management program by:

- Causing loss of trust and credibility.
- Wasting resources (money, time, and staff support) by focusing effort in areas that do not significantly affect quality outcomes, patient safety, and fiscal strength.
- Diminishing the role of risk management professionals by charging them with tasks that do not reduce risk or add value to the organization's bottom line. An understanding of this issue can best be reached by asking the following question: "What adds more value to the organization and promotes patient safety, a risk management professional charged with locating lost patient items (teeth, canes, glasses) or a risk management professional charged with reducing variability and risk within the labor and delivery unit?"

Although the primary business of health care is the delivery of safe and effective patient care, note that not all organizational risk management activities or programs should focus exclusively on clinical or patient-related risk. The identification and analysis of risk on an enterprise basis encourages the risk management professional to identify and analyze other areas of risk beyond what is referred to as operational or clinical risk. Those other areas include risks associated with the financial, human capital, legal and technological, regulatory, and hazard environments. For more information on Enterprise Risk Management, refer to Chapter 1 in this volume or Chapter 3 in Volume III in this series. This chapter is focused on identifying and analyzing patient-related risk. Information on other areas of risk is found throughout this series.

Risk Identification

Once the risk management professional understands the business of the organization and the risk inherent in its operations, the next step is to review existing early warning systems and implement new systems as necessary. Early warning systems alert the risk management professional to adverse events—preventable and unpreventable, incidents, occurrences, potentially compensable events, and claims. Systems for identifying potential risk and loss-producing incidents vary among organizations. Although risk can differ in frequency, complexity, and severity depending on the health care delivery setting (for example, the risk of pressure ulcers and elopement are greater in a long-term care setting than in an acute care hospital), the risk management process and need for a robust early warning system is the same. Internal early warning systems for the identification of risk can be formal or informal reporting and notification mechanisms. Reporting systems are used internally by the organization and externally for reporting to outside parties. Reporting systems can be mandatory or voluntary. The next section of this chapter will focus on internal warning systems.

Formal Reporting Methods—Internal

Formal risk identification systems are those that follow policies and procedures. Typically these systems are implemented to comply with requirements by commercial insurance carriers as a requisite for coverage, alternative risk financing arrangements such as programs of self-insurance (captives, risk retention groups, trusts, and so on), compliance with state statutes and other regulatory requirements, and to meet standards such as those promulgated by the Joint Commission on Accreditation of Healthcare Organizations (JCAHO), Utilization Review Accreditation Committee (URAC), Commission for Accreditation of Rehabilitation Facilities (CARF), and the National Committee for Quality Assurance (NCQA).

The Incident Report   Commercial insurance companies originally developed the incident report in the early 1960s as a means of event, claim, or loss notification. Most industries used incident reports to give notice to their carriers of an event that might give rise to a claim. In health care specifically, these reports were forms on which to record basic information about the patient, any other potential claimant(s), or third parties in the case of general liability claims. Included were name, other identifying information associated with the potential claimant, and a brief description of the incident. In addition, many forms required that "follow-up" information be recorded by the reporter confirming that the incident had been adequately addressed with appropriate intervention. Forms such as these were adopted for use in the majority of U.S. hospitals and other health care organizations. In fact, many insurance companies still provide the incident report forms and incident reporting protocols used in insured facilities today.

Traditionally, incident reporting has been the cornerstone of health care risk management. Generally, an incident is defined as any happening that is not consistent with the routine care of a particular patient or an event that is not consistent with the normal operations of a particular organization. Examples of incidents might include: a union strike, criminal acts such as a homicide or burglary, wrong-site or wrong-patient surgery, medication errors, or a physical disaster including, for example: hurricanes, bioterrorism threats, or the onset of mold contamination. The occurrence of an incident should trigger completion of a report to risk management and other necessary parties depending on the organization's policy and, as a general rule of thumb, on a "need to know" basis. The "need to know" standard must be reviewed annually for legal requirements to ensure that the confidentiality of incident report information is maintained and the "need" as defined still exists.

Incident report data should be collected, coded for study, and analyzed to determine whether there are any trends that represent real or potential problems in the delivery of care or service. The results of this analysis should be distributed and discussed with the individuals and departments involved and those authorized to promote changes in protocol, policy, and procedure. The analysis may reveal positive findings, which may be disseminated to employees or members of the medical staff, and issues of concern that should be addressed in a timely manner using the committee structures, problem resolution processes, and peer review mechanisms (if applicable) at the organization.

Long-term care (LTC) facilities, including skilled nursing facilities (SNF) and assisted living facilities (ALF), managed care organizations (MCO), and home health care organizations (HHC), have designed and implemented reporting mechanisms to capture event data necessary for risk management and loss prevention efforts. Historically, these organizations have placed less emphasis on true risk identification systems given their minimal medical professional liability experience. For example, over the past several years, the loss experience of long-term care organizations has increased both in terms of frequency and severity of claims. Leading causes of loss include: failure to provide adequate wound care, failure to monitor status of nutrition, elopement, pressure ulcers, abuse and neglect, and medication errors. The LTC industry has recently invested considerable time and effort to design and implement incident reporting systems for providers of care.

Electronic Incident Reporting   The public, including the organization's employee work force and patient population, are in many instances experienced users of technology. Personal use of home computers, cellular phones, and personal digital assistants (PDAs) are the norm today. Advances in technology, although somewhat slow in coming to health care documentation systems, are rapidly changing how and when care is delivered. With these changes, there has been a concomitant increase in use by risk management professionals for the computerization of risk management data. There are many commercially available prepackaged programs designed to track risk management data including front-end reporting, statistical analysis, claims management, and insurance schedules. There are many database management programs that can be used to customize an organization's risk management information needs.

By the end of 2005, there were twenty-three different risk management information systems (RMIS) available to risk management professionals. As with any new system or program, implementing an RMIS is not without risk. The development of policies and procedures that specifically address the risk associated with computerized systems is a priority. Specific issues of concern include computer failures, breaches of security, unauthorized access to data, authority and access levels, pass code protection, and compliance with the Health Insurance Portability and Accountability Act of 1996 (HIPAA) for electronic data that contains protected health information. For more information on HIPAA and Security, see Chapter 18 in Volume III of this series.

Many risk management information systems (RMIS) promote statistical analysis and offer graphic capabilities for benchmarking, allowing risk management professionals to compare their organization with similar organizations or significant national trends. Many risk management professionals find that implementing an RMIS decreases the common problems of under-reporting and lack of timeliness because those reporting are getting timely feedback through more comprehensive and understandable computer-generated reports.

An effective RMIS must have a data collection form or computer screens that allow information to be collected accurately, quickly, and in a manner that facilitates coding and entry. For example, incident report forms should be either pre-coded or designed for ease in coding. This will ensure fast and accurate entry and easy retrieval of information. These forms often contain check-off boxes and limited space for narrative descriptions. New technology, such as scanning software, promotes an easier means of converting paper documents to soft data, which can then be manipulated using the software.

Although a user-friendly input mechanism is vital to encourage reporting, the most important element of a successful computerized system is its ability to generate useful and readable reports. Without the capacity to produce aggregate reports and data trends, the value of a computerized system is minimal. The whole purpose of automating the data is to promote easy tracking and facilitate trend analysis, which can help the organization identify patterns and problems and by comparing current data with those of last month, last year, and perhaps the past five years.

Without meaningful data, it is easy to forget that the purpose of identification and analysis of incident report data is the development and implementation of systems and processes to minimize the potential for loss while enhancing patient care. Therefore, systems that generate clear and meaningful information are essential to risk control.

The kinds of variables related to occurrences that could be analyzed (regardless of the early warning system used) include:

- Date of the occurrence—Sometimes called *date of loss,* or *incident or event date.* This information is valuable for providing trending information to determine whether the number of occurrences has increased, decreased, or remained stable over time.

- Date of the report—Tracking the date of the occurrence in relationship to the date of the report is one metric by which risk management professionals can evaluate the effectiveness of the organization's early warning system. When a time lag in reporting is noted, systems, processes, policies, and procedures should be reviewed by the risk management professional to determine the reason for late notification. The goal is to receive few surprises in the future and for adverse events to be known at the time of their occurrence. Failure to report occurrences in a timely manner will not allow the risk management professional to implement risk control techniques to mitigate damages or to prevent future reoccurrences. The date of report also needs descriptors. Date of the report to whom? For risk management professionals who work in a corporate office for a large integrated system, does the date of report refer to when they received the report, or is it the date when the local facility risk management professional received the report or when the insurance carrier received the first report or notice of an event? When possible, RMIS should allow for the tracking of multiple dates to cover the scenario above.

- Date of lawsuit or notice of intent to file a lawsuit—Tracking the filing date of a lawsuit will allow the risk management professional to further evaluate the effectiveness of the organization's early warning systems by identifying how many lawsuits were based on occurrences not previously known and reported to the risk management professional. Key metrics to monitor include: time from the date of loss (DOL) to the date of report (DOR) to the date of filing a formal notice suit or intent to file suit. These dates are used to evaluate the timeliness and effectiveness of early warning systems.

- Type of occurrence—Looking at types of occurrences (for example, falls, medication-related occurrences, diagnosis-related occurrences, treatment-related occurrences, and so on) and their frequency is important when trying to prioritize loss prevention activities.

- Location of the occurrence—Analyzing where adverse occurrences are most likely to occur allows for targeted loss prevention activities. The effectiveness of these activities supports the generation of department-specific reports. These reports support departmental review and implementation of subsequent risk control activities.

- Severity of injury—By prioritizing loss prevention activities to address occurrences with the highest likelihood of severe injury, the risk management professional can respond to possible adverse events with the greatest potential for high cost. To review an index of categories of medical errors refer to the section on NCC-MERP reporting under Voluntary Reporting Systems later in this chapter.

In addition to those variables, other elements of the occurrence that can be examined for trends include:

- Patient demographics, such as age, gender, marital status, occupation, method of payment, and diagnosis

- Staff characteristics, such as name, title, employment status (for example, agency versus staff nurse) of all employees involved in the occurrence; or name, department, and specialty of all involved physicians

- Other occurrence-related data, such as time and shift of the occurrence, physical environment at the time of the occurrence such as wet floor, inoperative call light, location of occurrence within the organization, or the status of family training in home-care situations

The selection of a computerized RMIS is not an easy task. Expense, ease of use, and utility are important factors in choosing to either build or buy a system to manage reporting and data manipulation. Compatibility with the clinical and financial data systems currently in place at the organization is also a key decision element. To evaluate RMIS vendors and their products and services, risk management professionals might prepare an RMIS vendor request for proposals (RFP). The RFP process takes time and can be enhanced with the assistance of others in the organization with specialized skills, such as representatives from information technology (IT), the privacy officer, finance, legal, quality improvement, and nursing. By involving these resources, the risk management professional can also ensure that needs of key risk management program stakeholders are met. Risk management professionals should plan early as this process can take anywhere from three to six months at a minimum from the development of a RFP to the selection of a vendor. In addition, visiting other organizations that use the system being considered can provide valuable information. For more information on Request for Proposals refer to Chapter 13 in Volume III of this series. For more information on risk management information systems, see Volume III, Chapter 15 of this series.

Contents of the Incident Report   Today's incident report forms vary in content and structure and from organization to organization throughout the continuum of care. Recent emphasis has been placed on making forms "user friendly," less cumbersome, and a tool that employees are more likely to use, given the time constraints and staffing shortages that affect the nursing staff, which is a major contributor to reporting systems.

Although the majority of risk management programs use electronic risk management information systems, there are still programs that use a pencil and paper method and are effective reporting systems. Not all medical errors can be captured in an electronic system, and a paper-based portable tool might identify adverse events and incidents previously unknown. Manual incident report forms can, in some circumstances, be an effective method for gathering information. These manual forms might have only preprinted data elements for check-off, whereas others have extensive narrative portions including description of the event, steps taken after the event, follow-up, and action plans. Regardless of format, some basic information that is contained in most incident reports includes:

- Demographic information may include name, home address, and telephone number of the patient, visitor, or employee involved in the incident and medical record number, if the involved party is a patient. This information is used to identify the potential claimant and witnesses in case of litigation. Typically most forms, particularly those in acute care settings, will have a section in which a patient's identifier "plate" can be imprinted directly on the form.

- Facility-related information, such as admission or visit date, business number (a patient's medical record number does not change; however, each hospitalization generates a different business number for each admission), patient room number, and admitting diagnosis or presenting complaint. This information is used on an aggregate basis to determine whether certain units of the system are more incident-prone. Analyzing this information for trends promotes risk management interventions and action plans to manage the frequency of incidents reported.

- Socioeconomic data on the individual involved in the occurrence, such as age, gender, marital status, employment, and insurance status help assess the severity of any potential loss. For example, collecting employment status helps the risk management professional and legal counsel determine the potential for economic damages that includes loss of wages or salary.

- Description of the incident, and of the facts surrounding the event, such as location of the incident; type of incident such as medication error, treatment error, diagnostic error, slip and fall, lost property, elopement; extent of injury incurred; pertinent environmental findings like position of bed rails, condition of floor surfaces, physical defects in equipment; and results of any physical examination of the patient, visitor, or employee by clinical staff, is often provided by the staff in the emergency department.

Staff Participation in Incident Reporting

Incident reporting is the duty and responsibility of all staff, including employed and voluntary members of the medical staff, not just the nursing department. To enhance the effectiveness of the incident report as a tool for risk management, the risk management professional should encourage physicians, residents, interns, pharmacists, laboratory personnel, and other ancillary service personnel to report incidents. Working with these practitioners to identify the types of incidents to be reported is a worthwhile exercise.

For the risk management professional in an integrated delivery system (IDS), staff participation in incident reporting presents a significant challenge. The various organizations that encompass the IDS can be geographically distant from each other;

TABLE 20.1   Common Barriers to Incident Reporting

- Staff feels overworked with not enough time to report
- Reports are viewed as a non-clinical safety function and not for clinical events
- Staff are busy at the time of the incident, then forget
- Perception that completion of an incident report is a nursing function only
- Reporter fears embarrassment or wants to avoid embarrassing a co-worker
- Reporter does not want to be considered a *whistleblower* or *tattletale*
- No routine reminders or periodic education as to the importance of reporting
- Thought someone else would complete the incident report
- Non-physicians uncomfortable reporting physicians
- Lack of computer skills to complete form online

- Lack of confidentiality—anonymous reporting not allowed
- Reporting thought to be unnecessary due to lack of adverse outcome feedback or follow-up
- Fear of punishment, disciplinary action, or retribution
- Fear of lawsuits, having to testify, or "go to court"
- Uncertain of value in filing or completing incident reports
- Lack of administrative support
- Inadequate reporting policies and procedures
- Unclear definition as to what constitutes a reportable incident
- Difficulty in accessing computer or the unavailability of incident report forms
- Fear of placing the facility at risk

Roberta Carroll, 2006.

as a result, promoting the consistent and timely reporting of incidents demands effective staff education. Simplicity of the reporting system and easy accessibility to user training is especially important in encouraging staff members in widely dispersed locations to report incidents.[6] For these systems, risk management professionals should include training and development for home health care providers, private physician offices, ambulatory care centers, and mobile mammogram units, and so on. Many providers have turned to the Web or intranet-based programs to provide access to such training and development.

One of the greatest challenges risk management professionals face today is dealing with under-reporting and the negative perceptions of incident reports. Although organizations are changing the work environment and culture to eliminate the punitive aspects associated with incident reporting, the negative aspects continue nonetheless. Please refer to Table 20.1 for a list of common barriers to reporting.

These barriers result in no reporting or at best, slow reporting with delayed follow-up. By providing feedback on the results of investigation and problem resolution, the risk management professional can demonstrate the value of early and timely reporting. Once the staff sees the value of systematically identifying and addressing problems in patient care, they often are more motivated to participate in reporting incidents.

The incident report should not be used as either a punitive measure for disciplining employees or as a vehicle for airing interpersonal disagreements. The risk management professional should make every effort to ensure that incident reports are used properly. Unfortunately, if the culture of the organization is one in which these reports have been used and continue to be used as a disciplinary tool or in a punitive manner, the risk management professional will have to spend time trying to make incremental changes to the environment—no easy task. This is not to say that repeated medication errors that lead to patient injury from a single practitioner might not involve some form of discipline. Under these circumstances, the risk management professional should focus on, and employees must be clear on, the series of events in the practitioner's performance that is the reason for the discipline—not the completion of an incident report.

Incident report education should stress that the report is a factual account of what happened; no finger-pointing or accusatory language should be included. Incident reports are meant to collect "just the facts," avoiding subjective, hearsay, or third-party opinions of what did or did not happen. If a grievous error was made resulting in a severe outcome for the patient, an employee might require counseling regarding the incident and measures to prevent recurrence could be implemented. But the incident report should not be used as evidence against the employee in a disciplinary procedure and should not be included in the personnel file.

Effectiveness of the reporting process can be enhanced by written policies and procedures that clearly define a reportable incident. Incident reports have been used to report major categories of events including patient slips and falls, medication errors, intravenous infusion problems, and lost valuables, among others. Effectiveness has been limited due, in part, to the mistaken belief that the incident report is a document prepared for the facility's environment of care, or safety committee. Although events such as patient falls might occur frequently, claims studies clearly show that they are not the source of greatest payout in health care-related claims. By explaining the purpose and content of the incident report through in-service training, and a clear written definition of what constitutes a reportable incident, the risk management professional can broaden the types of incidents reported to include clinically related events.

Finally, staff should be encouraged to complete the incident report promptly, accurately, and completely. Ideally, the form should be completed at either the time of occurrence or immediately thereafter. Many organizations use a "twenty-four-hour rule" for reporting, and require reporting within twenty-four hours of the event or knowledge of the event. It is important that the risk management professional be aware of any mandated requirements, such as in Florida, that the incident report must be received within a specific timeframe. For accuracy's sake, the individual who has the most knowledge about the event—that is, the employee involved in the occurrence, an employee witness, or the employee to whom it was reported, should report the incident. If the incident report requires that follow-up information be entered directly onto the form, policies should ensure that this information is transmitted rapidly, perhaps by telephone to the risk management professional, and that the completed incident report is forwarded to risk management as soon as possible. Any delay in transmitting information could prevent the risk management professional from reacting immediately to the event and following up in a timely manner. Immediacy of information and follow-up action is particularly critical in those instances when the patient or other parties involved in the incident need medical attention to stabilize a condition brought on by the untoward or unanticipated event.

The analysis of incident reports will allow the risk management professional to evaluate processes, systems, protocols, and practices that give rise to loss. Efforts to mitigate loss can then be targeted and focused toward areas where incidents have been frequent or the resulting loss has been severe.

When educating staff on the policies and procedures for completing an incident report, the same questions that are asked during an interview are useful. What happened? How did it happen? When did the event take place? How can it be prevented in the future? Who was involved, and so on. Risk management professionals should highlight key points

TABLE 20.2   Key Points to Remember About Incident Reports

1. Notify risk management within twenty-four hours of an incident either in person, telephonically, or by using the formal incident reporting system.

2. Record only the facts related to the event.

3. Record the names of any witnesses and responsible parties with knowledge or involvement.

4. Record time and location of the incident.

5. For paper-based systems use blue or black ink ballpoint pens (no felt tip pens).

6. Use appropriate patient descriptors such as age, sex.

7. Record information on the condition of the patient, resident, or client after the incident such as "resident brought to radiology, findings negative for fracture."

8. Record in the patient's medical record a factual account of any unanticipated events involving patient injury.

9. Incident reports should go directly to risk management and not through any other department first.

10. Incident report forms should be received in a timely manner for review by the risk management professional. In some jurisdictions this time is mandated by law. For example, Florida Statute requires reporting within three business days to the risk manager or designee.[1] Receipt of incident reports should not be delayed for follow-up or extra review and signatures.

11. The clinical facts surrounding an incident should always be documented in the medical record. However, there should be no mention of the fact that a formal incident report has been completed.

12. Never place the incident report in the medical record. This is less of an issue as hospitals and other health care organizations move to electronic health records or use of an electronic incident reporting system. However, if the organization is using a paper-based incident report form, consider making the report form oversized so it will be noticeable if placed inadvertently in the medical record, printed in another color, or printed with a colored border or strip.

13. The medical record and incident report are not venues for professional infighting. Do not use accusatory, threatening, or inflammatory language. The assignment of blame or admitting liability or fault is not proper to place into the medical record.

14. Copying the incident report for any reason should not be permitted.

Roberta Carroll, 2006.

[1] Florida §395.0197(1) (e) The development and implementation of an incident reporting system based upon the affirmative duty of all health care providers and all agents and employees of the licensed health care facility to report adverse incidents to the risk manager, or to his or her designee, within three business days after their occurrence.

for participants such as members of the medical staff, office managers, and home health aides. For a listing of those key points refer to Table 20.2.

Guidelines for Preserving Incident Report Confidentiality

Although completed incident reports are statements of fact, and therefore contain readily available information from other sources, risk management professionals and staff should strive to maintain the confidentiality of these reports and related information. The preservation of confidentiality

- Encourages accurate and frequent reporting
- Ensures factual information and promotes honesty of reports
- Prevents the perception (usually introduced by plaintiff's counsel) that something "wrong" has occurred
- Supports a defense attorney's ability to provide for a proper defense

To protect the confidentiality of the document, one of two common approaches can be taken: to provide protection under state statutes regarding quality assurance studies and peer review activities, or to provide protection under the attorney-client privilege, also referred to as *work product protection.*

To maintain confidentiality, the original report should be sent to the risk management professional immediately upon completion. As mentioned previously, copies should never be made, and the report must never be made part of the medical record.

Frequently, a follow-up sheet is attached to the incident report form. This usually is completed by a departmental manager, the nursing supervisor, nursing home administrator, or other responsible administrator who has investigated the occurrence and, when possible, ascertained the fact pattern of events (cause) leading to the incident. It is important to protect the confidentiality of this addendum and other related information such as photographs, staffing records, and so on, in addition to the actual incident report.

If managers use incident reports to support quality improvement (QI) studies or insist on having the reports for any reason, risk management professionals should suggest that managers review the originals in the risk management office. Once again, it is important to ensure that copies are not made and the originals are not removed from the file.

If the incident report is best protected through assertion of attorney-client privilege, the incident report should be reviewed by legal counsel in a timely fashion and maintained in specifically identified files. If report confidentiality is best achieved through statutory protection afforded to QI data and peer review activities, the reports must be reviewed through the established QI program. This review can be accomplished when there is a distinct operational linkage between risk management and quality assurance (performance improvement) departments. It is best to discuss these options with legal counsel to determine the best method for preserving confidentiality, keeping in mind state statutes, regulations, and case law. Likewise, the risk management professional should consult with legal counsel regarding procedures for reviewing and maintaining the reports.

Risk management professionals and defense counsel have worked tirelessly to ensure protection of this type of information. However recently, health care organizations have found an increasing number of challenges to this protection by plaintiff attorneys and the courts. So remember that while organizations work diligently to protect this information, it must be assumed that all health care information is "discoverable" and that the health care organization cannot completely rely on evidentiary protections. Given that belief, it is of the utmost importance that only facts should be recorded on incident reports—the same facts or information that could be found in other documents including the medical record.

Risk management professionals should be aware of the efforts and advancement in patient safety, the promotion and requirements for the disclosure of unanticipated events, and the cultural emphasis on honesty in dealing with patients and families. While the practice of sequestering (or what might be perceived by patients as "hiding") incident reports might be perceived as undermining the cultural emphasis on disclosure, understand that incident reports are business records created for a specific purpose and are not part of the patient's medical record. This should not in any way diminish efforts to deal with patients in an open and honest manner with regard to issues that arise during the course of their care and treatment.

Contrasted with traditional incident reporting, many organizations are implementing anonymous hot lines. For example, one hospital reported that anonymous reporting resulted in many times the reporting of patient safety issues received with the traditional incident report.[7] The risk management professional will need a clear understanding of how the organization approaches these issues before developing relevant policies and procedures for incident reporting.

Occurrence Reporting   Focused-occurrence reporting gives staff clear guidelines and specific examples of reportable incidents. For example, these incidents might include:

- Occurrences of missed diagnosis or misdiagnosis that result in patient injury, such as failure to diagnose acute myocardial infarction, fractures, serious head trauma, or appendicitis
- Surgically related occurrences, such as the wrong patient being operated on, the wrong site operated on, the wrong procedure being performed, an incorrect instrument or sponge count, or an unplanned return to the operating room
- Treatment- or procedure-related occurrences, such as reactions to contrast material used in a diagnostic procedure, undesirable exposure to X-rays, or burns resulting from improper use of hot packs
- Blood-related occurrences, such as the wrong type of blood given to the patient, transmission of disease via infected blood, or improper use of blood or blood products
- Intravenous-related occurrences, such as the wrong solution being administered, infiltration of solution, or an incorrect infusion rate
- Medication-related occurrences
- Lack of adequate follow-up, such as failure to notify a patient of abnormal laboratory findings
- Falls

Given the recent attention that patient safety has been afforded via the media with the enactment of the Patient Safety and Quality Improvement Act of 2005, the Joint Commission International Center for Patient Safety and JCAHO's National Patient Safety Goals, medication safety has moved to the forefront of the risk management agenda. Medication safety programs are based on adverse event reporting systems, human factor analysis, and data analysis. Medication related claims can include:

- Wrong dosage
- Wrong route
- Wrong frequency (of rate for IV)
- Wrong medication
- Wrong choice of medication for condition
- Wrong time
- Wrong administration technique
- Wrong patient
- Missed dose
- Known drug-drug interaction
- Known allergy to drug
- Wrong reason

Ideally, the organization will implement a clinical area specific version of the event reporting system to focus on this important risk management area. Many organizations have designed clinical area-specific incident report forms for each clinical and operational department. The challenge of such reporting systems is to make certain that trends that cross department lines, such as medication errors in the radiology suite and the pharmacy, are identified and assessed.

Although the majority of these examples apply to the acute care setting, many are applicable to other parts of the health care continuum. Medication-related occurrences should be reported and tracked in all health care settings, including the private office setting.

Falls, which are a prevalent cause of injury in long-term care facilities, can occur in any setting, as can the development of pressure ulcers, nosocomial infections, patient elopement, and failure to refer. With the elderly, the resulting injury can be severe. Finally, as more primary care is provided in alternate settings such as in the home, providers of care in these settings must design incident reporting systems that track treatment variances and equipment malfunctions that lead to patient or client injury.

To further focus the reporting process, many health care organizations define reportable occurrences by designated location, such as the emergency department (ED), surgical suite, labor and delivery room, high-risk nursery, and so on. (Refer to Table 20.3, Emergency Department—Occurrence Reporting Criteria). For large integrated delivery systems (IDSs) and stand-alone alternate care settings, reportable occurrences are designed specifically to the type of service offered. By developing lists of specific adverse outcomes or events in these high-risk areas, the clinical focus of occurrence reporting is addressed, and the incidents that need to be reported are made clear. The risk management professional receives these reports directly. Because of the highly clinical nature of this data, most facilities will share this information with quality assurance, performance improvement, or the QI committee. The data can then be reviewed by peer review using root cause analyses. Action plans and incident follow-up will be implemented based on

TABLE 20.3   Emergency Department—Occurrence Reporting Criteria

- Any patient who leaves without being seen (LWBS)
- Any patient who leaves against medical advice (AMA)
- Any patient who returns to the Emergency Department without a scheduled re-visit within 72 hours
- Any discrepancy in reading the initial (wet read) X-ray from the final read
- Inappropriate EMTALA transfer received and transferred or discharged out
- Missing or inadequate discharge instructions
- Failure to deliver and act upon critical test results
- Failure to give patient ordered prescriptions
- Any incidents of assault or violence

- Patient falls
- Medication errors
- Any recognized failure to diagnose or misdiagnosis
- Failure to use or deliver thrombolytics in a timely manner
- Failure to initiate treatment in a timely manner
- Failure to remove a foreign body
- Inadequate staffing that affects patient care
- Long wait time to be seen that affects quality of care
- Misidentification of a patient
- Ineffective hand-off to other personnel, unit, or area
- Inadequate or missing medication reconciliation

Roberta Carroll, 2006.

such review. Aggregate reports of this information should be reported to the QI committee and risk management committees.

Generic or Occurrence Screening

Another method that attempts to identify adverse patient occurrences in clinical areas is the occurrence screening process, as originally developed by Joyce Craddick of Medical Management Analysis International. This system, and many others like it that followed, uses a clearly defined list of patient occurrences with which patient medical records are screened. The screeners are looking for deviations from practice, policy, and procedures. Criteria for the screens are established in areas that are considered to be either high risk, have a high number of incidents that have been reported as quality of care "red flags" to be further evaluated, or are areas where the effects of an untoward event occurring can have disastrous results from an injury standpoint. In the past, most screens were centered around clinical events and related administrative events, but they can just as well be used for regulatory and financial issues. Criteria are developed and exceptions are listed, if applicable. For example, in the operating room, one specific criterion that may be screened for is proper informed consent documentation. An exception to this criterion may be in a case of emergency surgery, where either the patient is unable to give consent or there is not time to obtain consent. Another criterion to screen for and evaluate, regardless of location in the health care setting, is an unexpected death. There are no exceptions to this criterion. In the emergency department, criteria may include misread X-rays or readmissions within twenty-four hours.

In an inpatient setting, all patient records are reviewed against the criteria within forty-eight to seventy-two hours of admission and every three or four days thereafter until the patient is discharged. The patient chart also is reviewed approximately two weeks after discharge to ensure that compliance with all criteria has been assessed.

Results of this screening process are prepared for each admission by trained data-retrieval personnel (screeners). The abstract is then forwarded to the QI office for follow-up and data collection. When identified, serious occurrences are reported immediately by the patient care reviewers to the correct person for action. All occurrences are aggregated to aid in identifying any trends that reflect patient care problems that require remedial action.

Occurrence screening also can be effective in other settings; ambulatory care organizations (ACOs), physician group practices, and medical clinics, in particular, have found this method useful in identifying sources of risk. Using a checklist, the staff reviews outpatient records for items such as documentation of patient allergies, prescription refills, patient notification of test results, and telephone communications. The records are also reviewed to see whether they are sufficient for another practitioner to continue the patient's care.[8]

Although occurrence screening is an effective method for identifying adverse occurrences, its implementation in most institutions is done entirely under the QI program. The major challenge of this system is how to ensure sufficient involvement of the risk management professional. In some institutions, the risk management professional is notified by having the patient care reviewer complete a separate risk management notification form for serious adverse patient occurrences. In other instances, the risk management professional is part of the quality management team and is apprised of the results of the occurrence screening through departmental or QI committee meetings.

Regardless of the method chosen, the risk management professional should have ready access to this data for the process to be useful to the risk management program. In addition, the risk management professional should play a key role in identifying and implementing action plans relating to abnormal and increasing negative data trends.

Failure Mode and Effects Analysis (FMEA)   Failure Mode and Effects Analysis (FMEA) is a risk control technique used to prevent the occurrence of loss by analyzing a situation which might create risk at a later time, such as a new morphine pump which has been purchased but not been placed in use. By conducting a *dry run* of pump protocols, the staff can identify risk issues that require attention before the pump is used. The purpose of FMEA is to identify ways in which that process might potentially fail. The goal is to eliminate or reduce the likelihood or outcome severity of such a failure.[9] FMEA is used before an adverse event or incident occurs, and it is considered to be a successful technique for *proactive* risk management.

A root cause analysis (RCA) is a structured analytic methodology used to examine the underlying contributors to an adverse event or condition. Because RCA is implemented after an event has occurred, it is considered a *reactive* risk management technique.

Health care organizations accredited by the Joint Commission are required to conduct a root cause analysis (RCA) in response to any sentinel event. JACHO Standard LD.5.2 requires facilities to select at least one high-risk process for proactive risk assessment each year. This selection is to be based, in part, on information published periodically by the JCAHO that identifies the most frequently occurring types of sentinel event. Organizations should also identify patient safety events and high-risk process for which an FMEA would be valuable.

Informal Reporting Methods—Internal   In addition to the more structured systems of risk identification, such as incident reporting, occurrence reporting, and occurrence screening and FMEA, there are many other sources of information available to the risk management professional for identifying actual loss-producing events and potential risks. Some of these include:

- Committee meeting minutes, such as from those dealing with performance improvement, quality assurance, safety, patient safety, infection control, and bioethics; and those from departmental committees such as morbidity and mortality, tissue review, pharmacy and therapeutics, and other quality- or risk-related committees.

- Claims data, including a review of both the facility's loss experience over a period of time and any national or regional trends as reported in various publications. For instance, risk management professionals will serve their organizations well by tracking regional or national loss trends even if those types of incidents have not occurred (nor been reported) in their organization. Planning and being proactive to avoid known risks is reflective of a mature risk management program.

- Survey reports, including those from the JCAHO, the National Committee on Quality Assurance (NCQA), the Commission on Accreditation of Rehabilitation Facilities (CARF), Occupational Safety and Health Administration (OSHA), the state fire marshal, state licensure surveys, broker or underwriter site assessments, consultant findings, and private review organization study results.

- Patient complaints and standardized patient satisfaction surveys can offer the risk management professional valuable information from the patient's perspective, a view not always ascertained in other reporting methods.

- Risk management walking rounds and patient safety walking rounds (commonly called "rounding") in which the risk management professional is visible and available to staff members, encourages the sharing of information that may be viewed by certain individuals as too sensitive for a written report. Having a routine presence on the units and availability in the office or by pager are important factors in the continuous effort to enhance the early reporting of incidents.

- MBWA, "management by walking around," does not have to be a formalized scheduled process. Risk management professionals need to be visible and available. If the staff does not know who they are, where they are located, and what they do, they will not likely call or report when they should.

Risk management professionals should contact legal counsel to determine how best to protect the confidentiality of any data collected, whether it be through evidentiary protection, through quality improvement activity, peer review, or risk management process protections offered in some states.

Ways to Enhance Reporting Effectiveness There are many ways to enhance the effectiveness of the reporting process. These include:

- Ensuring that departmental and medical staffs are involved in development of the list of reportable occurrences so that there is agreement as to the type of occurrences to report. Physician *buy-in* is very important in this process.

- Streamlining the reporting process so that the paperwork is not burdensome and reporting is easy. Because many of the items on the list of reportable incidents occur frequently (for example, patients leaving the ED against medical advice), objective checklists might be more useful than lengthy narrative reports. Again the intent and best practice at this time in health care is to improve and increase reporting. Simply increasing the number of reports is not the ultimate goal; rather receiving reports on events that require risk management review, and that afford an opportunity to reduce the likelihood of legal liability, is the hoped-for objective.

- Ensuring that the results of the reporting are given to the departments involved as quickly as possible for their review and consideration, thus emphasizing the utility of identifying problems in patient care rather than the punitive aspect of potential claims.

External Reporting

Risk management professionals have a wealth of available information from which they can develop risk management activities to eliminate or reduce loss. Much of this information is generated internally and used internally. There is however, a need for information by many groups outside the organization. These outside users of an organization's internal data are as varied as is the information they need or want. Many external reports are generated because of a legal mandate, whereas other information is reported voluntarily because of collaborative efforts to enhance patient safety.

Health care organizations as part of these collaborative arrangements have the reciprocal benefit of the identification and analysis of adverse events and occurrences on a larger scale than is possible with data generated only internally. In many circumstances, these outside data will direct the organizations to conduct their own FMEAs or initiate other proactive measures to eliminate loss prior to an occurrence.

The following will highlight a representative few of the external agencies and organizations with which health care organizations share data. This is not an exhaustive list, and is one that will continue to evolve over time.

JCAHO Sentinel Events   The JCAHO's Sentinel Event Policy is designed to encourage the self-reporting of medical errors to learn about the relative frequencies and underlying causes of sentinel events, share "lessons learned" with other health care organizations, thereby reducing the risk of future sentinel event occurrences. Accredited organizations must update their internal reporting systems to identify these types of events, which are fully described below.

According to the JCAHO, a sentinel event is any unexpected occurrence that involves death or serious physical or psychological injury, or the risk thereof. Serious injuries specifically include a loss of limb or function. The phrase "or the risk thereof" includes any process variation for which a recurrence would carry a significant chance of a serious adverse outcome.[10]

Anytime a sentinel event occurs, the accredited organization is expected to complete a RCA, implement improvements to reduce risk, and monitor the effectiveness of those improvements. Although the immediate cause of most sentinel events is due to human fallibility, the RCA is expected to dig down to underlying organizational systems and processes that can be altered to reduce the likelihood of human error in the future and to protect patients from harm when human error does occur.

A standard that creates explicit expectations regarding the internal identification and management of sentinel events was added to the leadership chapter of all accreditation manuals and became effective January 1, 1999.

Voluntary Self-Reporting of Sentinel Events   Under the Sentinel Event Policy, a defined subset of sentinel events is subject to review by the JCAHO and may be reported on a voluntary basis. Only those sentinel events that affect recipients of care (patients, clients, and residents) and that meet one of the following criteria fall into this category.[11]

- The event has resulted in an unanticipated death or major permanent loss of function, not related to the natural course of the patient's illness or underlying condition.
- The event is one of the following (even if the outcome was not death or major permanent loss of function unrelated to the natural course of the patient's illness or underlying condition).
  - Suicide of any individual receiving care, treatment, or services in a staffed around-the-clock care setting or within seventy-two hours of discharge.
  - Unanticipated death of a full-term infant.
  - Abduction of any individual receiving care, treatment, or services.
  - Discharge of an infant to the wrong family.
  - Rape.[12]
  - Hemolytic transfusion reaction involving administration of blood or blood products having major blood group incompatibilities.
- All events of surgery on the wrong patient or wrong body part are reviewable under the policy, regardless of the magnitude of the procedure.

- Unintended retention of a foreign object in an individual after surgery or other procedure.
- Severe neonatal hyperbillirubinemia (billirubin >30 milligrams/deciliter).
- Prolonged fluoroscopy with cumulative dose >1500 rads to a single field, or any delivery of radiotherapy to the wrong body region or >25 percent above the planned radiotherapy dose.

Sentinel Events That Are Not Self-Reported   Each accredited health care organization is encouraged, but not required, to report to the JCAHO any sentinel event that meets the aforementioned criteria for reviewable sentinel events. Or, the JCAHO might become aware of a sentinel event by some other means such as from a patient, family member, employee of the organization, or through the media.

Whether the organization voluntarily reports the event or the JCAHO becomes aware of the event by some other means, there is no difference in the expected response, time frames, or review procedures.

Response by the JCAHO   If the JCAHO becomes aware (either through voluntary self-reporting or otherwise) of a sentinel event that meets the definition of a reviewable sentinel event, the organization is required to:

- Prepare a thorough and credible RCA and action plan within forty-five calendar days of the event or of the organization becoming aware of the event.
- Submit its RCA and action plan or otherwise provide for JCAHO evaluation the organization's response to the sentinel event under an approved protocol, within forty-five calendar days of the known occurrence of the event.

Advantages to Reporting   There are several advantages to the organization that reports a sentinel event to the JCAHO. Some of those advantages are:

- Contributes to the general knowledge about sentinel events and the reduction of risk for such events in many other organizations.
- Gives the organization the opportunity to consult with the JCAHO staff while preparing the RCA and action plans.
- Enhances the public perception that the organization, by collaborating and working with the JCAHO, is doing everything possible to ensure that such an event will not happen again, understand how the event happened, and what can be done to reduce the risk of such an event occurring in the future.

Submission of RCA and Action Plan   The JCAHO has several procedures to protect the confidentiality of sentinel event information shared by accredited organizations and that are in the JCAHO's possession.

The JCAHO advises health care organizations not to provide patient or caregiver identifiers when reporting sentinel events.

An organization that experiences a sentinel event should submit two separate documents: (1) the RCA and (2) the resulting action plan. The RCA will be returned to the organization once information is abstracted and entered into the JCAHO database. If copies have been made for internal review, they will be destroyed after the review. Also, once the action plan has been implemented to the satisfaction of the JCAHO, it will be returned to the organization.

In addition, if the organization has concerns about increased risk of legal exposure as a result of sending the root cause analysis documents to the JCAHO, the following alternative approaches to review the organization's response to the sentinel event are acceptable.

1. An organization brings root cause analysis documents to the JCAHO headquarters for review and then takes the documents back on the same day.

2. A specially trained surveyor conducts an on-site visit to review the RCA and action plan.

3. A specially trained surveyor conducts an on-site visit to review the RCA and findings, without directly viewing the root cause analysis documents, through a series of interviews and review of relevant documentation.

4. Where the organization affirms that it meets specified criteria respecting the risk of waiving legal protection for RCA information shared with the JCAHO, a specially trained surveyor conducts an on-site visit to interview the staff and review relevant documentation to obtain information about:

   a. The process the organization uses in responding to sentinel events.

   b. The relevant policies and procedures preceding and following the organization's review of the specific event and the implementation thereof, sufficient to permit inferences about the adequacy of the organization's response to the sentinel event.[13]

Mandatory Reporting Systems

The reporting of adverse events by hospitals is legislated in twenty-five states as of September 2005.[14] In the vast majority of these states, reporting systems are mandatory. Many states have developed for the end users interpretive guidelines to clarify reporting requirements. States with electronic reporting guidelines may have developed Internet user guides for their systems. According to state officials, mandatory reporting systems play a vital role in hospital oversight by providing information about hospital patient safety practices. States use data to investigate individual events and ensure that corrective action is taken. Many states also share their data with other professional bodies such as licensure boards when professional standards may have been breached.[15]

Collaborative Arrangements

Publication of the 1999 Institute of Medicine Report *To Err is Human: Building a Safer Health System,* the advent of the JCAHO sponsored National Patient Safety Goals (NPSG) in 2003, and the prominence of organizations such as the National Patient Safety Foundation (NPSF) and the Institute for Safe Medication Practices (ISMP) prompted many organizations to develop complementary systems for risk identification particularly in the area of medication errors. These complementary systems broadened traditional incident reporting to involve other professionals not previously included in the reporting and analysis hierarchy, such as the hospital pharmacist. The use of technology such as bar coding, robotics for medication dispensing and packaging, and computerized physician (provider) order entry systems (CPOE) all have the potential to lower the risk profile associated with medication administration. In many organizations these professionals are now participating in front line risk management activities. These complementary systems might receive near-miss and error reports before review by the risk management professional. Internal collaboration is critical to ensure that the risk management professional is informed on a timely basis of the results and findings associated with these new systems. As discussed earlier, organizational risk should be assessed on an enterprise-wide basis. The risk management professional is the best person to fill that role.

••••••••••••

FOOD AND DRUG ADMINISTRATION (FDA)[16]

The federal Food and Drug Administration collects information in various categories that health care risk management professionals should be aware of and incorporate into their reporting plans. These are the Adverse Event Reporting System, the Vaccine Adverse Event Reporting System, the Special Nutritionals Adverse Event Reporting System, and the Manufacturers and User Facility Device Experience Database.

Adverse Event Reporting System (AERS)

AERS collects information about adverse events, medication errors, and product problems that occur after the administration of approved drugs and therapeutic biologic products. Quarterly (noncumulative) data files since January 2004 are available for downloading on the AERS Web site.

Vaccine Adverse Event Reporting System (VAERS)

VAERS is a cooperative program for vaccine safety of the Centers for Disease Control and Prevention (CDC) and the Food and Drug Administration (FDA). VAERS collects information about adverse events that occur after the administration of U.S. licensed vaccines. For more information on the Vaccine Adverse Event Reporting System go to [www.vaers.org].

The Special Nutritionals Adverse Event Monitoring System

This system is composed of adverse event (illness or injury) reports associated with the use of dietary supplements, infant formulas, and medical foods (1993–1998 data). For more information visit [www.fda.org].

Manufacturers and User Facility Device Experience Database (MAUDE)

Medical device reporting (MDR) is the mechanism used by the FDA to receive significant medical device adverse event reports from manufacturers, importers, and user facilities. Under the Safe Medical Devices Act of 1990 (SMDA), user facilities (hospitals, nursing homes) are required to report suspected medical device-related deaths to both the FDA and manufacturer. User facilities report medical device-related serious injuries only to the manufacturer unless the manufacturer is unknown, at which time the serious injury is reported to the FDA. For ease of reporting, the FDA has two forms: MedWatch 3500 for voluntary reporting and Medwatch 3500A for mandatory reporting. Refer to Exhibit 20.1, the MedWatch form 3500.[17]

MAUDE has search database information of all voluntary reports since June 1993, user facility reports since 1991, distributor reports since 1993, and manufacturer reports since August 1996 (MDR data files, 1992–1996).

EXHIBIT 20.1   MedWatch Form 3500 for Voluntary Reporting and Advice About Reporting

U.S. Department of Health and Human Services

MEDWATCH

The FDA Safety Information and
Adverse Event Reporting Program

For VOLUNTARY reporting of
adverse events, product problems and
product use errors

Page ____ of ____

Form Approved: OMB No. 0910-0291, Expires: 10/31/08
See OMB statement on reverse.

FDA USE ONLY

Triage unit
sequence #

PLEASE TYPE OR USE BLACK INK

A. PATIENT INFORMATION

1. Patient Identifier
2. Age at Time of Event, or Date of Birth:
3. Sex — ☐ Female ☐ Male
4. Weight ____ lb or ____ kg

In confidence

B. ADVERSE EVENT, PRODUCT PROBLEM OR ERROR

Check all that apply:

1. ☐ Adverse Event   ☐ Product Problem (e.g., defects/malfunctions)
   ☐ Product Use Error   ☐ Problem with Different Manufacturer of Same Medicine

2. Outcomes Attributed to Adverse Event (Check all that apply)
   ☐ Death: _____ (mm/dd/yyyy)
   ☐ Life-threatening
   ☐ Hospitalization - initial or prolonged
   ☐ Required Intervention to Prevent Permanent Impairment/Damage (Devices)
   ☐ Disability or Permanent Damage
   ☐ Congenital Anomaly/Birth Defect
   ☐ Other Serious (Important Medical Events)

3. Date of Event (mm/dd/yyyy)
4. Date of this Report (mm/dd/yyyy)

5. Describe Event, Problem or Product Use Error

6. Relevant Tests/Laboratory Data, Including Dates

7. Other Relevant History, Including Preexisting Medical Conditions (e.g., allergies, race, pregnancy, smoking and alcohol use, liver/kidney problems, etc.)

C. PRODUCT AVAILABILITY

Product Available for Evaluation? (Do not send product to FDA)
☐ Yes   ☐ No   ☐ Returned to Manufacturer on: _____ (mm/dd/yyyy)

D. SUSPECT PRODUCT(S)

1. Name, Strength, Manufacturer (from product label)
   #1
   #2

2. Dose or Amount | Frequency | Route
   #1
   #2

3. Dates of Use (If unknown, give duration) from/to (or best estimate)
   #1
   #2

4. Diagnosis or Reason for Use (Indication)
   #1
   #2

5. Event Abated After Use Stopped or Dose Reduced?
   #1 ☐ Yes ☐ No ☐ Doesn't Apply
   #2 ☐ Yes ☐ No ☐ Doesn't Apply

6. Lot # — #1, #2
7. Expiration Date — #1, #2

8. Event Reappeared After Reintroduction?
   #1 ☐ Yes ☐ No ☐ Doesn't Apply
   #2 ☐ Yes ☐ No ☐ Doesn't Apply

9. NDC # or Unique ID

E. SUSPECT MEDICAL DEVICE

1. Brand Name
2. Common Device Name
3. Manufacturer Name, City and State
4. Model # | Lot #
   Catalog # | Expiration Date (mm/dd/yyyy)
   Serial # | Other #
5. Operator of Device
   ☐ Health Professional
   ☐ Lay User/Patient
   ☐ Other: _____
6. If Implanted, Give Date (mm/dd/yyyy)
7. If Explanted, Give Date (mm/dd/yyyy)
8. Is this a Single-use Device that was Reprocessed and Reused on a Patient?
   ☐ Yes ☐ No
9. If Yes to Item No. 8, Enter Name and Address of Reprocessor

F. OTHER (CONCOMITANT) MEDICAL PRODUCTS

Product names and therapy dates (exclude treatment of event)

G. REPORTER (See confidentiality section on back)

1. Name and Address

Phone # | E-mail

2. Health Professional? ☐ Yes ☐ No
3. Occupation
4. Also Reported to:
   ☐ Manufacturer
   ☐ User Facility
   ☐ Distributor/Importer
5. If you do NOT want your identity disclosed to the manufacturer, place an "X" in this box: ☐

FORM FDA 3500 (10/05)   Submission of a report does not constitute an admission that medical personnel or the product caused or contributed to the event.

(Continued)

EXHIBIT 20.1   MedWatch Form 3500 for Voluntary Reporting and Advice About Reporting (*Continued*)

ADVICE ABOUT VOLUNTARY REPORTING

Detailed instructions available at: http://www.fda.gov/medwatch/report/consumer/instruct.htm

Report adverse events, product problems or productV use errors with:

- Medications *(drugs or biologics)*
- Medical devices *(including in-vitro diagnostics)*
- Combination products *(medication & medical devices)*
- Human cells, tissues, and cellular and tissue-based products
- Special nutritional products *(dietary supplements, medical foods, infant formulas)*
- Cosmetics

Report product problems - quality, performance or safety concerns such as:

- Suspected counterfeit product
- Suspected contamination
- Questionable stability
- Defective components
- Poor packaging or labeling
- Therapeutic failures (product didn't work)

Report SERIOUS adverse events. An event is serious when the patient outcome is:

- Death
- Life-threatening
- Hospitalization - initial or prolonged
- Disability or permanent damage
- Congenital anomaly/birth defect
- Required intervention to prevent permanent impairment or damage
- Other serious (important medical events)

Report even if:

- You're not certain the product caused the event
- You don't have all the details

How to report:

- Just fill in the sections that apply to your report
- Use section D for all products except medical devices
- Attach additional pages if needed
- Use a separate form for each patient
- Report either to FDA or the manufacturer *(or both)*

Other methods of reporting:

- 1-800-FDA-0178 -- To FAX report
- 1-800-FDA-1088 -- To report by phone
- www.fda.gov/medwatch/report.htm -- To report online

If your report involves a serious adverse event with a device and it occurred in a facility outside a doctor's office, that facility may be legally required to report to FDA and/or the manufacturer. Please notify the person in that facility who would handle such reporting.

If your report involves a serious adverse event with a vaccine call 1-800-822-7967 to report.

Confidentiality: The patient's identity is held in strict confidence by FDA and protected to the fullest extent of the law. FDA will not disclose the reporter's identity in response to a request from the public, pursuant to the Freedom of Information Act. The reporter's identity, including the identity of a self-reporter, may be shared with the manufacturer unless requested otherwise.

-Fold Here-   -Fold Here-

The public reporting burden for this collection of information has been estimated to average 36 minutes per response, including the time for reviewing instructions, searching existing data sources, gathering and maintaining the data needed, and completing and reviewing the collection of information. Send comments regarding this burden estimate or any other aspect of this collection of information, including suggestions for reducing this burden to:

Department of Health and Human Services *Food and Drug Administration - MedWatch* *10903 New Hampshire Avenue* *Building 22, Mail Stop 4447* *Silver Spring, MD 20993-0002*	*Please DO NOT* *RETURN this form* *to this address.*	*OMB statement:* *"An agency may not conduct or sponsor, and a person is not required to respond to, a collection of information unless it displays a currently valid OMB control number."*

U.S. DEPARTMENT OF HEALTH AND HUMAN SERVICES
Food and Drug Administration

FORM FDA 3500 (10/05) (Back)   Please Use Address Provided Below -- Fold in Thirds, Tape and Mail

In 1992, the FDA began monitoring medication error reports forwarded from several organizations, including the Institute for Safe Medication Practices (ISMP) and the United States Pharmacopeia (USP). MedWatch reports are also reviewed for possible medication errors. Additionally, medication errors are reported to the FDA by manufacturers with reports for adverse events that result in serious injury and for which a medication error may be a component.

INSTITUTE FOR SAFE MEDICATION PRACTICES (ISMP), UNITED STATES PHARMACOPEIA (USP), NATIONAL COORDINATING COUNCIL FOR MEDICATION ERROR REPORTING AND PREVENTION

Certain types of events have specific risks associated with them, due in large part to the complexity of the processes involved in delivering the care or providing the service. Medication ordering and administration is one such complex process. It involves many people, processes, and systems where failures can occur and can result in errors. Entire systems have been developed just to report, analyze, find trends in, and ultimately reduce the occurrence of medication events. One medication-specific external event reporting system is the Medication Errors Reporting (MER) program, a voluntary nationwide service operated by the U.S. Pharmacopeia in conjunction with the Institute for Safe Medication Practices. The MER program is designed to collect information about medication errors from physicians, pharmacists, and nurses and to share that information anonymously and develop educational services to prevent future errors. Information about the MER program can be found at [www. usp.org] or [www.ismp.org].

The National Coordinating Council for Medication Error Reporting and Prevention (NCC MERP) realized the need for a standardized categorization of errors. In 1996 the NCC MERP adopted a Medication Error Index that classifies an error according to severity of outcome. It is hoped that by creating a standardized index, health care institutions and practitioners will track medication errors in a consistent and systematic manner. The Council encourages the use of the index in all health care delivery settings.[18] Refer to the USP Medication Errors Reporting Program Form, the NCC MERP Index for Categorizing Medication Errors,[19] and the NCC MERP Index for Categorizing Medication Errors Algorithm[20] (Exhibits 20.2–4).

MEDICAL EVENT REPORTING SYSTEM—TRANSFUSION MEDICINE (MERS-TM)

Another example of a specialized area with complex processes involved is transfusion medicine. An online national reporting system for collecting and analyzing blood-transfusion errors, adverse events, and near misses recently became available. The voluntary reporting system, called Medical Event Reporting System—Transfusion Medicine (MERS-TM) is housed at Columbia University (New York). It allows participants to report anonymously and have access to a central aggregate database for comparative purposes. Information on MERS-TM is available at [www.mers-tm.net].

THE INTENSIVE CARE UNIT SAFETY REPORTING SYSTEM (ICUSRS)

Medical specialties are also initiating event reporting systems geared specifically to patient care issues inherent in that specialty. The Intensive Care Unit Safety Reporting System (ICUSRS), run by the Society for Critical Care Medicine and a team of investigators from Johns Hopkins University and funded by the Agency for Healthcare Research and Quality (AHRQ), is an external reporting system specifically for intensive care units. Its leaders intend to expand the program nationwide. The ICUSRS reporting form can be viewed at [www.icusrs.org].

PITTSBURGH REGIONAL HEALTHCARE INITIATIVE

What began in 1997 as a consortium of Pittsburgh-area medical, business, and civic leaders concerned about health care costs has become an innovator in patient safety initiatives. The Pittsburgh Regional Healthcare Initiative (PRHI) became one of the earliest community

EXHIBIT 20.2   USP Medication Errors Reporting Program Form

USP MEDICATION ERRORS REPORTING PROGRAM
Presented in cooperation with the Institute for Safe Medication Practices
USP is an FDA MEDWATCH partner

Reporters should not provide any individually identifiable health information, including names of practitioners, names of patients, names of healthcare facilities, or dates of birth (age is acceptable).

MEDI-CATION ERRORS

REPORTING PROGRAM

Date and time of event:

Please describe the error. Include description/sequence of events, type of staff involved, and work environment (e.g., code situation, change of shift, short staffing, no 24-hr. pharmacy, floor stock). If more space is needed, please attach a separate page.

Did the error reach the patient?   ☐ Yes ☐ No

Was the incorrect medication, dose, or dosage form administered to or taken by the patient?   ☐ Yes ☐ No

Circle the appropriate Error Outcome Category (select one—see back for details):   A   B   C   D   E   F   G   H   I

Describe the direct result of the error on the patient (e.g., death, type of harm, additional patient monitoring).

Indicate the possible error cause(s) and contributing factor(s) (e.g., abbreviation, similar names, distractions, etc.). _____

Indicate the location of the error (e.g., hospital, outpatient or community pharmacy, clinic, nursing home, patient's home, etc.). _____

What type of staff or healthcare practitioner made the initial error? _____

Indicate if other practitioner(s) were also involved in the error (type of staff perpetuating error). _____

What type of staff or healthcare practitioner discovered the error or recognized the potential for error? _____

How was the error (or potential for error) discovered/intercepted? _____

If available, provide patient age, gender, diagnosis. Do not provide any patient identifiers. _____

Please complete the following for the product(s) involved. (If more space is needed for additional products, please attach a separate page.)

	Product #1	Product #2
Brand/Product Name (If Applicable)		
Generic Name		
Manufacturer		
Labeler		
Dosage Form		
Strength/Concentration		
Type and Size of Container		

Reports are most useful when relevant materials such as product label, copy of prescription/order, etc., can be reviewed.
Can these materials be provided?   ☐ Yes ☐ No   Please specify:

Suggest any recommendations to prevent recurrence of this error, or describe policies or procedures you instituted or plan to institute to prevent future similar errors. _____

Name and Title/Profession	Telephone Number ( )	Fax Number ( )
Facility/Address and Zip		E-mail
Address/Zip (where correspondence should be sent)		

Your name, contact information, and a copy of this report are routinely shared with the Institute for Safe Medication Practices (ISMP). Copies of reports will be sent to third parties such as the manufacturer/labeler, and to the Food and Drug Administration (FDA). You have the option of including your name on these copies.

In addition to releasing my name and contact information to ISMP, USP may release my identity to these third parties as follows (check boxes that apply):

☐ The manufacturer and/or labeler as listed above   ☐ FDA   ☐ Other persons requesting a copy of this report   ☐ Anonymous to all third parties

Signature	Date

Return to: USP CAPS 12601 Twinbrook Parkway Rockville, MD 20852-1790	Submit via the Web at www.usp.org/mer Call Toll Free: 800-23-ERROR (800-233-7767) or FAX: 301-816-8532	Date Received by USP	File Access Number

WEPUF
©USPC 2003

PSF116C

EXHIBIT 20.3   NCC MERP Index for Categorizing Medication Errors

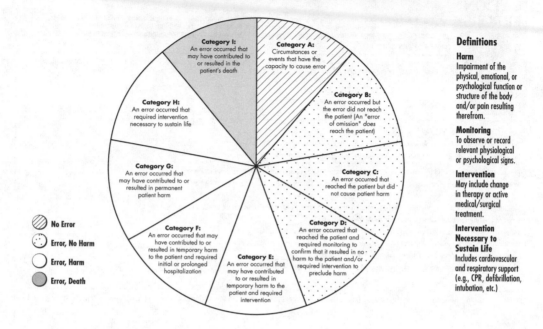

NCC MERP Index for Categorizing Medication Errors

Category I: An error occurred that may have contributed to or resulted in the patient's death

Category A: Circumstances or events that have the capacity to cause error

Category B: An error occurred but the error did not reach the patient (An "error of omission" *does* reach the patient)

Category H: An error occurred that required intervention necessary to sustain life

Category G: An error occurred that may have contributed to or resulted in permanent patient harm

Category C: An error occurred that reached the patient but did not cause patient harm

Category F: An error occurred that may have contributed to or resulted in temporary harm to the patient and required initial or prolonged hospitalization

Category E: An error occurred that may have contributed to or resulted in temporary harm to the patient and required intervention

Category D: An error occurred that reached the patient and required monitoring to confirm that it resulted in no harm to the patient and/or required intervention to preclude harm

No Error

Error, No Harm

Error, Harm

Error, Death

Definitions

Harm
Impairment of the physical, emotional, or psychological function or structure of the body and/or pain resulting therefrom.

Monitoring
To observe or record relevant physiological or psychological signs.

Intervention
May include change in therapy or active medical/surgical treatment.

Intervention Necessary to Sustain Life
Includes cardiovascular and respiratory support (e.g., CPR, defibrillation, intubation, etc.)

projects to experiment with transferring ideas from industry to improve safety and quality in health care.

PRHI and its partners are now starting to prove that improving quality of care not only benefits patients, but saves money. A template is emerging that confirms one of PRHI's foundational beliefs: that quality is the business case. For more information go to [www.prhi.org].

OTHER VOLUNTARY PROGRAMS

The Department of Veterans Affairs (VA) developed in collaboration with NASA a voluntary, confidential, non-punitive external learning system for employees of the Vin 2000. This system, called the Patient Safety Reporting System (PSRS) was implemented system-wide in 2002. It encourages the reporting of any issue or concern that affects patient safety. PSRS is modeled after NASA's successful and long-standing Aviation Safety Reporting System (ASRS), which it developed and has administered for the Federal Aviation Administration since 1976.

Part of the success of this program is not only the improved patient safety culture of the VA but the legal and procedural protection afforded under 38 USC 5705. For more information visit [www.psrs.arc.nasa.gov/flashsite/programoverview/index.html].

EXHIBIT 20.4   NCC MERP Index for Categorizing Medication Errors Algorithm

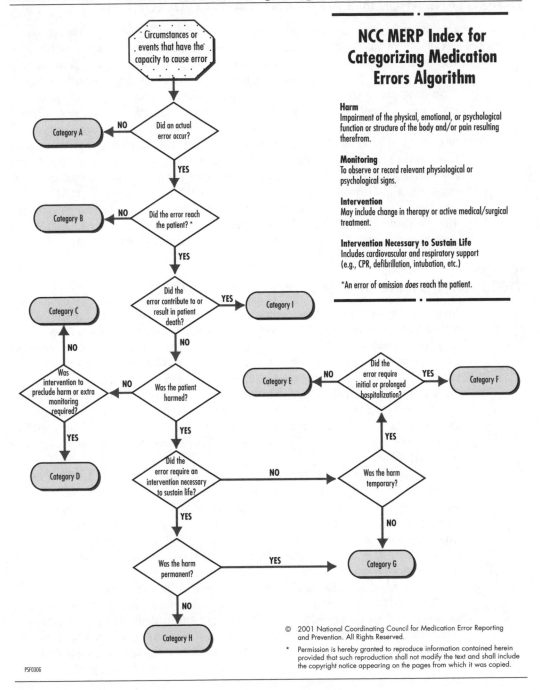

NCC MERP Index for Categorizing Medication Errors Algorithm

Harm
Impairment of the physical, emotional, or psychological function or structure of the body and/or pain resulting therefrom.

Monitoring
To observe or record relevant physiological or psychological signs.

Intervention
May include change in therapy or active medical/surgical treatment.

Intervention Necessary to Sustain Life
Includes cardiovascular and respiratory support (e.g., CPR, defibrillation, intubation, etc.)

*An error of omission *does* reach the patient.

PSF0306

. . . .

NQF: STANDARDIZING A PATIENT SAFETY TAXONOMY[21]

Until recently, there was no common method to classify or aggregate patient safety data because there was no standardized and consensus-driven definition of terms or language with which all institutions and providers of care could communicate effectively. The National Quality Forum (NQF) recently published a Consensus Report called *Standardizing a Patient Safety Taxonomy*. The NQF has endorsed this taxonomy and conveyed to it the special legal standing of a voluntary consensus standard. The Taxonomy is not a reporting system. It is a classification methodology by which data can be organized and analyzed. It is a tool to allow providers and organizations to turn data into information from which patient safety solutions can be developed and implemented. The report presents a set of four voluntary consensus standards around a specific patient safety taxonomy. This taxonomy is called the Patient Safety Event Taxonomy™ (PSET). It was developed by the JCAHO with the assistance of workgroups and the federal government. The effectiveness of the PSET will be its usefulness over time in providing better decision support at the point of care and with system design and policy development.

. . . .

THE PROTECTION OF SENSITIVE INFORMATION

Information assembled from medical error reporting systems does not have federal protection from discovery on a global basis. Although many states offer a level of protection through peer review, quality assurance, and risk management laws, attempts to implement a federal protection have not been successful to date. Organizations also rely on attorney-client privilege and work product protections to safeguard information regarding the investigation and analysis of the more serious patient events or catastrophic claims. Health care organizations shield sensitive information with several acceptable methods. Organizations fear the release of information gathered from early warning systems because such information could be used against them in the court of public opinion and in a court of law.

The reporting of catastrophic events to the Joint Commission on Accreditation of Healthcare Organizations under the JCAHO Sentinel Event Policy brought this issue to the forefront. Many hospitals determined that preparing RCA reports and reporting sentinel events to the JCAHO without explicit legal protection might place the organizations in jeopardy for the discovery of sensitive documents. The JCAHO being sensitive to their constituents' concerns created alternative methods to comply. See the earlier section on JCAHO Sentinel Event Reporting.

In November 2004, Floridians passed Amendment 7 by a large majority.[22]

Dr. Paul Barach, Associate Professor, Department of Anesthesiology and Medicine, Associate Dean for Patient Safety at the University of Miami Medical School explains that "Amendment 7, the 'Patients' Right To Know About Adverse Medical Incidents Act,' allows full access to all patient records related to adverse medical events, turning back twenty years of quality assurance (QA) and peer review protection. The broad definition of the new law allowed patients, families, and their attorneys access to all records kept by a facility, including all meetings, morbidity and mortality conferences, root cause analyses, and any other professional exchange of information related to a patient's injury or death.

In April 2005, the Florida legislature partly narrowed the application and interpretation of the new law, but damage to the health care system had been done. Reporting of events started to decline, and the fear of weakened peer review and QA protection had permeated the state. Anecdotal evidence suggests that morbidity and mortality conferences have either stopped or have been greatly sanitized; many now use fictitious data during case presentations. They have put a chill on the reporting of all patient events and have put a damper on patient safety and sensitive quality improvement research. The passage of Amendment 7 has led to an alarming wave of paranoia among health care providers and administration in discussing patient safety initiatives."[23]

The developments in Florida illustrate the difficulty that health care providers have with the reporting of medical errors. A primary cause for a hospital's failure to report adverse events might be in direct relationship to its inability to ensure data confidentiality. The only way to fully protect medical error reports from legal discovery is through legislation.[24]

Patient Safety and Quality Improvement Act of 2005

The National Patient Safety and Quality Improvement Act of 2005 signed into law July 29, 2005, by President George W. Bush was established to create a national database on medical errors, create and allow for the development of Patient Safety Organizations (PSO), and provide both a privilege and confidentiality protection for certain patient safety work product (PSWP) gathered under a patient safety evaluation system (PSES).

The Department of Health and Human Services (DHHS) will compile and maintain a list of PSOs whose certification has been accepted by the Secretary of the DHHS. To date there are no approved PSOs.

It is still too early to deliver concrete information about the implications and ramifications of this new Act. It is hoped that over time the language that now appears to be confusing and ambiguous will become clear. Currently, there seem to be more questions than answers:

- How will the Act interact with existing state mandatory reporting requirements for medical error?
- How will the Act interface with the Patient Safety Event Taxonomy?
- How will the Act interpret the confidentiality and privilege for each state?
- How will the Act further define patient safety work product and patient safety evaluation systems? Currently those definitions appear vague and ambiguous.

How these and other questions are resolved will determine the ease of implementing the PSQIA of 2005.

....

CONCLUSION

Risk management professionals confront challenges today unheard of just a few years ago. The requirements for data collection and information reporting are staggering. The complexity of risk and development and implementation of sophisticated solutions requires continuous education. How risk management professionals manage responsibilities and day-to-day activities is an accomplishment in its own right. Prioritizing and simplifying activities are therefore important steps in gaining and maintaining control. Assessing the organization for its exposure to loss and the development of a robust early warning system to identify risk will enable the risk management professional to prioritize and focus efforts on risk areas of greatest frequency and severity while advancing patient safety efforts.

Endnotes

1. American Institute for CPCU and Insurance Institute of America. Malvern, Pa. Information available at [www.aicpcu.org]. Accessed May 2006.

2. Membership information available for the American Society for Healthcare Risk Management at [www.ashrm.org].

3. Florida §395.0197 internal risk management programs (hospitals).

4. Florida §400.147 internal risk management and quality assurance program (LTC).

5. Florida §641.55 (2) Every organization which has an annual premium volume of $10 million or more and which directly provides health care in a building owned or leased by the organization shall hire a risk manager, certified under ss. 395.10971–395.10975, who shall be responsible for implementation of the organization's risk management program required by this section. A part-time risk manager shall not be responsible for risk management programs in more than four organizations or facilities. Every organization which does not directly provide health care in a building owned or leased by the organization and every organization with an annual premium volume of less than $10 million shall designate an officer or employee of the organization to serve as the risk manager. (HMO)

6. Maley, R. A. "Building Risk Management into Integrated Healthcare Delivery Systems." *Journal of Healthcare Risk Management,* 16(4), Fall 1996, pp. 31–40.

7. Gautam, N. "Ounce of Prevention–To Reduce Errors, Hospitals Prescribe Innovative Designs." *Wall Street Journal.* May 8, 2006 Vol. CCXLVII. No. 107, p. 1.

8. American Society for Healthcare Risk Management. *Mapping Your Risk Management Course in Ambulatory Care.* Chicago: ASHRM, 1995, pp. 12–13.

9. Medical Risk Management Associates, LLC. What is the difference between root cause analysis (RCA) and failure mode and effects analysis (FMEA)? Available online at [www.sentinel-event.com/rca-fmea.php]. Site accessed May 8, 2006.

10. JCAHO online available at [www.jointcommission.org/SentinelEvents/]. Site accessed May 7, 2006.

11. JCAHO sentinel event policy available on online at [www.jointcommission.org/ JointCommission/Templates/GeneralInformation.aspx?NRMODE= Published&NRORIGINALURL=%2fSentinelEvents%2fPolicyandProcedures% 2fse_pp%2ehtm&NRNODEGUID=%7bB37C3E00-728F-46AC-82AD-B6426A11ACCB% 7d&NRCACHEHINT=Guest#four]. Site accessed May 7, 2006.

12. *Ibid.* Rape, as a reviewable sentinel event, is defined as unconsented sexual contact involving a patient and another patient, staff member, or unknown perpetrator while being treated or on the premises of the health care organization, including oral, vaginal, or anal penetration or fondling of the patient's sex organ(s) by another individual's hand, sex organ, or object. One or more of the following must be present to determine reviewability:

    • Any staff witnessed sexual contact as described above

    • Sufficient clinical evidence obtained by the organization to support allegations of unconsented sexual contact

    • Admission by the perpetrator that sexual contact, as described above, occurred on the premises.

13. *Ibid.* JCAHO Sentinel Event Policy.

14. National Academy for State Health Policy. For a complete listing of states with adverse event reporting requirements visit [www.nashp.org]. Site accessed May 6, 2006.

15. Rosenthal J., M. Booth. Defining Reportable Adverse Events: A Guide for States Tracking Medical Errors, March 2003 GNL50 National Academy for State Health Policy [www.nashp.org].

16. Information available at [www.fda.gov]. Site accessed May 6, 2006.

17. For more information on mandatory reporting and to obtain the mandatory FDA form 3500A, go to [www.fda.gov/medwatch/REPORT/mtg.htm] for drugs/biologics, or [www.fda.gov.cdrh/mdr/] for devices.

18. Information available at [www.nccmerp.org/medErrorCatIndex.html]. Site accessed May 6, 2006.

19. Forms available online at [www.nccmerp.org/pdf/indexBW2001-06-12.pdf]. Site accessed May 6, 2006.

20. Form available online at [www.nccmerp.org/pdf/algorBW2001-06-12.pdf]. Site accessed May 6, 2006.

21. NQF Standardizing a Patient Safety Taxonomy—A Consensus Report ©2006 by the National Quality Forum. Washington D.C. [www.quality forum.org].

22. Vote Smart Florida available at [www.votesmartflorida.org/votesmarthw/hw.dll?page&file=trendbi].

2004	*Amendment Title*	*% of Turnout*	*Yes*
7	Patients' Right to Know About Adverse Medical Incidents	94.3%	5,849,125

23. Barach, P. Perspectives on Safety, The unintended consequences of Florida Medical Liability Legislation. AHRQ WebM&M available at [www.webmm.ahrq.gov/perspective.aspx?perspectiveID=14].

24. Implementation Planning Study for the Integration of Medical Event Reporting Input and Data Structure for Reporting to AHRQ, CDC, CMS, and FDA. Submitted by the Medstat Group, Santa Barbara, CA. June 2002 Final Report Volume 1. Technical Report, p. 5.

Glossary

Sources

The terms and definitions listed in this glossary have been compiled from the following sources:

1. ASHRM Barton Certificate in Healthcare Risk Management Program;
2. Iowa Hospital Association, "Common Health Care Abbreviations & Terminology";
3. Farmers Insurance Group, "Risk Management Definitions";
4. Risk Management Handbook for Health Care Organizations, Third and Fourth Editions

AAAASF	American Association for Accreditation of Ambulatory Surgery Facilities, Inc., http://www.aaaasf.org
AAAHC	Accreditation Association for Ambulatory Health Care, Inc., http://www.aaahc.org
AABB	American Association for Blood Banks, http://www.aabb.org
AAHP	American Association of Health Plans
AAHRPP	Association for the Accreditation of Human Research Protection Programs, Inc., http://www.aahrpp.org
AAMC	Association of American Medical Colleges, http://www.aamc.org
AANA	American Association of Nurse Anesthetists, http://www.aana.com
AAP	American Academy of Pediatrics, http://www.aap.org
AARP	American Association of Retired Persons
Abd.	Abdominal
ABMS	American Board of Medical Specialties, http://www.abms.org
Abuse	The willful infliction of injury, unreasonable confinement, intimidation, or punishment with resulting harm, pain, or mental anguish
	Definition (fraud and abuse) describes practices that result in unnecessary costs to the Medicare/Medicaid program and other payor sources. Patient abuse is deliberate, non-accidental contact or interaction that results in significant psychological harm, pain or physical injury.
"Access" problem	Issues relating to impediments that restrict or limit persons in need of specific healthcare services from receiving them, e.g., lack of health insurance
Accident (medical)	An unintended occurrence resulting in injury or death that is not the result of willful action. Generally an accident means that it resulted in some degree of injury or harm to the person(s) involved. In the medical field, the term "accident" is generally not used to describe an event associated with clinical care, but refers to other types of events.
	An event that involves damage to a defined system that disrupts the ongoing or future output of the system.
ACEP	American College of Emergency Physicians, http://www.acep.org
ACGME	Accreditation Council for Graduate Medical Education, http://www.acgme.org
ACHE	American College of Healthcare Executives, http://www.ache.org
ACLS	Advanced cardiac life support
ACS	American Cancer Society
ACOG	The American College of Obstetricians and Gynecologists, http://www.acog.org
Acquired Immune Deficiency Syndrome (AIDS)	Fatal, incurable disease caused by a virus that can destroy the body's ability to fight off illness resulting in recurrent opportunistic infections or secondary diseases afflicting multiple body systems

Acquisition	A business transaction in which one corporation or entity purchases or otherwise acquires all of the assets or stock of another entity or organization
ACR	American College of Radiology, http://www.acr.org
ACS	American College of Surgeons, http://www.facs.org
ACU	Ambulatory care unit
Active error	An error that occurs at the level of the frontline operator and whose effects are felt almost immediately
Actuarial analysis	A study performed by a professional known as an actuary aimed at predicting the frequency and severity of claims for a specific line of insurance coverage for a future time period. Such an analysis includes both an estimation of the ultimate value of known claims and an estimation of the number and value of claims that have occurred but have not yet been reported.
Actuarial study	An analysis performed by a recognized actuary that determines appropriate funding levels required for operation of a selfinsurance trust
Actuary	A person who uses statistics to compute loss probabilities to establish premiums for insurance companies and self-insurance trusts
Acuity	Degree or severity of illness
Acute Care Hospital	Typically a community hospital which has services designed to meet the needs of patients who require short-term care for a period of less than 30 days
ADA	See Americans With Disabilities Act
	Also American Diabetes Association
Additional insured	A person or entity added to an insurance policy by endorsement at the request of the named insured, often after the inception of the policy. Frequently required by contracts in order to give one contracting party the benefit of insurance coverage maintained by the other
ADE	Adverse Drug Event
ADEA	See Age Discrimination in Employment Act
Admission	An out of court statement made by a person who is a party to the action. Admissions are normally admissible into evidence at trial.
ADR	Alternative dispute resolution
Ad testificandum	Used to require recipient to give testimony
Advance Directives	A legal document that outlines a person's wishes concerning health-care services should the person be unable to communicate those wishes
	Written instructions recognized under law relating to the provision of health car when an individual is incapacitated. An advance directive takes two forms: living wills and durable power of attorney for health care
Adverse Drug Reports (ADRs)	A known or unknown, undesirable side effect or reaction to a medication. "An unintended act (either an omission or commission) or an act that does not achieve its intended outcome" (Lucian Leape)
Adverse event	A negative or bad result stemming from a diagnostic test, medical treatment or surgical intervention
	An injury resulting from a medical intervention

Adverse medication event	An unintended deviation from how one or more steps in the routine/regular medication prescribing, dispensing or administration processes is carried out. Under this definition, the patient may or may not have been harmed, and there may or may not be some degree of provider or system "fault" or negligence associated with the adverse medication event.
Adverse outcome	A clinical outcome that, while neither desirable nor necessarily anticipated, may still have been a known "possibility" associated with the treatment or procedure. Under this definition, using the term "adverse outcome" does not imply that any provider was negligent or any "error" in process or system factors contributed to the adverse outcome.
AED	Automatic External Defibrillator
AERS	Adverse Event Reporting System
Affidavit	A written statement made under oath, without notice to the adverse party. A written or printed declaration or statement of facts, made voluntarily, and confirmed by the oath, or affirmation of the party making it, taken before an officer having authority to administer such oath
Age Discrimination	The denial of privileges as well as other unfair treatment of employees on the basis of age. Age discrimination is prohibited by federal law under the Age Discrimination in Employment Act of 1978 to protect employees between the ages of 40 and 70 years of age
Age Discrimination in Employment Act	29 U.S.C. Section 621 et seq. The federal statute prohibiting certain types of employment discrimination on the basis of age
Agency by *estoppel*	See Ostensible Agency Doctrine
Aggregate limit	The maximum amount the insurer will pay during the policy period, irrespective of the policy's limit of liability
AHA	American Hospital Association, http://www.aha.org
	American Heart Association
AHCA	American Health Care Association, http://www.ahca.org
AHERA	Asbestos Hazard Emergency Response Act
AHRQ	Agency for Healthcare Research & Quality, http://www.ahrq.gov
	A component of the Public Health Services (PHS) responsible for research on quality, appropriateness, effectiveness, and cost of health care
AICPCU	American Institute for Chartered Property Casualty Underwriters, http://www.aicpcu.org
AIDS	Acquired immune deficiency syndrome
Allegation	The assertion, declaration or statement of a person setting out what the party to an action expects to prove. Made in a pleading.
Allied Health Professional	A specially trained non-physician health care provider. Allied health professionals include: paramedics, physician assistants (P:A), certified nurse midwives (CNM), phlebotomists, social workers, nurse practitioners (NP), and other caregivers who perform tasks that supplement physician services
Allocated Loss Adjustment Expense (ALAE)	Money paid in the claims resolution process. Includes defense attorney fees, court costs, expert witness fees and photocopy costs attributed directly to an individual claim.

Alternative Delivery Systems	Health services provided in other than an inpatient, acute care hospital, such as skilled and nursing facilities, hospice programs, and home health care
Alternative Dispute Resolution	Any method of resolving a dispute other than formal civil litigation. May include arbitration, mediation or "black box."
Alternative Risk Financing (or Funding) (ARF)	Any of a number of mechanisms employed by individuals or organizations to pay for claims other than through the use of traditional insurance programs, including various types of captive insurance companies, risk retention groups, self-insurance trust funds, etc.
Alternative Treatment Plan	Provision in managed care arrangements for treatment usually outside of a hospital
AMA	American Medical Association, http://www.ama-assn.org
AMAP	American Medical Accreditation Program
Ambulatory	Not confined to a bed—capable of moving
Ambulatory Care	Medical care provided on an outpatient basis
Americans with Disabilities Act	42 U.S.C. Section 12101 et seq. A federal statute aimed at prohibiting discrimination against individuals with certain mental and physical disabilities in the areas of employment and public accommodation
ANA	American Nurses Association, http://www.nursingworld.org
Ancillary	A term used to describe services that relate to a patient's care such as lab work, x-ray, and anesthesia.
Annuity	A fixed sum payable periodically, subject to the limitations imposed by the grantor
ANP	Advanced Nurse Practitioner
Answer	A document filed with the court in response to a Complaint or Petition. The Answer must generally (1) admit that the plaintiff's allegations are true; (2) deny that the plaintiff's allegations are true; or (3) state that the defendant does not have information regarding the truth or falsity of the allegations.
Anti-kickback statutes	Medicare-Medicaid Antikickback Statute (42 USC §1320a-7b) "Knowingly and willfully" seeking or receiving a bribe, rebate or kickback for a referral for a program, reimbursable item or service "Knowingly or willfully" seeking or receiving a bribe, rebate or kickback with the intent to induce a referral for a program, reimbursable item or service
Antitrust Laws	Generally, any law that is designed to discourage or prohibit restraints of free trade, to unfairly reduce or eliminate competition, or to unfairly prevent entrance into a marketplace
Any willing provider laws	Statutes in some jurisdictions prohibiting managed care organizations (MCOs) from discriminating among licensed providers of healthcare services and requiring that the MCO reimburse any licensed provider willing to accept the MCOs reimbursement schedule for the provision of covered services to a plan beneficiary
AOA	American Osteopathic Association, http://www.aoa-net.org
AONE	American Organizations of Nurse Executives

AORN	Association of Perioperative Registered Nurses, http://www.aorn.org
Apparent agency	See Ostensible Agency
Appeal	An action that is taken after the trial of a matter, or after a dispositive motion has been entered in a matter. An appeal may be taken for the purpose of correcting an error made by the trial court or to obtain a new trial.
	A resort to a higher court for the purpose of obtaining a review of a lower court decision and a reversal of the lower court's judgment or granting of a new trial
Appellate Court	A court that is empowered to hear appeals. There are normally two tiers of appellate courts: an intermediate appellate court (e.g., U.S. Circuit Courts of Appeal) and a supreme court (e.g., U.S. Supreme Court, New York Court of Appeals). Some states have only one tier of appellate court.
Arbiter	A neutral third party who issues a decision binding on the parties in a formal or informal hearing on a disagreement
Arbitration	The hearing and determination of a case in controversy by a person either chosen by the parties in opposition or by a person appointed under statutory authority
	A method of dispute resolution used as an alternative to litigation
	Submission by the parties of a dispute to one or more individuals who then decide the controversy. May be binding (final) or nonbinding (aggrieved party may appeal or pursue conventional civil litigation)
Arbitration Clause	A clause in a contract providing for arbitration of disputes arising under contract. Arbitration clauses are treated as separable part of the contract so that the illegality of another part of the contract does not nullify such agreement and a breach of repudiation of the contract does not preclude the right to arbitrate.
ARC	American Red Cross
Archiving	Retaining and organizing expired insurance policies or revised policies and procedures to facilitate the determination of provisions in place at a specific past point in time
ARM	Associate in Risk Management
ARM-P	Associate in Risk Management for Public Entities
ART	Accredited Record Technician
ASA	American Society of Anesthesiologists, http://www.asahq.org
ASC	Ambulatory surgery center
ASCP	The American Society for Clinical Pathology, http://www.ascp.org
ASHE	American Society for Healthcare Engineering, http://www.ashe.org
ASHP	American Society of Health-System Pharmacists, http://www.ashp.org
ASHRM	American Society for Healthcare Risk Management, http://www.ashrm.org
ASRS	Aviation Safety Reporting System
Assault	An intentional act that is designed to make the victim fearful and that produces reasonable apprehension of harm

Assignment	The act of transferring to another all or part of one's property, interest, or rights
Association	An unincorporated group of persons assembled for a specific purpose or to complete a specific project. Unless the state has a specific statute governing the liabilities of the members, each member may be liable for the debts and obligations of the association.
Association or Group Captive	Jointly owned by a number of companies that are usually affiliated through a trade, industry or service group
Assumption of Risk	Understanding the risks associated with a particular course of action and agreeing to accept those risks.
	An affirmative defense in a negligence case which alleges that the plaintiff knew of the danger involved in what he was doing, did nothing to prevent his own injury and therefore, as a result, must bear the consequences of the action and cannot ask for the defendant to pay for his injury.
ASTM	American Society for Testing and Materials, http://www.astm.org
ATLS	Advanced trauma life support
Attorney-client privilege	A legal doctrine recognized by both common and statutory law protecting certain confidential communications between an attorney and his or her client from discovery in a legal proceeding unless the privilege is waived by the client
	A confidential communication between an attorney and a client in the course of a professional relationship which cannot be disclosed without the consent of the client
Attorney work product privilege	A legal doctrine recognized by both common and statutory law protecting the documents generated, theories devised, legal strategies formulated, etc., by an attorney on behalf of a client from discovery in a legal proceeding unless the privilege is waived by the client
Automatic Dispensing Cabinet	A cabinet that by its design has certain controls and documentation features that dispense medications pursuant to individualized patient drug profiles, ordered by a physician, and confirmed by a pharmacist
AVP	Assistant Vice President
AWHONN	Association of Women's Health, Obstetric, and Neonatal Nurses
BAA	Business Associate Agreement
Back pay	In employment practices liability claims, a demand for or award of damages asking the defendant to pay the employee's wages from the time of the alleged improper act (such as wrongful termination) to the time of the settlement or judgment by the court in the employee's favor. In cases in which it is alleged that the employee was improperly denied a promotion or salary increase, back pay represents the difference in the wages actually earned by the employee and those that would have been earned had the promotion or salary increase not have been denied.
Bad outcome	Failure to achieve a desired outcome of care
Bar Code Technology	A computer identification system that uses unique bar-stripe code to identify specific items, medications or patients. Most often used with a scanning device to read, or verify, each code

Battery	The touching of one person by another without permission. See Medical Battery
BBA	Balanced Budget Act of 1997
BBRA	Balanced Budget Relief Act of 1999
BCAA	Blue Cross Association of America
Benchmarking	A comparative process used by organizations to collect and measure internal or external data that may ultimately be used for the purpose of developing, implementing, and sustaining quality improvements
	A process, which identifies best practices and performance standards, to create normative or comparative standards (benchmark) as a measurement tool. By comparing an organization against a national or regional benchmark, providers are able to establish measurable goals as part of the strategic planning and Total Quality Management (TQM) processes
Benevolent gesture	Actions taken to communicate a sense of compassion or compensation arising from humane feelings, when there is no implication (direct or implied) as to "fault" for having contributed to or caused the outcome
BI	See Business Interruption Insurance Coverage
BIPA	Benefits Improvement & Protection Act of 2000
BLS	Basic life support
BLS	Bureau of Labor Statistics
Board Certified	Describes a physician who is certified as a specialist in his/her area of practice. To achieve board certification, a physician must meet specific standards of knowledge and clinical skills within a specific field or specialty. Usually, this means completion of a supervised program of certified clinical residency and the physician passing both an oral and written examination given by a medical specialty group.
Board Eligible	Describes a physician who has graduated from a board-approved medical school, completed an accredited training program, practiced for a specified length of time, and is eligible to take a specialty board examination within a specific amount of time.
Boiler & Machinery Coverage	Provides protection for explosion of boilers and other pressure vessels and accidental damage to equipment
	Covers resulting damage to other property, including property in your care, for which you are liable
	Covers the cost of temporary repairs as well as the additional cost incurred to expedite repairs
	Coverage is written on a "cost to repair or replace" basis and is not subject to depreciation
Borrowed Servant	A person whose services an original employer loan, with his/her acquiescence or consent, to a second employer to whose control and direction he/she becomes wholly subject, free during the temporary period from the control of the original employer
BP	Blood pressure
Brain death	Total irreversible cessation of cerebral function, as well as spontaneous function of the respiratory and the circulatory systems

Breach of contract	Failure, without legal excuse, to perform any promise that forms the whole or part of a contract. Also, hindrance by a party regarding the required performance of the rights and duties identified in the contract
Broker	A person who represents a buyer of insurance in negotiations with the underwriter and who serves as a consultant on various aspects of the buyer's insurance program
BTLS	Basic trauma life support
BUN	Blood urea nitrogen
Business interruption insurance coverage	Insurance coverage typically provided as a part of a property insurance policy covering the lost revenues and extra operating expenses associated with a covered loss such as a fire Attempts to replace revenues lost due to covered loss
C-Section	Cesarean Section
CAA	Clean Air Act
CAAS	Commission on Accreditation of Ambulance Services
CABG	Coronary artery bypass graft
CAHPS	Consumer Assessment of Health Plans
CAMTS	Commission on Accreditation of Medical Transport Systems
CAP	College of American Pathologists
Capitation	In managed care contracts, a payment methodology in which a provider is paid a set fee, often per member per month, to provide designated healthcare services to individuals covered by the managed care plan. The fee remains constant regardless of how much or how little healthcare service is actually provided.
Captain of the Ship Doctrine	Doctrine that imposes liability on a surgeon in charge of an operation for the negligence of his assistants during the period when those servants are under the surgeon's control, even though those servants are also employees of the healthcare entity
Captive insurance company	An insurance company established to provide insurance coverage to a sponsoring entity as opposed to marketing and selling policies commercially to insureds. The sponsoring entity may be a parent corporation and its related subsidiaries, a professional association or other group.
CARF	See Commission on Accreditation of Rehabilitation Facilities
Cardiac Catheterization	A procedure used to diagnose disorders of the heart, lungs, and great vessels
CARME	Center for the Advancement of Risk Management Education
Case management	See Utilization Management.
	A managed care technique in which a patient with a serious medical condition is assigned an individual who arranges for costeffective treatment, often outside a hospital
CAT	Computerized axial tomography
	Diagnostic equipment which produces cross-sectional images of the head and/or body

Catastrophic protection	Protects against the adverse effects of large losses from natural forces or man-made disasters
Cause of Action	The fact or facts that give the plaintiff the legal grounds to seek damages from another person. It is necessary to have a cause (or causes) of action in order to bring and sustain a lawsuit.
CBC	Complete blood count
CBRN	Chemical, Biological, Radiological and Nuclear (countermeasures)
CCAC	Continuing Care Accreditation Commission
CCHSA	Canadian Council on Health Services Accreditation
CCRN	Certification in critical care nursing
CCU	Cardiac care unit
CDC	See Centers for Disease Control
Census	The number of inpatients who receive hospital care each day excluding newborns.
Centers for Disease Control	The arm of the U.S. Department of Health and Human Services, U.S. Public Health Service responsible for tracking mortality and morbidity statistics among the U.S. population and for making recommendations for a variety of public health measures, often focused on communicable diseases
Centers for Medicare and Medicaid Services	Formerly Health Care Financing Administration (HCFA) The federal agency responsible for administering Medicare, Medicaid and the State Children's Health Insurance Program (SCHIP)
CEO	See Chief Executive Officer
CERCLA	Comprehensive Environmental Response, Compensation and Liability Act
CERT	Centers for Education and Research in Therapeutics
Certificate of insurance	A standardized form, usually produced by the insurance agent or broker who arranged for the coverage, evidencing specific insurance in place, the insurance carrier, policy period, policy number, etc.
CFO	See Chief Financial Officer
CGL	See Commercial General Liability
CHAP	Community Health Accreditation Program
Chain of command	Mechanism approved by appropriate bodies (i.e.: administration, medical staff and nursing) that allows staff members a forum or process to air concerns and deal with difficult situations. It typically defines the route or hierarchy for pursuing such concerns.
Chain of evidence	Procedure to insure that the location and integrity of evidence (blood, clothing, weapons, etc.) collected is at all times accountable from when it is collected to when it is turned over to the police or court.
Charitable Immunity Doctrine	A doctrine that relieves a charity of liability in tort; long recognized, but currently most states have abrogated or restricted such immunity
Chemotherapy	In the treatment of disease, the application of chemical reagents which have a specific and toxic effect upon the disease-causing microorganism

Chief executive officer	The corporate officer charged with responsibility for the financial and operational performance of the company. Often the CEO also carries the title of president.
Chief financial officer	The corporate officer charged with responsibility for overseeing the finance and accounting functions of the company, including reporting financial information to the public and to regulatory agencies, and interfacing with independent financial auditors
Chief Operating Officer	The corporate officer charged with responsibility for the operations of the company
Chief risk officer	The corporate officer charged with responsibility for identifying and managing a variety of financial, legal, strategic and hazard risks faced by the organization. Distinguished from a traditional risk manager, whose role is generally confined to identifying and managing hazard risks
CICU	Cardiac intensive care unit
CISM	Critical incident stress management
Civil False Claims	Enables lawsuits by government or any individual ("qui tam relator") against one who submits a false claim to the government
Civil Law	The system of laws by which one person may bring an action against another person seeking compensatory or punitive damages, or injunctive relief. Also refers to the predominant theory of laws established by the governments of most western European countries (with the exception of the United Kingdom)
Civil Rights Act of 1964	42 U.S.C. Section 2000 et seq. Broad federal statute prohibiting discrimination on the basis of race, color, creed or national origin in a variety of settings, including employment
Claim	The amount of damage for which an insured seeks reimbursement from an insurance company. Once the amount has been determined, it becomes a loss.
Claimant	Someone who brings a claim for alleged injuries.
Claims-made insurance policy	An insurance policy covering claims that are made during the policy period and that occurred since the policy retroactive date. Although policy definitions vary somewhat, most claims-made insurance policies consider a claim to be made when it is first reported to the insurance company, subject to certain terms and conditions. Claims-made policies are common for professional liability and directors and officers liability insurance.
Claims management	A systemized approach to reducing the financial loss and negative community image of a healthcare organization in situations where prevention fails and injury occurs
Class actions	Lawsuits, frequently liability lawsuits, including a number of similarly situated plaintiffs whose cases are factually almost identical. Joining all of the plaintiffs into a single lawsuit expedites pretrial discovery and prevents multiple trials on the same issues and can provide a forum for plaintiffs whose individual damages may be quite small. Seen most frequently in products liability and employment practices litigation
CLIA	Clinical Laboratory Improvement Act
	Certification standards for laboratories established to consolidate the requirements for Medicare participation with rules for laboratories

engaged in interstate testing under the CLIA '67 program; standards contain new quality control and quality assurance, proficiency testing, and personnel requirements

Clinical Practice Guidelines
Also known as Clinical Pathways

Clinical research trials
Use of experimental drugs, devices or protocols on human subjects in a clinical setting under a set of prescribed procedures as part of the FDA approval process

CMP
Civil monetary penalties

CMS
See Centers for Medicare and Medicaid Services

CNM
Certified Nurse-Mid Wife

CNS
Central nervous system

COB
Coordination of benefits

Designates the anti-duplication provision designed by the group health insurance to limit benefits where there is multiple coverage in a particular case to 100 percent of the expenses covered, and to designate the order in which the multiple carriers are to pay benefits

COBRA
See the Consolidated Omnibus Budget Reconciliation Act of 1986

Co-defendant
A defendant who has been joined together with one or more other defendants in a single action.

Code Blue
Indicates an emergency situation has occurred and mobilizes staff to respond

COI
Certificate of Insurance

COLA
Commission of Office Laboratory Accreditation

Collateral-source benefits
Amounts that a plaintiff recovers from sources other than the defendant, such as the plaintiff's own insurance

Collective bargaining
Collective bargaining consists of negotiations between an employer and a group of employees so as to determine the conditions of employment. The result of collective bargaining procedures is a collective agreement. Employees are often represented in bargaining by a union or other labor organization.

Combined ratio
A measure of insurance company profitability calculated by adding the ratio of losses incurred/premium and the ratio expenses incurred/ premium

Commercial Auto Coverage
Protects against loss arising out of the ownership, maintenance, and use of automobiles and their equipment, both those you own, hire, or borrow, and those you don't own but may be responsible for, such as the personal car of an employee used to run a company errand

Commercial General Liability
Protects against financial loss resulting from liability to third parties arising out of the premises you own or occupy, acts of independent contractors hired by you, products you sell when they leave your premises and liability you assume under contract, subject to exclusions of the policy

Coverage applies to Bodily Injury, Property Damage and Personal Injury

Commission Error
Incorrect action performed, or an intended action that was improperly performed

Common cause
Factor that results from variation inherent in the process or system

Common Law	A system of laws in which the building blocks of the substantive law must be gleaned from decided cases, as opposed to statutory law
Compensatory damages	Damages sought or awarded to a plaintiff in a liability action to compensate him or her for losses, such as lost wages or medical expenses and for pain and suffering
Complaint	One of the initial filings with a court to begin a lawsuit. The Complaint normally recites all of the allegations against the defendant and theories upon which the plaintiff seeks to recover damages. May be called a Petition in some jurisdictions
Complementary medicine	Any of a number of therapies and treatment modalities, alone or in combination, utilized for the treatment or alleviation of specific symptoms or disease, which fall outside of those traditionally employed by physicians, surgeons and dentists, including acupuncture, massage therapy, herbal medicine, etc. Sometimes referred to as complementary and alternative medicine. Complementary and alternative medicine treatments often take a holistic approach to care and treatment and may include an emphasis on the spiritual dimensions of healing.
Complication	Undesired, unintended but often known negative clinical symptoms or physical injury that resulted from medical treatment. Also known as Clinical Complication
Computed Tomography Scan	The gathering of anatomical information from a cross-sectional plane of the body, presented as an image generated by a computer synthesis of x-ray transmission data obtained in many different directions through a given plane
Computer-aided Decision Support System	Computers with embedded knowledge (through software applications) that enhances clinicians' use of scientifically based patient care information
Computerized Practitioner Order Entry	A computerized system for prescriptions (or other orders) to be directly entered by the provider, thereby eliminating the transcription process. May or may not have CDSS embedded therein
CON	Certificate of need
Conditions of Participation	Requirements that hospitals must meet to participate in the Medicare and Medicaid programs
	Intended to protect patient health and safety and to assure that high quality care is provided to all patients
Confirmation Bias	The human tendency to prematurely form a conclusion based on a preconceived expectation
Consideration	In contract law, something of value exchanged for the promised performance of the other contracting party. Contracts frequently call for monetary consideration to be exchanged for the promise to provide specified goods or services.
The Consolidated Omnibus Budget Reconciliation Act of 1986	It provides in part for continuation of health coverage applicable to group health plans. Federal law thatrequires employers with more than 20 employees to extend group health insurance coverage for at least 18 months after employees leave their jobs. Employees must pay 100 percent of the premium
Constitution	A relatively short document enacted by a state or federal government that specifies the essential nature of governance by the elected legislature, and which generally restrains the actions of military or police forces, and the power exercised by regulatory agencies

Constructive termination	In employment law, a situation in which, even though an employee is not formally terminated from his or her position, the conditions of employment become so manifestly untenable that the employee had no choice but to quit and thus are treated by the court as a termination
Contingency fee	A fee for service, collectable only if the outcome is favorable to the payee
Contract	An agreement, either written or oral, involving an offer, the acceptance of the offer and an exchange of consideration
	An agreement between two or more persons that creates an obligation to do or not to do a particular thing. A promise or set of promises for the breach of which the law gives a remedy, or the performance of which the law in some way recognizes as a duty
Contributory Negligence	Conduct on the part of the plaintiff that falls below the standard to which he/she should conform for his/her own protection which is a legally contributing cause in addition to the negligence of the defendant
	If the claimant is himself negligent, and his negligence concurs with that of the health care provider to cause the injury, claimant cannot recover
COO	See Chief Operating Officer
COPs	See Conditions of Participation for Hospitals in Medicare and Medicaid. This term also applies to Skilled Nursing Facilities and Nursing Facilities.
Copayment	A type of cost sharing whereby a specified flat fee per unit of service or unit of time is charged to an enrollee for a service or supply. Many HMO's charge their members a nominal fee for all non-emergent ambulatory patient visits or for prescription medications
COR	Cost of Risk
Corporate compliance	As relates to healthcare fraud and abuse, any of number of programs and initiatives undertaken by providers to avoid civil and criminal investigations and charges related to improper billing procedures, inappropriate referrals, kickbacks and other prohibited activities under federal statutes such as the Anti-Kickback Act and the Stark I and Stark II amendments to the Medicare Act. Many healthcare providers have taken corporate compliance programs beyond these specific legislative and regulatory requirements to encompass broader corporate business ethics concerns.
Corporate liability	Holds the healthcare entity liable for the failure of administrators and staff to monitor and supervise properly the delivery of healthcare in that entity (i.e.: negligence in hiring, training, supervising, or monitoring).
Corporation	A legal entity that may be created by one or more persons or entities to carry out a business purpose. Corporations are persons in the eyes of the law and may sue and be sued. Except in extraordinary circumstances, the owners of the corporation—shareholders or members (in not-for-profit corporations)—are shielded from the liabilities of the corporation.
Cost benefit analysis	A method comparing the costs of a project to the resulting benefits, usually expressed in monetary value

Cost containment	Control or reduction of inefficiencies in the consumption, allocation or production of health care services
Counter-claim	A claim presented by the defendant in opposition to the claim of the plaintiff
CPA	Certified Public Accountant
CPCU	Chartered Property Casualty Underwriter
CPG	See Clinical Practice Guidelines or Critical Paths
CPHQ	Certified Professional in Healthcare Quality
CPHRM	Certified Professional In Healthcare Risk Management
CPI	Consumer price index
	An inflationary measure encompassing the cost of all consumer goods and services
CPOE	See Computerized Practitioner Order Entry
CPR	Cardiopulmonary resuscitation
CPT	Current procedural terminology
CQI	Continuous Quality Improvement
	An approach to organizational management that emphasizes meeting (and exceeding) consumer needs and expectations, use of scientific methods to continually improve work processes, and the empowerment of all employees to engage in continuous improvement of their work processes
Credentialing	The process of verifying and reviewing the education, training, experience, work history and other qualifications of an applicant for clinical privileges conducted by a healthcare facility or managed care organization. Typically performed for independent contractors such as physicians and allied health practitioners who are frequently not employed by the credentialing entity but who are granted specific clinical privileges to practice
Credentialing and Privileging	Process by which hospitals determine the scope of practice of practitioners providing services in the hospital; criteria for granting privileges or credentialing are determined by the hospital and include individual character, competence, training, experience, and judgment
Criminal False Claims	"Whoever makes or presents to any person or officer in the civil, military or naval service of the United States, or any department or agency thereof, any claim upon or against the United States, or any department or agency thereof, knowing such claim to be false, fictitious or fraudulent, shall be imprisoned not more than five years or shall be subject to a fine or both."
Criminal Law	The system of laws by which the state or federal governments may bring suit against an individual, which suit may result in the loss of freedom or the person's life
Critical Access Hospital (CAH)	Part of the Medicare Rural Hospital Flexibility Program created by BBA97. A critical access hospital is a limited service small rural hospital that receives cost based reimbursement for inpatient and outpatient care
Critical paths (CPG)	Clinical pathways, CareMaps, clinical path guidelines, and other variants
	Any of a number of processes employed to define the generally accepted course (or courses) of treatment for a specific medical

condition or illness. Generally deviations from the prescribed critical paths must be explained by existing co-morbidities, failure of prescribed treatments, etc.

CRNA Certified Registered Nurse Anesthetist

CRO See Chief Risk Officer

Cross-claim A claim brought by a defendant against a plaintiff in the same action or against a codefendant concerning matters related to the original petition. Its purpose is to discover facts that will aid the defense.

CSO Chief Security Officer

CT See Computed Tomography Scan

CVA Cerebrovascular accident, a stroke

CWA Clean Water Act

Cycle Time The time it takes to complete a defined process—for example, the length of stay for a patient in the ED from triage to final disposition (transfer to unit; discharge or transfer out) is the ED service cycle time

D&C Dilation and curettage

Damage cap A legislatively imposed upper limit on the amount of a specific type of damages that may be awarded to a plaintiff in a specific type of lawsuit. State tort reform legislation frequently places a cap on the non-economic damages that may be awarded to a plaintiff in a medical malpractice action.

Damages Monetary compensation for an injury

The injuries for which the plaintiff/claimant seeks compensation from the defendant/health care provider. May include economic losses, emotional distress, pain and suffering, disability, etc.

DBA See Doing Business As

DDS Doctor of Dental Surgery

DEA Drug Enforcement Authority

Declaration A "declaration" is a statement made out of court. An unsworn statement or narration of facts made by a party involved in a transaction or by someone who has an interest in the existence of the facts recounted. Recounts of statements made by a deceased person are admissible as evidence in some cases contrary to the general rule.

Deductible In insurance, the amount of loss that must be paid by the insured before the insurer starts to pay. The use of deductibles allows entities to avoid paying for coverage for smaller claims that it is capable of paying for itself.

Default judgment A judgment entered by the court in a civil case in favor of the plaintiff and against the defendant when the defendant has failed to file some appearance in response to a summons. Defendants failure to so file is deemed to be an admission that the demands of the plaintiff's complaint are valid.

Deemed status In order for a health care organization to participate in and receive payment from Medicare or Medicaid programs, it must be certified as complying with the Conditions of Participation, or standards, set forth in federal regulations.

Deep pocket	In claims, an informal term for the defendant having the most assets and/or available insurance coverage which becomes the target of the plaintiff. The "deep pocket" may have less responsibility for the plaintiff's injuries than other co-defendants but may be pursued more aggressively because of its financial resources.
Default judgment	May be entered for failure to plead (e.g., answer)
	May be entered on any claim in action
	May be set aside upon motion for good cause
Defendant	The person defending or defying; the party against whom relief or recovery is sought in an action or suit. In common usage, this term is applied to the party put upon his defense or summoned to answer a charge or complaint.
Defense	A denial, answer, or plea opposing the truth or validity of the plaintiff's case. This may be accomplished by cross-examination or demurrer. It is more often done by introduction of testimony of the plaintiff's case.
Demurrer	A generally archaic term (although still used in some jurisdictions) that essentially admits the truth of the allegations asserted by the plaintiff, but which seeks their dismissal due to legal insufficiency to state a cause of action. Has been largely replaced in the federal court system, and in jurisdictions following the federal court rules of civil procedure, by the Motion to Dismiss
Deposition	Testimony (under oath) of a witness taken upon interrogatories reduced to writing and used to support or substantiate testimony offered at trial. Depositions are a very important phase of the discovery process.
	A question and answer session in which the witness is interrogated, under oath, and the testimony is transcribed
DFASHRM	Distinguished Fellow of the American Society for Healthcare Risk Management
DHHS	Department of Health and Human Services (Federal)
Diagnosis-related Group	Methodology for establishing reimbursement to healthcare providers under federal Medicare programs, based on clinical diagnosis. Adapted for use by some managed care plans
	A resource classification system that serves as the basis of the method for reimbursing hospitals based on the medical diagnosis for each patient. Hospitals receive a set payment amount determined in advance based on the length of time patients with a given diagnosis are likely to stay in the hospital. Also used as the basis of the Medicare inpatient prospective payment system (PPS).
DIFF.	Differential blood count
Direct Insurance	A contractual arrangement involving the purchase of insurance by an "Insured" from an "Insurer"
Direct liability	Imposed upon party as a result of party's acts or omissions
Disclosure	Communication of information regarding the results of a diagnostic test, medical treatment or surgical intervention
Discovery	The process in litigation by which each party to the action seeks to learn all relevant facts that either: (1) support the plaintiff's cause(s) of action; or (2) support the defendant's asserted defenses or denials

	That period of time following the filing of a complaint during which the parties to the litigation attempt to gain information about all facts relevant to the litigation
	The process by which parties learn and disclose information about the facts and issues in a case
Dismissal with Prejudice	A dismissal of a defendant in a suit which bars any future action by the plaintiff
Dismissal without Prejudice	A dismissal that affects no right or remedy of the plaintiff to rejoin the dismissed party in the cause of action
DMAT	Disaster Medical Assistance Team
DME	Durable medical equipment
DNR	Do not resuscitate Do not report Department of Natural Resources
D.O.	Doctor of Osteopathy: a doctor who employs the diagnostic and therapeutic measures of ordinary medicine in addition to manipulative measures. This approach is based upon the idea that the normal body when in "correct adjustment" is a vital machine capable of making its own remedies against infections and other toxic conditions.
D&O	Directors & Officers (insurance coverage)
	Policies contain a two-part wrongful act definition: 1) any actual or alleged error or misstatement or misleading statement or act or omission or breach of duty by directors and officers while acting in their individual or collective capacities; 2) any matter claimed against them solely by reason of their being directors or officers of the company.
DOC	Date of closure
Documentation	The recording of pertinent facts and observations about an individual's health history including past and present illnesses, tests, treatments and outcomes The legal evidence of professional accountability. See Legal Health Record
DOE	Department of Education
DOI	Date of incident
Doing Business As	An entity organized under one name but carrying on a trade or business under another
DOJ	Department of Justice
DOL	Date of loss
DOL	Department of Labor
DOR	Date of report
DOT	Department of Transportation
DPM	Doctor of Podiatric Medicine
DPT	Diphtheria, pertussis, tetanus
DRG	See Diagnosis-Related Group
DRS	Designated Record Set
DSM-IV	Diagnostic and Statistical Manual of Mental Disorders—Fourth Edition
Dual capacity	In employer's liability, an individual or entity serving as both an injured party's employer in a workers' compensation claim and in some other role in which it is alleged to have caused injury, such as the manufacturer of a defective piece of equipment involved in the injury or as the provider of improper medical treatment for the injury

Duces tecum	Used to require production of documents and things
Due diligence	The review of an entity targeted for acquisition by the acquiring party to ascertain pertinent information about its financial and operating history and current status. Corporate staff are generally held to the legal standard of having performed the review with due diligence before making a recommendation to the board of directors as to whether to proceed with the acquisition.
Due Process	A procedural requirement that may be met by providing the affected party with: (1) adequate notice of the proceeding; (2) the right to be represented by counsel; (3) the opportunity to be heard; (4) the right to call and cross-examine witnesses; and (5) the right to a written transcript of the proceeding
Durable Power of Attorney for Health Care	Allows an individual to designate in advance another person to act on his/her behalf if he/she is unable to make a decision to accept, maintain, discontinue, or refuse any health care services
DVM	Doctor of Veterinary Medicine
DX	Diagnosis
EAP	Employee Assistance Program
ECF	Extended care facility
Economic damages (specific damages)	Damages sought by or awarded to a plaintiff to compensate for out-of-pocket expenses, such as medical treatment or housekeeping services and lost wages resulting from the injury, as distinguished from non-economic damages, such as pain and suffering and loss of consortium, for which a dollar value is more speculative
	Funds to compensate a plaintiff for the monetary costs of an injury, such as medical bills or loss of income
ECRI	Formerly the Emergency Care Research Institute
ED	Emergency Department
EEG	Electroencephalogram
EENT	Eye, ear, nose and throat
EEOC	See Equal Employment Opportunity Commission
"800"	Federal and State regulatory body toll free numbers for registering quality of care complaints
EKG, ECG	Electrocardiogram
EMC	Emergency Medical Condition
Emergency-prudent layman's definition	The determination by a reasonably prudent individual medical training that he or she (or a person for whom he or she is seeking medical care) has a medical condition requiring immediate care. In some jurisdictions, emergency evaluation and treatment must be covered by a health plan if a reasonably prudent layman would have determined that it was necessary, even if the medical condition is determined not to have been a true emergency based upon the evaluation performed by trained medical personnel.
Emergency Medical Treatment and Active Labor Act	See EMTALA
EMF	Electric and Magnetic Fields
EMG	Electromyogram

Employee Polygraph Protection Act	29 U.S.C. Section 2001 et seq. Federal statute limiting most employers' ability to use polygraph testing in applicant screening processes
Employers' liability	Any of a number of causes of action related to the employment relationship but falling outside of workers' compensation and employment practices liability insurance coverage, including dual capacity claims, spousal claims and third-party over claims
Employment-at-will	Legal doctrine in most jurisdictions that an employer may discharge an employee for any reason, unless specifically prohibited by law
Employment practices liability	Any of a number of violations by an employer, based on statute or common law, giving rise to damages outside of those covered by workers' compensation or similar statutes, including wrongful termination, discrimination and sexual harassment
Employment Retirement Income Security Act (ERISA)	42 U.S.C. Section 1002 et seq. Federal statute pertaining to protection of certain qualified employee pension and benefit plans A federal law that regulates retirement plans and health insurance plans. If a lawsuit is brought under ERISA against a health insurance plan, it may be removed to federal court and damages will include the value of services wrongfully withheld.
EMS	Emergency Medical Service
EMT	Emergency Medical Technician
EMTALA	42 U.S.C. Section 1395 et seq. The Emergency Medical Treatment and Active Labor Act. Federal statute prohibiting the "dumping" of patients presenting to the hospital with an emergent medical condition or in active labor and limiting a hospital's ability to transfer them to other facilities. EMTALA specifies when and how a patient may be: 1) refused treatment; or 2) transferred from one hospital to another when the patient is in an unstable medical condition.
ENT	Ear, nose and throat
Enterprise liability	Shift liability from individual physicians to the enterprise at which they practice
EOB	Explanation of benefits
EOC	Environment of Care
EPA	Environmental Protection Agency
EPL	See Employment Practices Liability
EPLI	Employment Practices Liability Insurance
Equal Employment Opportunity Commission	Federal agency charged with responsibility for enforcing several federal statutes prohibiting various types of employment discrimination. Under some statutes, administrative hearing procedures before the EEOC must be exhausted before an employee has access to the court system.
Equal Pay Act	29 U.S.C. Section 206 et seq. Federal statute requiring equal pay for equal work without regard to the gender of the worker
Equity	Cases brought in equity are cases in which the court has the power, without a jury, to determine the facts of the matter and to decide the case. The decision is less affected by precedent than are cases brought at law; it is generally based upon principles of fairness to the parties. Examples of actions in equity include most domestic

relations cases and cases for injunctive relief (restraining orders). Courts of equity have been merged with courts of law in the federal and most state systems.

ER/ED Emergency room/emergency department

ERISA See Employee Retirement Income Security Act

ERISA preemption A provision of ERISA that preempts state law governing qualified pension and benefit plans and makes the remedies provided for by ERISA exclusive. Generally interpreted as preempting malpractice actions against managed care plans which are governed by the Act

ERM Enterprise Risk Management

ERP Extended reporting period

Error Failure of a planned action to be completed as intended or use of a wrong plan to achieve an aim. The accumulation of errors results in accidents.

Errors and Omissions (E&O) insurance A type of insurance policy providing coverage for negligent advice or business services provided by an individual or entity not eligible for professional liability insurance coverage, such as medical billing companies, insurance brokers and managed care organizations

Essential job functions Under the Americans with Disabilities Act, those functions of a particular job that an applicant must be able to perform, either with or without accommodation, in order to perform the job

Ethics Committee Multi-disciplinary group which convenes for the purpose of staff education and policy development in areas related to the use and limitation of aggressive medical technology; acts as a resource to patients, family staff, physicians, and clergy regarding health care options surrounding terminal illness and assisting with living wills.

Event A happening or occurrence that is not part of the routine care of a particular patient or the routine operation of the healthcare entity

Event reporting A system in healthcare institutions by which employees use a standardized form to report any occurrence outside the routine so that the information can be used for loss prevention and claims management activities

Evergreen clause In contracts, a clause which makes the agreement perpetual and on-going unless terminated by one of the parties. Contracts with an evergreen clause have no set expiration date.

Evidence Evidence may be testimony, documents, things, pictures, recordings of sounds or other items that may prove that an occurrence did, or did not, occur. Such things may only be considered at trial if admitted into evidence by the court. Evidence may be excluded if it would unduly inflame the passions of the jury, if it is irrelevant, if it does not appear to be credible or probative, or for other reasons.

Evidence-based Recommended practices that are based on the best available scientific knowledge, that has generally gone through a rigorous review process by leading medical specialists

Excess and surplus lines carriers Insurance companies that specialize in providing cover-age over primary insurance policies or significant self-insured retentions. Under the insurance regulations of most states, such insurers may write coverage in the state according to certain specified conditions without going through the licensing provisions applicable to admitted insurance carriers.

Excess capacity

The difference between the number of hospital beds being used for patient care and the number of beds available

Excess insurance policy

An insurance policy providing coverage above the limits provided by a primary insurer or a self-insurance program. Some insurance programs feature multiple layers of excess insurance policies.

Expense

Costs incurred associated with the generation of revenues

Expenses within policy limits

A provision in some insurance policies that allocated loss-adjusting expenses paid by the insurer are included when determining the applicable limits of coverage. For example, if $900,000 is paid to a claimant to settle a claim, and expense costs total $300,000, and the occurrence is covered by an insurance policy having limits of $1 million that includes a provision for expenses within policy limits, the insurer will only pay $1 million. If the policy indicates that expenses are covered in addition to policy limits, the insurer will pay a total of $1.2 million. Expenses covered within policy limits are said to erode the limits.

Exposure

Term synonymous with risk: chance of loss and that potential for liability that is covered by insurance

A percentage, calculated by the attorneys and claims adjusters, which estimates the likelihood of losing a trial

Extended reporting endorsement (tail coverage)

An endorsement added to a claims-made insurance policy, generally for additional premium, extending the period of time that claims can be made under the policy past the policy expiration date, either for a specified time period or indefinitely

Extra expense

Attempts to replace additional expenses incurred due to covered loss

FAA

Federal Aviation Administration

Face value

A perception that the level of validity of a concept is high, even when there is no scientific evidence to support that hypothesis

FACHE

Fellow of the American College of Healthcare Executives

Factitious disorder by proxy

See Munchausen syndrome by proxy

Facultative

Usually covers a single transaction handled directly with a reinsurer

Failure Mode

Different ways that a process or sub-process can fail to provide the anticipated result (i.e. think of it as what could go wrong)

Failure Mode Cause

Different reasons as to why a process or sub-process would fail to provide the anticipated result (i.e. think of it as why it would go wrong)

Failure Mode Effects Analysis or Failure Mode Effects Criticality Analysis (FMECA)

A prospective assessment that identifies and improves steps in a process, thereby reasonably ensuring a safe and clinically desirable outcome

A systematic approach to identify and prevent product and process problems before they occur

A systematic process often used by engineers to identify the steps of a process that may be subject to failure, in order to design measures to either prevent or control such failures. If a Criticality phase is used in this process, the perceived level of criticality of each type of potential failure is identified, to aid in setting priorities for establishing control mechanisms.

Fair hearing plan	A document, either freestanding or part of the bylaws of a medical staff, describing the procedures applicable to denial, revocation and suspension of clinical privileges and other medical staff disciplinary issues. Such plans specify due process requirements such as the right to notice, hearings, representation by counsel, appeals, etc.
Fair Labor Standards Act	29 U.S.C. Section 201 et seq. Federal statute establishing the authority for the Department of Labor to promulgate wage and hour regulations and providing the framework for collective bargaining by employees
False Claims Act	Two separate statutes: 18 USC §287; [31 USC §3729(a) and 31 USC §3730 (a)-(b)]. See Civil False Claims and Criminal False Claims
Family Education Rights & Privacy Act	[20 U.S.C. § 1232G; 34 CFR Part 99] Federal legislation designed to protect the privacy of student education records. It is applicable to all schools that receive funds under designated U.S. Department of Education programs.
Family Medical Leave Act	29 U.S.C. Section 2611 et seq. Federal statute requiring certain employers to provide a period of unpaid leave to employees meeting specified criteria in order for them to receive medical treatment or to provide care to designated family members
FASHRM	Fellow of the American Society for Healthcare Risk Management
Fatigue factors	The degree to which a person's physical or mental fatigue contributed to an adverse event or outcome
Fault tree analysis	A total quality management technique in which a complex process is broken down into a series of simpler steps and then particular areas of vulnerability for system breakdown are identified in an effort to anticipate and thereby avoid problems
	An engineering tool designed to identify potential errors in a process
FDA	Food and Drug Administration
Federal Deemed Status	In order for healthcare organizations to participate in and receive payment from Medicare or Medicaid programs, it must be certified as complying with the Conditions of Participation, or standards, set forth in federal regulations.
Federal Emergency Management Agency (FEMA)	An independent response organization that reports directly to the President of the United States
Fee-for-service	A reimbursement mechanism that pays providers for each service or procedure they perform; opposite of capitation
FERPA	See Family Educational Rights and Privacy Act.
Fiduciary duty	A duty to act for someone else's benefit while subordinating one's personal interests to that of the other person. It is the highest standard of duty implied by law (e.g., trustee, guardian).
First-dollar coverage	Commercial insurance providing protection against the entire loss covered by the policy—without requiring the insured to pay a deductible

First party	Provides coverage for the insured's own property or person so that the insured will be restored to the same financial position that they had been in prior to the loss
Float staff	Hospital staff, either generally assigned to a specific patient care unit or not, made available to work on other units as required to yield appropriate staffing levels for a given patient volume and acuity
FLV (full liability value)	An estimate of the jury award if the plaintiff prevails on all issues.
FMEA	See Failure Mode Effects Analysis
FMLA	See Family Medical Leave Act
FOIA	Freedom of Information Act
Force Majuere	A clause found in some contracts making the contract, or specific provisions of the contract, inapplicable in times of natural disasters, such as earthquakes, hurricanes, etc., and sometimes other crises, such as war, riot and civil commotion
Forcing Function	A technological design feature that forces the user to conform to a certain process, usually for a safety reason (e.g., a car is designed to not permit ignition if the gear is in reverse)
Formulary system	A planned restriction on the inventory of medications stocked in a pharmacy, in order to limit the choice to essential drugs, in order to promote safety by virtue of increasing staff familiarity with a more limited range of stocked medications
For-profit hospital	A hospital operated for the purpose of making a profit for its owner(s); the initial source of funding is typically through the sale of stock; profits are paid to stockholders in dividends (also referred to as a proprietary or an investor-owned hospital)
Formulary	The list of prescription medications that may be dispensed by participating pharmacies without health plan authorization. The formulary is selected based on effectiveness of the drug, as well as its cost. The physician is requested or required to use only formulary drugs unless there is a valid medical reason to use a non-formulary drug. Formularies may be open or closed. Closed formularies are restricted by the number and type of drugs included in the list.
Forum non Conveniens	A forum that is not convenient for the parties for some reason. Such a forum will normally have jurisdiction over the matter, and the venue of the action is appropriate, but hearing and deciding the matter there will work a hardship upon the parties or the witnesses. Determining that a particular forum is not convenient is an exercise of the court's discretion.
FP	For Profit
FPO	Facility Privacy Official
Fraud	Making false statements or representations of material facts in order to obtain some benefit or payment for which no entitlement would otherwise exist
Fraud and abuse	Informal term for the various federal statutes and regulations regarding inappropriate billing, kickbacks, referrals, etc., related to the federal or state Medicare/Medicaid programs
Free Flow	The unrestricted flow of a fluid through an IV line
Freestanding Ambulatory Surgery Center	A medical facility which provides surgical treatment on an outpatient basis only

FTC	Federal Trade Commission
FTE	Full-time equivalent
Gag rule	An informal term for a provision found in some managed care contracts with physicians prohibiting the physicians from discussing treatment alternatives, such as experimental procedures, with managed care plan patients when such treatments are not covered by the plan
Garage Liability Policy	Covers loss resulting from premises exposure of parking areas, but excludes property in your care, custody and control
Gatekeeper	Term used to describe the coordination role of the primary care provider (PCP) who manages various components of a member's medical treatment, including all referrals for specialty care, ancillary services, durable medical equipment, and hospital services. The gatekeeper model is a popular cost-control component of many managed care plans because it requires a subscriber to first see their PCP and receive the PCP's approval before going to a specialist about a given medical condition (except for emergencies).
General liability insurance	Coverage for liability arising out of the hazards of the premises and operations
GI	Gastrointestinal
GL	General liability
GMP	Good manufacturing practice
GP	General practitioner
GU	genitourinary
Hard insurance market	Insurance market conditions characterized by rising premiums and shrinking availability of coverage. Hard markets typically prompt insureds to accept larger deductibles or self-insured retentions, reduce coverage limits and/or seek out alternative risk financing alternatives.
Hazard	A condition that increases the possibility of loss
Hazard Analysis	The process of collecting and evaluating information on hazards associated with the selected process. The purpose of the hazard analysis is to develop a list of hazards that are of such significance that they are reasonably likely to cause injury or illness if not effectively controlled.
Hazard Communication Standard	Also called the Employee Right-to-Know Rule
Hazardous Condition	"Any set of circumstances (exclusive of the disease or condition for which the patient is being treated) which significantly increases the likelihood of a serious adverse outcome" (JCAHO)
HAZWOPER	Hazardous Waste Operations and Emergency Response Standard
HCCA	See Health Care Compliance Association
HCFA	Health Care Financing Administration (currently known as the Centers for Medicare and Medicaid Services)
HCO	See Health Care Organization
HCQIA	See Health Care Quality Improvement Act
Health Care Compliance Association	The professional society for healthcare corporate compliance officers

Health Care Organization	Entity that provides, coordinates and/or ensures health and medical services for people
Health Care Quality Improvement Act	A federal law that requires reports to the National Practitioner Data Bank and which protects the confidentiality of peer review materials. 42 USC §11101et seq.
The Health Insurance Portability and Accountability Act of 1996	42 U.S.C. Section 201 et seq. Amendments to ERISA addressing a variety of healthcare-related issues including fraud and abuse and the portability of group healthinsurance benefits as well as mandating specific patient privacy protections.
	A federal law that resulted in the promulgation of several regulations including the HIPAA Privacy Rule. Full compliance with the privacy requirements is expected for covered entities by April 2003 with a one year extension for smaller health plans
Hearsay	An out-of-court statement made by a person not a party to the action, and who is not available to testify, that is offered to prove the truth of the matter asserted. Normally subject to numerous exceptions but, if not precluded by an exception to the rule, will act to preclude the admission of statements into evidence
HEDIS	Health Plan Employer Data and Information Set A standard data reporting system developed in 1991 to measure the quality and performance of health plans. A main goal of HEDIS is to standardize health plan performance measures for consumers and payers. HEDIS concentrates on four aspects of healthcare: (1) quality, (2) access and patient satisfaction, (3) membership and utilization, and (4) finance. Within each focus area is a specific set of HEDIS data measures (e.g., number of immunizations for pediatric enrollees, etc.). The National Committee for Quality Assurance (NCQA) is responsible for coordinating HEDIS and making changes each year.
H.E.I.C.S.	Hospital Emergency Incident Command System
HFAP	Health Care Facilities Accreditation Program (through the AOA)
HFMA	Healthcare Financial Management Association
Hgb.	Hemoglobin
HHS	The federal Department of Health and Human Services
HIAA	Health Insurance Association of America
Hierarchy Effect (steep hierarchy)	The effect that a perceived "pecking order" or relative stature/status differences have on the lower person's level of willingness to question a higher person's actions or decisions
High/Low Agreements	An agreement made between the plaintiff and defendant. The plaintiff will be entitled to at least the low amount and the defendant will be obligated to pay at least the low amount. The plaintiff will not be entitled to more than the high amount and the defendant will not be obligated to pay more than the high amount. If the jury returns a verdict between the low and high amounts, the case will settle for the amount of the verdict. A high/low agreement settles the case and no appeal may be taken.
HIM	Health information management
Hindsight bias	The tendency for a reviewer to focus most heavily on facts learned after an event and/or only the most obvious contributing factors, thereby failing to consider other, more subtle, contributing factors

HIPAA	See The Health Insurance Portability and Accountability Act of 1996
HIPDB	Health Integrity and Protection Data Bank
HIV	Human Immunodeficiency Virus
HMO	Health Maintenance Organization

A health care payment and delivery system involving networks of doctors and hospitals. Members must receive all their care from providers within the network

➤ *Staff Model HMO.* Physicians are on the staff of the HMO and are usually paid a salary

➤ *Group Model HMO.* The HMO rents the services of the physicians in a separate group practice and pays the group a per patient rate.

➤ *Network Model HMO.* The HMO contracts with two or more independent physician group practices to provide services and pays a fixed monthly fee per patient

Hold Harmless Provision	A contractual clause providing that one party agrees not to pursue a tort claim for vicarious liability against the other. Hold harmless provisions are usually found with indemnification provisions and are usually mutual.
Home Health Care	Health care services are provided in a patient's home instead of a hospital or other institutional setting; services provided may include nursing care, social services, and physical, speech, or occupational therapy
Hospice	An organization that provides medical care and support services (such as pain and symptom management, counseling, and bereavement services) to terminally ill patients and their families; may be a freestanding facility, a unit of a hospital or other institution, or a separate program of a hospital, agency, or institution
Hospitalists	A physician whose practice is caring for patients while in the hospital. A primary care physician (PCP) turns their patients over to a hospitalist, who becomes the physician of record and provides and directs the care of the patient while the patient is hospitalized and returns the patient to the PCP at the time of hospital discharge
HPL	Hospital Professional Liability (insurance)
HR	Human Resources (Department)
HRSA	Health Resources and Services Administration
Human Factors	Study of the interrelationship between humans, the tools they use, and the environment in which they live and work
Iatrogenic	Caused by medical treatment
IBNR	See Incurred But Not Reported
ICD-9-CM	International Classification of Diseases, 9th revision

The classification of disease by a diagnostic codification into sixdigit numbers. ICD-10, is under development and will use alphanumeric codes

ICF/MR	Intermediate care facility for the mentally retarded
ICS	Incident command system

ICU	Intensive Care Unit
I.D.	Identification
IDS	See Integrated Delivery System
IIA	Insurance Institute of America
IM	Intramuscular
IME	See Independent Medical Examination
Immediate Jeopardy	A situation in which the provider's noncompliance with one or more requirements of participation has caused, or is likely to cause, serious injury, harm, impairment or death to a resident
Immigration Reform and Control Act	8 U.S.C Section 1324 et seq. Federal legislation requiring employers to verify immigration status of prospective employees during hiring process
Improperly performed procedure or treatment	The appropriate procedure or treatment is done but is performed incorrectly. This is not to be confused with choosing the wrong procedure or treatment.
Inappropriate procedure or treatment	An incorrect procedure or treatment is provided. This usually involves medical judgment versus skills or techniques. This is not to be confused with performing the procedure incorrectly.
Incident	Any happening not consistent with the routine operations of the facility or routine care of a particular patient; an unexpected occurrence; an occurrence which leaves a patient, visitor or other person feeling, either rightly or wrongly, that he had been mistreated, neglected or injured in same manner.
Incident reporting	An early warning reporting system intended to identify risk situations or adverse events in a timely manner to trigger prompt investigation from a claims management perspective as well as corrective action to prevent similar future events
Incurred But Not Reported	Insurance and actuarial term for claims that have occurred but for which notification has not yet been received
Indemnification provision	A contractual clause in which one party agrees to accept the tort liability and legal defense of another. Indemnification provisions are usually found with hold harmless provisions and are usually mutual
Indemnify	To secure against loss, damage or expenses which may occur in the future; to insure.
Indemnity	An assurance or contract by one party to compensate for the damage caused by another; shifting an economic loss to the person responsible for the loss; the right which the person suffering the loss or damage is entitled to a claims; compensation given to make a person whole from a loss already received; settlements or awards made directly to plaintiffs as a result of the claims resolution process In regards to health care services: benefits in the form of cash payments rather than medical services.
Independent medical examination	Medical examination of a claimant by a practitioner other than the claimant's treating practitioner at the request of a defendant to verify the claimant's diagnosis and prognosis
Independent practice association	A group of independent physicians who have formed an association as a separate legal entity for contracting purposes. IPA physician providers retain their individual practices, work in separate offices, continue to see their non-managed care patients,

and have the option to contract directly with managed car plans. A key advantage of the IPA arrangement is that it helps its members achieve some of the negotiating leverage of a large physician group practice with some degree of flexibility for each provider. Also referred to as independent physician association.

Indicator

In quality improvement, a measurable objective standard against which performance is measured. Designed to be indicative of whether other care processes are also meeting established standards

Informed consent

Legal doctrine that patients generally have a right to be informed regarding proposed medical and surgical treatments, including anticipated benefits, risks and alternatives and to accept or reject such proposed treatments

Injunction

A court order prohibiting someone from doing some specified act or commanding someone to undo some wrong or injury

Insolvent

In reference to an insurance company, an insurer without the available financial resources to pay covered claims

Institute of Medicine

A division of The National Academy of Sciences, a private nonprofit organization of scholars dedicated to research and publications related to engineering and the sciences. Noted for its 1999 publication "To Err is Human: Building a Safer Health System," which focused in medical errors

Institutional review board

The body within a healthcare organization charged with establishing protocols for and overseeing clinical research trials and human experimentation

Insurance

Losses paid for with funds external to the organization

A contractual relationship which exists when one party (the insurer), for consideration (the premium), agrees to reimburse another party (the insured) for loss to a specified subject (the risk) caused by designated contingencies (hazards or perils)

Insurance schedule

A document or graphic showing all of the insurance coverages in place for a given insured, usually including the names of insurers, policy limits, deductibles and retentions, policy numbers, inception and expiration dates

Insured versus insured exclusion

A provision common in insurance policies excluding coverage for claims in which one insured makes a claim against another

Integrated care

A comprehensive spectrum of health services, from prevention through long-term care, provided via a single administrative entity and coordinated by a primary care "gatekeeper"

Integrated Delivery System

A healthcare system made up of various types of providers, including hospitals, ambulatory care centers, surgery centers, home health agencies, physician practices, etc., and frequently a managed care organization, such as a health maintenance organization or a preferred provider organization

An entity (corporation, partnership, association or other legal entity) that enters into arrangements with managed care organization; employs or has contracts with providers; and agrees to provide or arrange for the provision of health care services to members covered by the managed care plan

Intentional acts

In insurance policies, an exclusion for injuries caused by the intentional acts of an insured

Interrogatories	A written set of questions that is served upon the other party in litigation. All questions must be answered under oath and returned to the party that served the interrogatories.
Intravenously	Within the veins
IOM	See Institute of Medicine
IP	Internet Protocol
IPA	Independent practice association
IRB	See Institutional Review Board
IRMI	International Risk Management Institute
IRS	Internal Revenue Service
ISMP	Institute for Safe Medication Practices
IV	See Intravenously
IVP	Intravenous pyelogram (urogram)
JCAHO	See Joint Commission on Accreditation of Healthcare Organizations
JD	See Juris Doctor
Joint and Several Liability	A sharing of liabilities among a group of individuals collectively and also individually
	Liability in which each liable party is individually responsible for the entire obligation. Under joint-and-several liability, a plaintiff may choose to seek full damages from all, some, or any one of the parties alleged to have committed the injury. In most cases, a defendant who pays damages may seek reimbursement from nonpaying parties
Joint Commission on the Accreditation of Healthcare Organizations (JCAHO)	A voluntary nonprofit accreditation body which sets standards for hospitals and other types of healthcare organizations and conducts education programs and a survey process to assess organizational compliance
	The organization which evaluates and monitors the quality of care provided in hospitals based on standards established by the Joint Commission
Joint defense	Requires a defense of all defendants (e.g., physician and hospital) in an integrated response
Joint Venture	An undertaking by two or more entities to pursue business or other ventures. In many jurisdictions, entities cannot form partnerships; hence they are deemed to be joint venturers. Each joint venturer may be liable for the debts and obligations of the joint venture.
	An organization formed for a single purpose or undertaking which makes its membership liable for the organization's debts.
JUA	Joint Underwriting Agreement
Judgment	The official decision of a court that determines the relative legal rights and obligations of parties to a legal proceeding
Juris doctor	The educational degree awarded by law schools
Jurisdiction	The power of a court or other tribunal to hear and decide a legal matter. In common parlance, jurisdiction is often referred to as the physical locations from which courts are permitted to hear and decide cases.

Jury

A group of persons impaneled to hear a legal matter and to render a verdict. The jury typically finds the facts of the matter and the court applies the law to the facts. The number of jurors necessary to form a jury varies by jurisdiction and, possibly, by type of case.

Latent Error

Errors in the design, organization, training or maintenance that lead to operator errors and whose effects typically lie dormant in the system for lengthy periods of time

Law Courts

These are the courts that have jurisdiction to hear most civil lawsuits, such as suits for personal injury, breach of contract, etc. For almost all practical purposes, law courts have been merged with courts of equity, but differences in actions based in law versus actions based in equity still remain.

LCF

Loss Conversation Factor

LCL

See Lower Control Limit

LDF

Loss Development Factor

Leapfrog Group, The

A private business consortium for healthcare interests

Legal health record

The legal health record is the documentation of the healthcare services provided to an individual in any aspect of healthcare delivery by healthcare provider organizations. The legal health record is individually identifiable data, in any medium, collected and directly used in and/or documenting healthcare or health status. The term includes records of care in any health-related setting used by healthcare professionals while providing patient care services, for reviewing patient data, or documenting observations, actions or instructions.

Legally cognizable injury

An injury for which the law can provide redress

Length of stay

The period of hospitalization as measured in days billed; average length of stay is determined by discharge days divided by discharges.

LEP

Limited English Proficiency

Letter of intent

Formal notice to an organization that another organization is seeking to acquire or merge with it, setting due diligence in motion

Libel

Defamatory language expressed in print, writing, pictures or symbols tending to injure another's reputation, business or means of livelihood.

Limited Liability Companies

A limited liability company (LLC) may be formed by one or more persons or entities to carry out a business purpose. The LLC shields its owners (members) from liability but enjoys certain tax advantages not available to corporations.

Limits (policy limits)

In insurance, the maximum the insurer will pay, typically expressed either per occurrence (occurrence limit) or as an annual aggregate (the maximum insurer will pay for all claims covered under policy)

Living will

Document generated by a person for the purpose of providing guidance about the medical care to be provided in the person is unable to articulate those decisions (see Advance Directive).

LLC

See Limited Liability Companies

Long tail

An informal term for lines of insurance coverage in which there is frequently an extended period of time between the time an incident giving rise to a claim occurs and the time that the claim is reported.

	Medical professional liability is generally considered to be long tail insurance business.
Long term care	A continuum of maintenance, custodial, and health services to the chronically ill, disabled, or mentally handicapped
LOS	Length of stay
Loss	The reduction in the value of an asset
Loss control	Any of a number of programs and initiatives undertaken to prevent losses from occurring (loss prevention) or to decrease the severity of losses that do occur (loss reduction), including education and training, policy and procedure development, equipment maintenance, use of personal protective equipment, installation of sprinkler systems, etc.
Loss of consortium	Claim for damages relating to the loss of companionship, advice and sexual relationship with an injured party, typically filed by the injured party's spouse
Loss frequency	A measure of how many times a particular loss occurs or can be expected to occur in a given period of time
Loss prevention	Reduces an organization's losses by lowering their frequency
Loss reduction	A method to manage loss exposures. Actions taken to decrease severity of a loss
Loss run	A listing, usually generated by computer, of claims brought against an insured for a specific line of insurance coverage, that typically includes the name of the claimant, the date of occurrence, the date the claim was made, the status of claim (open or closed; suit, claim or occurrence), amounts paid and reserved for both indemnity and loss adjustment expenses, and a description of the facts giving rise to the claim
Loss severity	A measure of the size of an actual or expected loss; how much a loss will cost
Lower Control Limit	Used in statistical process control run charts
LPN	Licensed Practical Nurse
LPT	Licensed Physical Therapist
LTC	Long-term care
LTD	Long-term disability
LVN	Licensed Vocational Nurse
M. A.	Medical Assistant
M&A&D	Mergers, acquisitions and divestitures
Magnetic Resonance Imaging	Technology that utilizes magnetic fields to image the body's tissue
	A non-invasive diagnostic technique used to create images of body tissue and monitor body chemistry; uses radio and magnetic waves instead of radiation
Malfeasance	The wrongful or unjust doing of an act which the doer had no right to perform or which he had stipulated by contract not to do
Malpractice	Improper professional actions or the failure to exercise proper professional skills by a professional advisor, such as a physician, dentist, or healthcare entity. Also, professional misconduct, improper

discharge of professional duties, or failure to meet the standards of care of a professional, resulting in harm to another

Failure on one rendering professional services to exercise that degree of skill and learning commonly applied under all circumstances in the community by the average prudent reputable member of the profession with the result of injury, loss or damage to the recipient of those services or to those entitled to rely upon them

Managed care

A term that applies to the integration of health care delivery and financing. It includes arrangements with providers to supply health care services to members, criteria for the selection of health care providers, significant financial incentives for members to use providers in the plan, and formal programs to monitor the amount of care and quality of services

A healthcare organization, such as a health maintenance organization, that "manages" or controls what it spends on health care by closely monitoring how doctors and other medical professionals treat patients.

Managed care organization

Any of a number of organizations, such as health maintenance organizations and preferred provider organizations, which arrange for the provision of and payment for healthcare services with an eye toward reducing costs through managing access to specific providers

Mandatory Settlement Conference (MSC)

A court ordered meeting of the plaintiff and defendant held under the judges direction with the goal of resolving a claim. This meeting is not voluntary and the opposing parties must participate

MAR

See Medication Administration Record

Market-hard

See Hard Insurance Market

Maximum medical improvement (MMI)

In workers' compensation, the point in which the injured employee has recovered to the maximum extent medically expected (also called permanent and stationary, or P and S). When an employee reaches MMI, any residual disability, pain, etc., is expected to be permanent.

MBWA

Management by Walking Around

MCO

See Managed Care Organization

M.D.

Medical Doctor

MDR

Medical Device Reporting

MedPAC

Medicare Payment Advisory Commission

Mediation

Intervention between parties in conflict to promote reconciliation, settlement or compromise

Medicaid

A federal public assistance program enacted into law on January 1, 1966, under Title XIX of the Social Security Act, to provide medical benefits to eligible low income persons needing health care regardless of age. The program is administered and operated by the states which receive federal matching funds to cover the costs of the program. States are required to include certain minimal services as mandated by the federal government but may include any additional services at their own expense

Medical battery

Traditionally, a battery that occurs during the administration of medical care and procedures. May also include actions against medical care providers for prolonging the lives of patients who had previously requested for no "heroic measures" to be undertaken when faced with a medical emergency

Medical Malpractice Review Panel
A panel consisting of two lawyers, two health care providers, and a circuit court judge which, upon the request of any party, passes non-binding judgment on claims of alleged medical malpractice. May conclude that there was negligence, no negligence, or question of fact which must be decided by a jury.

Medical services
The furnishing of professional healthcare services, including the furnishing of food, medications or appliances, the postmortem handling of bodies or arising out of service by any persons as members of a formal accreditation review board

Medical technology
Techniques, drugs, equipment, and procedures used by healthcare professionals in delivering medical care to individuals and the systems within which such care is delivered

Medicare
A federally administered health insurance program for persons aged 65 and older and certain disabled people under 65 years old. Created in 1965 under Title XVIII of the Social Security Act, Medicare covers the cost of hospitalization, medical care, and some related services for eligible persons without regard to income. Medicare has two parts. Medicare Part A: Hospital Insurance (HI) Program is compulsory and covers inpatient hospitalization costs. Medicare Part B: Supplementary Medical Insurance Program is voluntary and covers medically necessary physicians' services, outpatient hospital services, and a number of other medical services and supplies not covered by Part A. Part A is funded by a mandatory payroll tax. Part B is supported by premiums paid by enrollees.

Medication Administration Record
The record of all medications ordered and when each has been administered, maintained by nursing staff

Medication Error
"A medication error is any preventable event that may cause or lead to inappropriate medication use or patient harm while the medication is in the control of the healthcare professional, patient, or consumer. Such events may be related to professional practice, healthcare products, procedures, and systems, including prescribing; order communication; product labeling, packaging, and nomenclature; compounding; dispensing; distribution; administration; education; monitoring; and use." Source: National Coordinating Council for Medication Error Reporting and Prevention

"An unintended act, either by omission or commission, or an act that does not achieve its intended outcome" (JCAHO)

MEq.
millequivalent

MER
Medical Error Reporting (system)

Merger
A combination of business entities in which two or more organizations join assets and stock if applicable

Union of two or more organizations by the transfer of all assets to one organization that continues to exist while the other(s) is (are) dissolved.

MERS-TM
Medical Event Reporting System for Transfusion Medicine

MHA
Master of Hospital (Health) Administraton

MHSA	Master of Health Services Administration
MO	Myocardial infarction
	Mitral insufficiency
	Mental institution
Micro-system	Organizational unit built around the definition of repeatable core service competencies. Elements of a micro-system include: 1) a core team of healthcare professionals; 2) a defined population of patients; 3) carefully designed work processes; and 4) an environment capable of linking information on all aspects of work and patient or population outcomes to support ongoing evaluation of performance.
Misrepresentation	Any manifestation by words or other conduct by one person to another that, under circumstances, amounts to an assertion not in accordance with the facts. An untrue statement of fact
M&M	Morbidity and mortality
MOB	Medical office building
Morbidity	Associated negative consequences relating to a clinical treatment or procedure, e.g., complication
	Incidence and severity of illness and accidents in a well-defined class or classes of individuals
Mortality	Death rate
	Incidence of death in a well-defined class or classes of individuals
Motion	A filing with a court or other tribunal that requests that the court perform some function. The party seeking the relief in question "moves" the court to perform the act.
Motion for Judgment Notwithstanding the Verdict	In a trial process, the court normally enters judgment on a jury's verdict, and thus gives effect to the verdict. This motion seeks to have the jury verdict set aside and judgment entered by the court that is not in accord with the verdict. Usually granted for the appearance of bias, prejudice, or possible misconduct by the jury
Motion for New Trial	A motion that seeks to invalidate the original trial and declare that the matter must be re-tried. Usually granted when the verdict is contrary to the manifest weight of the evidence, or when there is a scant amount of evidence to support the jury's verdict
Motion for Summary Judgment	A motion that seeks to have a lawsuit decided (have judgment rendered) because there are no genuine issues of material fact for the jury to decide
Motion *in Limine*	A motion to preclude the admission of certain facts, testimony, items or proofs at trial. May be granted on the grounds that the evidence is not relevant, is redundant or duplicative of other evidence, will unduly arouse or inflame the jury, etc.
Motion to Dismiss	A motion that seeks to have a lawsuit dismissed because the Complaint or Petition fails to state a cause of action upon which relief may be granted. The filing of a Motion to Dismiss often stays the period in which an Answer must be filed.
Motion to Strike	Motion to eliminate a cause of action in the Complaint or Petition or to preclude the defendant from mounting a defense based upon a certain theory
MPA	Master of Public Administration

MPH	Master of Public Health
MQSA	Mammography Quality Standards Act
MRI	See Magnetic Resonance Imaging
MSN	Master of Science in Nursing
MSO	Management service organization
MSW	Master of Social Work
MT	Medical Technologist
Multi-hospital system	Two or more hospitals owned, leased, contract managed, or sponsored by a central organization; they can be either not-forprofit or investor-owned
Munchausen syndrome by proxy	A form of factitious disorder where one person, usually a parent, exaggerates or feigns illness in a child or deliberately causes or exacerbates actual medical problems the patient is experiencing
NASA	National Aeronautics and Space Administration
National Center for Complementary and Alternative Medicine	An agency of the National Institutes of Health developed to study and provide information about complementary and alternative medicine treatments and therapies
National Committee for Quality Assurance	A private nonprofit accrediting body for managed care organizations
National Labor Relations Act	The main body of law governing collective bargaining Explicitly grants employees the right to collectively bargain and join trade unions
	Originally enacted by Congress in 1935 under its power to regulate interstate commerce
National Practitioner Data Bank	A data bank maintained by the federal government containing reports on certain individual practitioners. A report must be made by any entity that pays money on behalf of a practitioner to settle a legal claim asserted against the practitioner. Reports must also be made by hospitals that restrict, suspend or terminate a practitioner's privileges to examine or treat patients at the hospital.
NB	Newborn
NBC emergencies	Disaster scenarios involving nuclear, bioterrorism or chemical warfare agents
NCC-MERP	National Coordinating Council for Medication Error Reporting and Prevention
NCI	National Cancer Institute
NCQA	See National Committee for Quality Assurance
NCVIA	National Childhood Vaccine Injury Act, U.S. Code 42 U.S.C. 300, established the National Vaccine Injury Compensation Program
NDS	National Disaster Medical System
Near Miss	"Used to describe any process variation which did not affect the outcome, but for which a recurrence carries a significant chance of a serious adverse outcome. Such a near miss falls within the scope of the (JCAHO's) definition of a sentinel event, but outside the scope of those sentinel events that are subject to review by the Joint Commission under its Sentinel Event Policy" (JCAHO)

Neglect	Failure to provide goods and services necessary to avoid physical harm, mental anguish or mental illness
Negligence	A legal conclusion that is reached when it has been determined that: (1) the defendant owed a duty of care to the plaintiff; (2) the defendant breached the duty of care; (3) the plaintiff was injured as a result of the breach of the duty of care; and (4) legally cognizable damages resulted from the injury
	Carelessness, failure to act as an ordinary prudent person or action contrary to that of a reasonable party. Or failure to use such care as a reasonably prudent and careful person would demonstrate under similar circumstances
	A violation of a duty to meet an applicable standard of care
Neonatal	The part of an infant's life from the hour of birth through the first 27 days, 23 hours and 59 minutes; the infant is referred to as newborn throughout this period
NESHAP	National Emission Standard for Hazardous Air Pollutants
Network	Self-contained, fully integrated system of providers
NF	Nursing Facility
NFP	Not-For-Profit
NICU	Neonatal intensive care unit
NIH	National Institute for Health
NIMH	National Institute of Mental Health
NIOSH	National Institute of Occupational Safety and Health
NLRA	See National Labor Relations Act
NLRB	National Labor Relations Board
NMHPA	Newborns' and Mothers' Health Protection Act
No-fault system	A system of compensation for injured parties that is not based on the fault or negligence of the party causing the injury. Examples include the workers' compensation system and the personal injury protection (PIP) automobile insurance mandated or available in some jurisdictions.
Nomenclature	A naming classification system, e.g., FDA's choice of new medication names
Non-economic damages (general damages)	Damages asserted by or awarded to a claimant for pain and suffering, loss of consortium, loss of enjoyment of life, etc., for which no objective dollar value exists Damages payable for items other than monetary losses, such as pain and suffering. The term technically includes punitive damages, but those are typically discussed separately
Non-Insurance transfer	The transfer of the financial obligations to pay for defense, expenses, verdicts, awards and settlements
	Reduces the transferor's loss exposure by contractually shifting legal responsibility for a loss through leases, contracts and agreements (exculpatory clauses)
Nonsuit	A privilege granted to plaintiffs in Virginia that allows them to withdraw a civil lawsuit at any time before decision, without prejudice to their right or ability to bring it one more time
NORA	National Occupational Research Agenda
Nose coverage	See Prior Acts Coverage

Nosocomial infection	A type of infection acquired during treatment/admission within a healthcare facility
	Infection acquired in a hospital
Notice of Claim	A letter from or on behalf of a claimant, addressed to a health care provider, which puts the health care provider on notice that a claim of alleged medical negligence is being made, and which triggers certain rights of the parties to request a medical malpractice review panel
NPDB	See National Practitioner Data Bank
NPSF	National Patient Safety Foundation
NPSG	National Patient Safety Goals (JCAHO)
NQF	National Quality Foundation
NRC	Nuclear Regulatory Commission
NTSB	National Transportation Safety Board
Nuclear medicine	The use of radioisotopes to study and treat disease, especially in the diagnostic area
Nurse practitioner	A licensed nurse who has completed a nurse practitioner program at the master's or certificate level and is trained in providing primary care services. NPs are qualified to conduct expanded health care evaluations and decision making regarding patient care, including diagnosis, treatment and prescriptions, usually under a physician's supervision and, generally, they provide services at a lower cost than PCPs. NPs may also be trained in medical specialties, such as pediatrics, geriatrics, and midwifery. Legal regulations in some states prevent NPs from qualifying for direct Medicare and Medicaid reimbursement, writing prescriptions, and admitting patients to hospital. Also called advance practice nurse (APN).
OASIS	Outcomes and Assessment Information Set
OBE	Occupied Bed Equivalent
OBRA	Omnibus Budget Reconciliation Act
OBS	Office-based surgery
OB-GYN	Obstetrics and gynecology
Obstetrics (OB)	The medical specialty concerned with the care of women during pregnancy and childbirth
Occupational Safety and Health Act/ Administration	29 U.S.C. Section 651 et seq. Federal statute (and agency created by it) charged with responsibility for promulgating standards and enforcement mechanisms governing worker safety for most industries
Occurrence insurance policies	Insurance policies for which coverage is provided for claims which occur during the policy period, regardless of when the claim is made
Occurrence reporting	An unexpected patient medical intervention, intensity of care or healthcare impairment
Occurrence Screen Reports	A systematic review of medical records/cases (either retrospectively or concurrently conducted) using predetermined screening criteria, conducted for the purpose of identifying cases that may warrant

closer PI review. Example criteria: unplanned returns to the ED within 72 hours of admission or prior treatment for a similar condition

OCR	Office of Civil Rights
OD	Doctor of Optometry
O.D.	Right eye
OIG	Office of Inspector General, www.oig.hhs.gov
Older Workers' Benefit Protection Act	29 U.S.C. Section 621 et seq. Amendments to the Age Discrimination in Employment Act restricting employers from making certain age-based distinctions in employee benefits plans
OMB	Office of Management and Budget
Omission Error	Failure to carry out an intended action, or failure to recognize that an action should have been carried out
OPDRA	Office of Post Marketing Drug Risk Assessment
Operating margin	Margin of net patient care revenues in excess of operating expenses
Operating Room	Surgical suite
OPO	Organ Procurement Organization
OR	See Operating Room
Ordinance	A legislative enactment typically enacted by the elected legislative body of a city, town, county or other such minor political subdivision
ORYX™	The trademarked terms JCAHO used for its approach to integrate performance measures into the accreditation process. A key component of ORYX is the use of standardized core measures.
O.S.	Left eye
OSCAR	Online Survey Certification and Reporting Database
OSHA	See Occupational Safety and Health Act/Administration
OSHA general duty clause	OSHA's general requirement that employers maintain a safe work environment. OSHA inspectors may cite the general duty clause whenever an unsafe workplace condition or work practice is identified, but no specific OSHA regulation applies.
Ostensible agency doctrine	The doctrine of ostensible agency, sometimes referred to as apparent agency, permits a finding of liability on a hospital where there is the appearance of an employment relationship with an independent contractor.
	In the absence of employer-employee relationship, a managed care organization (MCO) may still be held vicariously liable for the acts of provider physicians if the patient had a reasonable belief that the physician was the MCO's agent and that this belief was based upon representations made by the MCO to that effect. The burden is on the plaintiff to prove that he or she detrimentally relied on the fact that the MCO held the physician out as its agent.
OT	Occupational therapy
OTC	Over-the-counter
Out-of-plan (or out-of-network) services	In managed care, healthcare services required by a plan participant which are either not provided for by the plan (such as most experimental procedures) or which must be provided for outside of the plan network (such as an emergency department visit for a participant who is traveling out of town)

Outcomes	The end result of medical care, as indicated by recovery, disability, functional status, mortality, morbidity, or patient satisfaction
Outcomes measurement	The process of systematically tracking a patient's clinical treatment and responses to that treatment using generally accepted outcomes or quality indicators, such as mortality, morbidity, disability, functional status, recovery, and patient satisfaction. Such measures are considered by many health care researchers as the only valid way to determine the effectiveness of medical care
Outpatient care	Treatment provided to a patient who is not confined in a health care facility. Outpatient care includes services that do not require an overnight stay, such as emergency treatment, same-day surgery, outpatient diagnostic tests, and physician office visits. Also referred to as ambulatory care.
Over-the-counter	Drugs that may be obtained without a written prescription from a physician
Overuse	A healthcare quality problem involving the application or performance of unnecessary procedures or the provision of unnecessary services for patients
PA	Physician Assistant also posterior-anterior
PALS	Pediatric advanced life support
Paradigm	A conceptual framework that aids in the explanation of a complex phenomena or field of inquiry
Parallel processes	Two or more processes being performed simultaneously
Partnership	An entity formed by two or more persons to undertake a business purpose for profit. Each partner is liable for the obligations and liabilities of the partnership. Income to the partnership is considered income to the partners; there is no taxation at the level of the partnership.
Patient safety	Freedom from accidental injury. Ensuring patient safety involves the establishment of operational systems and processes that minimize the likelihood of errors and maximizes the likelihood of intercepting them when they occur.
Patient Self-Determination Act	42 U.S.C. Section 1395 et seq. Federal statute requiring certain healthcare organizations, including hospitals and HMOs, to provide patients with information regarding advanced directives
PC	See Professional Corporation
PCA	Patient Controlled Analgesia
PCE	See Potentially Compensable Event.
Peer review	A process whereby possible deviations from the standard of patient care are reviewed by an individual or committee from the same professional discipline to determine whether the standard of care was met and to make recommendations for improving patient care processes. Most jurisdictions provide at least a limited protection from discovery in civil actions for peer review activities.
	An evaluation of the appropriateness, effectiveness, and efficiency of medical services ordered or performed by practicing physicians or professionals by other practicing physicians or clinical professionals. A peer review focuses on the quality of services that are performed

	by all health personnel involved in the delivery of the care under review and how appropriate the services are to meet the patients' needs.
***Per diem* staff**	Staff of a healthcare provider called in to work on an "as needed" basis depending on patient volume and acuity, as opposed to having their work schedules determined in advance
Peril	The cause of the loss
Perinatal	The care of a woman before conception, of the woman and her fetus through pregnancy, and of the mother and her neonate until 28 days after childbirth
PET	Positron emission tomography
Petition	See Complaint. Also used to denote the written instrument that initiates certain proceedings, such as bankruptcy
Pharmacy patient profile	The specific record created for each patient in the pharmacy that typically notes the patient's name, diagnoses, weight, allergy history and medications prescribed and dispensed
PHI	See Protected Health Information
PHN	Public health nurse
PHO	Physician hospital organization
PHRP	Program for Human Research Protection
PHS	Public Health Services
Physician Hospital Organization	A type of integrated delivery system that links hospitals and a group of physicians for the purpose of contracting directly with employers and managed care organizations. A PHO is a legal entity which allows physicians to continue to own their own practices and to see patients under the terms of a professional services agreement. This type of arrangement offers the opportunity to better market the services of both physicians and hospitals as a unified response to managed care
Physician's assistant	A specially trained and licenses allied health professional, who performs certain medical procedures previously reserved to the physician. PAs practice under the supervision of a physician
PI	Performance Improvement (also known as process improvement)
PIAA	Physician Insurers Association of America
PICU	Pediatric intensive care unit
PIP	Personal injury protection
PL	Professional liability
Plaintiff	A person who brings a civil lawsuit
Pleadings	The formal allegations by the parties involved in a lawsuit that delineate the claims and defenses of each party and that request judgment by the court prior to resolution
PM	Preventive maintenance
PMA	Pre-market approval application
Policy	A predetermined course of action established as a guide toward accepted business strategies and objectives
	The formal, approved description of how a governance, management, or clinical-care process is defined, organized and carried out (JCAHO CAMH Manual, 2002)

POS	Point of service
Positron Emission tomography	An imaging technique, which tracks metabolism and responses to therapy. Used in cardiology, neurology, and oncology; particularly effective in evaluating brain and nervous system disorders
Post-loss damage control	Any of a number of initiatives taken after a potentially compensable event to build rapport with the patient and family and to decrease the likelihood or severity of a subsequent claim
Potentially Compensable Event	An occurrence of the type for which a claim can be reasonably anticipated but for which no claim has yet been asserted
	An adverse event for which there are grounds or contributing factors found after investigation, worthy of compensation being awarded the patient
P&P	Policy and procedure
PPE	Personal protective equipment
PPO	Preferred provider organization
PPS	Prospective payment system
Practice guidelines	Formal procedures and techniques for the treatment of specific medical conditions that assist physicians in achieving optimal results. Practice guidelines are developed by medical societies and medical research organization, such as the American Medical Association (AMA) and the Agency for Health Care Policy and Research (AHCPR), as well as many HMOs, insurers, and business coalitions. Practice guidelines serve as educational support for physicians and as quality assurance and accountability measures for managed care plans.
Precedent	A previously decided case that turned upon the same facts, circumstances or legal theory as presented in the case under consideration. Lower courts are bound to follow precedents set by higher courts in the jurisdiction in which the lower court is located. Cases decided by courts in other jurisdictions may be considered "persuasive authority" by the court rendering judgment in a given case. In this case the court may follow the decision of the other court, although not legally required to do so. The doctrine requiring the binding effect of precedent is called *stare decisis.*
Preemption	Doctrine adopted by the U.S. Supreme Court holding that certain matters are of such a national, as opposed to local, character that federal laws preempt or take precedence over state laws
Preexisting condition	A physical or mental condition that an insured has prior to the effective date of coverage. Policies may exclude coverage for such condition for a specified period of time
Preferred provider organization	A plan that contracts with independent providers at a discount for services. Generally, the PPO's network of providers is limited in size. Patients usually have free choice to select other providers but are given strong financial incentives to select one of the designated preferred providers. Unlike an HMO, a PPO is not a prepaid plan but does use some utilization management techniques. PPO arrangements can be either insured or self-funded. An insurersponsored PPO combines a large network of providers, utilization management programs, administrative sponsored PPO combines a large network of providers, utilization management programs,

administrative services, and health care insurance. A self-funded PPO generally excludes administrative and insurance services from the plan package. However, employers can purchase these services separately.

Preventable Adverse Event	An adverse event that could have been avoided, if actions were taken prior to the final step of the process
Primary care	Basic care including initial diagnosis and treatment, preventive services, maintenance of chronic conditions, and referral to specialists
Prior acts coverage	In insurance, coverage that extends a claims-made policy to claims that occurred before the inception date of the policy but subsequent to a specified retroactive date for which a claim is made during the policy period. Sometimes referred to as "nose coverage"
Privileged communication	Communications, which occur in the context of legal or other, recognized professional confidentiality. Privileged communication allows participants to resist legal pressure to disclose its contents. A breach in such communication can result in a civil suit or tort.
Privileging (delineation of clinical privileges)	The process of granting specific clinical privileges, based on training, experience and current competence, for individuals credentialed to provide healthcare services under medical staff bylaws
PRN	"On an as-needed basis"
PRO	Peer Review Organization. See Quality Improvement Organization
Procedure	A method by which a policy can be accomplished; it provides instructions necessary to carry out a policy statement
Professional Corporation	A corporation formed by professional persons to undertake their profession (e.g., by physicians to practice medicine). The professional corporation (PC) is typically licensed to practice the profession of the owners. Only members of the profession can be owners (shareholders) of the professional corporation.
Professional liability insurance	Coverage for liability arising from the rendering of or failure to render professional services
Promulgation	The process for creation of rules or regulations. The process typically involves the announcement of the proposed regulation by the agency, allowance of a reasonable public comment period, consideration of the comments received, and the announcement of the final regulation.
Property Coverage	Covers your buildings, contents, attached equipment and building service equipment used for cleaning and maintenance
Prospective payment system	Also called prospective pricing; a payment method in which the payment a hospital will receive for patient treatment is set up in advance; hospitals keep the difference if they incur costs less than the fixed price in treating the patient and they absorb any loss if their costs exceed the fixed price.
Protected concerted activity	A group activity that seeks to modify wages or working conditions
Protected health information	Medical record information and other individually identifiable information for which privacy protection is afforded under HIPAA

Provider sponsored organization	Public or private entities established or organized and operated by a health provider or a group of affiliated health care providers that provide a substantial proportion of services under the Medicare+Choice contract and share substantial financial risk
PSA	Prostate specific antigen
PSDA	See Patient Self-Determination Act
PSO	Provider sponsored organization
PT	Physical therapy
PTO	Paid Time Off
Punitive damages (exemplary damages)	Damages sought or awarded to punish or deter the defendant or to deter others from similar conduct rather than to compensate the injured party. Generally require a showing of gross negligence or willful and wanton misconduct. Not insurable in some jurisdictions and may be excluded by insurance policies
	Damages awarded to the plaintiff over and above what will barely compensate him for his property loss, where the wrong done to him was aggravated by circumstances of violence, oppression, malice, fraud or wanton and wicked conduct on the part of the defendant and are intended to solace the plaintiff for mental anguish or to punish the defendant or make an example of him
	Damages awarded in addition to compensatory (economic and noneconomic) damages to punish a defendant for willful and wanton conduct
QA	Quality assurance
QAPI	Quality Assessment and Performance Improvement Program (Conditions of Participation)
QI	Quality improvement
QIO	See Quality Improvement Organization
QS	Quality System regulation for medical devices (21 CFR Part 820)
Quality assurance	Term that describes attempts by managed care organizations to measure and monitor the quality of care delivered
Quality Improvement Organization	Successor name for PROs. The Centers for Medicare and Medicaid Services (CMS) administers the Peer Review Organization (PRO) program that is designed to monitor and improve utilization and quality of care for Medicare beneficiaries. The program consists of a national network of fifty-three PROs (also known as Quality Improvement Organizations) responsible for each U.S. state and territory and the District of Columbia
	Federally funded physician organizations, under contract to the Department of Health and Human Services, that review quality of care, determine whether services are necessary and payment should be made for care provided under the Medicare and Medicaid programs
Quality of care	The degree to which health services for individuals and populations increase the likelihood of desired health outcomes and are consistent with current professional knowledge
	A desired degree of excellence in the provision of health care. The health care delivery processes which are thought to be determinants of

quality include: structural adequacy, access and availability, technical abilities of practitioners, practitioner communication skills and attitudes, documentation of services provided, coordination and follow-up, patient commitment and adherence to a therapeutic regimen, patient satisfaction, and clinical outcome

QuIC	Quality Interagency Coordinating Committee
Quid pro quo	"This for that"
***Qui Tam* Plaintiff**	A plaintiff in an action under the False Claims Act that is brought on behalf of the federal government. The False Claims Act prohibits the presentation of false claims for remuneration to the federal government.
Qui Tam Relator	One who brings an action on behalf of the government (originally on behalf of the king)
RAC	See Rent-A-Captive
RBC	Red blood count
RCA	See Root Cause Analysis
RCRA	Resource Conservation and Recovery Act
Release	A document executed by the plaintiff, usually in exchange for a monetary settlement, which releases the defendant from any further obligation or threat of suit
Reasonable accommodation	Under the Americans with Disabilities Act, those actions required by an employer to allow an otherwise qualified individual with a disability to perform a specific job. Reasonable accommodations include modifications to work processes and schedules and to physical facilities that are not "unduly burdensome."
Reconstruction Civil Rights Acts	42 U.S.C. Section 1981 and 1983. Post-Civil War federal legislation prohibiting certain types of racial discrimination
Regulation	An enactment issued (promulgated) by a regulatory (non-elected) agency. Regulations must be promulgated pursuant to a statute that gives the agency the authority to do so and typically must go through a promulgation process
Rehab Act	Section §504 of this 1973. Federal law prohibiting discrimination on the basis of handicap
Reinsurance	A contractual arrangement involving the purchase of insurance by an "Insurer" from "Another Insurer"—i.e., insurance for the insurance company
	A type of insurance purchased by providers and health plans to protect themselves from extraordinary losses. Types of reinsurance coverage include: individual stop loss, aggregate stop loss, out-of-area protection, and insolvency protection. Reinsurance is a transaction between and among insurers for the assumption of risk in exchange for a premium. Usually, a primary insurer will cede only a portion of its total risk and premium payments to a reinsurer, either as a percentage of total premiums or only for losses above a particular threshold
Release	A written instrument that normally concludes a legal proceeding and precludes the initiation or re-initiation of a further legal proceeding against the released party(s) with respect to the released claims

	A document executed by the plaintiff, usually in exchange for a monetary settlement, which releases the defendant from any further obligation or threat of suit
Rent-A-Captive	Owned by investors rather than insureds and organized to insure or re-insure third-party risks
Request for Admission	A set of questions served upon a party in litigation during discovery that requests the party served to admit or deny the truth of the requested question
Request for Production	A written set of requests served upon a party in litigation during discovery that asks the party to produce tangible things (e.g., records, photographs, equipment, etc.)
Reserves	Estimates of the amount ultimately required to settle a claim or pay a judgment (indemnity reserve) and to provide for a defense and pay other allocated expenses related to managing a claim (expense reserve)
	The amount of money the insurance company sets aside to satisfy a claim, based on the insurance company's estimate of what it will take to satisfy a settlement or verdict
Res Ipsa Loquitur	"The thing speaks for itself"; arises upon proof that the instrumentality was in defendant's exclusive control and that the accident was one which ordinarily does not happen in absence of negligence.
	A legal theory, which translated from Latin means "the thing speaks for itself" which applies in situations where the fact that a particular injury occurred allows an inference of negligence
Respondeat superior	Legal doctrine that the employer is responsible for the act and omissions of employees in the course and scope of employment. While the employee is also generally liable for his or her own negligence, the employer remains vicariously liable.
	"Let the master answer"—a doctrine of law under which the employer is responsible for the legal consequences of the acts of the servant or employee who is acting within the scope of employment
Restraint, chemical	A drug used as a restraint is a medication used to control behavior or to restrict the patient's freedom of movement and is not a standard treatment for the patient's medical or psychiatric condition.
Restraint, physical	A physical restraint is any manual method or physical or mechanical device, material, or equipment attached or adjacent to the patient's body that he or she cannot easily remove that restricts freedom of movement or normal access to one's body.
Retrospective premium plans	In insurance, a policy for which an initial deposit premium is paid with the ultimate premium determined based on the loss experience of the insured. Some plans adjust the premium based on losses incurred (which include reserves for claims not yet settled), while others make adjustments based on paid losses only. Common in workers' compensation insurance programs
Reuse	Most often used in the context of processing a single use device (SUD) in order to permit it to be used again
Reviewable sentinel event	The event has resulted in an unanticipated death or major permanent loss of function not related to the natural course of the patient's illness or underlying condition.
RFP	Request for Proposal

Risk	The chance of loss. Pure risk is uncertainty as to whether loss will occur. Speculative risk is uncertainty about an event that could produce loss. Pure risk is insurable, but speculative risk usually is not.
Risk acceptance	The decision not to transfer an identified risk but instead to assume its financial consequences
Risk adjusted (data)	The process of matching different groups in a manner that takes into account significant differences and equalizes them prior to performing comparisons. For example, prior to comparing mortality rates of different physicians, the patient population groups are "risk adjusted" to equalize for age and other clinical status differences.
Risk analysis	The process used by the person or persons assigned risk management functions to determine the potential severity of the loss from an identified risk, the probability that the loss will happen, and alternatives for dealing with the risk
Risk avoidance	The decision not to undertake a particular activity because the risk associated with the activity is unacceptable
	The only risk control technique that completely eliminates the possibility of loss from a given exposure. This technique reduces the possibility of a loss to zero by the conscious choice not to engage in or avoid a specific activity or operation.
Risk control techniques	Those techniques designed to prevent the likelihood of an occurrence or reduce the frequency of occurrences that give rise to losses or to minimize at the least possible cost those losses that strike an organization
Risk financing	Any of a number of programs implemented to pay for the costs associated with property and casualty claims and associated expenses, including insurance, self-insurance, captive insurance companies, etc.
Risk identification	The process of identifying problems or potential problems that can result in loss; recognizing the potential for loss
Risk Management	The process of making and carrying out decisions that will assist in prevention of adverse consequences and minimize the adverse effects of accidental losses upon an organization. Making these decisions requires the five steps in the decision process. Carrying out these decisions requires the risk management professional to perform the four functions in the management process. These include planning, organizing, leading and controlling.
	A systematic and scientific approach in the empirical order to identify, evaluate, reduce, or eliminate the possibility of an unfavorable deviation from expectation and, thus, to prevent the loss of financial assets resulting from injury to patients, visitors, employees, independent medical staff, or from damage, theft, or loss of property belonging to the healthcare entity or persons mentioned. The definition includes transfer of liability and insurance financing relative to the inability to reduce or eliminate intolerable deviations. Originally defined by the American Hospital Association as the "science for the identification, evaluation, and treatment of the risk of financial loss." Risk management now also encompasses the evaluation and monitoring of clinical practice to recognize and prevent patient injury.

Risk purchasing group	Any group that decides to buy, on a group basis, liability insurance in compliance with the Federal Risk Retention Act
	Domestic organization formed to purchase commercial market liability insurance on a group basis for members engaged in similar activities
Risk reduction	Reduces the severity of those losses that other risk control techniques do not prevent
Risk Retention Group	Liability-only domestic insurance captive for group whose members are engaged in similar activities
Risk transfer	The procedure of shifting risk of loss to another party who agrees to accept it
RMIS	Risk management information system
RN	Registered Nurse
Root Cause Analysis	A multi-disciplinary process of study or analysis that uses a detailed, structured process to examine factors contributing to a specific outcome (e.g., an adverse event)
	A process for identifying the basic or causal factors that underlie variation in performance, including the occurrence or possible occurrence of a sentinel event
RPG	See Risk Purchasing Group
RPLU	Registered Professional Liability Underwriter
RRG	See Risk Retention Group
RX	Prescription
Safe Medical Devices Act	21 U.S.C. Section 360 et seq. Federal statute governing the tracking of certain implantable medical devices and requiring reporting of patient deaths and serious injuries involving the use of medical devices or equipment
Sarbanes-Oxley Act	Applies to public companies that are required to file periodic Securities and Exchange Commission (SEC) Reports under Sections 12 or 15(d) of the Security Exchange Act of 1934 or if the public company has filed a registration statement that has not yet become effective under the Securities Act of 1933
SBS	Sick building syndrome
SC	Subcutaneous
SCCM	Society of Critical Care Medicine, www.sccm.org
SCHIP	State Children's Health Insurance Program
SE	Sentinel event
SEC	Securities and Exchange Commission
Segregation	Segregation of exposure units reduces the uncertainty of losses by increasing the predictability of both loss frequency and severity
Self-governing	As pertains to the hospital medical staff, a requirement contained in JCAHO standards that the medical staff elect its own officers and approve its own bylaws and rules and regulations
Self-insurance trust fund	A mechanism for funding claims and related expenses under a program of self-insurance whereby the insured establishes a segregated fund, administered by a trustee, which is replenished from time to time according to actuarially determined estimates of future loss costs

Self-insured retention	In insurance, that portion of a claim that the insured is required to pay before the insurer begins to pay. Similar to a deductible, but frequently funded through a mechanism such as a self-insurance trust fund and larger than a deductible. The insured generally manages claims falling entirely within the SIR (or contracts with a third party to do so), so that the insurer is only involved if the amount of the claim exceeds or is anticipated to exceed the amount of the retention. Common in hospital professional liability programs
Sentinel event	The JCAHO term for an unexpected occurrence involving death or serious physical or psychological injury or the risk thereof, including loss of limb or function. The phrase "or risk thereof" includes any process variation for which a recurrence would carry a significant chance of a serious adverse outcome. The JCAHO has a policy to encourage the voluntary self-reporting of sentinel events by accredited organizations in order to gather and publish information about the relative frequencies and underlying causes of such occurrences.
Settlement	An agreement between the parties in which consideration is passed and the matter is concluded as to those parties. Settlement may occur at any time. A compromise achieved by the adverse parties in a civil suit before final judgment
Severance agreement	A contract between an employer and a terminated employee. Generally severance agreements provide a lump sum payment or a period of salary continuation in return for the employee's agreement not to make certain claims against the employer.
Sexual harassment	Any of a number of statutorily prohibited kinds of sexually oriented and unwanted contact, remarks and comments or conditions of employment. In quid pro quo sexual harassment, participation in sexual activity or performance of sexual favors is made an explicit or implicit condition of employment. In a hostile environment, sexual harassment, jokes, comments, cartoons or touching of a sexual nature permeate the workplace, interfering with an employee's ability to perform his or her job comfortably.
SICU	Surgical intensive care unit
SIDS	Sudden infant death syndrome
Single Payer System	A financing system such as Canada's in which a single entity-usually the government-pays for all covered health care services
Single Point Weakness	A step in the process so critical that its failure would result in system failure or in an adverse event
SIR	See Self-Insured Retention
Skilled Nursing Facility	A facility, either freestanding or part of a hospital, that accepts patients in need of rehabilitation and medical care. To qualify for Medicare coverage, SNFs must be certified by Medicare and meet specific qualifications, including 24-hour nursing coverage and availability of physical, occupational, and speech therapies.
Slander	The speaking of base and defamatory words tending to prejudice.
Slips	Unintended human errors, usually during an activity that the person is proficient in and is performing on an "automatic mode" basis
SMDA	See Safe Medical Devices Act

SNF	Skilled Nursing Facility, a certain level of care provided to nursing home residents
SOB	Short of breath
Special cause	Factor that intermittently and unpredictably induces variation over and above that inherent in the system
Specials	Those elements of a plaintiff's damages which can be computed with relative precision. Includes lost wages, medical expenses, future expenses, etc.
SSA	Social Security Act
SSI	Supplemental security income, also ServiShare
SSN	Social security number
Standard	A minimum level of acceptable performance or results or excellent levels of performance or the range of acceptable performances on results. The American Society for Testing and Materials (ASTM) defines six types of standards: 1) standard test methods—a procedure for identifying, measuring, and evaluating a material, product or system; 2) standard specification—a statement of a set of requirements to be satisfied and the procedures for determining whether each of the requirements are satisfied; 3) standard practice—a procedure for performing one or more specific operations or functions; 4) standard terminology—a document comprising terms, definitions, descriptions, explanations, abbreviations, or acronyms; 5) standard guide—a series of options or instructions that do not recommend a specific course of action; 6) standard classification—a systematic arrangement or division of products, systems, or services into groups based on similar characteristics.
Standard of Care	In medical malpractice cases, a standard of care is applied to measure the competence of the professional. The traditional standard for doctors is that they exercise the average degree of skilled care and diligence exercised by members of the same profession, practicing in the same or similar locality in light of the present state of medical and surgical science. With increasing specialization, however, certain courts have disregarded geographical considerations holding that, in the practice of a boardcertified medical or surgical specialty, the standard should be that of a reasonable specialist practicing medicine or surgery in the same specialty.

In a legal proceeding, the standard against which the defendant's conduct is measured. The defendant is expected to act as an ordinary, prudent person with similar training and skill would have acted in a similar situation. If the defendant's conduct falls below this standard, the defendant may be determined to have acted negligently. |
Standing	The right or authority by which a person may bring and sustain a legal proceeding. It is normally conferred upon a person who has suffered an injury. It may also be possessed by someone who has been given the legal right to bring suit on behalf of someone who has suffered an injury.
Stark (#)	Physician referral laws-part of OBRA '89 ("Stark I") and '93 ("Stark II")
Stark I	Enacted initially in 1989 and took effect in 1992. Focus was on referrals involving provision of clinical laboratory services

Stark II	Broadened scope of prohibited designated health services
Stat.	Immediately
Statement of fault	A statement acknowledging responsibility for a specific event or outcome
Statute	A legislative enactment that has typically been enacted by the elected legislature of a state or the federal government
Statute of limitations	The time period defined by law in which a claimant must file a claim for damages or be barred from so doing. Most jurisdictions extend the allowable time period for individuals who are injured as minors, and many include a discovery rule extending the time period for individuals whose injuries were not readily discoverable.
	A statute that requires, absent good cause for delay, that a person bring suit within a certain period of time. The running of the statute may be stayed (tolled) for a number of reasons, such as incompetence, infancy, disability, etc. The effect of a statute of limitations may also be stayed if the plaintiff can prove late discovery of the injury, a continuing course of treatment, or active misrepresentation of the plaintiff's condition.
	A statute specifying the period of time after the occurrence of an injury or in some cases, after the discovery of the injury-or of its cause-during which any suit must be filed
Statute of Repose	A statute that sets a maximum period of time in which a suit may be brought. This statute is always longer than the statute of limitations, and generally is subject to fewer, if any, exceptions or tolling provisions.
STD	Short-term disability
	Sexually transmitted disease
Stop loss	Insurance coverage for healthcare and managed care organizations that have agreed in advance to accept financial risk for the provision of healthcare services under capitated managed care contracts. Stop loss policies limit the losses experienced by such entities when utilization of services exceeds estimates.
Sub-acute care	A level of care that is between acute care and long-term care
Subpoena	"Under penalty"
	A process to cause to cause a witness to appear and give testimony, commanding him to lay aside all pretenses and excuses and appear before the court named at a time mentioned to testify for the party named or experience a penalty.
	A document, issued by the court at the request of a party, which compels an individual to produce documents and/or attend a deposition or trail and give testimoney
Subpoena duces tecum	A process by which the court commands a witness who has in his possession or control some document or paper that is pertinent to the issues of a pending controversy, to produce it at the trial.
Subrogation	The process of collecting from the person responsible for damages. Allows the insurer making a payment to the insured to assume the insured's right of recovery against the third party responsible for the loss.
SUDs	Single Use Devices

Summary judgment	Procedural device available for prompt and expeditious disposition of controversy without trial when there is no dispute as to either material fact or inferences to be drawn from undisputed facts, or if only a question of law is involved
Summons	Usually a brief (one-page) document commanding defendant(s) to appear and answer before a court
Supreme Court	The highest appellate court within a given jurisdiction. Appeals taken from the trial of a lawsuit are ultimately heard by this tribunal.
Surety bonds	A three-part contract in which two parties, the surety and the principal (or obligor), agree to be bound by a promise to a third party, the obligee. If the principal defaults on the promise, the surety, for a premium paid in advance by the principal, steps in and fulfils the obligation. Surety bonds typical in the healthcare setting include patient trust fund bonds (to ensure that patient funds and valuables held by hospitals and nursing homes are appropriately safeguarded), performance bonds (to ensure that construction projects are completed as agreed upon) and various license bonds (to ensure appropriate performance of the licensee's duties). Once the surety fulfills the obligations to the obligee, it may seek reimbursement from the principal.
Surge capacity	Reserve capacity in terms of staff, space, equipment and supplies built into a healthcare provider's operations to accommodate emergency situations in which the demand for services may be greatly increased over normal levels
Surgicenter	A health care facility that is physically separate from a hospital and provides prescheduled surgical services on an outpatient basis, generally at a lower cost than inpatient hospital care. Also called a Free-Standing Outpatient Surgery Center
Swing beds	Acute care hospital beds that can also be used for long-term care, depending on the needs of the patient and the community; only those hospitals with fewer than 100 beds and located in a rural community, where long-term care may be inaccessible, are eligible to have swing beds.
System	Set of interdependent elements interacting to achieve a common aim. These elements may be both human and nonhuman (equipment, technologies, etc.).
Systemic or system-related issue	An issue that arises due to some design, process or any other operational aspect of a complex, multiple entity "system" or multistep process
T&A	Tonsillectomy and adenoidectomy
Tail	The delay between an actual incident of malpractice or alleged action and the filing of a claim is called the long tail. An insurance company underwriting occurrence policies will be covering claims for many years after the policy has expired due to this long tail. In contrast, the claims-made policy covers only those claims that are actually made during tenure of the policy. Therefore, if you cancel your claims-made policy, and wish to have continued coverage, you must purchase an extended reporting endorsement or tail coverage.
Tail coverage	See Extended Reporting Endorsement.
TB	Tuberculosis

Teaching hospitals	Hospitals that have an accredited medical residency training program and are typically affiliated with a medical school
Telehealth	See Telemedicine
Telemedicine	The use of telecommunications to provide medical information and services
	The provision of healthcare consultation and education using telecommunications networks to communicate information; medical practice across distance via telecommunications and interactive video technology (American Medical Association's Council on Medical Education and Medical Services)
	The use of electronic information and communications technologies to provide and support healthcare when distance separates the participants (Institute of Medicine)
Tertiary care	Refers to highly technical services for the patient who is imminent danger of major disability or death
Therapeutic Privilege	A decision by a doctor that a patient should not have access to certain parts of the patient's medical records, out of a concern that the patient will not be able to cope with the information contained therein
Third party	Provides coverage to a party other than the insured to make that person whole for loss or injury caused by the insured
Third-party administrator	An independent organization that contracts to provide claims management services to a self-insured entity
	A firm outside the insuring organization, which handles the administrative duties such as collecting premiums, claims processing, claims payment, membership services, utilization review, for employee health benefit plans and managed care plans. Third party administrators are used by organizations that actually fund the health benefits but find it not cost effective to administer the plan themselves. If claims payment is one of the services, the TPA is considered a third party payer. Unlike insurance carriers, TPAs do not underwrite the insurance risk.
Third-party over claim	A claim by an injured employee against a party other than his or her employer, such as the manufacturer of a machine involved in the injury, in which the third party brings in the employer as an additional defendant, such as for failure to properly maintain the machine. Third-party over claims are a type of claim by an injured worker against his or her employer that fall outside of workers' compensation coverage and are generally covered by employers' liability policies.
Threat envelope	In disaster planning, the analysis of those types of occurrences most likely to occur, as well as those less likely but having particularly serious consequences for a community or organization for which it determines it must prepare
Tight coupling	An engineering term to describe when the steps of a process follow so closely to one another that a variation in the first step cannot be recognized and responded to or corrected, prior to a variance or adverse consequence resulting from the first step thereby affecting the second step, and the entire, desired outcome
Tomography	A diagnostic technique using x-ray photographs which do not show the shadows of structures before and behind the section under scrutiny

Tort	A private or civil wrong or injury for which the court will provide a remedy in the form of an action for damages
Tortfeasor	Party to direct liability as a result of party's acts or omissions
Total Quality Management	A systematic set of processes and tools designed to improve quality on an ongoing basis
	A philosophy and system for achieving constant performance improvement at every level. Key elements of TQM include company wide continuous quality improvement (CQI) efforts (sometimes called a quality improvement program), self-directing work teams, employee involvement programs, flexible service delivery processes, quick change over and adaptability, customer focus, supplier integration, and production cycle time reduction. Many health care organizations implement TQM programs as a competitive strategy
TPA	See Third-party Administrator
TPO	Treatment, payment and operations
TQI	Total quality improvement
TQM	Total Quality Management
Transitional duty (alternative duty, light duty, modified duty)	The assignment of an injured employee to work differently than what he or she ordinarily performs in terms of duties, work environment or duration during a period of recovery
Transparency	A practice of full disclosure to the consumer/patient, as opposed to providing limited information or a policy of secrecy
Treaty	The reinsurer agrees in advance to accept certain classes of exposures as outlined in a "treaty." The insurer assumes underwriting authority on behalf of the reinsurer.
Triage	Evaluation of patient conditions for urgency and seriousness and the establishment of a priority list in order to direct care and ensure the efficient use of medical and nursing staff and facilities. Triaging patients occurs in situations with multiple victims
Trial Court	Usually the lowest level court within a given jurisdiction and the court in which the actual trial of the matter will be conducted
TSCA	Toxic Substances Control Act
TX	A charting abbreviation for "treatment."
UCL	See Upper Control Limit
Ultrasound	Refers to sound that has different velocities in tissues which differ in density and elasticity from others; this property permits the use of ultrasound in outlining the shape of various tissues and organs in the body
UM	See Utilization Management
Umbrella	In insurance, an excess insurance policy providing limits above more than one type of primary policy, such as professional and general liability and auto liability. Umbrella policies may also include some specific coverages not found in the underlying policies.
Unanticipated outcome	A result that differs significantly from what was anticipated to be the result of the treatment or procedure
Under use	A quality problem involving the failure to provide a healthcare service or procedure for persons for whom it was clinically indicated or needed

Underwriter	An insurance company employee who makes determinations regarding the acceptability of a given risk for insurance coverage and for specific terms, conditions and pricing of such coverage
Underwriting	The process of identifying, evaluating, and classifying the potential level of risk represented by a group seeking insurance coverage, in order to determine appropriate pricing, risk involved, and administrative feasibility. The chief purpose of underwriting is to make sure the potential for loss is within the range for which the premiums were established. Underwriting can also refer to the acceptance of risk
Universal access	The provision of coverage for health care services to all citizens
Upper Control Limit	Used in statistical process control run charts
UR	Utilization review
URAC	Utilization Review Accreditation Commission, also known as American Accreditation HealthCare Commission
URL	Uniform Resource Locator (also known as web address)
Urgent Care	Care for injury, illness, or another type of condition (usually not life threatening) which should be treated within 24 hours. Also refers to after-hours care, and to a health plan's classification of hospital admissions as urgent, semi-urgent, or elective
USC	U.S. Code
USERRA	The Uniformed Services Employment and Reemployment Rights Act
USP	U.S. Pharmacopeia, a non-governmental organization that promotes the public health by establishing standards to ensure the quality of medicines and other healthcare technologies
U.S. Patriots Act	Federal legislation that enhances the ability of law enforcement to deter and detect acts of terrorism, including cyber-intelligence gathering, wire-tapping and other means of gathering needed information from designated privacy records
USPHS	United States Public Health Service
Utilization	Patterns of usage for a particular medical services such as hospital care or physician visits
Utilization Management	The function of monitoring the utilization of healthcare resources by individual patients, e.g., to verify that surgical cases justify criteria for performing that procedure; to verify that the length of stay in a hospital is justified, etc. Also referred to as case management
Utilization review	An evelution of the care and services that patients receive which is based on pre-established criteria and standards
VAHRPAP	Veterans Administration Human Research Protection Accreditation Program
VBAC	Vaginal Birth After Cesarean Section
VDRL	Serology
Venue	The physical location, or the tribunal within such location, in which a legal proceeding may be brought. Usually the place in which the injury is alleged to have occurred
Verdict	The formal decision or definitive answer of a jury impaneled to hear and decide the facts of a legal proceeding, which is reported to the court

VHA	Veterans Health Administration
Vicarious Liability	The imposition of liability on one person for the actionable conduct of another, based solely on a relationship between the two persons. Indirect or imputed legal responsibility for the acts of another, e.g., the liability of an employer for the acts of an employee. A principle for torts and contracts of an agent
VIP	Very important person
Voir Dire	The process of questioning jurors, prior to seating them, to determine if any jurors have knowledge of the case, personally know or know of the parties, or may otherwise have preconceptions that would prevent them from hearing and deciding the case impartially
Volume-outcome relationship	The theory that for certain procedures, higher volume (by either a specific provider or a hospital) is associated with better health outcomes
Waiver of subrogation	A contractual provision in which one party agrees not to seek indemnification by the other in the event of a subsequent loss for which the second party may bear responsibility
War risk exclusion	A exclusion found in many types of insurance policies excluding losses caused by acts of war or military action
WC	Workers' compensation
Whistleblower	An individual, frequently an employee or former employee, who reports unlawful activity, such as healthcare fraud and abuse or OSHA violations, to the government or an administrative agency. Some statutes provide for the whistleblower to receive a share of fines levied against the organization for making the report. Most statutes prohibit retaliatory discharge or other discriminatory actions against an employee who makes such a report.
WHO	World Health Organization
WIC	Women and Infant Children Program
Withholds	A provision in some managed care contracts withholding a portion of a healthcare provider's reimbursement until the end of a specific time period. If certain utilization targets are met for the period, the provider then receives the withheld reimbursement payments.
WBC	White blood count
WMD	Weapons of mass destruction
Workers' compensation	Statutory obligation requiring employers to provide compensation to employees for injuries arising out of, and in the course of, their employment
Working memory	The concentrated short-term memory used by persons when learning any new task, process
Worried well	Individuals who, in a disaster, contact healthcare providers for information or present at treatment sites for reassurance, even though they have no specific injuries or symptoms, inhibiting the provider's ability to assess and treat those truly in need of medical services

Index

incident reporting mechanisms, 497
staffing, 434
Hoopes, D., 309n2, 309n4
Horn, Stephen, 98–99
hospice care, 33–34
hospital emergency incident command system (HEICS),
468–470
hostile environment sexual harassment, 27
Howard, S., 11n3
human capital, 9
human resources, 92, 438
See also employment issues; staffing issues
human subjects protections, 170–172, 185n8
Belmont Report, 171–172, 190–200
Nuremburg Code, 171, 201–202
On the Protection of Human Subjects, 203–211
Humana Medical Plan v. Fischman, 287–288

identification of risk, 97–100
anonymous reporting, 504–505
confidentiality standards, 503–507
contract and lease reviews, 100
external reporting, 508–519
failure mode and effects analysis (FMEA), 508
five-step decision-making process, 493
formal reporting methods, 496–500
generic/occurrence screening, 97, 507–509
identification procedures, 494–496
incident reports, 496–507
informal internal reporting, 508–509
occurrence reporting, 505–507
outside consultants, 99
patient complaints/patient surveys, 98, 508–509
patient safety classification taxonomy (PSET), 520
prior claims analysis, 98–99
program scope, 493–494
protection of sensitive information, 520–521
regulatory agency reporting systems, 513–519
role of "smart" technology, 512–513
staff participation in incident reporting, 500–503
survey processes, 99
voluntary reporting systems, 518–520
walking rounds (rounding) and walking around, 509
incident command system (ICS), 468–471
incident investigations, 292, 338–339
incident reports, 292, 496–507, 509
common barriers to reporting, 501
confidentiality standards, 369, 503–507
contents, 499–500
electronic systems, 379, 497–499
mandatory reporting systems, 512
medical records, 282–283
occurrence reporting, 505–507
protection of sensitive information, 520–521
regulatory agency reporting systems, 513–521
staff participation in reporting, 500–503
staff training, 438–439, 502–503
incompetent patients, 34–35
independent practice associations (IPAs), 424–425, 497

individual case method, 306–307
individual practice association HMOs, 38
infection control programs, 91, 100
information. *See* communication; confidentiality standards;
health information management; information technology
information technology, 250, 308, 335–353
clinical information systems, 343–345
computerized physician order entry (CPOE), 269, 295,
343–345
electronic health records (EHR), 275, 335–336,
340–343, 373–379, 512–513
e-mail, 340–341, 380, 392n93
guidelines for transmission of information,
374–375, 380
internet technology, 340–341
interoperable systems, 340
online databases, 250, 308
personal health records (PHRs), 341–342
point of care technology, 347
redundancy features, 345–346, 349n8, 375
report production, 339–340
risk management information systems (RMIS), 338–340
security methods, 345–346, 376–377, 380–382,
392n90
"smart" technology, 347, 512–513
telemedicine, 347–348
terminology, 350–353
See also health information management
informed consent, 17, 174, 175, 223–224
Institute for Healthcare Improvement (IHI), 165
Institute for Safe Medical Practices (ISMP), 515–516
medication management, 512–513
unacceptable terms list, 236
institutional biosafety committees, 176
institutional review boards (IRBs), 171–180
insurance, 400–404, 407–432
academic medical centers, 131
acute care hospitals, 128, 130
all risk policies, 419
ambulatory care organizations, 139
analysis of coverage, 412, 416
automobile liability insurance, 315, 426–427
aviation insurance, 430
binding of coverage, 413
brokers and agents, 410–411
captive insurance, 399
claims management, 300
claims-made policies, 414–415, 423
commercial general liability insurance, 423–424
crime insurance, 421
deductibles, 417
defense cost, 416–417
definition, 407–410
directors' and officers' (D&O) liability insurance,
427–428, 460
electronic data processing (EDP) insurance, 420–421
employee benefit legal insurance, 429
employee health and welfare insurance, 430
employment practices liability insurance, 428